ADVANCED UNDERSTANDING OF NEURODEGENERATIVE DISEASES

Edited by **Raymond Chuen-Chung Chang**

Advanced Understanding of Neurodegenerative Diseases
Edited by Raymond Chuen-Chung Chang

Published by InTech

Janeza Trdine 9, 51000 Rijeka, Croatia

Publishing Process Manager Ivana Zec

Technical Editor Teodora Smiljanic

Cover Designer InTech Design Team

Additional hard copies can be obtained from orders@intechopen.com

Advanced Understanding of Neurodegenerative Diseases,
Edited by Raymond Chuen-Chung Chang
p. cm.
ISBN 978-953-307-529-7

For EU product safety concerns:
IN TECH d.o.o., Prolaz Marije Krucifikse Kozulić 3, 51000 Rijeka, Croatia,
info@intechopen.com or visit our website at intechopen.com.

Meet the editor

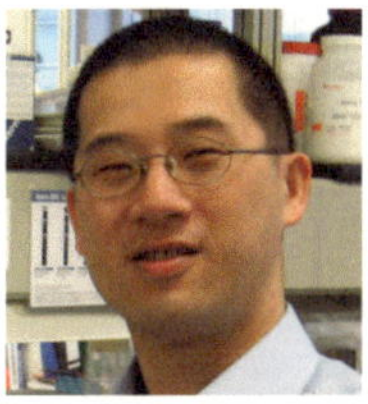

Dr Chang did his BSc training in Biochemistry in Hong Kong. Then he furthered his MPhil training in neurochemistry and neuroanatomy at the same university. He received a research scholarship by German Academic Exchange Service (DAAD) to pursue his doctoral training in neurophysiology and clinical neuroscience at the University of Munich, Germany. Afterwards, he continued his postdoctoral training in neuropharmacology and molecular neuroscience at NIH, USA. He has published over 80 peer-reviewed papers and book chapters in neurodegeneration, neuroimmunology and drug discovery in these areas. Dr Chang is now the Scientific Advisory Board member in International AD/PD Symposium, Scientific Review Committee for Alzheimer Association in USA, editorial board member in many different journals including Journal of Alzheimer's Disease. Dr. Chang's research interest is to investigate molecular mechanisms of neurodegeneration in Alzheimer's disease, Parkinson's disease, ALS, glaucoma and aging-related macular degeneration (AMD) so that pharmacological targets can be found.

Contents

Preface

The main focus in editing this book was to discuss different neurodegenerative diseases in depth. The book concentrates not only on pathological mechanisms, but also on the protective methods. Different chapters attempt to illustrate how different systems/organs, different foods an individual susceptibility affect the progression of diseases.

Of all the different neurodegenerative diseases, Alzheimer's disease (AD) is the most common one and has consequentially received much attention. In this book a thorough elaboration is given on its etiology, mechanisms, clinical intervention, drug screening and protection. Dr Babusikova et al. give the definition of AD and its etiology. Dr Balin et al. then challenge the general concept of developing AD by providing evidence to show that AD may be developed following an infectious disease. Dr Sun and Dr Zhang give an overview of Aβ hypothesis and AD. Dr Walsh and Dr Sharpe discuss the structure-toxicity of Aβ oligomer. Dr Kawahara et al. discuss and provide evidence about calcium dysfunction in AD. Dr Kumar explains the molecular changes of different toxic molecules in AD. Dr Martorana et al. give an overview of the clinical profile of AD, while Dr Wang et al. describe the drug screening platform for a new drug. Dr Herrera-Rivero and Dr Aranda-Abreu discuss therapeutic interventions in AD. Apart from AD, Dr Schlachetzki gives an overview of Frontotemporal dementia. Dr Wobst and Dr Wade-Martins discuss different tauopathies.

In the Parkinson's disease (PD) section, Dr Bayliss et al. discuss about how PD is affected by hormonal control and how hormonal control can serve for therapeutic intervention. Dr Dzhambazova et al. further discuss how food and food supplements modulate the progression of neurodegenerative diseases.

The third section discusses the problem of a devastating disease - prion disease. Dr Zhang uses the computational method to analyze the structure stability of the rabbit prion protein. Dr Yang et al. discuss the use of trimethyamine N-oxide on the stability of prion protein. By reading these two chapters, we may gain an insight of how to tackle the problem of prion proteins by modulating the stability of the protein.

The last section of this book discusses the problems in different motor neurons diseases. Dr Bebee and Dr Chandler give an overview of SMA in a mouse model. Dr Mietto et al. discuss the pathological mechanisms of Wallerian degeneration as one process of neurodegeneration. Dr Dasari et al. explain how to use mesenchymal cells as stem cells in spinal cord injury. Dr Vereyken et al. describe pathological mechanisms of multiple sclerosis, while Dr Shin et al. give an overview of amyotrophic lateral sclerosis.

To sum up, this book can give us a comprehensive overview of different neurodegenerative diseases. It is hoped that we can provide a wide scope of neurodegeneration in a book to illustrate its principles. I am very proud to have acted as the editor of this book.

Raymond Chuen-Chung CHANG, PhD
Assistant Professor and Laboratory Head
Laboratory of Neurodegenerative Diseases
Department of Anatomy
The University of Hong Kong Alzheimer's Disease Research Network
Research Centre of Heart, Brain, Hormone and Healthy Aging
LKS Faculty of Medicine
State Key Laboratory of Brain and Cognitive Sciences
The University of Hong Kong
Pokfulam, Hong Kong SAR,
China

Part 1

Alzheimer's Disease & Dementia

1

Alzheimer's Disease: Definition, Molecular and Genetic Factors

Eva Babusikova[1], Andrea Evinova[1],
Jana Jurecekova[1], Milos Jesenak[2] and Dusan Dobrota[1]
Comenius University in Bratislava, Jessenius Faculty of Medicine in Martin,
[1]Department of Medical Biochemistry
[2]Department of Paediatrics
Slovakia

1. Introduction

Frequency of neurodegenerative diseases increase significantly with the age. One of the most frightening and devastating of all neurological disorders is the dementia that occurs in the elderly. Dementia is a common name for progressive degenerative brain syndromes which affect memory, thinking, behaviour and emotions. Dementia mainly affects older people, although there is a growing incidence of the cases that start before the age of 65. After age 65, the likelihood of developing dementia roughly doubles every five years. Dementia affects 1 - 6% of human population over 65 years and 10 - 20% over 80 years. In the present, average age is increasing and the number of people over 60 years increases as well. Although Ageing is a physiological process, however it seems to be linked with an increasing risk of origin and development of several diseases including neurodegenerative disorders. Dementia is characterised by the loss of or decline in memory and other cognitive abilities. It is caused by various diseases and conditions resulting in damaging brain cells. Different types of dementia (Alzheimer`s disease, vascular dementia or post-stroke dementia, mixed dementia, dementia with Lewy bodies, Parkinson`s disease, frontotemporal dementia, Creutzfeld-Jacob disease, normal pressure hydrocephalus) have been associated with distinct symptom patterns and distinguishing microscopic brain abnormalities. Alzheimer's disease (AD) is the most common cause of dementia and this disease represents 60 - 80% of all dementia. Alzheimer's disease is age-related disease and it is characterized by a range of changes in brain anatomy, biochemistry, genetic, and function. According to Alzheimer`s disease International in 2010, there were an estimated 35.6 million people with dementia worldwide. This means a 10 percent increase over previous global dementia prevalence reported in 2005 in The Lancet. Number of people with dementia will be increasing to 65.7 million by 2030 and 115.4 million by 2050.

Hallmark abnormalities of Alzheimer`s disease are deposits of the protein fragment β-amyloid (plaques) and twisted strands of the protein tau (tangles). Protein oxidation and generation of protein aggregates may be caused by loss of cell function alike a decreased ability of old organisms to resist the physiological stresses and oxidative damage. The relationship between protein aggregation, oxidative damage and neurodegenerative diseases is still unclear. Study of the ageing process is very important because this process is a cause of onset of many neurodegenerative diseases which occurrence is raising with increasing age. Epidemiological studies have indicated that several genetic and environmental risk factors are associated with AD. Neuropathological, genetic and molecular biologic data suggest central roles for age-related changes in the metabolism of amyloid precursor protein and tau protein.

Ageing is a universal process which started with a life origin billions years ago and in the present we still did not find the way how to defeat our own ageing. Nobody can say when and where ageing is starting. Biologic, epidemiological and demographic data represent base for a lot of theories which try to identify a cause of ageing or to explain the ageing process and its consequence death. Exact mechanisms of ageing are still unclear but experimental evidences support a hypothesis that ageing changes are consequences of increasing oxidative damage of organs, tissues, cells and biomolecules. Oxidative damage is elevated when production of reactive oxygen species is increased compared to the physiological condition or a defence ability of organism against an attack of reactive oxygen species is decreased. Oxidation of specific proteins can play a key role in age associated damage. A relationship between protein aggregation, oxidative stress and neurodegeneration remains unclear. One of the basic problems is the analysis of mechanisms that are base of damage. Both localisation and kind of damage are necessary for understanding of neurodegeneration. Neurodegenerative diseases are connected with an origin of protein deposits. It assumes that protein oxidation and generation of protein aggregates generates a base for a loss of cell function and a reduced ability aged organisms to resist to physiological stress.

2. Alzheimer's disease

Ageing is the main risk factor of neurodegenerative disorders such as Alzheimer`s disease and Parkinson`s disease. Approximately 5% of people in age 65 years have AD and the prevalence of this disease increases with increasing age from 19% to 30% after 75 years of age. Overall, 90-95% of Alzheimer`s disease represents a sporadic form and 5-10% represents familiar form. Alzheimer`s disease is neurodegenerative disorder characterised by cognitive failures, impairment of memory and by dramatic chenges in behaviour. AD symptoms may include:

- loss of memory,
- difficulty in finding the right words or understanding what people are saying,
- difficulty in performing previously routine tasks, and activities,
- problems with language,
- personality and mood changes.

AD is the most wide-spread progressive neurological disorder in men after 65 years of age and it becomes very serious all-society problem in consequence of increasing of average age. Although the cause or causes of Alzheimer's disease are not yet known, most experts agree that AD, like other common chronic conditions, probably develops as a result of multiple factors rather than a single cause. Risk factors for AD are:

- age,
- gender,
- gene polymorphism,
- hypercholesterolemia,

- diabetes mellitus,
- stroke,
- brain injuries,
- education,
- alcohol and smoking.

The greatest risk factor for Alzheimer's disease is advancing age, but AD is not a normal part of ageing. There is none available effective treatment or a preventive therapy of AD today and a definitive diagnosis is still established *post mortem* through the histopatological analyse of patient's brain.

Alois Alzheimer in 1906 described neuropsychiatric disorder affecting older people (Alzheimer, 1907). Nowadays this disorder is called Alzheimer`s disease. He did *post mortem* analysis of 51 years old woman (Auguste D.) who suffered from progressive pre-senile dementia (rapid loss of memory, disorientation in time and space) and she died four and half years after beginning of the disease. Alois Alzheimer observed brain atrophy with obvious neurofibrillar pathology and unusual deposits. For Alzheimer`s disease many neurochemical and pathological changes are characteristic such as gliosis, tissue atrophy caused by loss of synapses which is the most striking in frontal and temporal parts of brain cortex (fig. 1.) and by formation of **two main protein clusters** in extracellular and intracellular region of brain. **Extracellular deposits** or senile amyloid plaques occur the most frequently in neocortex. Primary they are consisting of 4 kDa, 40-42 amino acid polypeptide chain called **amyloid β peptide** (Aβ) (Glenner and Wong, 1984). **Intracellular deposits** represent neurofibrillar tangles which are generated from filaments of microtubullar hyperphosphorylated tau protein (Alonso et al., 2008; Grundke-Iqbal et al., 1986; Lee et al., 1991). **Tau protein** is a neuronal microtubullar associated protein which is primary localized in axons. It is assumed that microtubullar associated proteins play a major role in conserve shape of cells and in a axonal transport (Buée et al., 2000). Tau induces *in vivo* packing and stabilization of cell microtubules, tightens and keeps polarity of neuronal cells. Amyloid plaques are example of a specific damage that is characteristic for AD while neurofibrillar tangles are present in different neurodegenerative pathological situations (Robert & Mathuranath, 2007). Created aggregates are involved in a process which leads to progressive degeneration and to neuron death. In the past decade, a significant body of evidence has pointed the attention to the amyloid processing of amyloid precurcor protein - "**amyloid cascade**". This event is the major causative factor in AD.

Pathogenesis of AD is complex and involves many molecular, cellular, biochemical and physiological pathologies. Alzheimer`s disease is a characteristic process with identifiable clinical state which are in a continuity with normal ageing process. It is a multifactorial disease and **genetic** as well as **environmental** factors are included in its pathogenesis. Whereas majority of AD is sporadic 5% is caused by mutations (familiar AD). There was observed a large loss of synapses and a neuronal death in a part of brain which is crucial for cognitive function including cerebral cortex, entorhinal cartex and hippocampus. Senile plaques created by deposits of amyloid fibres were localized in the brain. Intranerve clusters were estimated by electron microscopy and it was shown that they are made by paired spiral fibres (thin fibres, diameter 10 nm) (Kurt et al., 1997). A protein component core of paired spiral fibres was identified as a microtubular protein tau (Grundke-Iqbal et al., 1986).

In the last years, two main hypothesis explaining a cause of AD development were proposed: **hypothesis of amyloid cascade** – a neurodegenerative process is a serie of events started by an abnormal processing of amyloid precursor protein (APP) (Hardy & Higgins,

1992), and hypothesis of **neuronal cytoskeletal degeneration** (Braak & Braak, 1991) – cytoskeletal changes are the starting events of AD.

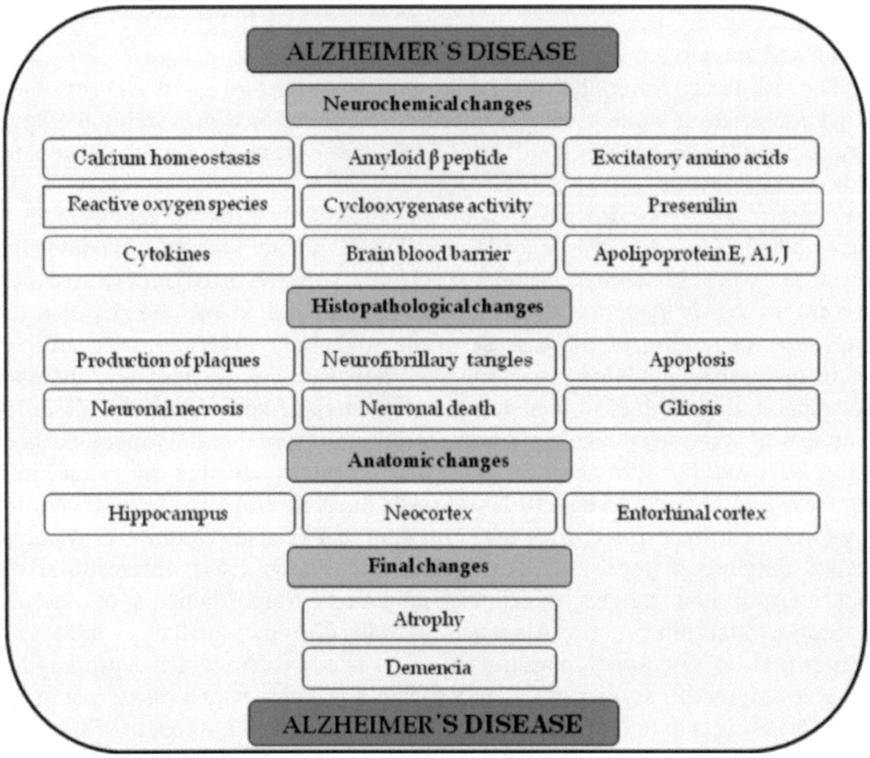

Fig. 1. Typical changes in patients with Alzheimer`s disease

2.1 Amyloid precursor protein

Amyloid precursor protein (APP) is an integral type I transmembrane family of glycoproteins (Kang et al., 1987) and it is expressed under normal physiological condition in brain but its function is unknown so far. It is expressed in several kinds of cells. Gene for amyloid precursor protein contains 18 exons (170 kb) (Yoshikai et al., 1990). N-terminus of amyloid precursor protein is localized toward to extracellular domain or may be localized in the lumen of intracellular vesicles, such as endoplasmic reticulum, Golgi apparatus or intracellular endosomes (Neve & McPhie, 2000). C-terminal of APP lies in cytoplasmic domain (Kang et al., 1987). There are known three different forms of APP mRNA: APP695, APP751 and APP770 that code three isoforms of APP with 695, 751 or 770 amino acids in the chain. The dominant form of APP is APP with 770 amino acids. It is encoded by 18 exons, where exon 17 resembles the membrane-spanning domain. APP695 lacking exon 7 and exon 8 is primarily expressed by neurons and it is the most abundant APP transcript in the brain (Neve et al., 1988). APP751 is lacking exon 8. A part coding of Aβ sequence contain a fraction of exon 16 and exon 17 and contains 40- to 42-amino acids residues that extend from ecto domain to transmembrane domain of protein. N-terminal part of Aβ originates by cleaving of bound between Met-Asp at the position 671-672. This process is catalysed by protease known as β-secretase.

Amyloid precursor protein is sensitive to proteolysis and *in vivo* can be processed by two different pathways: **amyloid** and **non-amyloid processing**, with the contribution of three kinds of proteases (α-, β-, γ-secretase) (fig. 2.). Beta and γ secretase are responsible for the amyloid processing and production of $A\beta_{40}$ or $A\beta_{42}$ variant with significantly higher ability of self aggregate (Citron et al., 1996) and carboxyl-terminal fragments of amyloid precursor protein which are included in the pathogenesis of AD (Selkoe, 1999; Suh, 1997). Alpha secretase is responsible for non-amyloid processing of amyloid precursor protein.

In dominant non-amyloid processing APP is cleaved first by α-secretase within Aβ domain. There are produced two fragments: soluble extracellular fragment (sAPPα) and 83-residue COOH-terminal fragment (C83). Later C83 can be cleaved by γ-secretase. It is unusual hydrolysis in the middle of transmembrane domain and produces small 3 kDa peptid called p3 and C57-59 (amyloid intracellular domain - AICD).

Cleaving of amyloid precursor protein starts by β-secretase in amyloid processing of APP and soluble extracellular fragment (sAPPβ) and 99-residue COOH-terminal fragmet (C99) are produced. C99 is still membrane-bounded and it is substrate for γ-secretase which releases 4 kDa amyloid β peptide and AICD. Proteolysis by γ-secretase is heterogeneous. It can be produced 40-residue peptide ($A\beta_{40}$) (main product) but also a small part of 42-residue COOH-terminal variant ($A\beta_{42}$). Longer and more hydrofobic $A\beta_{42}$ peptide is much more prone to the production of plaques than $A\beta_{40}$ (Jarret et al., 1993). It is assumed that $A\beta_{42}$ is a minority form of amyloid β peptide and it is a main form of amyloid β peptide found in cerebral plaques (Iwatsubo a kol., 1994). Both pathways of APP processing occurr during physiological conditions and therefore it is supposed that all APP fragments including Aβ may be a part of current unknown normal processes.

Alpha-secretase shows characteristics of membrane-bound metalloproteinases. Non-amyloid processing of APP is the main pathway of APP processing which cleaves end part of 16 amyloid β sequence generating C83 (fig. 2.) (Esch et al., 1990). Gamma-secretase subsequently releases a small peptide (p3) which contains C-terminus of Aβ (fig. 2.). A biological importance of p3 and its role, if there is any, in the amylogenesis is still mystery. Sequence of Aβ is disturbed by non-amyloid processing of APP. It is assumed that α-secretase pathway reduces production of amyloid plaques however it has not been yet clearly demonstrated. In addition sAPPα, which is released by α-secretase, has trophic effects (Esch et al., 1990) which can act against neurotoxic effects of aggregated Aβ (Mok et al., 2000). The localisation of α-secretase is unknown. However trans-Golgi (Kuentzel et al., 1993) was suggested as a place of α-cleaving. It has been found that membrane-bound endoprotease on the cell surface has similar activity as α-secretase. Obscurity for α-secretase localisation can be explained by possibility that this enzyme can be made more by than one protein and enzyme. Activity of α-secretase has constitutive and inducible components. A constitutive activity was not identified but an inducible α-secretase activity is probably controlled by protein kinase C (Sinha and Lieberburg, 1999). It is shown that several proteases are responsible for α-secretase activity - member of ADAM (a disintegrin and metalloprotease) family ADAM9, ADAM10, ADAM 17/tumor necrotic factor-α (TNF-α)-converting enzyme (TACE) and pro-protein convertase PC7 (Brou et al., 2000; Fahrenholz & Postina, 2006; Lopez-Perez et al., 2001).

Beta-site amyloid precursor protein cleaving enzyme - **β-secretase** - (BACE1, Asp2) was identified in 1999 as an unusual member of pepsine family of the transmembrane aspartic proteases (Hussain et al., 1999; Lin et al., 2000; Sinha & Lieberburg, 1999; Yan et al., 1999).

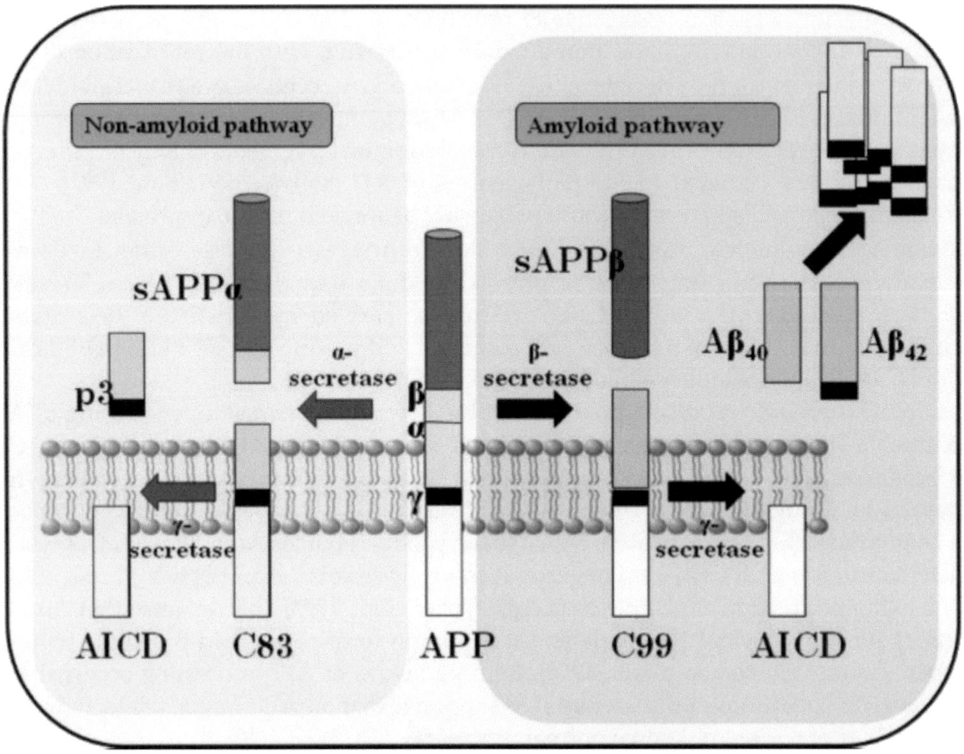

Fig. 2. Processing of amyloid precursor protein (APP). Non-amyloid processing of APP starts by α-secretase cleavage and continues by γ-secretase. A soluble fragment of amyloid precursor protein (sAPPα), a small peptide (p3) and amyloid intracellular domain (ACID) are produced. Amyloid pathway of APP starts with β–secretase cleavage and after that it continues by γ–secretase. A soluble fragment of amyloid precursor protein (sAPPβ), amyloid β peptide and amyloid intracellular domain are generated. Amyloid β peptide can be degradated or accumulated and therefore can be responsible for generation of amyloid plaques

BACE1 has N-terminal catalytic domain containing two important aspartate residues which are bounded to 17-residue transmembrane domain and a short C-terminal cytoplasmic end (Lin et al., 2000; Yan et al., 1999). Beta-secretase activity is present in most of the cells and tissues (Haass et al., 1992) and the highest activity was found in the neural tissue and in the neural cell lines (Seubert et al., 1993). This enzyme contains four potentially N-bond glycosylation sites and peptide sequence at N-terminal. It is phosphorylated inside its cytoplasmic domain at serine residue 498 by casein kinase 1 and phosphorylation is happened exclusively after BACE1 maturation by pro-peptide cleaving and N-glycosylation (Walter et al., 2001). Gene for β-secretase is localised on chromosome 11. BACE1 is an authentical β-secretase (Hussain et al., 1999; Yan et al., 1999). Related transmembrane aspartyl protease (BACE2 or Asp1) (Yan et al., 1999) has similar substrate specificity (Farzan et al., 2000) but it is not very expressed in the brain (Bennett et al., 2000). Beta-secretase is expressed with APP in several regions of the brain. Recent studies demonstrate that BACE1 levels and activity are increased in *post mortem* AD brains (Fukumoto et al., 2002; Harada et al., 2006), suggesting a role of this enzyme in AD.

Residual carboxyl fragments C83 and C99 which are generated after APP cleaving by α- and β-secretase undergo proteolysis inside their domain in a cytoplasmatic membrane. It is regulated intramembrane proteolysis. An intracellular part goes to the nucleus where can influence transcription of several genes. Cleaving of C99 fragment by **γ-secretase** is a final step in the production of Aβ. The right position of cleaving by γ-secretase is determining for development of AD. Gamma-secretase which catalyses secondary cleavage of APP has pharmacological characteristics of aspartyl protease and a specific uncertain sequential specificity for its substrate because many mutations in APP near γ-secretase place are responsible for the production of Aβ in transfected cells (Lichtenthaler et al., 1997; Maruyama et al., 1996). It indicates that γ-secretase represents a multimer enzyme complex and contains at least four proteins: presenilin 1 (PS1), presenilin 2 (PS2), anterior pharynx defective 1 (Aph-1) and nicastrin.

2.1.1 Gene family of amyloid precursor protein

Amyloid precursor protein belongs to the family of genes which has three members in mammals: **amyloid precursor protein** (APP), **amyloid precursor-like protein 1** (APLP1) and **amyloid precursor-like protein 2** (APLP2). Homologues of amyloid precursor protein were found in *Drosophila melanogaster* and *Caenorhabditis elegans* - amyloid like protein (APL1) (de Strooper & Annaert, 2000). All the three proteins are type of I transmembrane proteins with a large extracellular domain (~ 624-700 amino acids), one transmembrane domain (~ 25 amino acids) and a short intracellular domain (~ 46 amino acids). Proteins have similar sequences but the main difference is in an absence of Aβ sequence in two APP similar proteins (fig. 3). No mutations associated with AD were observed in *APLP1* and *APLP2* genes and it supports a hypothesis that Aβ is connected with AD.

The physiological function of APP and its homologues remains unclear. It has been suggested that APP plays a trophic role in neuronal cells (Neve & McPhie, 2000; Qiu et al., 1995). Gene for amyloid precursor protein undergoes a complex alternative exon splicing (Selkoe, 2001a, 2001b; Tanaka et al., 1988). Other heterogenity of APP is reached by series of controlled posttranslational modifications such as N- and O-glycosylation, phosphorylation and sulfation. N-terminal domain shows a homology with Kunitz-type of serine protease inhibitors (KPI) (Kitaguchi et al., 1988; Ponte et al., 1988). Amyloid precursor protein may also participate in cell adhesion, cell proliferation, and synaptogenesis and could have neurotrophic and neuroprotective properties (Caillé et al., 2004; Coulson et al., 2000; Kirazov et al., 2001). Kamal et al. (2000) suggested that APP may serve as a membrane axonal transport receptor for kinesin 1. This hypothesis is interesting because several studies suggest that abnormal processing of APP may play a role in the pathogenesis of AD (Selkoe, 1999; Sinha & Lieberburg, 1999). It assumes that amyloid precursor protein could modulate signal transduction connected with G protein (Nishimoto et al., 1993).

Amyloid precursor protein maps to chromosome 21 in humans. Pathological mutations in sequence which is for amyloid β peptide and for *APP* gene are responsible for increasing production of Aβ and grow in amyloid β peptide self aggregation and production of plaques deposits (Seubert et al., 1993). Deletion of *APP* gene in mouse is without any significant impact to their life and no higher morbidity was revealed. Nevertheless small changes were observed in mobility and in old animals gliosis was found (Zheng et al., 1995). Amyloid β peptide is accumulated in some regions of brain such as *cerebellum, striatum* and *thalamus* and it is clearly contained in clinical signs of Alzheimer`s disease (Selkoe, 2001b).

Domain	Present in	Location
Amyloid β peptide	APP	Exons 16, 17
AICD	APP, APLP-1, APLP-2	Exons 16, 17, 18
Signal peptide	APP, APLP-1, APLP-2	Exon 1
Transmembrane	APP, APLP-1, APLP-2	
Heparin-binding I	APP, APLP-2	Exon 3
Cu^{2+}-binding	APP, APLP-2	Exon 4
Zn^{2+}-binding	APP, APLP-1, APLP-2	Exon 5
KPI	APP, APLP-2	Exon 7
OX-2	APP	Exon 8
Heparin-binding II	APP, APLP-1, APLP-2	Exon 9
Growth-promoting	APP	Exon 9
Collagen-binding	APP, APLP-2	Exon 13
Chondroitin (SO_4)-binding	APP, APLP-2	Exon 15
G0 binding	APP, APLP-1, APLP-2	Exon 17
Clarithin	APP, APLP-1, APLP-2	Exon 18

Fig. 3. Functional domains in amyloid precursor protein superfamily (Adapted by Marks & Berg, 2008). APP - amyloid precursor protein, APLP - amyloid precursor protein-like protein, AICD - amyloid intracellular domain, KPI - Kunitz protease inhibitor, OX-2 - thymocyte MRC antigen

2.1.2 Amyloid β peptide

Amyloid β peptide which is produced in amyloid pathway during APP processing preserves and accumulates whereby generates amyloid plaques in AD (fig. 4). Amyloid β peptide contains 40 ($A\beta_{40}$) or 42 amino acids ($A\beta_{42}$) (Younkin, 1998). It is physiological peptide which is produced in the brain continuosly. Its level is determined by balance between anabolic and catabolic activities (Saido, 1998; Selkoe, 1993). Amyloid β peptide is toxic for the cells in cell lines (Yankner et al., 1989) by different pathways and its toxicity correlates with the level of its aggregation. This peptide is able to influence a lot of metabolic pathways in brain. It is able to activate caspases, effectors of apoptosis, to affect calcium homeostasis by increasing intracellular calcium concentration (Mattson et al., 1993), and to induce neuron death.

Neurotoxicity of Aβ can be mediated through the ability of amyloid β peptide participate in the production of reactive oxygen species and increased oxidative damage of biomolecules (fig. 4). Methionine residue 35 plays an important role in this process. Damage induced by Aβ can be modulated by superoxide dismutase. Aβ induces production of superoxide anion radical by stimulation of NADPH oxidase. Hydrogen peroxide arises in the presence of amyloid β peptide through reduction of the copper and the iron. Neurotoxicity is caused also by binding to nicotine acetylcholine receptor, forming calcium and potassium channels in cell membranes, decreasing glucose transport and releasing of chemokines and cytokines.

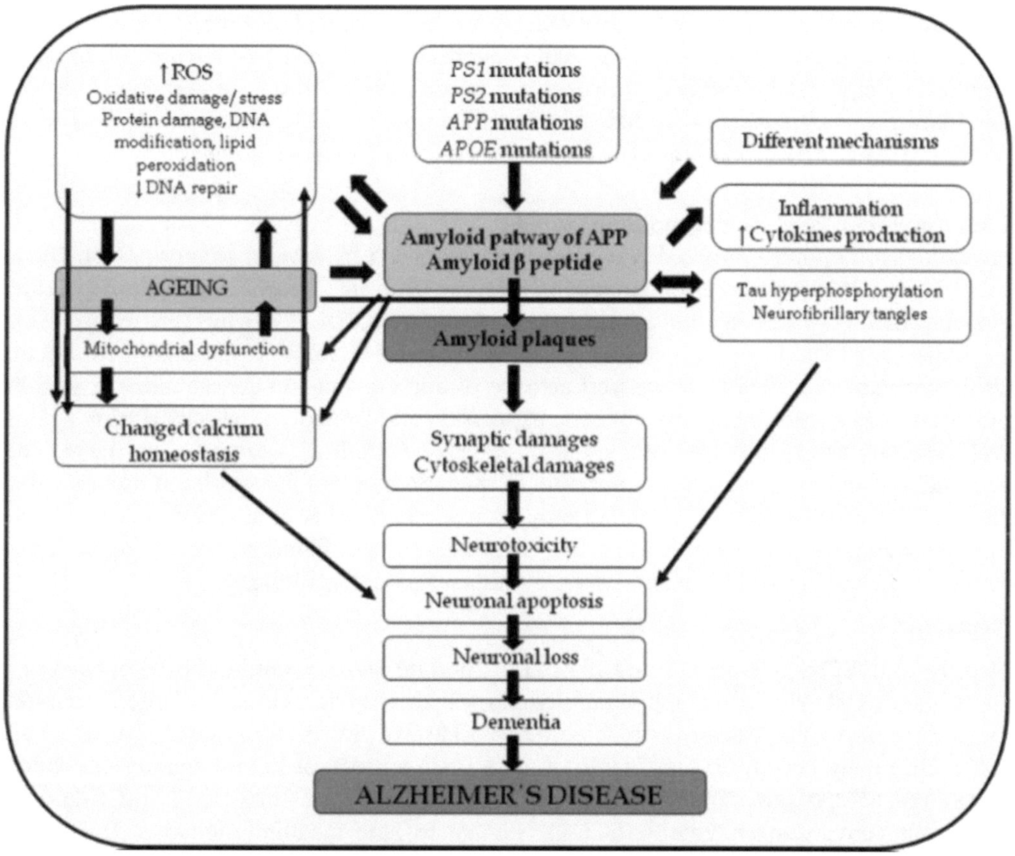

Fig. 4. Relationship between amyloid β peptide (Aβ), the ageing process, oxidative damage and Alzheimer's disease. ROS-reactive oxygen species, PS - presenilin, APP-amyloid precursor protein, APOE-apolipoprotein E

Oxidative modification of glutamate transporter and glutamate synthetase oxidation can be caused by Aβ as well. In AD patients was observed mitochondrial dysfunction and reduced energetic metabolism in brain. The main pathway of glucose oxidation is Krebs cycle in mitochondria. Oxidative decarboxylation of pyruvate (product of glycolysis) is catalysed by pyruvate dehydrogenase complex and offers acetyl CoA initiating Krebs cycle. Pyruvate dehydrogenase complex is formed by three enzymes: pyruvate dehydrogenase (EC 1.2.4.1, E1), dihydrolipoyl transacetylase (EC 2.3.1.12, E2) and dihydrolipoyl dehydrogenase (EC 18.1.4, E3). Rate limiting steps in Krebs cycle are reactions catalysed by pyruvate dehydrogenase complex and by oxoglutarate dehydrogenase complex. Oxoglutarate dehydrogenase complex is compact of three enzymes: oxoglutarate dehydrogenase (EC1.2.4.2), dihydrolipoyl succinyltransferase (EC 2.3.1.61) and dihydrolipoyl dehydrogenase (EC 1.8.1.4). AD patients had decreased concentration of these enzymes. Calcium modulates a lot of metabolic processes including synaptic plasticity and apoptosis. In the pathogenesis of AD play an important role dysregulation of intracellular calcium signalling. It is assumed that neurodegeneration induced by Aβ and protein tau can be mediated by changes in calcium homeostasis. Permanent changes in calcium homoeostasis are proximal reason of neurodegeneration in AD patients (Khachaturian, 1989).

Amyloid β peptide is metabolised very quickly in the brain. Its half time is 2 hours and 10 minutes in the plasma (Betaman et al., 2006) nevertheless it is resistant towards elimination (Jankowsky et al., 2005). Several proteases can participate in Aβ conversion. However one dominant protease is not known today. A lots of proteases cleave monomer Aβ in several positions (Eckman and Eckman, 2005; Rangan et al., 2003; Tucker et al., 2000).

2.1.3 Amyloid β peptide degrading enzymes

Physiological peptide - amyloid β peptide is metabolised by several enzymes. **Neprilysin** (NEP; EC 3.4.24.11), **endothelin-converting enzyme** (ECE; EC 3.4.24.71), **insulin-degrading enzyme** (IDE; EC 3.4.24.56), and probably also **plasmin** (EC 3.4.21.7) which are expressed in the brain contribute to the proteolysis of Aβ in the brain (Eckman et al., 2003; Iwata et al., 2000; Shirotani et al., 2001). Decreased activity of any enzymes in consequence of genetic mutation or as a result of changes in gene expression and proteolytic activity during ageing and diseases may increase risk of AD. Insulin-degrading enzyme, neprilysin and endothelin-converting enzyme are not able to degrade amyloid β deposits. It assumes that amyloid β aggregates can be degraded only by plasmin (Tucker et al., 2000). **Plasmin** is an important enzyme present in blood where degrades a lot of blood plasma proteins. It is a serine proteinase derived from an inactive zymogen called plasminogen.

Neprilysin

Neprilysin (NEP) is a 90 to 110 kDa plasma membrane glycoprotein that is composed of a short N-terminal cytoplasmic region, a membrane-spanning domain and a large C-terminal extracellular, catalytic domain, which contains a HexxH zinc-binding motif (Turner et al., 2001). Originally neprilysin was identified as a main antigen of kidney membranes thirty years ago. Neprilysin together with endothelin-converting enzyme 1 (ECE-1) and endothelin-converting enzyme 2 (ECE-2) belongs to zinc metalloproteinases, II. type of integral membrane peptidase – M13 family.

Neprilysin has several roles in the central nervous system, liver, lungs, musles, and bones. It participates in cardiovascular regulation, inflammation, neuropeptide metabolism, cell migration, and proliferation (Harrison et al., 1995; Turner & Tanzawa, 1997). Neprilysin cleaves peptide bound of small regulatory peptides and degrades a variety of bioactive peptides (Turner & Tanzawa, 1997). Studies of Aβ catabolism using inhibitors of metalloproteinases and neprilysin knock out mice (Iwata et al., 2000) showed that neprilysin is enzyme degrading amyloid β peptide. Expression and activity of neprilysin is regulated by several factors that are related to AD, and age.

Recently a homologue of neprilysin was discovered and named neprilysin 2 (NEP2). Unlike neprilysin and endothelin-converting enzyme 1, which are expressed in the central nervous system and periphery, NEP2 was found to be almost exclusively expressed only in selected population of neurons and spinal cord (Turner at al., 2004). This enzyme may also degrade Aβ (Shirotani et al., 2001).

Endothelin-converting enzyme

Endothelin-converting enzyme (ECE) plays an important role in the metabolism of Aβ. Endothelin-converting enzyme is a homologue of neprilysin and it is a zinc metalloproteinase. The enzyme catalyses a change of inactive molecule of big endothelin (bET) to a very effective vasoconstrictor endothelin 1 (ET-1) (Xu et al., 1994). Endothelin-converting enzyme was discovered in neurons and glial cells in the brain and it is localised both intra- and extra-cellularly (Barnes & Turner, 1997). The enzyme is able to hydrolyse some biological active peptides such as bradykinin, neurotesin, substantion P and oxidized chain of insulin B (Johnson et al., 1999). Ability of endothelin-converting enzyme to degrade amyloid β peptide has been discovered in experiments with a metallopreoteinase inhibitor - phosphoramid and then its positive effect was verified in human brain (Funalot et al., 2004).

Insulin-degrading enzyme

Insulin-degrading enzyme (IDE) is a zinc metalloproteinase. It is primarily located in the cytosol but it is also found in peroxisomes (Seta & Roth, 1997). A fraction of IDE can be found in the plasma membrane (Vekrellis et al., 2000). Insulin-degrading enzyme is able to cleave *in vitro* several physiological substrates, including insulin, glucagon, atriopoetin, amylin, Aβ. Insulin-degrading enzyme has physiological functions in insulin metabolism. It can degrade amyloid β peptide and it is selective for amyloid β peptide monomer (Farris et al., 2003; Vekrellis et al., 2000). Farris et al. (2003) and Miller at al. (2003) showed that endogenous levels of $A\beta_{40}$ and $A\beta_{42}$ were increased in the brain of IDE transgenic mice. Some *post mortem* analysis showed that decreased levels of insulin-degrading enzyme in patients with Alzheimer`s disease (Cook et al., 2003). Products that are produced by IDE cleaving of amyloid β peptide are not toxic.

2.2 Genetic risk factors for Alzheimer's disease

Alzheimer`s disease is a multifactorial disease and genetic as well as environmental factors are included in AD pathology. In the last decades, several genes involved in AD have been identified. There is no single gene responsible for an origin of Alzheimer`s disease. Mutations in amyloid precursor protein, presinilin 1 and presinilin 2 are liable for familiar AD. Mutations and polymorphisms in multiple genes contribute to sporadic AD.

2.2.1 Familiar form of Alzheimer's disease

Familiar form of Alzheimer`s disease is responsible for 5-10% of all cases of AD. It is characterized by early manifestation of dementia (sometimes in patients 40 years old) (Rosenberg, 2000). Mutations in three genes - gene for **amyloid precursor protein** on chromosome 21q21, gene for **presenilin 1** on chromosome 14q24.2 and gene for **presenilin 2** on chromosome 1q42.13 - increase production of $A\beta_{42}$ peptide and play a role in an autosomal dominant hereditary of Alzheimer`s disease (Goate et al., 1991; Levy-Lahad et al., 1995; Schellenberg et al., 1992). It is described 23 mutations of *APP* gene and 155 mutations of *PS1* gene and 9 mutations of *PS2* gene (www.alzforum.org). In familiar form of AD is increased level of amyloid β peptide years before any clinical symptoms of Alzheimer`s disease are observed. Interestingly, mutations in the tau gene are not associated with AD.

Amyloid precursor protein

Missense mutations in *APP* gene causing familiar form of AD are clustered around secretese cleavage sites. These mutations are responsible for increased production of Aβ which can cumulate and form amyloid plaques. Concentration of Aβ is increased in patients with Down syndrome. Most of these patients have neuritic plaques and tangles in their 40s. Gene for *APP* is located on chromosome 21 and patients with Down syndrome have trisomy 21, and this fact can be cause of AD development. Over 23 different *APP* mutations have been observed (Campion et al., 1999; Cruts & van Broeckhoven, 1998; de Jonghe et al., 2001).

Presenilins

Presenilins are main candidates for γ-secretase and they are contained in amyloid processing of APP. The human *PS1* and *PS2* mutations are linked to early onset AD. Presenilin 1 occurs in a normal processing of APP. Many different *PS1* mutations have been identified in 390 families. Mutations of presenilin 1 may be responsible for missing cleaving of APP and production of $A\beta_{42}$ the most aggressive variant for generation of amyloid plaques in the human brain (Xia et al., 1997). Moreover presenilin 1 acts together with glycogen synthase kinase (GSK3b). Glycogen synthase kinase is one of the critical protein kinases included in tau phosphorylation. In some cases of familiar Alzheimer`s Disease mutations of presenilin 1 cause an unusual interaction of PS1 with GSK3b and it can lead to increased hyperphosphorylation of tau protein and this form of tau protein then does not play its physiological roles (Takashima et al., 1998). Mutations in *PS2* are a much rarer than in *PS1* mutations. *PS2* mutations have been already described in 6 families.

2.2.2 Sporadic form of Alzheimer's disease

Despite numerous efforts, our knowledge of the heredity of AD remains incomplete. No consensus exists about the involvement of gene polymorphisms in risk of AD sporadic form. Genes for alfa-2-macroglobulins (Blacker et al., 1998), apolipoprotein E (*ApoE* ε4 variant) (Poirier et al., 1996), component of oxoglutarate dehydrogenase complex (Ali a kol., 1994), glycogen synthase kinase (*GSK3B*) (Schaffer et al., 2008), and some mitochondrial genes may be involved in familiar AD as well. Genes of secretases and amyloid β peptide degrading enzymes have been suggested as candidate genes for AD because they play a crucial role in a process of formation of senile plaques. The *BACE1* promoter polymorphisms may contribute to sporadic AD (Wang & Jia, 2009). Polymorphisms in the neprilysin gene (Helisalmi et al., 2004), and insulin-degrading enzyme (Vepsäläinen et al., 2010) increase the risk for AD. Angiotensin-converting enzyme (ACE) gene insertion/deletion polymorphism is considered as a biomarker for AD. Insertion/deletion and other *ACE* polymorphisms have a statistically significant effect on the risk of AD (Helbecque et al., 2009; Yang & Li, 2008; Wang et al., 2006). Oxidative damage is one of the mechanisms which results in stimulation of the amyloid pathway of APP processing therefore genes of antioxidant enzymes could present another group of candidate genes. Catalase (EC 1.11.1.6) is a common antioxidant enzyme found in all organisms. Catalase gene polymorphism does not confirm a protective role in AD patients (Capurso et al., 2008). Glutathione transferases (GSTs, EC 2.5.1.18) may play an important role as risk factors for AD because GSTs detoxify products of oxidative damage. Polymorphisms of *GSTs* can be therefore implicated in AD (Pinhel et al., 2008; Spalletta et al., 2007).

Apolipoprotein E

The most important genetic risk factor for sporadic AD is the *ApoE* gene, its ε4 allele, and is linked to familial late onset AD as well. ApoE is essential for a normal metabolism of lipoproteins, cholesterol and triacylgylcerols. Gene for ApoE is located on chomosome 19q13.2-13.3 and consists of 4 exons and 3 introns and is approximately 3.7 kb in length. *ApoE* has three isoforms: *ApoE* ε2 variant, *ApoE* ε3 variant, and *ApoE* ε4 variant. *ApoE* ε4 variant increased the risk of AD compared to *ApoE* ε2 variant, and ε3 variant (Carter, 2005; Fernandez & Scheibe, 2005; Poirier et al., 1993). ApoE may be connected to Aβ production and to increased aggreagation of Aβ. Polymorphism in *ApoE* promoter may be a risk factor for AD as well (Bizzarro et al., 2009).

Cytokines

Cytokines are secretory proteins that mediate intracellular communication in the immune system. However, they regulate a variety of processes in the central nervous system and may be involved in AD because neurodegeneration is accompanied by inflammation (so-called neuroinflammation). Inflammatory mediators are overexpressed and present in AD lesions (Selkoe, 2001a). Polymorphims in the promoter of IL-6, IL-10, and TNFα gene were suggested to be a risk factors for AD (Candore et al., 2007; Gnjec et al., 2008; Vural et al., 2009).

Methylenetetrahydrofolate reductase

5, 10-Methylenetetrahydrofolate reductase (MTHFR, EC 1.5.1.20) is a pivotal enzyme for DNA synthesis and homocysteine remethylation. Increased plasma homocysteine level is a risk factor for the development of AD (Seshadri et al., 2002). Two common genetic polymorphisms in the *MTHFR* gene C677T (Kang et al., 1988) and A1298T (van der Put et al., 1998) were discovered. *MTHFR* polymorphism causes decreased enzymatic activity of MTHFR and increased of the plasma total homocysteine level. Mutation in *MTHFR* is slightly associated with the onset of senile dementia (Nishiyama et al., 2000). Genotypes and haplotypes of the MTHFR have important implication for the pathogenesis of AD (Bi et al., 2009; Dorszewska et al., 2007; Gorgone et al., 2009; Kim et al., 2008; Wakutani et al., 2004). The MTHFR is a component of one carbon metabolism therefore it may interact with dietary intake of methionine, vitamins B6, B12, and folic acid in associations with AD.

2.2.3 Epigenetics and Alzheimer's disease

Recent evidence has suggested that histone acetylation and DNA methylation are implicated in the etiology of AD. Changes in chromatin structure are a prominent pathological feature of neurodegenerative diseases. Gene-environment interactions underlie neuropsychiatric disorders and epigenetics is involved in human processes (Figure 5). Epigenetic mechanisms refer to the processes that modify gene expression without altering the genetic code itself. Important epigenetic mechanisms include covalent modifications of two core component of chromatin: histone proteins - posttranslational modifications: histone acetylation, methylation, phosphorylation and the DNA - methylation, nucleosome positioning, higher order chromatin remodeling, deployment of numerous classes of short and long non-protein-coding RNAs, RNA editing and DNA recoding. Epigenetic mechanisms may play a crucial role in the interplay of genetic and environmental factors in determining a subject's phenotype (Reichenberg at al., 2009). Epigenetics may represent a basic molecular genetic mechanism in the pathophysiology of AD. The most frequently studied epigenetic mechanisms are DNA methylation and histone modification. These phenomena have been recognized as important permissive and submissive factors in controlling the expressed genome via gene transcription.

DNA methylation

DNA methylation is performed by the addition of a methyl group from S-adenosyl methionine to CpG islands by DNA methyltransferases (Mehler, 2008). Usually are methylated CpG islands near promoter regions of genes and DNA methylation generally represses transcription and so is associated with gene silencing. DNA methylation is dependent on the methylation potential and is closely related to the one-carbon metabolism. Methylenetetrahydrofolate reductase is a key enzyme in the one-carbon metabolism. The enzyme is coded by the gene *MTHFR* on chromosome 1 location p36.3 in humans (Goyette et al., 1994).

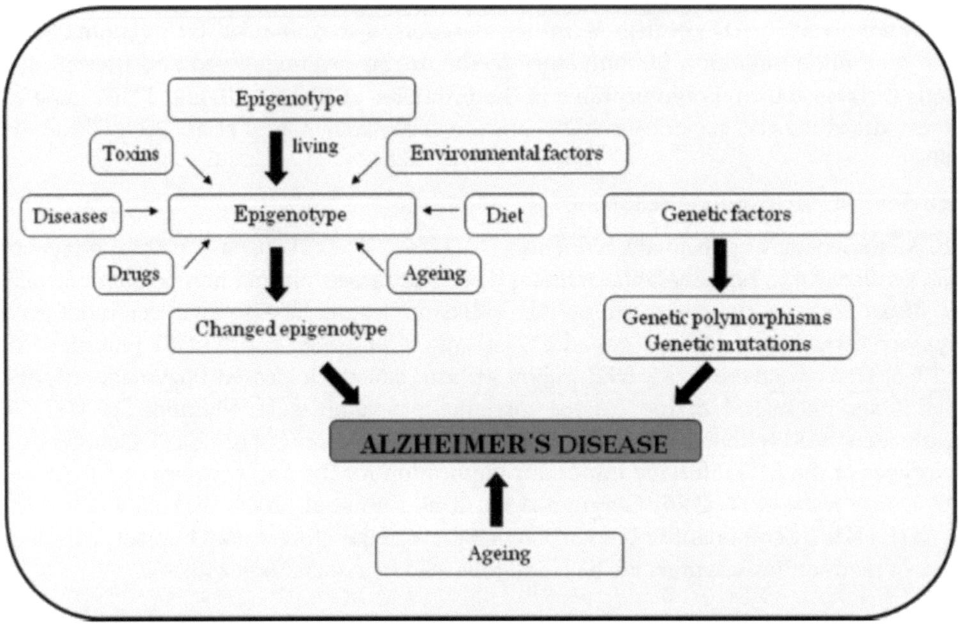

Fig. 5. Implication of epigenetic, genetic and environmental factors to Alzheimer`s disease origin

Histone modifications

The covalent modification of histones is happened at distinct amino acid residues on their amino terminal fails (Felsenfeld & Groudine, 2003). Histone acetylation, methylation, phosphorylation, ubiquitylation are the most common histone modifications. Histone acetylation is linked to transcriptional activation, while deacetylation is related to transcriptional repression (Berger, 2007).

Epigenetic modifications contribute to the phenotype's differences. DNA methylation was examined in monozygotic twins discordant for AD. In AD twin was observed decreased DNA methylation compared to non AD twin (Mastroeni et al., 2009). Amyloid precursor protein has been shown to be normally methylated, and hypomethylated with age (Tohgi at al., 1999) and in AD patients (West et al., 1995), which subsequently enhanced production of Aβ. Hypomethylation occurs with age and Aβ may be involved in the generation of amyloid β peptide itself. Amyloid β peptide causes global DNA hypomethylation and neprilysin hypermethylation, which consequently suppresses its expression in mRNA and protein level (Chen et al., 2009). In cell culture and in human post-mortem study, hypomethylation of the promoter region of *PS1* was found to increase presenilin expression, and enhance amyloid β generation (Scarpa et al., 2003, Wang et al., 2008). *PS1* and *BACE* are expressed at high levels in brain cells and both genes are unmethylated in brain (Fuso et al., 2005). AD may be associated with an increased in histone acetylation. Altered gene transcripton in AD has been associated with alterations in histone acetylation profiles (Kilgore et al., 2010). Amyloid intracellular domain (AICD) can interact *in vitro* with the histone acetyltransferase Tip60 and co-act as a transcriptional activator (Cao & Sudhof, 2001).

3. Conclusion

Neurological diseases, including AD are very serious medical problems. More than 150 million people suffer from neurodegenerative and neurological diseases. The average age of the world population is increased as a result of better knowledge, advances in diagnosis and treatment of various diseases. Unfortunately, age represents a key risk factor for development of age-related diseases, such as AD. Molecular and genetic analyses represent a new potential for AD studying. The role of mentioned gene polymorphisms and many others gene polymorphisms as risk factors for the occurrence of AD is still controversial. We still need new studies for clear determination gene polymorphisms which are related to AD. Moreover multiple genotype analyses are necessary as well because a single gene polymorphism can be without relationship to increased risk of AD but the combination of gene polymorphisms may have significant effect for AD development. Every person is unique and dementia affects people differently - no two people will have symptoms that develop in exactly the same way. An individual's personality, general health and social situation are all important factors in determining the impact of Alzheimer`s disease on him or her.

4. Acknowledgment

The work was supported by grant of Ministry of Health SVK, MZ SR 2007/57-UK-17.

5. References

Ali, G., Wasco, W., Cai, X., Szabo, P., Sheu, K.F., Cooper, A.J., Gaston, S.M., Gusella, J.F., Tanzi, R.E., & Blass, J.P. (1994). Isolation, characterisation, and mapping of gene encoding dihydrolipoyl succinyltransferase (Ek2) of human alpha-ketoglutarate dehydrogenase complex. *Somatic Cell and Molecullar Genetetics*, Vol.20, No.2, (March 1994), pp. 99-105

Alonso, A.C., Li, B., Grundke-Iqbal, I., & Iqbal, K. (2008). Mechanis, of tau-induced neurodegeneration in Alzheimer disease and related tauopathies. *Current Alzheimer Research*, Vol.5, No.4, (August 2008), pp. 375-384

Alzheimer A. (1907). Über eine eigenartige Erkrankung der Hirnrinde. *Allgemeine Zeitschrift fur Psychiatrie Psychisch-Gerichtliche Medizin*, Vol.64, (1907), pp. 146-148

Barnes, K., & Turner, A.J. (1997). The endothelin system and endothelin-converting enzyme in the brain: molecular and cellular studies. *Neurochemical Research*, Vol.22, No.8, (August 1997), pp. 1033-1040

Bennett, B.D., Babu-Khan, S., Loeloff, R., Louis, J.C., Curran, E., Citron, M., & Vassar, R. (2000). Expression analysis of BACE2 in brain and peripheral tissues. *The Journal of Biological Chemistry*, Vol.275, No.28, (July 2000), pp. 20647-20651

Berger, S.L. (2007). The complex language of chromatin regulation during transcription. *Nature*, Vol.447, No.7143, (May 2007), pp. 407-412

Betaman, R.J., Munsell, L.Y., Morris, J.C., Swarm, R., Yarasheski, K.E., & Holtzman, D.M. (2006). Human amyloid-beta synthesis and clearance rates as measered in cerebrospinal fluid in vivo. *Nature Medicine*, Vol.12, No.7, (July 2006), pp. 856-861

Bi, X.H., Zhao, H.L., Zhang, Z.X., & Zhang, J.W. (2009). Association of RFC1 A80G and MTHFR C677T polymorphisms with Alzheimer`s Disease. *Neurobiological Aging*, Vol.30, No.10, (October 2009), pp. 1601-1607

Bizzarro, A., Seripa, D., Acciarri, A., Matera, M.G., Pilotto, A., Tiziano, F.D., Brahe, C., & Masullo, C. (2009). The complex interaction between APOE promoter and AD: an Italian case-control study. *European Journal of Human Genetetics*, Vol.7, No.7, (July 2009), pp. 938-945

Blacker, D., Wilcox, M.A., Laird, N.M., Rodes, L., Horvath, S.M., Go, R.C., Perry, R., Watson, B. Jr., Bassett, S.S., McInnis, M.G., Albert, M.S., Hyman, B.T., & Tanzi, R.E. (1998). Alpha-2 macroglobulin is genetically associated with Alzheimer disease. *Nature Genetetics*, Vol.19, No.4, (August 1998), pp. 3357-3360

Braak, H., & Braak, E. (1991). Neuropathological stageing of Alzheimer-related changes. *Acta Neuropatholocica*, Vol.82, No.4, (September 1991), pp. 239-259

Brou, C., Logeat, F., Gupta, N., Bessia, C., LeBail, O., Doedens, J.R., Cumano, A., Roux, P., Black, R.A., & Israël, A. (2000). A novel proteolytic cleavage involved in Notch signaling: the role of the disintegrin-metalloprotease TACE. *Molecular Cell*, Vol.5, No.2, (February 2000), pp. 207-216

Buée, L., Bussière, T., Buée-Scherrer, V., Delacourte, A., & Hof, P.R. (2000). Tau protein isoforms, phosphorylation and role in neurodegenerative disorders. *Brain Research. Brain Research Reviews*, Vol.33, No.1, (August 2000), pp. 95-130

Caillé, I., Allinquant, B., Dupont, E., Bouillot, C., Langer, A., Müller, U., & Prochiantz, A. (2004). Soluble form of amyloid precursor protein regulates proliferation of progenitors in the adult subventricular zone. *Development*, Vol.131, No.9, (May 2004), pp. 2173-2181

Campion, D., Dumanchin, C., Hannequin, D., Dubois, B., Belliard, S., Puel, M., Thomas-Anterion, C., Michon, A., Martin, C., Charbonnier, F., Raux, G., Camuzat, A., Penet, C., Mesnage, V., Martinez, M., Clerget-Darpoux, F., Brice, A., Frebourg, T. (1999). Early-onset autosomal dominant Alzheimer disease: prevalence, genetic heterogeneity, and mutation spectrum. *American Journal of Human Genetics*, Vol.65, No.3, (September 1999), pp. 664-670

Candore, G., Balistreri, C.R., Grimaldi, M.P., Listì, F., Vasto, S., Chiappelli, M., Licastro, F., Colonna-Romano, G., Lio, D., & Caruso, C. (2007). Polymorphisms of pro-inflammatory genes and Alzheimer`s Disease risk: A phatmacogenomic approach. *Mechanisms of ageing and development*, Vol.128, No.1, (January 2008), pp. 67-75

Cao, X., & Südhof, T.C. (2001), A transcriptionally [correction of transcriptively] active complex of APP with Fe65 and histone acetyltransferase Tip60. *Science*, Vol.293, No.5527, (July 2001), pp. 115-120. Erratum in: *Science*, Vol.293, No.5534, (August 2001), pp. 1436

Capurso, C., Solfrizzi, V., D'Introno, A., Colacicco, A.M., Capurso, S.A., Bifaro, L., Menga, R., Santamato, A., Seripa, D., Pilotto, A., Capurso, & A., Panza, F. (2008). Short arm of chromosome 11 and sporadic Alzheimer`s Disease: catalase and cathepsin D gene polymorphisms. *Neuroscience Letters*, Vol.432, No.3, (February 2008), pp. 237-242

Carter, D.B. (2005). The interaction of amyloid-beta with ApoE. *Subcellular Biochemistry*, Vol.38, (2005), pp. 255-272

Citron, M., Diehl, T.S., Gordon, G., Biere, A.L., Seubert, P., & Selkoe, D.J. (1996). Evidence that the 42 and 40-amino acid forms of amyloid beta protein are generated from the beta-amyloid precursor protein by different protease activities. *Proceedings of the*

National Acadademy of the Sciences of the United States of America, Vol.93, No.23, (November 1996), pp. 13170-13175

Cook, D.G., Leverenz, J.B., McMillan, P.J., Kulstad, J.J., Ericksen, S., Roth, R.A., Schellenberg, G.D., Jin, L.W., Kovacina, K.S., & Craft, S. (2003). Reduced hippocampal insulin-degrading enzyme in late-onset Alzheimer`s Disease is asssociated with the apolipoprotein E-epsilon4 allele. *The American Journal of Pathology*, Vol.162, No.1, (January 2003), pp. 313-319

Coulson, E.J., Paliga, K., Beyreuther, K., & Masters, C.L. (2000). What the evolution of te amyloid protein precursor supergene family tells us about its function. *Neurochemistry International*, Vol.36, No.3, (March 2000), pp. 175-184

Cruts, M., & Van Broeckhoven, C. (1998). Molecular genetics of Alzheimer`s Disease. *Annals of Medicine*, Vol.30, No.6, (December 1998), pp. 560-565

De Jonghe, C., Esselens, C., Kumar-Singh, S., Craessaerts, K., Serneels, S., Checler, F., Annaert, W., Van Broeckhoven, C., & De Strooper, B. (2001). Pathogenetic APP mutations near the gamma-secretase cleavage site differentially affect Abeta secretion and APP C-terminal fragment stability. *Human Molecular Genetics*, Vol.10, No.16, (August 2001), pp. 1665-1671

De Strooper, B., & Annaert, W. (2000). Proteolytic processing and cell biological functions of the amyloid precursor protein. *Journal of Cell Science*, Vol.113, Pt11, (June 2000), pp. 1857-1870

Dorszewska, J., Florczak, J., Rozycka, A., Kempisty, B., Jaroszewska-Kolecka, J., Chojnacka, K., Trzeciak, W.H., & Kozubski, W. (2007). Oxidative DNA damage and level of thiols as related to polymorphisms of MTHFR, MTR, MTHFD1 in Alzheimer`s Disease and Parkinson`s disease. *Acta Neurobiologiae Experimentalis (Wars)*, Vol.67, No.2, (2007), pp. 113-129

Eckman, E.A., & Eckman, C.B. (2005). Abeta-degradating enzymes: modulators of Alzheimer`s Disease pathogenesis and targets for therapeutic intervention. *Biochemical Society Transactions*, Vol.33, Pt5, (November 2005), pp. 1101-1105

Eckman, E.A., Watson, M., Marlow, L., Sambamurti, K., & Eckman, C.B. (2003). Alzheimer`s Disease beta-amyloid peptide is increased in mice deficient en endothelin-converting enzyme. *The Journal of Biological Chemistry*, Vol.278, No.4, (January 2003), pp. 2081-2084

Esch, F.S., Keim, P.S., Beattie, E.C., Blacher, R.W., Culwell, A.R., Oltersdorf, T., McClure, D., & Ward, P.J. (1990). Cleavage of amyloid beta peptide during constitutive processing of its precursor. *Science*, Vol.248, No.4959, (June 1990), pp. 1122-1124

Fahrenholz, F., & Postina, R. (2006). α-secretase activation – an approach to Alzheimer`s Disease therapy. *Neuro-degenerative Diseases*, Vol.3, No.4-5, (October 2006), pp. 255-261

Farris, W., Mansourian, S., Chang, Y., Lindsley, L., Eckman, E.A., Frosch, M.P., Eckman, C.B., Tanzi, R.E., Selkoe, D.J., & Guenette, S. (2003). Insulin-degrading enzyme regulates the levels of insulin, amyloid beta-protein, and the beta-amyloid precursor protein intracellilar damain in vivo. *Proceedings of the National Acadademy of the Sciences of the United States of America*, Vol.100, No.7, (April 2003), pp. 4162-4167

Farzan, M., Schnitzler, C.E., Vasilieva, N., Leung, D., & Choe, H. (2000). BACE2, a beta-secretase homolog, cleaves at the beta site and within the amyloid-beta region of the amyloid-beta precursor protein. *Proceedings of the National Acadademy of the Sciences of the United States of America,* Vol.97, No.17, (August 2000), pp. 9712-9717

Felsenfeld, G., & Groudine, M. (2003). Controlling the double helix. *Nature,* Vol.421, No.6921, (January 2003), pp. 448-453

Fernandez, L.L., & Scheibe, R.M. (2005). Is MTHFR polymorphism a risk factor for Alzheimer`s Disease like APOE? *Arquivos de Neuro-psiquiatria,* Vol.63, No.1, (March 2005), pp. 1-6

Fukumoto, H., Cheung, B.S., Hyman, B.T., & Irizarry, M.C. (2002). Beta-secretase protein and activity are increased in the neocortex in Alzheimer disease. *Archives of Neurology,* Vol.59, No.9, (September 2002), pp. 1381-1389

Funalot, B., Ouimet, T., Claperon, A., Fallet, C., Delacourte, A., Epelbaum, J., Subkowski, T., Léonard, N., Codron, V., David, J.P., Amouyel, P., Schwartz, J.C., & Helbecque, N. (2004). Endothelin-converting enzyme 1 is expressed in human cerebral cortex and protects against Alzheimer`s Disease. *Molecullar Psychiatry,* Vol.9, No.12, (December 2004), pp. 1122-1128

Fuso, A., Seminara, L., Cavallaro, R.A., D'Anselmi, F., & Scarpa, S. (2005). S-adenosylmethionine/homocysteine cycle alterations modify DNA methylation status with consequent deregulation of PS1 and BACE and beta-amyloid production. *Molecular and Cellular Neuroscience,* Vol.28, No.1, (January 2005), pp.195-204. Erratum in: *Molecular and Cellular Neuroscience;* Vol.32, No.4, (August 2006), pp. 419

Glenner, G.G., and Wong, C.W. (1984). Alzheimer`s Disease: initial report of the purification and characterization of a novel cerebrovascular amyloid protein. *Biochemical and Biophysical Research Communications,* Vol.120, No.3, (August 1984), pp. 885-889

Gnjec, A., D'Costa, K.J., Laws, S.M., Hedley, R., Balakrishnan, K., Taddei, K., Martins, G., Paton, A., Verdile, G., Gandy, S.E., Broe, G.A., Brooks, W.S., Bennett, H., Piguet, O., Price, P., Miklossy, J., Hallmayer, J., McGeer, P.L., & Martins, R.N. (2008). Association of alleles carried at TNFA-850 and BAT1 -22 with Alzheimer`s Disease. *Journal of Neuroinflammation,* Vol.20, No.5, (August 2008), pp. 36

Goate, A., Chartier-Harlin, M.C., Mullan, M., Brown, J., Crawford, F., Fidani, L., Giuffra, L., Haynes, A., Irving, N., James, L., Mant, R., Newton, P., Rooke, K., Roques, P., Talbot, Ch., Pericak-Vance, M., Roses, A., Williamson, R., Rossor, M., Owen, M., & Hardy, J. (1991). Segregation of a missense mutation in the amyloid precursor protein gene with familial Alzheimer`s Disease. *Nature,* Vol.349, No.6311, (February 1991), pp. 704-706

Gorgone, G., Ursini, F., Altamura, C., Bressi, F., Tombini, M., Curcio, G., Chiovenda, P., Squitti, R., Silvestrini, M., Ientile, R., Pisani, F., Rossini, P.M., & Vernieri, F. (2009). Hyperhomocysteinemia, intima-media thickness and C677T MTHFR gene polymorphism: a correlation study in patiens with cognitive impairment. *Atherosclerosis,* Vol.206, No.1, (September 2009), pp. 309-313

Goyette, P., Sumner, J.S., Milos, R., Duncan, A.M., Rosenblatt, D.S., Matthews, R.G., & Rozen, R. (1994). Human methylenetetrahydrofolate reductase: isolation of cDNA, mapping and mutation identification. *Nature Genetetics*, Vol.7, No.2, (June 1994), pp. 195-200. Erratum in: *Nature Genetetics*, Vol.7, No.4, (August 1994), pp. 551

Grundke-Iqbal, I., Iqbal, K., Tung, Y.C., Quinlan, M., Wisniewski, H.M., & Binder, L.I. (1986). Abnormal phosphorylation of the microtubule-associated protein tau (tau) in Alzheimer cytoskeletal pathology. *Proceedings of the National Acadademy of the Sciences of the United States of America,* Vol.83, No. 13, (July 1986), pp. 4913-4917

Haass, C., Schlossmacher, M.G., Hung, A.Y., Vigo-Pelfrey, C., Mellon, A., Ostaszewski, B.L., Lieberburg, I., Koo, E.H., Schenk, D., Teplow, D.B., & Selkoe, D.E. (1992). Amyloid beta-peptide is produced by cultured cells during normal metabolism. *Nature,* Vol.359, No.6378, (June 1992), pp. 322-325

Harada, H., Tamaoka, A., Ishii, K., Shoji, S., Kametaka, S., Kametani, F., Saito, Y., & Murayama, S. (2006). Beta-site APP cleaving enzyme 1 (BACE1) is increased in remaining neurons in Alzheimer`s Disease brains. *Neuroscience Research,* Vol.54, No.1, (January 2006), pp. 24-29

Hardy, J.A., & Higgins, G.A. (1992). Alzheimer`s Disease: the amyloid cascade hypothesis. *Science,* Vol.56, No.5054, (April 1992), pp. 184-185

Harrison, N.K., Dawes, K.E., Kwon, O.J., Barnes, P.J., Laurent, G.J., & Chung, K.F. (1995). Effects of neuropeptides on human lung fibroblast proliferation and chemotaxis. *The American Journal of Physiology,* Vol.268, No.2 Pt1, (February 1995), pp. L278-L283

Helbecque, N., Codron, V., Cottel, D., & Amouyel, P. (2009). An age effect on the association of common variants of ACE with Alzheimer`s Disease. *Neuroscience Letters,* Vol.461, NO.2, (September 2009), pp. 181-184

Helisalmi, S., Hiltunen, M., Vepsäläinen, S., Iivonen, S., Mannermaa, A., Lehtovirta, M., Koivisto, A.M., Alafuzoff, I., & Soininen, H. (2004). Polymorphisms in neprilysin gene affect the risk of Alzheimer`s Disease in Finnish patients. *Journal of Neurology, Neurosurgery, and Psychiatry,* Vol.75, No.12, (December 2004), pp. 1746-1748

Hussain, I., Powell, D., Howlett, D.R., Tew, D.G., Meek, T.D., Chapman, C., Gloger, I.S., Murphy, K.E., Southan, C.D., Ryan, D.M., Smith, T.S., Simmons, D.L., Walsh, F.S., Dingwall, C., & Christie, G. (1999). Identification of a novel aspartic protease (Asp 2) as beta-secretase. *Molecular and Cellular Neurosciences,* Vol.14, No.6, (December 1999), pp. 419-427

Chen, K.L., Wang, S.S., Yang, Y.Y., Yuan, R.Y., Chen, R.M., & Hu, C.J. (2009). The epigenetic effects of amyloid-beta(1-40) on global DNA and neprilysin genes in murine cerebral endothelial cells. *Biochemical and Biophysical Research Communications,* Vol.378, No.1, (January 2009), pp. 57-61

Iwata, N., Tsubuki, S., Takaki, Y., Watanabe, K., Sekiguchi, M., Hosoki, E., Kawashima-Morishima, M., Lee, H.J., Hama, E., Sekine-Aizawa, Y., & Saido, T.C. (2000). Identification of the major Abeta 1-42 degrading catabolic pathway in brain parenchyma: suppression leads to biochemical and pathological deposition. Nature Medicine, Vol.6, No. 2, (February 2000), pp. 143-150

Iwatsubo, T., Odaka, A., Suzuki, N., Mizusawa, H., Nukina, N., & Ihara, Y. (1994). Visualization of A beta 42 (43) and A beta 40 in senile plaques with end-specific A beta monoclonals: evidence that an initially deposited species is A beta 42(43). *Neuron,* Vol.13, No.1, (July 1994), pp. 45-53

Jankowsky, J.L., Slunt, H.H., Gonzales, V., Savonenko, A.V., Wen, J.C., Jenkins, N.A., Copeland, N.G., Younkin, L.H., Lester, H.A., Younkin, S.G., & Borchelt, D.R. (2005). Persistent amyloidosis following suppression of Abeta production in a transgenic model of Alzheimer disease. *PloS Medicine*, Vol.2, No.12, (Decmber 2005), e355

Jarret, J.T., Berger, E.P., & Lansbury, P.T. Jr. (1993). The carboxy terminus of the beta amyloid protein is critical for the seeding of amyloid formation: implications for the pathogenesis of Alzheimer`s Disease. *Biochemistry*, Vol.32,No.18, (May 1993), pp. 4693-4697

Johnson, G.D., Stevenson, T., & Ahn, K. (1999). Hydrolysis of peptide hormones by endothelin-converting enzyme-1. A comparison with neprilysin. *The Journal of Biological Chemistry*, Vol.274, No. 7, (February 1999), pp. 4053-4058

Kamal, A., Stokin, G.B., Yang, Z., Xia, C.H., & Goldstein, L.S. (2000). Axonal transport of amyloid precursor protein is mediated by direct binding to the kinesin light chain subunit of kinesin-I. *Neuron*, Vol.28, No2., (November 2000), pp. 449-459

Kang, J., Lemaire, H.G., Unterbeck, A., Salbaum, J.M., Masters, C.L., Grzeschik, K.H., Multhaup, G., Beyreuther, K., & Müller-Hill, B. (1987). The precursor of Alzheimer`s Disease amyloid A4 protein resembles a cell-surfase receptor. *Nature*, Vol.325, No.6106, (February 1987), pp. 733-736

Kang, S.S., Zhou, J., Wong, P.W., Kowalisyn, J., & Strokosch, G. (1988). Intermediate homocysteinemia: a thermolabile variant of methylenetetrahydrofolate reductase. *The American Journal of Human Genetetics*, Vol.43, No.4, (October 1988), pp. 414-421

Khachaturian, Z.S. (1989). Calcium, membranes, aging, and Alzheimer`s Disease. Introduction and overview. *Annals of the New York Academy of Science*, Vol.568, (December 1989), pp. 1-4

Kilgore, M., Miller, C.A., Fass, D.M., Hennig, K.M., Haggarty, S.J., Sweatt, J.D., & Rumbaugh, G. (2010). Inhibitors of class 1 histone deacetylases reverse contextual memory deficits in a mouse model of Alzheimer`s Disease. *Neuropsychopharmacology*, Vol.35, No.4, (March 2010), pp. 870-880

Kim, J.M., Stewart, R., Kim, S.W., Yang, S.J., Shin, I.S., Shin, H.Y., & Yoon, J.S. (2008). Methylenetetrahydrofolate reductase gene and risk of Alzheimer`s Disease in Koreans. *International Journal of Geriatric Psychiatry*, Vol.23, No.5, (May 2008), pp. 454-459

Kirazov, E., Kirazov, L., Bigl, V., & Schliebs, R. (2001). Ontogenetic changes in protein level of amyloid precursor protein (APP) in growth cones and synaptosomes from rat brain and prenatal expression pattern of APP mRNA isoforms in developing rat embryo. *International Journal of Development Neuroscie*, Vol.19, No.3, (June 2001), pp. 287-296

Kitaguchi, N., Takahashi, Y., Tokushima, Y., Shiojiri, S., & Ito, H. (1988). Novel precursor of Alzheimer`s Disease amyloid protein shows protease inhibitory activity. *Nature*, Vol.331, No.6156, (February 1988), pp. 530-532

Kuentzel, S.L., Ali, S.M., Altman, R.A., Greenberg, B.D., & Raub, T.J. (1993). The Alzheimer beta-amyloid protein precursor/protease necin-II is cleaved by secretase in a trans-Golgi secretory compartment in human neuroglioma cells. *The Biochemical Journal*, Vol.295, Pt2, (October 1993), pp. 367-378

Kurt, M.A., Davies, D.C., & Kidd, M. (1997). Paired helical filament morphology varies with intracellular location in Alzheimer`s Disease brain. *Neuroscience Letters*, Vol.239, No.1, (December 1997), pp. 41-44

Lee, V.M., Balin, B.J., Otvos, L. Jr., & Trojanowski, J.Q. (1991). A68: a major subunit of paired helical filaments and derivazed forms of normal Tau. *Science*, Vol.251, No.4994, (February 1991), pp. 675-678

Levy-Lahad, E., Wijsman, E.M., Nemens, E., Anderson, L., Goddard, K.A., Weber, J.L., Bird, T.D., & Schellenberg, G.D. (1995). A familial Alzheimer`s Disease locus on chromosome 1. *Science*, Vol.269, No.5226, (August 1995), pp. 970-973

Lichtenthaler, S.F., Ida, N., Multhaup, G., Masters, C.L., & Beyreuther, K. (1997). Mutations in the transmembrane domain of APP altering gamma-secretase specificity. *Biochemistry*, Vol.36, No.49, (December 1997), pp. 15396-15403

Lin, X., Koelsch, G., Wu, S., Downs, D., Dashti, A., & Tang, J. (2000). Human aspartic protease memapsin 2 cleaves the beta-secretase site of the beta-amyloid precursor protein. *Proceedings of the National Acadademy of the Sciences of the United States of America*, Vol.97, No.4, (February 2000), pp. 1456-1460

Lopez-Perez, E., Zhang, Y., Frank, S.J., Creemers, J., Seidah, N., & Checler, F. (2001). Constitutive alpha-secretase cleavage of the beta-amyloid protein in the furin-deficient LoVo cell line: involvement of the pro-hormone convertase 7 and the disintegrin metalloprotease ADAM 10. *Journal of Neurochemistry*, Vol.76, No.5, (March 2001), pp. 1532-1539

Marks, N., & Berg, M.J. (2008). Neurosecretases provide strategies to treat sporadic and familial Alzheimer disorders. *Neurochemistry International*, Vol.52, No.1-2, (January 2008), pp. 184-215

Maruyama, K., Tomita, T., Shinozaki, K., Kume, H., Asada, H., Saido, T.C., Ishiura, S., Iwatsubo, T., & Obata, K. (1996). Familiar Alzheimer`s Disease-linked mutations at Val717 of amyloid precursor protein are specific for the increased secretion of A beta 42(43). Biochemical and Biophysical Research Communications, Vol.227, No.3, (October 1996), pp. 730-735

Mastroeni, D., McKee, A., Grover, A., Rogers, J., & Coleman, P.D. (2009). Epigenetic differences in cortical neurons from a pair of monozygotic twins discordant for Alzheimer`s Disease. *PLoS One*, Vol.4, No.8, (August 2009), e6617

Mattson, M.P., Tomaselli, K.J., & Rydel RE. (1993). Calcium-destabilizing and neurodegenerative effects of aggregated beta-amyloid peptide are attenuated by basic FGF. *Brain Research*, Vol.621, No.1, (September 1993), pp. 35-49

Mehler, M.F. (2008). Epigenetics and the nervous system. *Annual Neurology*, Vol.64, No.6, (December 2009), pp. 602-617

Miller, B.C., Eckman, E.A., Sambamurti, K., Dobbs, N., Chow, K.M., Eckman, C.B., Hersh, L.B., & Thiele, D.L. (2003). Amyloid-beta peptide levels in brain are inversely correlated with insulysin activity levels in vivo. *Proceedings of the National Acadademy of the Sciences of the United States of America*, Vol.100, No.10, (May 2003), pp. 6221-6226

Mok, S.S., Clippingdale, A.B., Beyreuther, K., Masters, C.L., Barrow, C.J., & Small, D.H. (2000). A beta peptides and calcium influence secretion of the amyloid protein precursor from chick sympathetic neurons in cell culture. *Journal of Neuroscience Research*, Vol.61, No.4, (August 2000), pp. 449-457

Neve, D.L., & McPhie, Y.C. (2000). Alzheimer`s Disease: a dysfunction of the amyloid precursor protein. *Brain Research*, Vol.886, No.1-2, (December 2000), pp. 54-66

Neve, R.L., Finch, E.A., & Daves, L.R. (1988). Expression of the Alzheimer amyloid precursor gene transcripts in the humans. *Neuron*, Vol.1, No.8, (October 1988), pp. 669-677

Nishimoto, I., Okamoto, T., Matsuura, Y., Takahashi, S., Okamoto, T., Murayama, Y., & Ogata, E. (1993). Alzheimer amyloid protein precursor complexes with brain GTP-binding protein G(o). *Nature*, Vol.362, No.6415, (March 1993), pp. 75-79

Nishiyama, M., Kato, Y., Hashimoto, M., Yukawa, S., & Omori, K. (2000). Apolipoproteine E, methylenetetrahydrofolate reductase (MTHFR) mutation and the risk of senile dementia—an epidemiological study using the polymerase chain reaction (PCR) method. *Journal of Epidemiology*, Vol.10, No.3, (May 2000), pp. 163-172

Pinhel, M.A., Nakazone, M.A., Cação, J.C., Piteri, R.C., Dantas, R.T., Godoy, M.F., Godoy, M.R., Tognola, W.A., Conforti-Froes, N.D., & Souza, D. (2008). Glutathione S-transferase variants increase susceptibility for late-onset Alzheimer`s Disease: association study and relationship with apolipoprotein E epsilon 4 allele. Clinical Chemistry and Laboratory Medicine, Vol.46, No.4, (2008), pp. 439-445

Poirier, J. (1996). Apolipoprotein E in the brain and its role in Alzheimer`s Disease. *Journal of Psychiatry and Neuroscience*, Vol.21, No.2, (March 1996), pp. 128-134

Poirier, J., Davignon, J., Bouthillier, D., Kogan, S., Bertrand, P., & Gauthier, S. (1993). Apolipoprotein E polymorphism and Alzheimer`s Disease. *Lancet*, Vol.342, No.8873, (September 1993), pp- 697-699

Ponte, P., Gonzales-DeWhitt, P., Schilling, J., Miller, J., Hsu, D., Greenberg, B., Davis, K., Wallace, W., Lieberburg, I., Fuller, F., & Gordell, B. (1988). A new A4 amyloid mRNA contains a domain homologous to serine protease inhibitor. *Nature*, Vol.331, No.6156, (February 1988), pp. 525-532

Qiu, W.Q., Ferreira, A., Miller, C., Koo, E.H., & Selkoe, D.J. (1995). Cell-surface beta-amyloid precursor protein stimulates neurite outgrowth of hippocampal neurons in an isoform-dependent manner. *The Journal of Neuroscience*, Vol.15, No.3Pt2, (March 1995), pp. 2157-2167

Rangan, S.K., Liu, R., Brune, D., Planque, S., Paul, S., & Sierks, M.R. (2003). Degradation of beta-amyloid by proteollytic antibody light chains. *Biochemistry*, Vol.42, No.48, (December 2003), pp. 14328-14334

Reichenberg, A., Mill, J., & MacCabe, J.H. (2009). Epigenetics, genomic mutations and cognitive function. *Cognitive Neuropsychiatry*, Vol.14, No.4-5, (2009), pp. 377-390

Robert, M, & Mathuranath, P.S. (2007). Tau and tauopathies. *Neurology India*, Vol.55, No.1, (January-March 2007), pp. 11-16

Rosenberg, R.N. (2000). The molecular and genetic basis of AD: the beginning: the 2000 Wartenberg lecture. *Neurology*, Vol.54, No.11, (June 2000), pp. 2045-2054

Saido, T.C. (1998). Alzheimer`s Disease as proteolytic disorders: anabolism and catabolism of beta-amyloid. *Neurobiology of Aging*, Vol.19, 1 Suppl. (January-February 1998), pp. S69-S75

Scarpa, S., Fuso, A., D'Anselmi, F., & Cavallaro, R.A. (2003). Presenilin 1 gene silencing by S-adenosylmethionine: a treatment for Alzheimer`s Disease? *FEBS Letters*, Vol.541, No.1-3, (April 2003), pp. 145-148

Selkoe, D.J. (1993). Physiological production of the beta-amyloid protein and the mechanism of Alzheimer`s Disease. *Trends in Neurosciences*, Vol.16, No.10, (October 1993), pp. 403-409

Selkoe, D.J. (1999). Translating cell biology into therapeutic advances in Alzheimer`s Disease. *Nature*, Vol.399, 6738 Suppl., (June 1999), pp. A23-A31

Selkoe, D.J. (2001a). Alzheimer`s Disease: genes, proteins, and therapy. *Physiological Reviews*, Vol.81, No.2, (April 2001), pp. 741-766

Selkoe, D.J. (2001b). The genetics and molecular pathology of Alzheimer`s Disease: roles of amyloid and the presenilins. *Neurologic Clinics*, Vol.18, No.4, (November 2001), pp. 903-922

Seshadri, S., Beiser, A., Selhub, J., Jacques, P.F., Rosenberg, I.H., D'Agostino, R.B., Wilson, P.W., & Wolf, P.A. (2002). Plasma homocysteine as a risk factor for dementia and Alzheimer`s Disease. *The New England Journal of Medicine*, Vol.346, No.7, (February 2002), pp. 476-483

Seta, K.A., & Roth, R.A. (1997). Overexpression of insulin degrading enzyme: cellular localization and effects on insulin signaling. *Biochemical Biophysisal Research Communications*, Vol.231, No.1, (February 1997), pp. 167-171

Seubert, P., Oltersdorf, T., Lee, M.G., Barbour, R., Blomquist, C., Davis, D.L., Bryant, K., Fritz, L.C., Galasko, D., Thal, L.J., & Schenk, D.B. (1993). Secretion of beta-amyloid precursor protein cleaved at the amino terminus of the beta-amyloid peptide. *Nature* Vol.361, No.6049, (January 1993), pp. 260-263

Shirotani, K., Tsubuki, S., Iwata, N., Takaki, Y., Harigaya, W., Maruyama, K., Kiryu-Seo, S., Kiyama, H., Iwata, H., Tomita, T., Iwatsubo, T., & Saido, T.C. (2001). Neprilysin degrades both amyloid beta peptides 1-40 and 1-42 most rapidly and efficiently among thiorphan- and phosphoramidon-sensitive endopeptidases. *The Journal of Biological Chemistry*, Vol.276, No.4, (June 2001), pp. 21895-21901

Schaffer, B.A., Bertram, L., Miller, B.L., Mullin, K., Weintraub, S., Johnson, N., Bigio, E.H., Mesulam, M., Wiedau-Pazos, M., Jackson, G.R., Cummings, J.L., Cantor, R.M., Levey, A.I., Tanzi, R.E., & Geschwind, D.H. (2008). Association of GSK3B with Alzheimer disease and frontotemporal dementia. *Archives of Neurology*, Vol.64, No.10, (October 2008), pp. 1368-1374

Schellenberg, G.D., Bird, T.D., Wijsman, E.M., Orr, H.T., Anderson, L., Nemens, E., White, J.A., Bonnycastle, L., Weber, J.L., & Alonso, M.E. (1992). Genetic linkage evidence for a familial Alzheimer`s Disease locus on chromosome 14. *Science*, Vol.258, No.5082, (October 1992), pp. 668-671

Sinha, S., & Lieberburg, I. (1999). Cellular mechanisms of beta-amyloid production and secrection. *Proceedings of the National Acadademy of the Sciences of the United States of America*, Vol.96, No.20, (September 1999), pp. 11049-11053

Spalletta, G., Bernardini, S., Bellincampi, L., Federici, G., Trequattrini, A., Ciappi, F., Bria, P., Caltagirone, C., & Bossù, P. (2007). Glutathione S-transferase P1 and T1 gene polymorphisms predict longitudinal course and age at onset of Alzheimer disease.

The American Journal of Geriatriatric Psychiatry, Vol.15, No.10, (October 2007), pp. 879-887

Suh, Y.H. (1997). An etiological role of amyloidogenic carboxy-terminal fragments of the beta-amyloid precursor protein in Alzheimer`s Disease. *Journal of Neurochemistry,* Vol.68, No.5, (May 1997), pp. 1781-1791

Takashima, A., Murayama, M., Murayama, O., Kohno, T., Honda, T., Yasutake, K., Nihonmatsu, N., Mercken, M., Yamaguchi, H., Sugihara, S., & Wolozin, B. (1998). Presenilin 1 associates with glycogen synthase kinase-3beta and its substrate tau. *Proceedings of the National Acadademy of the Sciences of the United States of America,* Vol.95, No.16, (August 1998), pp. 9637-9641

Tanaka, S., Nakamura, S., Ueda, K., Kameyama, M., Shiojiri, S., Takahashi, Y., Kitaguchi, N., & Ito, H. (1988). Three types of amyloid protein precursor mRNA in human brain: their differential expression in Alzheimer`s Disease. *Biochemical Biophysical Research Communications,* Vol.157, No.2, (December 1988), pp. 472-479

Tohgi, H., Utsugisawa, K., Nagane, Y., Yoshimura, M., Ukitsu, M., & Genda, Y. (1999). The methylation status of cytosines in a tau gene promoter region alters with age to downregulate transcriptional activity in human cerebral cortex. *Neuroscience Letters,* Vol.275, No.2, (November 1999), pp. 89-92

Tucker, H.M., Kihiko, M., Caldwell, J.N., Wright, S., Kawarabayashi, T., Price, D., Walker, D., Scheff, S., McGillis, J.P., Rydel, R.E., & Estus, S. (2000). The plasmin system is induced by and degrades amyloid-beta aggregates. *The Journal of Neuroscience,* Vol.20, No.11, (June 2000), pp.3937-3946

Turner, A.J., & Tanzawa, K. (1997). Mammalian membrane metallopeptidase: NEP, ECE, KELL, and PEX. *The FASEB Journal,* Vol.11, No.5, (April 1997), pp. 355-364

Turner, A.J., Fisk, L., & Nalivaeva, N.N. (2004). Targeting amyloid-degrading enzymes as therapeutic strategies in neurodegeneration. *Annals of the New York Academy of Science,* Vol.1035, (December 2004), pp. 1-20

Turner, A.J., Isaac, R.E., & Coates, D. (2001). The neprilysin (NEP) family of zinc metallendopeptidase: genomics and function. *Bioessays,* Vol.23, No.3, (March 2001), pp. 261-269

van der Put, N.M., Gabreëls, F., Stevens, E.M., Smeitink, J.A., Trijbels, F.J., Eskes, T.K., van den Heuvel, L.P., & Blom, H,J. (1998). A second common mutation in the methylenetetrahydrofolate reductase gene: an additional risk factor for neural-tube defects? *The American Journal of Human Genetetics,* Vol.62, No.5, (May 1998), pp. 1044-1051

Vekrellis, K., Ye, Z., Qiu, W.Q., Walsh, D., Hartley, D., Chesneau, V., Rosner, M.R., & Selkoe, D.J. (2000). Neurons regulate extracellular levels of amyloid beta-protein via proteolysis by insulin-degrading enzyme. *The Journal of Neuroscience,* Vol.20, No.5, (March 2000), pp. 1657-1665

Vepsäläinen, S., Helisalmi, S., Mannermaa, A., Pirttilä, T., Soininen, H., & Hiltunen, M. (2009). Combined risk effects of IDE and NEP gene variants on Alzheimer disease. *Journal of Neurology, Neurosurgery, and Psychiatry,* Vol.80, No.11, (November 2009), pp. 1268-1270

Vural, P., Değirmencioğlu, S., Parildar-Karpuzoğlu, H., Doğru-Abbasoğlu, S., Hanagasi, H.A., Karadağ, B., Gürvit, H., Emre, M., & Uysal, M. (2009). The combination of

TNFalpha-308 and IL-6 -174 or IL-10 -1082 genes polymorphisms suggest an association with susceptibility to sporadic late-onset Alzheimer`s Disease. *Acta Neurologica Scandinavica,* Vol.120, No.6, (December 2009), pp. 396-401

Wakutani, Y., Kowa, H., Kusumi, M., Nakaso, K., Yasui, K., Isoe-Wada, K., Yano, H., Urakami, K., Takeshima, T., & Nakashima, K. (2004). A haplotype of the methylenetetrahydrofolate reductase gene is protective against late-onset Alzheimer`s Disease. *Neurobiological Aging,* Vol.25, No.3, (March 2004), pp. 291-294

Walter, J., Fluhrer, R., Hartung, B., Willem, M., Kaether, C., Capell, A., Lammich, S., Multhaup, G., & Haass, C. (2001). Phosphorylation regulates intracellular trafficking of beta-secretase. *The Journal of Biological Chemistry,* Vol.276, No.18, (May 2001), pp. 14634-14641

Wang, B., Jin, F., Yang, Z., Lu, Z., Kan, R., Li, S., Zheng, C., & Wang, L. (2006). The insertion polymorphism in angiotensin-converting enzyme gene associated with the APOE epsilon 4 allele increases the risk of the late-onset Alzheimer disease. *Journal of Molecular Neuroscie,* Vol.30, No.3, (2006), pp. 267-271

Wang, S., & Jia, J. (2010). Protomer polymorphisms which modulate BACE1 expression are associated with sporadic Alzheimer`s Disease. *American Journal of Medical Genetics, Part B, Neuropsychiatric Genetics,* Vol. 153B, No.1, (January 2010), pp. 159-166

Wang, S.C., Oelze, B., & Schumacher, A. (2008). Age-specific epigenetic drift in late-onset Alzheimer`s Disease. *PLoS One,* Vol.3, No.7, (July 2008), e2698

West, R.L., Lee, J.M., & Maroun, L.E. (1995). Hypomethylation of the amyloid precursor protein gene in the brain of an Alzheimer`s Disease patient. *Journal of Molecular Neuroscience,* Vol.6, No.2, (1995), pp. 141-146

Xia, W., Zhang, J., Perez, R., Koo, E.H., and Selkoe, D.J. (1997). Interaction between amyloid precursor protein and presenilins in mammalian cells: implications for the pathogenesis of Alzheimer disease. *Proceedings of the National Acadademy of the Sciences of the United States of America,* Vol.94, No.15, (July 1997), pp. 8208-8213

Xu, D., Emoto, N., Giaid, A., Slaughter, C., Kaw, S., deWit, D., & Yanagisawa, M. (1994). ECE-1: a membrane-bound metalloprotease that catalyzes the proteolytic activation of big endothelin-1. *Cell,* Vol.78, No.3, (August 1994), pp. 473-485

Yan, R., Bienkowski, M.J., Shuck, M.E., Miao, H., Tory, M.C., Pauley, A.M., Brashier, J.R., Stratman, N.C., Mathews, W.R., Buhl, A.E., Carter, D.B., Tomasselli, A.G., Parodi, L.A., Heinrikson, R.L., & Gurney, M.E. (1999). Membrane-anchored aspartyl protease with Alzheimer`s Disease beta-secretase activity. *Nature,* Vol.402, No.6761, (December 1999), pp. 533-537

Yang, Y.H., & Liu, C.K. (2008). Angiotensin-converting enzyme gene in Alzheimer`s Disease. *The Tohoku Journal of Experimental Medicine,* Vol.215, No.4, (August 2008), pp. 295-298

Yankner, B.A., Dawes, L.R., Fisher, S., Villa-Komaroff, L., Oster-Granite, M.L., & Neve, R.L. (1989). Neurotoxicity of a fragment of the amyloid precursor associated with Alzheimer`s Disease. *Science,* Vol.245, No.4916, (July 1989), pp. 417-420

Yoshikai, S., Sasaki, H., Doh-ura, K., Furuya, H., & Sakaki, Y. (1990). Genomic organization of the human amyloid beta-protein precursor gene. *Gene,* Vol.87, No.2, (March 1990), pp. 257-263; Erratum in: *Gene* (1991) Vol.102, No.2, (June 1991), pp. 291-292

Younkin, S.G. (1998). The role of A beta 42 in Alzheimer`s Disease. *Journal of Physiology Paris,* Vol.192, No.3-4, (july-August 1998), pp. 289-292

Zheng, H., Jiang, M., Trumbauer, M.E., Sirinathsinghji, D.J., Hopkins, R., Smith, D.W., Heavens, R.P., Dawson, G.R., Boyce, S., Conner, M.W., Stevens, K.A., Slunt, H.H., Sisoda, S.S., Chen, H.Y., & Van der Ploeg, L.H. (1995). beta-Amyloid precursor protein-deficient mice show reactive gliosis and decreased locomotor activity. *Cell,* Vol.81, No.4, (May 1995), pp. 525-531

2

Evidence for an Infectious Etiology in Alzheimer's Disease

Brian Balin, Christine Hammond,
C. Scott Little, Denah Appelt and Susan Hingley
Philadelphia College of Osteopathic Medicine, Center for Chronic Disorders of Aging, United States of America

1. Introduction

The possibility of an infectious etiology of several chronic diseases, including Alzheimer's Disease, has long been debated. More than a century ago Alois Alzheimer studied neurological infection with *Treponema pallidum*, the causative agent of syphilis, a spirochete later associated with dementia (Noguchi and Moore, 1913). There are many chronic diseases for which there is strong evidence of an infectious etiology (see table 1), and numerous chronic diseases for which there is suspicion of infection as the etiologic agent for that disease (see table 2) (Tables 1 and 2 are adapted from a colloquium sponsored by the American Academy of Microbiology from June 2004). Koch's postulates, that can, in some cases, provide absolute proof that a particular microorganism causes a particular disease, have been invaluable in the prevention and treatment of many diseases as well as in advancing microbiology. However, the postulates do not hold for most chronic diseases of microbial etiology, particularly those occurring late in life. Furthermore, they do not hold true for those of possible viral etiology, or for those that are multi-factorial in origin. In diseases of relatively old age, microbes acting earlier in life might operate by a "hit-and-hide" mechanism, or could over time be present at an extremely low level, so that searches for the organism might not reveal the culprit until long after damage has been initiated. In viral diseases and for those involving unique organisms such as obligate intracellular bacteria (eg, Chlamydia), the postulates requiring isolation and growth in pure culture cannot be met completely as these organisms reproduce only within living cells. In multi-factorial diseases, a causative organism might not be readily apparent, as other factors may be more prominent. However, absence of evidence is not proof of absence; in several cases when overwhelming experimental evidence was obtained, the pathogen concept had to be accepted even though it had met with great opposition initially. Two examples, among many, are the involvement of viruses in certain types of cancer such as human papillomavirus in cervical cancer, and of the bacterium *Helicobacter pylori* in stomach ulcers.
Alzheimer's Disease(AD) is a neurodegenerative disease that is considered to be the single most significant cause of dementia in the elderly (Keefover, 1996). There are two major categories of AD, familial and sporadic late-onset. The familial form of AD accounts for approximately 5% of total cases and usually presents in individuals in their 40's and 50's. This form of disease is caused by rare mutations in genes associated with β-amyloid

production and processing resulting in β-amyloid deposition into senile plaques. The genes code for transmembrane proteins including β-amyloid precursor protein, presenilin 1 and presenilin 2 (Scheuner et al., 1996). In contrast, the sporadic late-onset form of AD accounts for ~95% of total cases, displays similar pathological accumulations such as amyloid and tau as occurs in familial disease, but does not exhibit mutations in the genes of familial disease. However, at least one genetic risk factor, the APOE ε4 genotype, has been linked with

INFECTION	CHRONIC DISEASE(S)
Human T-cell Lymphotrophic virus type I	Adult T cell leukemia
	Tropical spastic paraparesis
Human papilloma virus (HPV)	Cervical carcinoma
	Larynginal papilloma
Epstein-Barr virus (EBV)	Burkitt's lymphoma in Africa
	Nasopharyngeal carcinoma
	Hodgkin's disease
Hepatitis B virus (HBV)	Hepatocellular carcinoma, chronic hepatitis
Hepatitis C virus (HCV)	
HBV and delta virus	
HBV	Polyarteritis nodosa
HCV	Mixed cryoglobulinemia
Measles	Sub acute sclerosing panencephalitis
Kaposi's sarcoma-associated herpes virus	Lymphoma
	Kaposi's sarcoma
Parvovirus B19	Anemia; arthritis
Rubella	Post-rubella arthritis syndrome
	Congenital rubella syndrome
Prions	Creutzfeld Jacob disease
	Kuru
Helicobacter pylori	Gastric lymphoma
	Peptic ulcer disease (PUD)
Histoplasmosis	Chronic pericarditis
Syphilis	Tertiary & neurosyphilis
Borellia burgdorferi	Lyme disease
Group A *Streptococcus*	Post-streptococcal glomerulonephritis
Chlamydia trachomatis	Reiter's syndrome & reactive arthritis
Tropheryma whippleii	Whipple's disease
Mycobacterium leprae	Leprosy
Mycobacterium tuberculosis	Tuberculosis
Campylobacter jejuni	Guillan-Barre syndrome
Chlamydia trachomatis	Pelvic inflammatory disease
Osteomyelitis	Squamous cell carcinoma
***Escherichia coli* O157:H7**	Hemolytic-uremic syndrome
Cytomegalovirus	Post-transplant accelerated atherosclerosis

Table 1. Chronic diseases for which there is strong evidence of an infectious etiology

DISEASE	SUSPECTED AGENT(S), IF ANY
Primary biliary cirrhosis	*Helicobacter pylori*, retrovirus
Mesothelioma	Simian virus 40
Multiple sclerosis	Epstein-Barr Virus
Tics and Obsessive Compulsive Disorder	Group A *Streptococcus agalactiae*
Obsessive compulsive disorder	Group A *Streptococcus agalactiae*
Crohn's disease	*Mycobacterium paratuberculosis*
Alzheimer's Disease	*Chlamydia pneumoniae*
Diabetes	Enteroviruses
Sjogren's disease	*H. pylori*
Sarcoidosis	*Mycobacterium* species
Atherosclerosis	*Chlamydia pneumoniae,* CMV
Bell's palsy	Herpes Simplex Virus
Schizophrenia	Intrauterine exposure to Influenza
ALS	Prions
Chronic fatigue	HTLV-1; EBV
Prostate cancer	BK virus

Table 2. Chronic diseases for which there is suspicion of an infectious etiology

late-onset disease (Roses, 1996). For late onset AD, there appears to be interplay between genetic risk(s) and environmental insult, but the exact etiology has yet to be clearly delineated.

Sporadic late-onset AD is thought to arise from a multi-factorial interplay between genetic and environmental factors. Speculation as to which environmental factors may have a great impact on the pathogenesis of this disease has led to studies of infectious disease. This is a rational approach as different types of infections have been associated with dementing illnesses, including infection with *Treponema pallidum,* mentioned previously, as well as other infections such as measles virus (Frings et al., 2002) and HIV (Zhou et al., 2010). Early studies of infection directly related to AD attempted to correlate viral infection with late-onset disease (Pogo, et al. 1987). The viruses considered were: Herpes Simplex 1 and 2, cytomegalovirus, measles virus, poliovirus, adenoviruses, hepatitis B virus, and the influenza A and B viruses. No association with disease was established for these viruses. More recent studies have found evidence for direct brain infection in AD with HSV1 (Itzhaki et al., 1997), *Borrelia burgdorferi* (Miklossy, 1993), and *Chlamydia pneumoniae* (Balin et al., 1998; Gerard et al., 2006). There are some reports indicating that systemic infections may correlate with increased incidence of AD and infection with *Helicobacter pylori,* the agent of gastric ulcers, and *Porphyromonas gingivalis,* an agent of periodontitis, have been studied in late-onset disease (Honjo et al., 2009; Kim et al., 2007). Given these reports and the need to identify and understand causative factors for sporadic late-onset AD, further investigations are required to determine the mechanisms by which these different infections might initiate and participate in the pathogenesis of AD.

Interestingly, when one considers factors that may drive the accumulation of amyloid and tau in AD, infectious triggers are some of the most significant and logical choices. In particular, the organisms likely to be involved in AD are those that can evade host defenses, gain entry to specific selectively vulnerable regions of the brain, and establish chronic/persistent and/or latent infection. Upon considering the other risk factors associated with AD, infection may be the central hub connecting these factors. Currently, evidence from research on *Chlamydia pneumoniae*, Herpes Simplex Virus 1, and *Borrelia burgdorferi* in the AD brain, links numerous risk factors in the pathogenesis of AD with infection. Linkage has been recognized for risk factors such as ApoEε4 expression, chronic neuroinflammation, autoimmune mechanisms, oxidative and mitochondrial damage, cardiovascular factors, diabetes with insulin resistance, trauma to the blood brain barrier, and selectively vulnerable brain insult (Itzhaki et al., 2004; Miklossy, 2008). Thus, infection actually may be the overarching "unifying hypothesis" for sporadic late-onset AD, rather than other more mainstream hypotheses.

2. Alzheimer's Disease and Herpes Simplex Virus 1

Studies have implicated Herpes Simplex Virus type 1 (HSV1) as a potential etiologic agent for AD (Itzhaki and Wozniak, 2008). HSV1 is ubiquitous and produces latent infection in neurons, initially in the trigeminal ganglia of the peripheral nervous system. Reactivation and transport along axons allows access to the central nervous system (CNS), with latency and periodic reactivation possible in the CNS. While productive infection in the CNS may be mild and asymptomatic, it can also result in encephalitis. In fact, HSV1 is the leading cause of sporadic acute encephalitis in people. Interestingly, regions in the brain that are affected in herpes simplex encephalitis, namely the frontal and temporal cortices and the hippocampus, are also the areas associated with Alzheimer pathology (Ball, 1982). The chronic nature of this infection, with periodic reactivation of productive infection, may contribute to the gradual accumulation of pathology associated with AD.

Epidemiologic studies linking HSV1 with AD are difficult because the virus is ubiquitous and a large percentage of the population is exposed to this virus. However, in support of this connection, HSV1 DNA has been detected in a high proportion of elderly individuals, both AD patients and non AD patients, relative to younger individuals (Jamieson et al., 1991). Studies have also detected HSV1 antibodies in the cerebral spinal fluid (CSF) of elderly, but not younger, individuals (Wozniak et al., 2005), and elevated anti-HSV1 IgM antibodies in CSF of AD patients (Letenneur et al., 2008). These data indicate that reactivation of HSV1 occurs in the CNS and implies that reactivation is more likely to occur in older individuals.

While HSV1 is present in the brains of many elderly people, only a subset of these individuals will develop AD. Thus, it is reasonable to expect that host factors also play a role in determining one's risk of developing AD. For example, a recent study has shown that HSV1-infected individuals who are carriers of the APOE ε4 allele are at greater risk of developing AD than those carriers who are not infected with HSV1 (Itzhaki et al., 1997). Consistent with the idea that APOE might influence susceptibility to CNS infection by HSV1 are several studies by Burgos et al. using transgenic mice expressing either the human APOE ε4 allele or the APOE ε3 allele (Burgos et al., 2003). These investigators show that entry into the brain and viral load in the brain of HSV1-infected mice is greater in animals expressing the APOE ε4 allele than in those expressing the APOE ε3 allele.

Mechanistically, the role that HSV1 plays in the etiology of AD requires direct and/or indirect insult leading to the pathology associated with the disease. Herpesvirus DNA has been detected in plaques in AD brains, suggesting that HSV1 may be involved in AD disease progression (Wozniak et al., 2009b). Further, HSV1 has been shown to associate with the amyloid precursor protein (app) during anterograde transport of viral capsids to the cell surface (Cheng et al., 2011). This results in an abnormal distribution of APP in infected cells, which might influence cleavage of this protein and the generation of β-amyloid. APP levels also have been reported to decrease in cultured neuronal cells infected with HSV1, while several secreted and intracellular fragments of APP, including the neurotoxic β-amyloid peptides, 1-40 and 1-42, have been detected upon infection with HSV1 (De Chiara et al., 2010; Shipley et al., 2005; Wozniak et al., 2007). The decrease in levels of APP is likely the result of HSV1-induced down-regulation of host protein synthesis, as well as an increase in abnormal processing of APP in HSV1-infected cells. At least some of the altered APP processing observed in HSV1-infected human neuroblastoma cells is due to cleavage by host proteases, including β-secretase (also known as β-site APP cleaving enzyme 1, or BACE1), γ-secretase and caspase-3-like enzymes (De Chiara et al., 2010). In addition to the detection of novel fragments of APP in HSV1-infected cells, increased levels of BACE1 and nicastrin, a component of the γ-secretase complex, have been detected upon HSV1 infection of human neuronal cells (Wozniak et al., 2007). Furthermore, HSV1 produces an envelope glycoprotein, gpB, with homology to a segment of β-amyloid. Peptides synthesized from this region form fibrils *in vitro* that resemble β-amyloid and are able to seed the formation of neurotoxic amyloid plaques (Cribbs et al., 2000). Therefore, reactivation of HSV1 in the brain of AD patients can potentially contribute to the formation of β-amyloid and senile plaques, which in turn would exacerbate the disease process.

HSV1 can also be linked to the second major pathological feature of AD, neurofibrillary tangles (NFT), that form as a consequence of hyperphosphorylation of tau proteins. Infection of neuronal cells by HSV1 results in hyperphosphorylation of tau, resulting in neuronal damage and loss of viability (Wozniak et al., 2009a; Zambrano et al., 2008). In addition, cleavage of tau by caspase 3 has been demonstrated in HSV1-infected cells, an event which accelerates the aggregation of tau (Lerchundi et al., 2011). HSV1 also encodes an enzyme homologous to protein kinase A (PKA), one of the enzymes involved in phosphorylation of tau; this viral protein is functionally similar to PKA and could potentially phosphorylate tau and contribute to NFT formation (Benetti and Roizman, 2004). Thus, there is evidence that supports the hypothesis that HSV1 infection can contribute to both tau-mediated and β-amyloid-mediated neurodegenerative pathologies associated with AD.

Autophagy is a process involving clearance of abnormal proteins and cellular organelles by lysosomal proteases. Disruption of this process has been implicated in neurodegenerative disorders such as AD (Chu, 2006). Autophagosomes are known to accumulate in dystrophic neurites of damaged neurons in AD, and impairment of the autophagic pathway could account for the intracellular deposits of β-amyloid seen in this disease (Nixon, 2007). Furthermore, β-amyloid and enzymes responsible for processing of APP have been recognized in autophagosomes (Yu et al., 2004), which could enhance cleavage of APP into toxic fragments. While the accumulation of autophagic vacuoles could be the result of increased induction of autophagy, Boland et al. suggest that the AD pathology attributed to disruption of autophagy is due to impaired clearance of autophagosomes by lysosomal cathepsins (Boland et al., 2008). A recent study by Santana et al presents evidence linking the accumulation of β-amyloid and disruption of autophagy with HSV1 infection (Santana et al., 2011). These investigators demonstrate that infection of neuroblastoma cells with HSV1 results in an accumulation of intracellular β-amyloid 1-40 and 1-42 peptides in autophagosomes. Furthermore, the data indicate that autophagosomes do not fuse with lysosomes in HSV1-infected cells, and β-amyloid co-localizes with a marker for autophagosomal membranes (LC3) but not with a marker for lysosomes (CD63). While Santana et al did not observe any significant change in secretases involved in APP processing in HSV1-infected cells, as observed in other studies (De Chiara et al., 2010; Wozniak et al., 2007), their results indicate a mechanism whereby infection with HSV1 might contribute to the intracellular accumulation of β-amyloid by inhibiting the autophagocytic pathway.

Additional evidence that autophagy may be a key feature in AD pathogenesis with HSV1 infection involves another cellular process that has been implicated in AD pathology. This process is activation of protein kinase R (PKR) and subsequent phosphorylation of elongation initiation factor 2α (eIF2α), which ultimately results in inhibition of protein synthesis (Peel, 2004). PKR can be activated by the presence of dsRNA, which many viruses, including HSV1, generate during their replication cycle; this activation of PKR is a cellular defense mechanism to protect against these infections. HSV1, however, expresses a protein, US11, that binds dsRNA and prevents activation of PKR (Cassady and Gross, 2002). HSV1 also expresses a protein called infected cell polyprotein 34.5 (ICP34.5) that activates a cellular protein to dephosphorylate eIF2α (He et al., 1997), thus allowing protein synthesis to occur. While these observations seem to contradict how the PKR pathway is affected in AD, it has been shown that HSV1 inhibition of PKR and eIF2α phosphorylation disrupts autophagy (Talloczy, et al. 2002). Thus, the deleterious effects of disrupting autophagy might overshadow any advantage to inhibiting the PKR pathway especially since disruption of autophagy occurring in HSV1-infected cells has been associated with an accumulation of β-amyloid, a key ingredient in AD pathogenesis.

3. Alzheimer's Disease and Spirochetes

Spirochetes are gram negative bacteria. These microorganisms have life cycles both external to and within the human host. Once they have established an infection within the human host, they can spread throughout the periphery and enter the central nervous system. Infection by these bacteria can cause many human diseases and disorders. For example, *Treponema pallidum* is known to cause syphilis which, in later stages of the disease, can have neurologic components (Miklossy, 2008). Additionally, the genus Borrelia includes spirochetes capable of causing many human diseases. In the Northern hemisphere, *Borrelia burgdorferi* sensu lato cause Lyme disease. The organism is transmitted from tick saliva during a bite. The infection begins in the human host as a localized acute infection that then spreads systemically. Once the bacteria have entered the human host, changes occur within the bacteria to allow evasion of the human immune system (Rupprecht et al., 2008). MacDonald has described life cycle/phases of Borrelia within the human host which have different morphologic appearances, such as corkscrew, cysts, and granular forms (MacDonald, 2006). Other changes occur in the expression of surface proteins on the Borrelia which prevent complete elimination of the organism and help to establish a more chronic infectious state. Further, Borrelia can infect the immune cells such as monocytes allowing further dissemination via a blood route. Borrelia cross the blood brain barrier into the central nervous system where they cause Lyme neuroborreliosis (Rupprecht et al., 2008). An *in vitro* model has shown that Borrelia can cross the blood brain barrier by affecting calcium signaling in endothelial cells of the blood brain barrier (Grab et al., 2009).

In 1987, MacDonald and Miranda described a well documented case of Alzheimer's dementia that had symptoms of a tertiary stage Borrelia neurospirochetosis. The damage from the infection occurred in the frontal cortex where the damage from AD is located. They suggested that there may be a link between chronic infection due to Borrelia and AD (MacDonald and Miranda, 1987). Miklossy in 1993 presented a study of 27 autopsy cases of which 14 had an AD diagnosis and the other 13 cases were non AD age matched cases. They used sterile post-mortem brain biopsy material. All 14 AD cases were positive for spirochetes. Further, from these 14 AD cases they were able to isolate motile coiled spirochetes from the sterile CSF and blood samples. One of the 14 cases had both a Lyme disease and an AD diagnosis. In this case, *Borrelia burgdorferi* immunoreactivity was found in senile plaques and neurons (Miklossy, 1993; Miklossy et al., 2004). The report by MacDonald and Miranda and the studies by Miklossy et al have established a link between tertiary neurospirochetosis and AD pathology.

To examine whether Borrelia could induce the amyloid and tau pathologies seen in AD, *in vitro* studies were performed. Miklossy et al exposed mammalian neuronal, astrocytic and microglial cells in culture to *Borrelia burgdorferi* for 2-8 weeks. They also infected mixtures of primary rat cells from the telencephalon. They were able to show by Western blot analysis that there were increased levels of beta amyloid precursor protein and hyperphosphorylated tau in extracts of the cells that had been exposed to the bacteria or to the bacterial product lipopolysaccharide when compared to uninfected or untreated cell cultures. Furthermore, they were able to show formation of plaque- like structures when they infected cells with Borrelia. The amyloid deposits that formed were extracellular and reacted with antibodies to β-amyloid and stained with thioflavin S. They analyzed these aggregates with Synchrotron InfraRed MicroSpectroscopy to examine the secondary structure of the proteins and were able to determine that the amyloid was similar to the beta sheet structure seen in AD senile plaques. Additionally, the neuronal cells showed morphological changes similar to the neurofibrillary tangles observed in AD. These "tangle-like" structures were immunoreactive with anti-Borrelia antibodies. The spirochetes and bacterial lipopolysaccharide alone induced the AD-like pathology (Miklossy et al., 2006).

In addition to stimulating the production and aggregation of amyloid, bacterial products, such as lipopolysaccharide, can cause an inflammatory response (Miklossy et al., 2006). In this regard, the bacterial lipopolysaccharide and the induced amyloid plaque formation could induce neuroinflammation similar to that seen in AD. This self perpetuating cycle of production of amyloid and inflammation leading to more amyloid may start in the early stages of a neuroborreliosis, which then perpetuates and exacerbates as it becomes more chronic. Thus, a chronic inflammatory state could be initiated by infection with Borrelia which could explain, in part, the neuroinflammation observed in AD.

4. Alzheimer's Disease and *Chlamydia pneumoniae*

Chlamydia pneumoniae is an atypical bacterium classified as an obligate intracellular pathogen that most commonly infects the human respiratory tract (Grayston et al., 1990). First classified in 1989 (Grayston et al., 1990), the organism has been determined to be ubiquitous in the human population (Leinonen, 1993) and infects mucosal epithelial cells in the nasal passages and the pulmonary tract (Hahn et al., 2002). *Chlamydia pneumoniae* often will spread to the systemic circulation following infection of monocytes in lung tissues (Moazed et al., 1998). The organism exhibits a distinctive biphasic life cycle similar to that of other chlamydia. In this regard, there is an infectious elementary body form as well as an actively metabolizing reticulate body form of the organism. The organism typically attaches to host cells and is endocytosed into a vacuole in which the elementary bodies convert into reticulate bodies that will replicate by binary fission. After 48 to 72 hrs of infection, the organism reorganizes into the elementary body form and is released from the host cell either following host cell lysis or exocytosis.

Some investigations have demonstrated that under certain host cell conditions such as nutrient deprivation, a persistent form of *Chlamydia pneumoniae* develops (Byrne et al., 2001). These organisms exhibit aberrant phenotypes as well as unusual transcriptional characteristics and are thought to contribute to the chronicity of disease recognized in numerous chlamydia-associated conditions (Hogan et al., 2004) including both respiratory and non-respiratory diseases such as chronic obstructive pulmonary disease and atherosclerosis, respectively(Rosenfeld et al., 2000).

The initial report of an association of *Chlamydia pneumoniae* in AD demonstrated that 90% of sporadic late-onset AD brains contained DNA from the organism as determined by polymerase chain reaction (Balin et al., 1998); in contrast, 5% of control brains were positive. These data were corroborated using other tests including: immunohistochemistry, *in vitro* culturing, electron microscopy, immunoelectron microscopy, and reverse transcriptase polymerase chain reaction. All tests utilized brain tissues from regions of the brain typically affected in AD, including those of the pre-frontal cortex, entorhinal cortex, hippocampus, and the parietal cortex. The cerebellum was analyzed also as an internal control since this region is far less affected in this disease. PCR analysis demonstrated that 17 of 19 AD brains were positive for *Chlamydia pneumoniae* in regions with distinct neuropathology, whereas only 4 brains were positive for the organism in the cerebellum. The organism was shown to be present in perivascular macrophages, microglia, and astroglia. In later studies (Gerard et al., 2006), the organism also was shown to infect approximately 20% of neurons in the AD brain. Further analysis of the brain samples indicated that 64% of the polymerase chain reaction-positive samples contained at least one allele for the apoE ε4 isoform which is consistent with earlier findings of the APOE ε4 allele conferring risk for developing sporadic late-onset AD (Roses, 1996).

Interestingly, in a separate and non-brain related study of reactive arthritis, 68% of individuals who demonstrated infection in synovial tissues with *Chlamydia pneumoniae* were carriers of at least one APOE ε4 allele (Gerard et al., 1999). As these percentages were consistent with what had been determined by Roses for risk in AD, further analysis of the relationship of apoE with infection with *Chlamydia pneumoniae* as it would apply to AD was undertaken. Analysis of late-onset disease brains with in situ hybridization for *Chlamydia pneumoniae* that were ε4-containing as compared to those that were ε2 or ε3 indicated that more cells were positive for the organism in the ε4 brains that those of the other two (Gerard et al., 2005). Real time polymerase chain reaction revealed that the ε4 brains contained significantly higher bacterial loads than did the ε2 or ε3 brains. These data are consistent with previous findings that the ε4 positive individuals have both a higher risk of developing AD, and a higher likelihood of exhibiting a faster progression of cognitive dysfunction (Roses, 1996). Mechanistically, apoE appears to bind to the *Chlamydia pneumoniae* elementary body and to enhance the attachment of the organism to the host cell (Gerard et al., 2008). The apoE and *Chlamydia pneumoniae* complex is thought to utilize the low density lipoprotein receptor protein for uptake. This receptor is the normal receptor for the apoE glycoprotein. Thus, the apoE ε4 isoform appears to interact with *Chlamydia pneumoniae* to promote infection, and in this way, may contribute as a risk factor to the development of infection-related AD.

4.1 Analysis of *Chlamydia pneumoniae* cultured from the brain

Culturing of *Chlamydia pneumoniae* from the late-onset AD brain has been performed from multiple AD brain samples (Balin et al., 1998; Dreses-Werringloer et al., 2009), two of which were obtained from different geographic regions in North America. Organisms from these two brains were detectable after passaging in HEp-2 cells (Dreses-Werringloer et al., 2009). Using PCR assays for *Chlamydia pneumoniae*-specific genes Cpn0695, Cpn1046, and tyrP, both isolates were demonstrated to be *Chlamydia pneumoniae*. The omp1 gene from each isolate was sequenced from DNA prepared from several brain tissue samples shown to be PCR-positive for *Chlamydia pneumoniae*. This sequencing revealed that the chlamydial populations from the two brains were genetically diverse. In addition, the brain isolates carried different numbers of copies of the tyrP gene indicating that the brain isolates were more closely related to respiratory strains of *Chlamydia pneumoniae* than to vascular or atheroma strains.

4.2 Entry of *Chlamydia pneumoniae* into the brain

Chlamydia pneumoniae typically infects through the respiratory tract. This route of entry allows Chlamydia access to the brain through the olfactory system since olfactory neuroepithelial cells in the nasal passages can be infected with this pathogen (Little et al., 2004). The olfactory pathway has been shown to be affected early in AD (Kovacs et al., 2001), and this may be the single most vulnerable site for which a respiratory pathogen, like *Chlamydia pneumoniae,* can gain access to the brain. Evaluation of the olfactory bulbs from late-onset AD using PCR and reverse transcriptase PCR techniques has revealed *Chlamydia pneumoniae*-specific sequences at this site (Balin et al., 1998). Since olfactory bulbs contain some of the earliest pathology occurring in the AD brain, even prior to pathology observed in the entorhinal cortex, the suggestion has been made that olfaction is actually damaged with alterations in the sense of smell as a preclinical event prior to incipient AD (Kovacs et al., 2001). As damage progresses from the olfactory bulbs into the entorhinal cortex, layers II and III demonstrate neurofibrillary tangles (Braak and Braak, 1997). Neural projections arise from these layers to pass through the perforant pathway to innervate the hippocampal formation. Our studies have shown that *Chlamydia pneumoniae* was also present in the AD entorhinal cortex, hippocampus, and other areas of the temporal cortex (Balin et al., 1998; Gerard et al., 2006; Hammond et al., 2010), thus implicating *Chlamydia pneumoniae* infection of the olfactory pathway in the early pathological changes observed in AD, ie, damage to the mesial temporal cortex. For some time, pathogen entry into the brain following infection of the olfactory path has been well-recognized (Flexner and Clark, 1912; Morales et al., 1988). Whether there is direct damage to this pathway leading to changes in the sense of smell and pathology in the brain proper or whether the path is just a conduit for deeper brain infection must be addressed for each individual pathogen. As stated above, we have observed the presence of *Chlamydia pneumoniae* in this pathway and brain regions connected directly to this pathway (Balin et al., 1998; Hammond et al., 2010). However, we have not correlated infection with changes in the sense of smell at this time, although this appears reasonable and will be tested in the future. Furthermore, our animal model studies, in which the normal BALB/c mouse has been inoculated intranasally, have demonstrated the organism in the olfactory neuroepithelia, olfactory bulb, and in deeper brain structures, as well as concordant amyloid pathology (Little et al., 2004), suggesting that the infection induces pathological change consistent with what is observed in the AD brain.

The other likely pathway by which *Chlamydia pneumoniae* can enter the brain is through the blood brain barrier. *Chlamydia pneumoniae* can be engulfed by monocytes that circulate within the lung vasculature following inhalation into the lungs (Boman et al., 1998). Following uptake of the organism into monocytes, the monocytes can traffic the organism throughout the circulation for potential penetration into the brain, much like what is observed for HIV infection in HIV-dementia cases (Roberts et al., 2010). In the AD brain, *Chlamydia pneumoniae* was revealed in glial cells, perivascular macrophages, and monocytes within and around blood vessels (Balin et al., 1998; MacIntyre et al., 2003), suggesting that indeed the organism can enter the AD brain by this mechanism. We have obtained experimental evidence for this occurrence using an *in vitro* model of the blood-brain barrier. This model analyzed the transmigration of *Chlamydia pneumoniae*-infected monocytes through an intact monolayer of infected human brain microvascular endothelial cells (MacIntyre et al., 2003). Up-regulation of ICAM-1 and VCAM-1 on the endothelial cells, and up-regulation of integrin molecules on the monocyte surface were detected. This would allow enhanced binding of monocytes to the endothelial cell monolayers and could account for the observed 3-fold increase in transmigrated cells. Further support for this occurrence followed analysis of the junctional molecules maintaining the adherens and tight junctional complexes between the endothelial cells (MacIntyre et al., 2002). Transient up-regulation of expression was observed for N-cadherin and β-catenin, two proteins involved in the adherens junctional assembly complex. In contrast, down-regulation occurred for occludin, a tight-junctional protein, with recovery of expression by 72 hr post-infection. These data suggest that a compensatory response to infection was evident in the endothelial cells, and that transient opening of the tight junctions between endothelial cells would allow transmigration of infected monocytes through the barrier.

Consequences of monocyte infection and subsequent entry into the brain can result in further damage and spread throughout the central nervous system. The chronic nature of *Chlamydia pneumoniae* infections could lead to significant immunopathology resulting in neuronal cell damage and death. Evidence for spread in the human nervous system also has been reported by others who evaluated whether *Chlamydia pneumoniae* DNA was present in the cerebrospinal fluid of individuals diagnosed with AD and vascular dementia as compared to control, non-demented individuals (Paradowski et al., 2007). This investigation used polymerase chain reaction techniques to determine that the prevalence of the organism in the AD brains was 43.9% (N = 57 patients). This prevalence was much higher than that for vascular dementia which was 9.5% (N = 21 patients) and for controls which was 0.6% (N = 47 patients). From these data, the odds ratio for persons having *Chlamydia pneumoniae* in their cerebrospinal fluid and also having AD was 7.21, thus indicating a significant association of this infection with AD. In an unrelated report, the presence of *Chlamydia pneumoniae* was examined in atherosclerotic arteries from various vascular regions including the brain (Rassu et al., 2001). Seven of 9 (78%) patients were PCR-positive in brain samples. Interestingly, none of these patients were diagnosed with late-onset AD at the time of death, but all had severe atherosclerosis. Atherosclerosis is considered a risk factor for the development of late-onset AD, although the risk has more often been attributed to cholesterol processing abnormalities than to infection (de la Torre, 2006). Ironically, this conclusion fails to consider that *Chlamydia pneumoniae* infection in blood vessels has been shown to result in the development of foam cells containing abnormal accumulations of cholesterol (Kalayoglu and Byrne, 1998).

4.3 Association of neuroinflammation with *Chlamydia pneumoniae*

Neuroinflammation has been well-documented in the AD brain and is thought to arise as a result of glial cell exposure to toxic forms of β-amyloid (Lue et al., 1996). While this eventuality is likely, there is a gap in our understanding of how, why, and when the toxic forms of β-amyloid arise in disease pathogenesis. In this regard, infection with *Chlamydia pneumoniae* may be a trigger or stimulus for neuroinflammation that actually precedes the processing of β-amyloid into toxic entities. Immunopathogenesis as a result of chronic inflammation is a hallmark of infection with *Chlamydia pneumoniae* and typically involves inflammatory cells such as monocytes and macrophages (Rasmussen et al., 1997). Components of chlamydia such as heat shock protein 60, outer membrane proteins, and lipopolysaccharide elicit strong inflammatory responses in tissues. The inflammatory response is usually pro-inflammatory with the production of interleukins IL-1β, IL- 6, IL-12, tumor necrosis factor-α, and reactive oxygen species. These inflammatory molecules have been found in the AD brain and are thought to promote nerve cell damage (Lue et al., 1996). The cell types in the brain involved with secreting these inflammatory molecules are microglia, astroglia, and perivascular macrophages. All of these cell types in the AD brain have been shown to be infected with *Chlamydia pneumoniae* (Balin et al., 1998; Gerard et al., 2006; Hammond et al., 2010). In addition, approximately 20% of neurons in the hippocampal formation also have been shown to be infected (Gerard et al., 2006). Intriguingly, all of these infected cells were found in areas of amyloid deposition. The relationship of these infected cells to pathology has been investigated with *in vitro* studies in which *Chlamydia pneumoniae*-infected murine microglial cells were shown to secrete several pro-inflammatory cytokines including MCP-1, IL-6, and tumor necrosis factor-α. Neurons exposed to the supernatants containing these cytokines exhibited an increase in cell death as compared to those exposed to mock infected supernatants (Boelen et al., 2009). Thus, the pro-inflammatory response to *Chlamydia pneumoniae* infections may result in neurodegeneration in the immediate environment and in the neuropathology such as amyloid deposition characteristic of Alzheimer's Disease.

Neuronal cell death in AD may occur through several mechanisms that lead to the characteristic amyloid and tau pathologies. There is increasing evidence to suggest that dysregulation of apoptosis and autophagy may be the interconnecting link in the abnormal cellular processing that occurs in AD. The initiation of the apoptotic process and mitochondrial dysfunction which may play a central role in neurodegeneration, have been observed in AD brains (Pereira et al., 2004). Autophagy has been linked to Alzheimer's pathogenesis through its merger with the endosomal-lysosomal system, which also has been shown to play a role in aberrant amyloid processing. Contents of an autophagosome are degraded as a result of the autophagosome fusing with the lysosome. Research has demonstrated that the activity of the lysosomal system is enhanced in patients with AD (Nixon et al., 2000). The lysosomal system is also related to the endosomal pathway since early endosomes that are formed fuse with late endosomes or lysosomes. Neurons from AD brains have been found to exhibit an increase in the number of enlarged early endosomes. This is significant in the development of AD because early endosomes sequester proteins such as apolipoprotein E and app, and studies have demonstrated that Aβ is formed in early endosomes (Nixon et al., 2000). From these observations, the data suggest that aberrant autophagy induction may result in an accumulation of autophagic vacuoles in the AD brain containing β-amyloid. With regards to infection, apoptosis and autophagy are common pathways by which infected cells, incapable of eliminating the infectious agent, undergo cell death. *Chlamydia pneumoniae* has been shown to inhibit apoptosis in neuronal cells and monocytes thereby prolonging cell viability (Appelt et al., 2008), and previous work from other laboratories has demonstrated that chlamydiae-infected host cells are resistant to proapoptotic stimuli (Fischer et al., 2001). Inhibition of apoptotic activity may be important in the earlier stages of infection. This anti-apoptotic activity may block cytochrome c release from the mitochondrial membrane and subsequent activation of caspases that would promote apoptosis. *Chlamydia pneumoniae* infection has been shown to modulate the pro-apoptotic cytoplasmic proteins, such as caspase-3 and cytochrome c, as well as the anti-apoptotic mitochondrial protein Bcl-2 and the anti-apoptotic nuclear protein NF-κB (Fischer et al., 2001). Interestingly, intracellular pathogens, such as Chlamydia, have been shown to alter the apoptosis pathway and interfere with the autophagy pathway to ensure survival of the host cell (Al-Younes et al., 2004). We have demonstrated that infection with *Chlamydia pneumoniae* results in changes in gene expression in the apoptotic and autophagic pathways (unpublished observations) consistent with previous work by others, suggesting that infection may be altering these pathways in AD.

4.4 Approaches to prove causation of AD by infection with *Chlamydia pneumoniae*

4.4.1 Clinical trial to treat for CNS infection with *Chlamydia pneumoniae*

Investigations to prove that chronic infection with *Chlamydia pneumoniae* can be causative for late-onset AD have used clinical trial approaches and animal modeling. Anti-microbial treatment may be feasible in combating infection-initiated AD. One reported clinical trial has used an antibiotic combination approach for treatment of late-onset disease (Loeb et al., 2004). Patients with probable late-onset disease and/or mild to moderate dementia were treated for 3 months with doxycycline and rifampin. Primary and secondary outcomes were assessed. Primary outcome was any change in the Standardized AD Assessment Scale cognitive subscale (SADAScog) at 6 months and secondary outcomes were any change in SADAScog at 12 months along with analysis of dysfunctional behavior, depression, and functional status. There was significantly less decline at 6 months in the antibiotic group as compared to placebo for SADAScog ($p = .034$), whereas the same score at 12 months was not significantly different. However, the antibiotic group showed significantly less dysfunctional behavior ($p = .028$), and less decline in mini-mental status scores ($p = .032$). There was no correlation that could be determined for change in *Chlamydia pneumoniae* infection based on serum antibody titers in blood or by PCR of blood samples. Although the correlation to change in infection was not apparent based on these limited measures, there was some limited improvement in patient status. Future studies must include better measures of Chlamydial infection in the CNS (ie, tests of cerebrospinal fluid) to better understand how antibiotics may be affecting change in CNS infection, in addition to possibly using delivery adjuvants with antibiotics to obtain better concentration effects in the CNS.

4.4.2 Experimental animal models to study AD

As mentioned previously, AD has an early onset form that is primarily driven by autosomal dominant genetic alterations in genes encoding app, as well as the loci encoding presenilins-1 and 2. Genetically modified mouse models have taken advantage of these genes to induce enhanced β-amyloid production and subsequent deposition of β-amyloid (Wisniewski and Sigurdsson, 2010). One important issue that cannot be addressed using these model systems is how to target the early initiating events in sporadic late-onset AD and not just the "tombstone lesions that are the result of a long chain of pathological processes" (Wisniewski and Sigurdsson, 2010). Transgenic animals serve as models for early onset AD, which accounts for ~5 % of all reported cases.

Animal models that mimic the sporadic late-onset form of AD have been hampered by the lack of understanding of the primary factors that promote the deposition of β-amyloid. Currently, models that experimentally induce AD-like pathology use bacterial toxins such as streptozotocin (Labak et al., 2010), chronic stress (Alkadhi et al., 2010), or colchicine to chemically induce damage (Kumar et al., 2007) to the CNS to initiate pathology. Several infectious agents, including *Chlamydia pneumoniae*, have been proposed to play a causal role in AD. Animal models based on this infection as well as on infections with other organisms such as Herpes Simplex Virus-1 and *Borrelia burgdorferi* (Itzhaki et al., 2004) are being pursued, but at this time are limited. The paucity of experimental animal systems that model sporadic late-onset AD leaves the scientific community with few options to address key questions related to the initiation/progression of late-onset disease.

4.4.3 Experimental induction of progressive AD-like pathology following infection with *Chlamydia pneumoniae*

The identification of *Chlamydia pneumoniae* in AD brain tissue (Balin et al., 1998) was a stimulus to investigate the potential role *Chlamydia pneumoniae* plays in the induction and progression of late-onset disease. In addition to utilizing cell culture systems to investigate changes in particular cell populations, we have established a mouse model to investigate induction of AD-like pathology following infection with *Chlamydia pneumoniae* (Little et al., 2004). In this experimental system, BALB/c mice were infected with *Chlamydia pneumoniae* isolated from human AD brain autopsy tissue. The isolate of *Chlamydia pneumoniae*, 96-41, was propagated in HEp-2 cells and then introduced into 3 month old BALB/c mice via intranasal inoculation; brain tissue was analyzed at monthly time points following infection. In mice infected with *Chlamydia pneumoniae*, β-amyloid deposits were identified as early as two months post-infection, with the greatest number of deposits identified at three months post-infection. The number and size of amyloid deposits increased over time, thus the development of AD-like pathology was progressive.

The experimental induction of mouse derived β-amyloid deposits in inbred BALB/c mice (not genetically modified) at 5 and 6 months of age (2 and 3 months post-infection) indicates that infection can trigger the production and deposition of β-amyloid in the mouse brain. In transgenic mouse models used to study AD, 6 months of age is very early to observe substantial amyloid deposits, yet we observed substantial pathology 2 months after introduction of the infectious agent into non-transgenic animals. *Chlamydia pneumoniae* is a respiratory pathogen and was introduced into mice via an intranasal inoculation. This is the natural route of infection and the organism is responsible for an acute respiratory illness in mice. The respiratory infection precedes dissemination to other organ systems (Little et al., 2005) and age is an important factor in the host's ability to control the dissemination, with even greater spread with the advent of immunosenescence.

The first study to utilize a human AD-brain isolate of *Chlamydia pneumoniae* to induce AD-like pathology in non-transgenic mice (Little et al., 2004) was designed to address Koch's postulates. The first postulate requires that the infectious organism be isolated from autopsy brain tissue of an affected individual. In this particular case, the first postulate is satisfied, but for other cases of the disease this issue is still debated (Itzhaki et al., 2004). To satisfy Koch's second postulate, the pathogen must be isolated from a diseased organism and grown in pure culture. *Chlamydia pneumoniae* was isolated, post mortem, from human AD-brain tissue and grown in culture. Third, the organism was introduced into a mouse, and induced pathology consistent with AD, while uninfected mice did not display the same pathology. Fourth, the organism was identified in the tissues of affected mice, but was not re-isolated from the tissue. Thus, Koch's postulates were used as a general guide, and although difficult to use in their purest sense when addressing any intracellular infection, our findings support the hypothesis that *Chlamydia pneumoniae* infection can induce β-amyloid deposition and contribute directly to pathogenesis.

All experimental animal models of human disease have limitations. In this experimental model, tau pathology was not noted, though due to the relatively short duration of the experiment, amyloid was the primary AD pathology expected to develop. In addition, no learning/memory deficits were measured following infection with *Chlamydia pneumoniae*. The pathology was noted in multiple regions of the brain, and subsequent experiments using the respiratory/laboratory isolate of *Chlamydia pneumoniae*, AR-39, have determined that a majority of the amyloid deposition co-localized in the same area as chlamydia antigen (unpublished observations). Substantial AD-like pathology was noted at three months post-infection, although to determine the full extent of pathology induced and to further characterize the progressive nature of infection with the human AD-brain isolate (96-41) of *Chlamydia pneumoniae*, additional time points still need to be analyzed and evaluated for amyloid and tau pathology. BALB/c mice have an average lifespan of 22-24 months and analysis of brain tissue at six, nine, twelve, and fifteen months post-infection (that is 18 months old) would help to determine the degree of AD-like pathology induced over the course of a persistent *Chlamydia pneumoniae* infection. Similar to any animal model for human disease this system has limitations, but this model of experimentally induced AD-like pathology in the brains of BALB/c mice is well-suited to address key early events in the initiation of pathology associated with sporadic late-onset disease.

4.4.4 Experimental induction of non-progressive AD-like pathology following infection with respiratory isolates of *Chlamydia pneumoniae*

One investigation designed to replicate the initial report of experimental induction of AD-like pathology in BALB/c mice did not identify substantial AD-like pathology following infection with the respiratory isolate/laboratory strain of *Chlamydia pneumoniae* (TWAR 2043) (Boelen et al., 2007). Boelen and co-workers infected BALB/c mice, via intranasal inoculation and examined brain tissue at one and three months post infection, based upon the assumption that TWAR 2043 and the human AD brain isolate 96-41 would both induce a progressive pathology following infection. The number of amyloid beta deposits was not given in this study, but the researchers indicated that *Chlamydia pneumoniae* was not detected in the CNS at 1 month or 3 months post-infection. In addition, both mock-infected and *Chlamydia pneumoniae*-infected mice displayed no difference in amyloid deposits. The clear difference noted in our study of number and size of deposits was notably different than in this report. The researchers noted that these discrepancies could be due to the fact that the TWAR 2043 *Chlamydia pneumoniae* strain used may have different virulence properties than the human AD-brain isolate, 96-41.

Given that TWAR 2043 and 96-41 display different phenotypes with respect to both the ability to establish a persistent infection and the subsequent induction of pathology within the brains of BALB/c mice, we initiated experiments to address these issues using the respiratory isolate/laboratory strain of *Chlamydia pneumoniae* AR-39. In our laboratory, BALB/c mice were given a single intranasal inoculation, in an identical manner to our initial report with the respiratory isolate/laboratory strain. Brains were analyzed at 1, 2, 3, and 4 months post-infection by immunohistochemistry with antibodies specific for Chlamydia antigen and antibodies specific for β-amyloid 1-42. Similar to the initial report utilizing the 96-41 human AD-brain isolate, no substantial amyloid deposits were observed at 1 month post-infection and a limited degree of AD-like pathology was identified at 2 months post-infection with AR-39. In contrast to the study utilizing the 96-41 isolate of *Chlamydia pneumoniae,* at 3 months post-infection, AD-like pathology was comparable to that observed in uninfected mice (at all time points) or infected mice at 1 month post-infection. The degree of pathology had decreased between 2 and 3 months post-infection. In contrast to infection with the 96-41 isolate, at 3 and 4 months post-infection amyloid deposits in the brains of mice infected with AR-39 resembled that of uninfected controls. Identification and quantitative analysis of Chlamydia antigen burden indicated that peak Chlamydia antigen burden preceded peak amyloid deposition. The greatest Chlamydia antigen burden, in brains of infected BALB/c mice, was noted at 1 month post infection (a mean of 51 immunoreactive sites per mouse), and decreased at 2 months (45), 3 months (30), and 4 months (25) post-infection. Taken together, the burden of Chlamydia antigen and number of amyloid deposits suggests that *Chlamydia pneumoniae* infection serves as the primary stimulus for β-amyloid processing and deposition. Host immune responses that limit or reduce *Chlamydia pneumoniae* replication and antigen burden effectively decrease the primary stimulus for the production of β-amyloid in this experimental system. We propose that the difference in progressive versus non-progressive pathologic profiles of amyloid deposits are due to as yet uncharacterized differences between the human AD-brain adapted isolate (96-41) and respiratory isolates/laboratory strains (TWAR 2043 and AR-39). This implies that there are different virulence factors including tissue tropism for different strains of *Chlamydia pneumoniae.* The ability of the organism to persist in the central nervous system and elicit a chronic inflammatory response may be critical to the initiation of AD pathogenesis.

4.4.5 Experimental induction of progressive AD-like pathology following multiple inoculations with a respiratory isolate/laboratory strain of *Chlamydia pneumoniae*

Exposure to *Chlamydia pneumoniae* is a common event, and over the course of an individual's life, one may be infected multiple times (Leinonen, 1993). We assessed the potential consequences of multiple exposures and infections with *Chlamydia pneumoniae* using BALB/c mice that were intranasally inoculated, at monthly intervals, once (day 0), twice (days 0 and 30), or three times (days 0, 30 and 60) with the respiratory *Chlamydial* isolate/laboratory strain, AR-39. The brain tissue of experimentally infected and control mice was isolated at day 90, processed in an identical manner as previously described (Little et al., 2004) and analyzed by light microscopy following immunohistochemistry using amyloid-specific antibodies. The total number and size of amyloid deposits was quantified and compared with uninfected BALB/c mice as well as BALB/c mice receiving only a single inoculation with *Chlamydia pneumoniae.* BALB/c mice inoculated twice with *Chlamydia pneumoniae* strain AR-39 displayed 68 amyloid deposits/mouse. In contrast, the brains of BALB/c mice inoculated 3 times had 177 amyloid deposits/mouse. Mice receiving only a single intranasal inoculation had fewer than 10 deposits per mouse, which was comparable to uninfected control mice. Based upon these findings, we concluded that the primary stimulus for the induction of amyloid deposition is the extent or continuous exposure of *Chlamydia pneumoniae* infection.

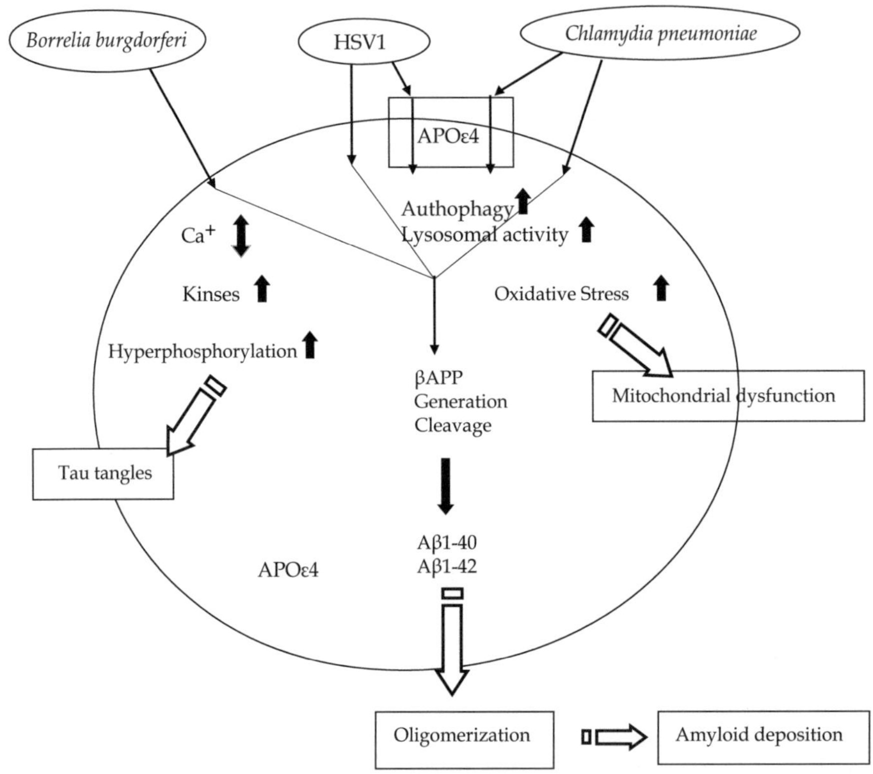

Fig. 1. The diagram illustrates a proposed process of AD pathology development following infectious insult. There are common cellular processes that appear to be activated by all three infectious agents (ie, Herpes, Borrelia, Chlamydia), although the particular activation pathways may differ between the different organisms. In any event, data have been obtained for all three infectious agents that support the contention that infection can initiate changes in the human brain resulting in AD pathology. Thus, specific infections may be primary factors in the pathogenesis of sporadic late-onset Alzheimer's Disease

Based on the isolate of *Chlamydia pneumoniae* used to experimentally induce AD-like pathology in BALB/c mice we have observed progressive as well as non-progressive amyloid pathology. The human AD-brain isolate, 96-41, establishes a persistent infection and promotes chronic inflammation leading to a progressive accumulation of amyloid deposits (Little et al., 2004). Experimental evidence suggests that the respiratory isolates/laboratory strains are able to infect the CNS and induce substantial amyloid deposits (comparable to that of the human AD-brain isolate) at day 60 post infection, but fail to establish a persistent infection and do not promote amyloid deposition at later times. As the burden of *Chlamydia pneumoniae* antigen decreases the number of amyloid deposits also decreases. This model of experimentally induced AD-like pathology in the brains of BALB/c mice supports a role for infection in the induction of AD-pathology, and will enable the Alzheimer's research community to address key early events in the initiation of pathology associated with sporadic late-onset AD.

5. Conclusion

New concepts of infectious disease are evolving with the realization that pathogens are key players in the development of progressive chronic diseases that originally were not thought to be infectious. Infection is known to be associated with numerous neurological diseases and its role in inducing pathologic effects has been well documented (Johnson, 1996). What has remained unclear, however, has been the role of infection as a causative agent or risk factor in the development of chronic neurodegenerative diseases, in particular, Alzheimer's Disease. In this regard, numerous studies over the past 20 years have investigated whether there is an association between various infectious agents and Alzheimer's Disease, the most prevalent neurodegenerative condition accounting for dementia in the elderly. Of the pathogens being considered in sporadic late-onset Alzheimer's Disease, Herpes Simplex Virus 1 (HSV-1) (Itzhaki et al., 1997; Itzhaki and Wozniak, 2008), Borrelia species (Miklossy, 1993), and *Chlamydia pneumoniae* (Balin et al., 1998; Gerard et al., 2006) have garnered significant attention. Work from other laboratories on systemic infectious disease (Kamer et al., 2008) has also led to further interest in the role that infection may play in contributing to the neurodegenerative process in older populations. Data from these investigations are intriguing, and have led to a renewed interest in investigating the role(s) of pathogens in the etiology of sporadic late-onset Alzheimer's Disease. Furthermore, there is renewed interest in challenging long-held hypotheses in the Alzheimer's research arena as investigations are uncovering more novel features of the amyloid protein, as well as the inflammatory response, associated with this disease. Manifestations of chronic disorders are more and more frequently being attributed to a consequence of chronic infection, and infections must be considered as significant contributors to the morbidity and mortality of Alzheimer's Disease.

6. Acknowledgment

We would like to acknowledge the families for the magnanimous donations of Alzheimer's Disease and normal brain tissues for our ongoing research. We also thank all of our students and research support personnel for their contributions to this work. Finally, we thank our funding agencies that have supported our work over the years. These include: Adolph and Rose Levis Foundation (BJB & DMA), Alzheimer's Association (BJB), Center for Chronic Disorders of Aging (endowed by the Osteopathic Heritage Foundation) (BJB, DMA, STH), Foundation for Research into Diseases of Aging (BJB & CSL), PHS/NIH (BJB), and National Foundation for Infectious Diseases (DMA).

7. References

Alkadhi, K. A., Srivareerat, M. & Tran, T. T. (2010). Intensification of Long-Term Memory Deficit by Chronic Stress and Prevention by Nicotine in a Rat Model of Alzheimer's Disease. *Molecular and Cellular Neurosciences,* 45(3), 289-296. 1095-9327; 1044-7431

Al-Younes, H. M., Brinkmann, V. & Meyer, T. F. (2004). Interaction of Chlamydia Trachomatis Serovar L2 with the Host Autophagic Pathway. *Infection and Immunity,* 72(8), 4751-4762. 0019-9567; 0019-9567

Appelt, D. M., Roupas, M. R., Way, D. S., Bell, M. G., Albert, E. V., Hammond, C. J. & Balin, B. J. (2008). Inhibition of Apoptosis in Neuronal Cells Infected with Chlamydophila (Chlamydia) Pneumoniae. *BMC Neuroscience,* 9, 13. 1471-2202; 1471-2202

Balin, B. J., Gerard, H. C., Arking, E. J., Appelt, D. M., Branigan, P. J., Abrams, J. T., Whittum-Hudson, J. A. & Hudson, A. P. (1998). Identification and Localization of Chlamydia Pneumoniae in the Alzheimer's Brain. *Medical Microbiology and Immunology,* 187(1), 23-42. 0300-8584; 0300-8584

Ball, M. J. (1982). "Limbic Predilection in Alzheimer Dementia: Is Reactivated Herpesvirus Involved?". *The Canadian Journal of Neurological Sciences.Le Journal Canadien Des Sciences Neurologiques,* 9(3), 303-306. 0317-1671; 0317-1671

Benetti, L. & Roizman, B. (2004). Herpes Simplex Virus Protein Kinase US3 Activates and Functionally Overlaps Protein Kinase A to Block Apoptosis. *Proceedings of the National Academy of Sciences of the United States of America,* 101(25), 9411-9416. 0027-8424; 0027-8424

Boelen, E., Stassen, F. R., van der Ven, A. J., Lemmens, M. A., Steinbusch, H. P., Bruggeman, C. A., Schmitz, C. & Steinbusch, H. W. (2007). Detection of Amyloid Beta Aggregates in the Brain of BALB/c Mice After Chlamydia Pneumoniae Infection. *Acta Neuropathologica,* 114(3), 255-261. 0001-6322; 0001-6322

Boelen, E., Steinbusch, H. W., Bruggeman, C. A. & Stassen, F. R. (2009). The Inflammatory Aspects of Chlamydia Pneumoniae-Induced Brain Infection. *Drugs of Today (Barcelona, Spain: 1998),* 45 Suppl B, 159-164. 1699-3993; 1699-3993

Boland, B., Kumar, A., Lee, S., Platt, F. M., Wegiel, J., Yu, W. H. & Nixon, R. A. (2008). Autophagy Induction and Autophagosome Clearance in Neurons: Relationship to Autophagic Pathology in Alzheimer's Disease. *The Journal of Neuroscience: The Official Journal of the Society for Neuroscience,* 28(27), 6926-6937. 1529-2401; 0270-6474

Boman, J., Soderberg, S., Forsberg, J., Birgander, L. S., Allard, A., Persson, K., Jidell, E., Kumlin, U., Juto, P., Waldenstrom, A. & Wadell, G. (1998). High Prevalence of Chlamydia Pneumoniae DNA in Peripheral Blood Mononuclear Cells in Patients with Cardiovascular Disease and in Middle-Aged Blood Donors. *The Journal of Infectious Diseases,* 178(1), 274-277. 0022-1899

Braak, H. & Braak, E. (1997). Diagnostic Criteria for Neuropathologic Assessment of Alzheimer's Disease. *Neurobiology of Aging,* 18(4 Suppl), S85-8. 0197-4580; 0197-4580

Burgos, J. S., Ramirez, C., Sastre, I., Bullido, M. J. & Valdivieso, F. (2003). ApoE4 is More Efficient than E3 in Brain Access by Herpes Simplex Virus Type 1. *Neuroreport,* 14(14), 1825-1827. 0959-4965; 0959-4965

Byrne, G. I., Ouellette, S. P., Wang, Z., Rao, J. P., Lu, L., Beatty, W. L. & Hudson, A. P. (2001). Chlamydia Pneumoniae Expresses Genes Required for DNA Replication but Not Cytokinesis during Persistent Infection of HEp-2 Cells. *Infection and Immunity,* 69(9), 5423-5429. 0019-9567

Cassady, K. A. & Gross, M. (2002). The Herpes Simplex Virus Type 1 U(S)11 Protein Interacts with Protein Kinase R in Infected Cells and Requires a 30-Amino-Acid Sequence Adjacent to a Kinase Substrate Domain. *Journal of Virology,* 76(5), 2029-2035. 0022-538X; 0022-538X

Cheng, S. B., Ferland, P., Webster, P. & Bearer, E. L. (2011). Herpes Simplex Virus Dances with Amyloid Precursor Protein while Exiting the Cell. *PloS One,* 6(3), e17966. 1932-6203; 1932-6203

Chu, C. T. (2006). Autophagic Stress in Neuronal Injury and Disease. *Journal of Neuropathology and Experimental Neurology*, 65(5), 423-432. 0022-3069; 0022-3069

Cribbs, D. H., Azizeh, B. Y., Cotman, C. W. & LaFerla, F. M. (2000). Fibril Formation and Neurotoxicity by a Herpes Simplex Virus Glycoprotein B Fragment with Homology to the Alzheimer's A Beta Peptide. *Biochemistry (John Wiley & Sons)*, 39(20), 5988-5994. 0006-2960

De Chiara, G., Marcocci, M. E., Civitelli, L., Argnani, R., Piacentini, R., Ripoli, C., Manservigi, R., Grassi, C., Garaci, E. & Palamara, A. T. (2010). APP Processing Induced by Herpes Simplex Virus Type 1 (HSV-1) Yields several APP Fragments in Human and Rat Neuronal Cells. *PloS One*, 5(11), e13989. 1932-6203; 1932-6203

de la Torre, J. C. (2006). How do Heart Disease and Stroke Become Risk Factors for Alzheimer's Disease? *Neurological Research*, 28(6), 637-644. 0161-6412; 0161-6412

Dreses-Werringloer, U., Bhuiyan, M., Zhao, Y., Gerard, H. C., Whittum-Hudson, J. A. & Hudson, A. P. (2009). Initial Characterization of Chlamydophila (Chlamydia) Pneumoniae Cultured from the Late-Onset Alzheimer Brain. *International Journal of Medical Microbiology: IJMM*, 299(3), 187-201. 1618-0607

Fischer, S. F., Schwarz, C., Vier, J. & Hacker, G. (2001). Characterization of Antiapoptotic Activities of Chlamydia Pneumoniae in Human Cells. *Infection and Immunity*, 69(11), 7121-7129. 0019-9567

Flexner, S. & Clark, P. F. (1912). A Note on the Mode of Infection in Epidemic Poliomyelitis. *Proceedings of the Society for Experimental Biology and Medicine, 10*(1), 1-2. 1535-3699

Frings, M., Blaeser, I. & Kastrup, O. (2002). Adult-Onset Subacute Sclerosing Panencephalitis Presenting as a Degenerative Dementia Syndrome. *Journal of Neurology*, 249(7), 942-943. 0340-5354; 0340-5354

Gerard, H. C., Dreses-Werringloer, U., Wildt, K. S., Deka, S., Oszust, C., Balin, B. J., Frey, W. H.,2nd, Bordayo, E. Z., Whittum-Hudson, J. A. & Hudson, A. P. (2006). Chlamydophila (Chlamydia) Pneumoniae in the Alzheimer's Brain. *FEMS Immunology and Medical Microbiology*, 48(3), 355-366. 0928-8244

Gerard, H. C., Fomicheva, E., Whittum-Hudson, J. A. & Hudson, A. P. (2008). Apolipoprotein E4 Enhances Attachment of Chlamydophila (Chlamydia) Pneumoniae Elementary Bodies to Host Cells. *Microbial Pathogenesis*, 44(4), 279-285. 0882-4010

Gerard, H. C., Wang, G. F., Balin, B. J., Schumacher, H. R. & Hudson, A. P. (1999). Frequency of Apolipoprotein E (APOE) Allele Types in Patients with Chlamydia-Associated Arthritis and Other Arthritides. *Microbial Pathogenesis*, 26(1), 35-43. 0882-4010

Gerard, H. C., Wildt, K. L., Whittum-Hudson, J. A., Lai, Z., Ager, J. & Hudson, A. P. (2005). The Load of Chlamydia Pneumoniae in the Alzheimer's Brain Varies with APOE Genotype. *Microbial Pathogenesis*, 39(1-2), 19-26. 0882-4010

Grab, D. J., Nyarko, E., Nikolskaia, O. V., Kim, Y. V. & Dumler, J. S. (2009). Human Brain Microvascular Endothelial Cell Traversal by Borrelia Burgdorferi Requires Calcium Signaling. *Clinical Microbiology and Infection: The Official Publication of the European Society of Clinical Microbiology and Infectious Diseases*, 15(5), 422-426. 1469-0691; 1198-743X

Grayston, J. T., Campbell, L. A., Kuo, C. C., Mordhorst, C. H., Saikku, P., Thom, D. H. & Wang, S. P. (1990). A New Respiratory Tract Pathogen: Chlamydia Pneumoniae Strain TWAR. *J Infect Dis*, 161(490203703), 618-625.

Hahn, D. L., Azenabor, A. A., Beatty, W. L. & Byrne, G. I. (2002). Chlamydia Pneumoniae as a Respiratory Pathogen. *Frontiers in Bioscience [Computer File]: A Journal and Virtual Library*, 7, e66-76. 1093-4715

Hammond, C. J., Hallock, L. R., Howanski, R. J., Appelt, D. M., Little, C. S. & Balin, B. J. (2010). Immunohistological Detection of Chlamydia Pneumoniae in the Alzheimer's Disease Brain. *BMC Neuroscience*, 11, 121. 1471-2202; 1471-2202

He, B., Gross, M. & Roizman, B. (1997). The Gamma(1)34.5 Protein of Herpes Simplex Virus 1 Complexes with Protein Phosphatase 1alpha to Dephosphorylate the Alpha Subunit of the Eukaryotic Translation Initiation Factor 2 and Preclude the Shutoff of Protein Synthesis by Double-Stranded RNA-Activated Protein Kinase. *Proceedings of the National Academy of Sciences of the United States of America*, 94(3), 843-848. 0027-8424; 0027-8424

Hogan, R. J., Mathews, S. A., Mukhopadhyay, S., Summersgill, J. T. & Timms, P. (2004). Chlamydial Persistence: Beyond the Biphasic Paradigm. *Infection and Immunity*, 72(4), 1843-1855. 0019-9567

Honjo, K., van Reekum, R. & Verhoeff, N. P. (2009). Alzheimer's Disease and Infection: Do Infectious Agents Contribute to Progression of Alzheimer's Disease? *Alzheimer's & Dementia: The Journal of the Alzheimer's Association*, 5(4), 348-360. 1552-5279

Itzhaki, R. F., Lin, W. R., Shang, D., Wilcock, G. K., Faragher, B. & Jamieson, G. A. (1997). Herpes Simplex Virus Type 1 in Brain and Risk of Alzheimer's Disease [See Comments]. *Lancet*, 349(904797167222), 241-244.

Itzhaki, R. F., Wozniak, M. A., Appelt, D. M. & Balin, B. J. (2004). Infiltration of the Brain by Pathogens Causes Alzheimer's Disease. *Neurobiology of Aging*, 25(5), 619-627. 0197-4580

Itzhaki, R. F. & Wozniak, M. A. (2008). Herpes Simplex Virus Type 1 in Alzheimer's Disease: The Enemy within. *Journal of Alzheimer's Disease: JAD*, 13(4), 393-405. 1387-2877; 1387-2877

Jamieson, G. A., Maitland, N. J., Craske, J., Wilcock, G. K. & Itzhaki, R. F. (1991). Detection of Herpes Simplex Virus Type 1 DNA Sequences in Normal and Alzheimer's Disease Brain using Polymerase Chain Reaction. *Biochemical Society Transactions*, 19(2), 122S. 0300-5127; 0300-5127

Johnson, R. T. (1996). Microbiology of the Nervous System. In S. Baron (Ed.), *Medical Microbiology* 4th ed., The University of Texas Medical Branch at Galveston. 0963117211

Kalayoglu, M. V. & Byrne, G. I. (1998). A Chlamydia Pneumoniae Component that Induces Macrophage Foam Cell Formation is Chlamydial Lipopolysaccharide. *Infection and Immunity*, 66(11), 5067-5072. 0019-9567; 0019-9567

Kamer, A. R., Dasanayake, A. P., Craig, R. G., Glodzik-Sobanska, L., Bry, M. & de Leon, M. J. (2008). Alzheimer's Disease and Peripheral Infections: The Possible Contribution from Periodontal Infections, Model and Hypothesis. *Journal of Alzheimer's Disease: JAD*, 13(4), 437-449. 1387-2877; 1387-2877

Keefover, R. W. (1996). The Clinical Epidemiology of Alzheimer's Disease. *Neurol Clin*, 14(296424714), 337-351.

Kim, J. M., Stewart, R., Prince, M., Kim, S. W., Yang, S. J., Shin, I. S. & Yoon, J. S. (2007). Dental Health, Nutritional Status and Recent-Onset Dementia in a Korean

Community Population. *International Journal of Geriatric Psychiatry*, 22(9), 850-855. 0885-6230; 0885-6230

Kovacs, T., Cairns, N. J. & Lantos, P. L. (2001). Olfactory Centres in Alzheimer's Disease: Olfactory Bulb is Involved in Early Braak's Stages. *Neuroreport*, 12(2), 285-288. 0959-4965; 0959-4965

Kumar, A., Seghal, N., Naidu, P. S., Padi, S. S. & Goyal, R. (2007). Colchicines-Induced Neurotoxicity as an Animal Model of Sporadic Dementia of Alzheimer's Type. *Pharmacological Reports: PR*, 59(3), 274-283. 1734-1140; 1734-1140

Labak, M., Foniok, T., Kirk, D., Rushforth, D., Tomanek, B., Jasinski, A. & Grieb, P. (2010). Metabolic Changes in Rat Brain Following Intracerebroventricular Injections of Streptozotocin: A Model of Sporadic Alzheimer's Disease. *Acta Neurochirurgica. Supplement*, 106, 177-181. 0065-1419; 0065-1419

Leinonen, M. (1993). Pathogenetic Mechanisms and Epidemiology of Chlamydia Pneumoniae. *European Heart Journal, 14 Suppl K*, 57-61. 0195-668X; 0195-668X

Lerchundi, R., Neira, R., Valdivia, S., Vio, K., Concha, M. I., Zambrano, A. & Otth, C. (2011). Tau Cleavage at D421 by Caspase-3 is Induced in Neurons and Astrocytes Infected with Herpes Simplex Virus Type 1. *Journal of Alzheimer's Disease: JAD*, 23(3), 513-520. 1875-8908; 1387-2877

Letenneur, L., Peres, K., Fleury, H., Garrigue, I., Barberger-Gateau, P., Helmer, C., Orgogozo, J. M., Gauthier, S. & Dartigues, J. F. (2008). Seropositivity to Herpes Simplex Virus Antibodies and Risk of Alzheimer's Disease: A Population-Based Cohort Study. *PloS One*, 3(11), e3637. 1932-6203; 1932-6203

Little, C. S., Bowe, A., Lin, R., Litsky, J., Fogel, R. M., Balin, B. J. & Fresa-Dillon, K. L. (2005). Age Alterations in Extent and Severity of Experimental Intranasal Infection with Chlamydophila Pneumoniae in BALB/c Mice. *Infection and Immunity*, 73(3), 1723-1734. 0019-9567

Little, C. S., Hammond, C. J., MacIntyre, A., Balin, B. J. & Appelt, D. M. (2004). Chlamydia Pneumoniae Induces Alzheimer-Like Amyloid Plaques in Brains of BALB/c Mice. *Neurobiology of Aging*, 25(4), 419-429. 0197-4580

Loeb, M. B., Molloy, D. W., Smieja, M., Standish, T., Goldsmith, C. H., Mahony, J., Smith, S., Borrie, M., Decoteau, E., Davidson, W., McDougall, A., Gnarpe, J., O'DONNell, M. & Chernesky, M. (2004). A Randomized, Controlled Trial of Doxycycline and Rifampin for Patients with Alzheimer's Disease. *Journal of the American Geriatrics Society*, 52(3), 381-387. 0002-8614

Lue, L. F., Brachova, L., Civin, W. H. & Rogers, J. (1996). Inflammation, A Beta Deposition, and Neurofibrillary Tangle Formation as Correlates of Alzheimer's Disease Neurodegeneration. *J Neuropathol Exp Neurol, 55*(1097010972), 1083-108.

MacDonald, A. B. (2006). A Life Cycle for Borrelia Spirochetes? *Medical Hypotheses*, 67(4), 810-818. 0306-9877; 0306-9877

MacDonald, A. B. & Miranda, J. M. (1987). Concurrent Neocortical Borreliosis and Alzheimer's Disease. *Human Pathology*, 18(7), 759-761. 0046-8177; 0046-8177

MacIntyre, A., Abramov, R., Hammond, C. J., Hudson, A. P., Arking, E. J., Little, C. S., Appelt, D. M. & Balin, B. J. (2003). Chlamydia Pneumoniae Infection Promotes the Transmigration of Monocytes through Human Brain Endothelial Cells. *Journal of Neuroscience Research*, 71(5), 740-750. 0360-4012

MacIntyre, A., Hammond, C. J., Little, C. S., Appelt, D. M. & Balin, B. J. (2002). Chlamydia Pneumoniae Infection Alters the Junctional Complex Proteins of Human Brain Microvascular Endothelial Cells. *FEMS Microbiology Letters*, 217(2), 167-172. 0378-1097

Miklossy, J. (1993). Alzheimer's Disease--a Spirochetosis? *Neuroreport*, 4(7), 841-88.

Miklossy, J. (2008). Chronic Inflammation and Amyloidogenesis in Alzheimer's Disease -- Role of Spirochetes. *Journal of Alzheimer's Disease: JAD*, 13(4), 381-391. 1387-2877; 1387-2877

Miklossy, J., Khalili, K., Gern, L., Ericson, R. L., Darekar, P., Bolle, L., Hurlimann, J. & Paster, B. J. (2004). Borrelia Burgdorferi Persists in the Brain in Chronic Lyme Neuroborreliosis and may be Associated with Alzheimer Disease. *Journal of Alzheimer's Disease: JAD*, 6(6), 639-49; discussion 673-81. 1387-2877; 1387-2877

Miklossy, J., Kis, A., Radenovic, A., Miller, L., Forro, L., Martins, R., Reiss, K., Darbinian, N., Darekar, P., Mihaly, L. & Khalili, K. (2006). Beta-Amyloid Deposition and Alzheimer's Type Changes Induced by Borrelia Spirochetes. *Neurobiology of Aging*, 27(2), 228-236. 0197-4580; 0197-4580

Moazed, T. C., Kuo, C. C., Grayston, J. T. & Campbell, L. A. (1998). Evidence of Systemic Dissemination of Chlamydia Pneumoniae Via Macrophages in the Mouse. *The Journal of Infectious Diseases*, 177(5), 1322-1325. 0022-1899

Morales, J. A., Herzog, S., Kompter, C., Frese, K. & Rott, R. (1988). Axonal Transport of Borna Disease Virus Along Olfactory Pathways in Spontaneously and Experimentally Infected Rats. *Medical Microbiology and Immunology*, 177(2), 51-68. 0300-8584; 0300-8584

Nixon, R. A. (2007). Autophagy, Amyloidogenesis and Alzheimer Disease. *Journal of Cell Science*, 120(Pt 23), 4081-4091. 0021-9533; 0021-9533

Nixon, R. A., Cataldo, A. M. & Mathews, P. M. (2000). The Endosomal-Lysosomal System of Neurons in Alzheimer's Disease Pathogenesis: A Review. *Neurochemical Research*, 25(9-10), 1161-1172. 0364-3190; 0364-3190

Noguchi, H. & Moore, J. W. (1913). A Demonstration of Treponema Pallidum in the Brain in Cases of General Paralysis. *The Journal of Experimental Medicine*, 17(2), 232-238. 0022-1007; 0022-1007

Paradowski, B., Jaremko, M., Dobosz, T., Leszek, J. & Noga, L. (2007). Evaluation of CSF-Chlamydia Pneumoniae, CSF-Tau, and CSF-Abeta42 in Alzheimer's Disease and Vascular Dementia. *Journal of Neurology*, 254(2), 154-159. 0340-5354; 0340-5354

Peel, A. L. (2004). PKR Activation in Neurodegenerative Disease. *Journal of Neuropathology and Experimental Neurology*, 63(2), 97-105. 0022-3069; 0022-3069

Pereira, C., Ferreiro, E., Cardoso, S. M. & de Oliveira, C. R. (2004). Cell Degeneration Induced by Amyloid-Beta Peptides: Implications for Alzheimer's Disease. *Journal of Molecular Neuroscience: MN*, 23(1-2), 97-104. 0895-8696; 0895-8696

Pogo, B. G., Casals, J. & Elizan, T. S. (1987). A Study of Viral Genomes and Antigens in Brains of Patients with Alzheimer's Disease. *Brain*, 110(Pt 488001484), 907-915.

Rasmussen, S. J., Eckmann, L., Quayle, A. J., Shen, L., Zhang, Y. X., Anderson, D. J., Fierer, J., Stephens, R. S. & Kagnoff, M. F. (1997). Secretion of Proinflammatory Cytokines by Epithelial Cells in Response to Chlamydia Infection Suggests a Central Role for Epithelial Cells in Chlamydial Pathogenesis. *J Clin Invest*, 99(197148774), 77-87.

Rassu, M., Cazzavillan, S., Scagnelli, M., Peron, A., Bevilacqua, P. A., Facco, M., Bertoloni, G., Lauro, F. M., Zambello, R. & Bonoldi, E. (2001). Demonstration of Chlamydia Pneumoniae in Atherosclerotic Arteries from various Vascular Regions. *Atherosclerosis,* 158(1), 73-79. 0021-9150

Roberts, T. K., Buckner, C. M. & Berman, J. W. (2010). Leukocyte Transmigration Across the Blood-Brain Barrier: Perspectives on neuroAIDS. *Frontiers in Bioscience: A Journal and Virtual Library,* 15, 478-536. 1093-4715; 1093-4715

Rosenfeld, M. E., Blessing, E., Lin, T. M., Moazed, T. C., Campbell, L. A. & Kuo, C. (2000). Chlamydia, Inflammation, and Atherogenesis. *J Infect Dis, 181 Suppl 3,* S492-7.

Roses, A. D. (1996). Apolipoprotein E Alleles as Risk Factors in Alzheimer's Disease. *Annu Rev Med,* 4796266653, 387-400.

Rupprecht, T. A., Koedel, U., Fingerle, V. & Pfister, H. W. (2008). The Pathogenesis of Lyme Neuroborreliosis: From Infection to Inflammation. *Molecular Medicine (Cambridge, Mass.),* 14(3-4), 205-212. 1076-1551; 1076-1551

Santana, S., Recuero, M., Bullido, M. J., Valdivieso, F. & Aldudo, J. (2011). Herpes Simplex Virus Type I Induces the Accumulation of Intracellular Beta-Amyloid in Autophagic Compartments and the Inhibition of the Non-Amyloidogenic Pathway in Human Neuroblastoma Cells. *Neurobiology of Aging,* 1558-1497; 0197-4580

Scheuner, D., Eckman, C., Jensen, M., Song, X., Citron, M., Suzuki, N., Bird, T. D., Hardy, J., Hutton, M., Kukull, W., Larson, E., Levy-Lahad, E., Viitanen, M., Peskind, E., Poorkaj, P., Schellenberg, G., Tanzi, R., Wasco, W., Lannfelt, L., Selkoe, D. & Younkin, S. (1996). Secreted Amyloid Beta-Protein Similar to that in the Senile Plaques of Alzheimer's Disease is Increased in Vivo by the Presenilin 1 and 2 and APP Mutations Linked to Familial Alzheimer's Disease. *Nature Medicine,* 2(8), 864-870. 1078-8956; 1078-8956

Shipley, S. J., Parkin, E. T., Itzhaki, R. F. & Dobson, C. B. (2005). Herpes Simplex Virus Interferes with Amyloid Precursor Protein Processing. *BMC Microbiology,* 5, 48. 1471-2180; 1471-2180

Talloczy, Z., Jiang, W., Virgin, H. W. 4th, Leib, D. A., Scheuner, D., Kaufman, R. J., Eskelinen, E. L. & Levine, B. (2002). Regulation of Starvation- and Virus-Induced Autophagy by the eIF2alpha Kinase Signaling Pathway. *Proceedings of the National Academy of Sciences of the United States of America,* 99(1), 190-195. 0027-8424; 0027-8424

Wisniewski, T. & Sigurdsson, E. M. (2010). Murine Models of Alzheimer's Disease and their use in Developing Immunotherapies. *Biochimica Et Biophysica Acta,* 1802(10), 847-859. 0006-3002; 0006-3002

Wozniak, M. A., Frost, A. L. & Itzhaki, R. F. (2009a). Alzheimer's Disease-Specific Tau Phosphorylation is Induced by Herpes Simplex Virus Type 1. *Journal of Alzheimer's Disease: JAD,* 16(2), 341-350. 1387-2877; 1387-2877

Wozniak, M. A., Itzhaki, R. F., Shipley, S. J. & Dobson, C. B. (2007). Herpes Simplex Virus Infection Causes Cellular Beta-Amyloid Accumulation and Secretase Upregulation. *Neuroscience Letters,* 429(2-3), 95-100. 0304-3940; 0304-3940

Wozniak, M. A., Mee, A. P. & Itzhaki, R. F. (2009b). Herpes Simplex Virus Type 1 DNA is Located within Alzheimer's Disease Amyloid Plaques. *The Journal of Pathology,* 217(1), 131-138. 1096-9896

Wozniak, M. A., Shipley, S. J., Combrinck, M., Wilcock, G. K. & Itzhaki, R. F. (2005). Productive Herpes Simplex Virus in Brain of Elderly Normal Subjects and

Alzheimer's Disease Patients. *Journal of Medical Virology*, 75(2), 300-306. 0146-6615; 0146-6615

Yu, W. H., Kumar, A., Peterhoff, C., Shapiro Kulnane, L., Uchiyama, Y., Lamb, B. T., Cuervo, A. M. & Nixon, R. A. (2004). Autophagic Vacuoles are Enriched in Amyloid Precursor Protein-Secretase Activities: Implications for Beta-Amyloid Peptide Over-Production and Localization in Alzheimer's Disease. *The International Journal of Biochemistry & Cell Biology*, 36(12), 2531-2540. 1357-2725; 1357-2725

Zambrano, A., Solis, L., Salvadores, N., Cortes, M., Lerchundi, R. & Otth, C. (2008). Neuronal Cytoskeletal Dynamic Modification and Neurodegeneration Induced by Infection with Herpes Simplex Virus Type 1. *Journal of Alzheimer's Disease: JAD*, 14(3), 259-269. 1387-2877; 1387-2877

Zhou, L., Diefenbach, E., Crossett, B., Tran, S. L., Ng, T., Rizos, H., Rua, R., Wang, B., Kapur, A., Gandhi, K., Brew, B. J. & Saksena, N. K. (2010). First Evidence of Overlaps between HIV-Associated Dementia (HAD) and Non-Viral Neurodegenerative Diseases: Proteomic Analysis of the Frontal Cortex from HIV+ Patients with and without Dementia. *Molecular Neurodegeneration*, 5, 27. 1750-1326; 1750-1326

3

Amyloid Hypothesis and Alzheimer's Disease

Xiaqin Sun and Yan Zhang
Laboratory of Neurobiology and State Key Laboratory of Biomembrane and Membrane Biotechnology, College of Life Sciences, Peking University, Beijing, China

1. Introduction

This chapter reviews the major hypotheses in Alzheimer's disease (AD) research with the focus on amyloid hypothsis. Since amyloid hypothesis of AD pathology was proposed, extracellular amyloid β (Aβ) toxicity and its role of inducing synaptic plasticity and memory function has been studying intensively. Accumulating evidence indicates that Aβ also exists inside the neurons in AD. Intracellular Aβ has great impact on a variety of cellular events from protein degradation, axonal transport, neuronal firing, autophagy to apoptosis, suggesting an important role of Aβ in AD development, especially in the early stage. This chapter overviews the studies on the presence, production, metabolism and toxicity of extracellular and intracellular Aβ. Therapeutics targeting Aβ could be a new and effective treatment for early AD.

2. Overview of Alzheimer's disease

Alzheimer's disease (AD) is a progressive neurodegenerative disorder characterized by age-related impairment in cognition and memory. The first AD case was reported in 1907 in Germany by Dr. Alois Alzheimer of a middle-aged woman who developed memory deficits and progressive loss of cognitive abilities. Many AD patients show clinical symptoms of severe memory loss and progressive cognitive difficulty in their 60's or 70's except the familial AD (FAD) patients who usually show clinical symptoms in their 40's (Price and Sisodia, 1998). These clinical symptoms include abnormalities of learning, memory, problem solving, speaking, calculation, judgment and planning (McKhann et al., 1984). The development of AD is progressive and can sometimes last for over decades. The development of AD can be divided into three stages according to clinical symptoms (Boller et al., 2002). In the mild stage of AD, patients first lose their short-term memory. They tend to forget the recent events, while they still remember the events that happened many years ago. Simple calculation and daily organization become more and more difficult. They become more and more passive for social activities and some of them develop depression and anxiety. In this stage, most of the patients can still maintain normal daily activities. The mild stage usually lasts for 2-3 years (Boller et al., 2002). The second stage of AD is the moderate stage. In this stage, patients cannot recognize family members. They are not able to communicate well with others since they lose thought flow or words during speaking. The daily self-care and housekeeping events of patients require more and more help from others. Since the daily activities, such as feeding, cooking, dressing and bathing become more and more difficult, the patients are depressed and paranoid more easily (Boller et al., 2002). In the late stage of AD, patients completely lose the abilities to speak, solve problems and make decisions. Daily activities can be affected greatly and everyday life of patients totally depends on caregivers (Price and Sisodia, 1998; Boller et al., 2002).

3. AD pathological hallmarks

AD affects neurons in the neocortex, including the frontal lobe and the temporal lobe (Mann et al., 1985; Mesulam and Geula, 1988; Gomez-Isla et al., 1997), the entorhinal cortex and the hippocampus (Samuel et al., 1994; West et al., 1994; Gomez-Isla et al., 1997). Subcortical limbic areas such as the cholinergic neurons in the basal forebrain (Struble et al., 1986) and the neurons in the amygdala, the anterior nucleus of the thalamus, the raphe, and the locus coeruleus (Price and Sisodia, 1998), are also affected. It is suggested that the first area affected in the brain is the entorhinal cortex and then neurodegeneration progresses to the hippocampus and then to the cortex (Price and Sisodia, 1998).

3.1 Senile plaques

Senile plaques (SPs) are the extracellular proteinacous deposits found in AD patient brains. Deteriorated neurons are often seen near the SP area in the brain (McKhann et al., 1984; Morris et al., 1991; Defigueiredo et al., 1995; Price and Sisodia, 1998; Tseng et al., 1999; Urbanc et al., 1999; Alorainy, 2000). In the SPs, there are dystrophic neuritis. Astrocytes and microglia are often associating with the amyloid deposits (Defigueiredo et al., 1995; Tseng et al., 1999; Urbanc et al., 1999; Alorainy, 2000). The primary proteinacous material of SPs is amyloid β peptide (Aβ), a fibrillar peptide containing 40 to 42 amino acids derived from amyloid precursor protein (APP) (Glenner and Wong, 1984; Masters et al., 1985; Mori et al., 1992; Roher et al., 1993). There are four types of SPs often found in AD brains according to morphology (Defigueiredo et al., 1995; Gearing et al., 1995; Tseng et al., 1999; Urbanc et al., 1999; Alorainy, 2000): (1) Diffuse plaques are usually 10-200 μm in diameter with irregular shapes, in which Aβ is not aggregated into fibrils or deposits. Near these plaques, there are less NFTs and dystrophic neurites. The diffuse plaques are not detectable by Congo red or silver staining, but can be stained by Aβ antibodies. The diffuse plaques are close to neuronal cell bodies, that raises the possibility that the diffuse plaques may originate within the cell body as intracellular Aβ peptides (D'Andrea et al., 2001). The diffuse plaques appear in the DS patients, younger AD patients and other head injury patients (Defigueiredo et al., 1995; Gearing et al., 1995; Tseng et al., 1999; Urbanc et al., 1999; Alorainy, 2000; D'Andrea et al., 2001). All the above evidence suggests that diffuse plaques might be the earliest amyloid aggregates appearing in AD development and the origin of these diffuse plaques might be intracellular amyloid. (2) Primitive plaques are 20-60 μm in diameter, in which Aβ starts to form fibrils and NFTs that are detectable near these plaques. The primitive plaques associate less with the neuronal cell bodies, but more with astrocytes and glial cells. The primitive plaques appear in the older AD patients (Defigueiredo et al., 1995; Gearing et al., 1995; Tseng et al., 1999; Urbanc et al., 1999; Alorainy, 2000). (3) Classic plaques are the most significant type of plaques in AD brains. These plaques are also 20-60 μm in diameter and Aβ peptides form clearly visible aggregates and deposits of fibrils. These aggregates often induce a central dense core structure surrounded by dystrophic neurites and a large amount of glial cells. The classic plaques are located throughout the hippocampus and the neocortex in advanced and older AD patient brains (Defigueiredo et al., 1995; Gearing et al., 1995; Tseng et al., 1999; Urbanc et al., 1999; Alorainy, 2000). (4) Compact plaques are similar to the classic plaques, with 5-15 μm in diameter, but lack the surrounding dystrophic neurites (Defigueiredo et al., 1995; Gearing et al., 1995; Tseng et al., 1999; Urbanc et al., 1999; Alorainy, 2000). Congo red and silver staining are the common cytochemical detectors for SPs. The Congo red dye forms non-polar hydrogen bonds with amyloid fibrils (Braak et al., 1989). The red to green birefringence occurs when viewed by polarized light due to parallel alignment of the dye molecules on the linearly arranged amyloid fibrils (Braak et al., 1989). Silver staining, on the other hand, detects pre-plaques or presumed early SPs, which cannot be stained by the conventional Congo red staining (Braak et al., 1989).

In addition to human, extracellular SPs are also found in other long-lived mammals, such as some non-human primates like Cheirogelidae, Callitricadae, Cebidae and Pogidae (Struble et al., 1984; Gearing et al., 1995; Gearing et al., 1997), domestic dogs (Cummings et al., 1996; Tekirian et al., 1996), cats (Cummings et al., 1996) and polar bears (Cork et al., 1988; Tekirian et al., 1996). However, common laboratory rats and mice do not have natural accumulation of amyloid with age (Jucker et al., 1994). SPs are often found in the amygdala, the hippocampus and the neocortex (Gearing et al., 1995).

3.2 Neurofibrillary tangles

In AD brains, besides SPs, another striking pathological feature is intracellular neurofibrillary tangles (NFTs). The affected neurons often show intracellular accumulations of single straight filaments and paired helical filaments and neuropil threads (Arnold et al., 1991; Braak and Braak, 1994; Gold, 2002). The major component of these poorly soluble filaments is hyperphosphorylated tau, a 68 kDa microtubule-associated protein (Lee et al., 1991; Gomez-Isla et al., 1996; Hardy, 2003; Roder, 2003). The diseases with tau-based neurofibrillary pathology include: AD, Down's syndrome (DS), amyotrophic lateral sclerosis/parkinsonism-dementia complex, Creutzfeldt-Jakob disease, frontotemporal dementia, Pick's disease and argyrophilic grain dementia. Among these diseases, amyotrophic lateral sclerosis and frontotemporal dementia have the most significant neurofibrillary pathology (Michaelis et al., 2002; Hardy, 2003; Roder, 2003). Furthermore, besides human, tau immunoreactivity and deposition-like structures are also found in rhesus monkeys (Garver et al., 1994; Hartig et al., 2000). NFTs can be detected by anti-tau antibody or silver staining. In AD, NFTs are found in the hippocampus, the entorhinal cortex, the association cortex and some other subcortical areas, such as the nucleus basalis of Meynert, the amygdala and the dorsal raphe (Arnold et al., 1991; Braak and Braak, 1994).

In vitro exposure of non-phosphorylated recombinant tau to high concentrations of sulfated glycosaminoglycans leads to the formation of paired helical filaments and single-strand filaments (Goedert et al., 1996). These results suggest that tau phosphorylation as well as the interaction of tau and glycosaminoglycans may play a role in abnormal filament formation *in vivo*. Phosphorylated tau has reduced ability to bind microtubules, which changes the stability of microtubules. In addition, phosphorylated tau may also affect intracellular transportation, cellular geometry and neuronal viability (Lassmann et al., 1995; Smale et al., 1995; Troncoso et al., 1996).

3.3 Synaptic and neuronal loss

3.3.1 Synaptic loss

In AD, a significant synaptic loss ranging from 20% to 50% is reported. Biochemistry, electron microscopy and immunocytochemistry have shown a decrease in synaptic density, presynaptic terminals, synaptic vesicle and synaptic protein markers in AD brains compared with the normal aged controls (Terry et al., 1991; Geula, 1998; Larson et al., 1999; Yao et al., 1999; Ashe, 2000; Baloyannis et al., 2000; Terry, 2000; Masliah, 2001; Masliah et al., 2001b; Price et al., 2001; Scheff and Price, 2001; Scheff et al., 2001; Stephan et al., 2001; Callahan et al., 2002; Chan et al., 2002; Dodd, 2002). Although synaptic loss is remarkable in AD, it is not specific to AD. Reduction in synaptic density is also found in Pick's disease, Huntington's disease, Parkinson's disease as well as in vascular dementia (Geula, 1998; Larson et al., 1999; Yao et al., 1999; Ashe, 2000; Baloyannis et al., 2000; Terry, 2000; Masliah, 2001; Masliah et al., 2001b; Price et al., 2001; Scheff and Price, 2001; Scheff et al., 2001; Stephan et al., 2001; Callahan et al., 2002; Chan et al., 2002; Dodd, 2002).

Since one of the most important physiological functions of synapses is to release and accept neurotransmitters, the changes of activity of these neurotransmitters in neurodegenerative diseases have also been intensively studied (Terry, 2000). In AD, most significant lesions happen in the cholinergic, adrenergic and serotoninergic systems (Davies and Maloney, 1976; Geula, 1998; Larson et al., 1999; Yao et al., 1999; Ashe, 2000; Baloyannis et al., 2000; Terry, 2000; Masliah, 2001; Masliah et al., 2001b; Price et al., 2001; Scheff and Price, 2001; Scheff et al., 2001; Stephan et al., 2001; Callahan et al., 2002; Chan et al., 2002; Dodd, 2002). Some other peptidergic neurotransmitters also decrease in AD, such as somatostatin, neuropeptide Y and substance P (Terry, 2000).

Synaptic loss might be one of the first events in AD development (Terry et al., 1991; Terry, 2000; Selkoe, 2002). Decrease in presynaptic terminals, synaptic vesicle and synaptic protein markers occur in very early stage of AD (Ashe, 2000; Terry, 2000; Masliah et al., 2001b; Price et al., 2001; Scheff et al., 2001; Callahan et al., 2002; Chan et al., 2002; Dodd, 2002). In the transgenic mice with FAD mutations, synaptophysin, marker for presynaptic protein, decreases before the appearance of Aβ deposits and formation of plaques (Hamos et al., 1989; Masliah et al., 1989; Selkoe, 2002). Most importantly, the decline of function of synaptic transmission occurs even before synaptic structural changes (Masliah, 2001; Scheff and Price, 2001; Chan et al., 2002; Selkoe, 2002). Long-term potentiation (LTP) is commonly accepted as a measurement for capacity of synaptic plasticity, which is the basis of learning, memory and complex information processing. The incidence and duration of LTP formation are used as an indication for formation and maintenance of working memory. Several lines of FAD mutant transgenic mice show a decline in the formation of LTP and synaptic excitation before the appearance of synaptic loss, plaques and other AD pathology (Geula, 1998; Ashe, 2000; Masliah, 2001; Masliah et al., 2001b; Scheff and Price, 2001; Callahan et al., 2002; Chan et al., 2002; Selkoe, 2002). In summary, synaptic loss seems to appear earlier than all other pathological markers and the functional loss of synapses may be responsible for the initiation of cognitive decline in AD patients.

3.3.2 Neuronal loss

Synaptic loss and degeneration induce neuronal dysfunction and cell body loss. Neuronal loss in the cerebral cortex and the hippocampus is a hallmark feature of AD. Some of AD patients at late stage of the disease can have a severe decrease in brain volume and weight due to either neuronal loss or atrophy (Smale et al., 1995; Cotman and Su, 1996; Gomez-Isla et al., 1996; Gomez-Isla et al., 1997; Li et al., 1997; Su et al., 1997; Gomez-Isla et al., 1999). Assumption-based and design-based unbiased stereological cell counting shows decreased density of neurons in the cerebral cortex, the entorhinal cortex, the association cortex, the basal nucleus of Meynert, the locus coeruleus and the dorsal raphe of AD brains (Bondareff et al., 1982; Lippa et al., 1992; Gomez-Isla et al., 1996; Gomez-Isla et al., 1997; Gomez-Isla et al., 1999; Colle et al., 2000). Profound neuronal loss is especially observed in the entorhinal cortex in the mild AD brains (Gomez-Isla et al., 1996; Gomez-Isla et al., 1997; Gomez-Isla et al., 1999). Besides AD, significant neuronal loss is also observed in the entorhinal cortex in very mild cognitive impairment patient brains (Gomez-Isla et al., 1996; Gomez-Isla et al., 1997; Gomez-Isla et al., 1999). These data suggest that neuronal loss may be one of the early events before formation of SPs and NFTs in AD development.

The loss of cholinergic neurons in AD is widely studied. The hippocampus and cortex receive major cholinergic input from the basal forebrain nuclei (Hohmann et al., 1987). Decrease of choline acetyltransferase activity and acetylcholine synthesis correlate well with the degree of cognitive impairment in AD patients (Mesulam, 1986; Hohmann et al., 1987; Pearson and Powell, 1987). Cholinergic neuronal lesion can be detected in the patients that have showed clinical memory loss symptoms for less than one year (Whitehouse et al., 1981; Whitehouse et al., 1982; Francis et al., 1993; Weinstock, 1997). However, markers for dopamine, γ-aminobutyric acid (GABA), or somatostatin are not altered (Whitehouse et al., 1981; Whitehouse et al., 1982; Francis et al., 1993). These results suggest that cholinergic neuronal loss is probably one of the early events in AD.

3.4 Correlation of AD pathology to dementia levels

Besides the main pathology discussed above, some other pathologies of AD include granulovacuolar degeneration, cerebral amyloid angiopathy, blood-brain barrier disorder, white matter lesions, neuropil thread and gliosis (Jellinger, 2002a; Jellinger, 2002b, c; Jellinger and Attems, 2003). Because of a lack of diagnostic markers for live AD patients, the definite diagnosis of AD depends on cognitive tests and a quantitative assessment of numbers of SPs and NFTs in the postmortem brain tissues. However, studies of the relationship of the major AD pathological markers with clinical dementia levels suggest that the best correlation with dementia is neither SPs nor NFTs. The extent of neuronal and synaptic loss correlates better with the severity of clinical disease than the neuropathological lesions, SPs and NFTs (De Kosky and Scheff, 1990; Terry et al., 1991), suggesting that neuronal loss has a closer and more direct relationship to clinical dementia.

4. Aβ and Aβ hypothesis in AD

4.1 Production of Aβ

4.1.1 APP

One of the most remarkable pathological features of AD is extracellular deposition of SPs containing Aβ peptide aggregates derived from amyloid precursor protein (APP). APP, cloned in 1987 (Kang et al., 1987), is a type-1 transmembrane glycoprotein with ten isoforms generated by alternative mRNA splicing. APP is encoded by a single gene at human chromosome 21 containing 18 exons (Kang et al., 1987; Goate et al., 1991). APP has a signal peptide, a large extracellular N terminal domain and a small intracellular C terminal domain, a single transmembrane domain and an endocytosis signal at the C terminal (Golde et al., 1992; Haass et al., 1992a; Haass et al., 1992b; Haass et al., 1994; Lai et al., 1995) (Figure 1A). Among ten isoforms of APP ranging from 563 to 770 amino acids, the major ones are APP_{770}, APP_{751} and APP_{695}. Isoforms APP_{751} and APP_{770} are expressed in both peripheral neural and non-neural tissues and have a protease inhibitor domain in the extracellular regions (Kitaguchi et al., 1988; Ponte et al., 1988). Isoform APP_{695}, which lacks the KPI domain, is expressed at high levels in the brain (Yamada et al., 1989; Kang and Muller-Hill, 1990; LeBlanc et al., 1991). Since the CNS neurons are mostly affected in AD, intensive efforts have been made to focus on the APP_{695} isoform (Sinha and Lieberburg, 1999).

Under physiological conditions, newly synthesized APP matures in the endoplasmic reticulum and the Golgi, acquiring N- and O-linked glycosylation and phosphorylation. The function of APP phosphorylation is not known yet. APP is located in the neuronal cell bodies as well as axons. Cellular APP is transported by the fast anterograde system (Koo et al., 1990; Sisodia et al., 1993), therefore, it is suggested that APP may play a role in neurite

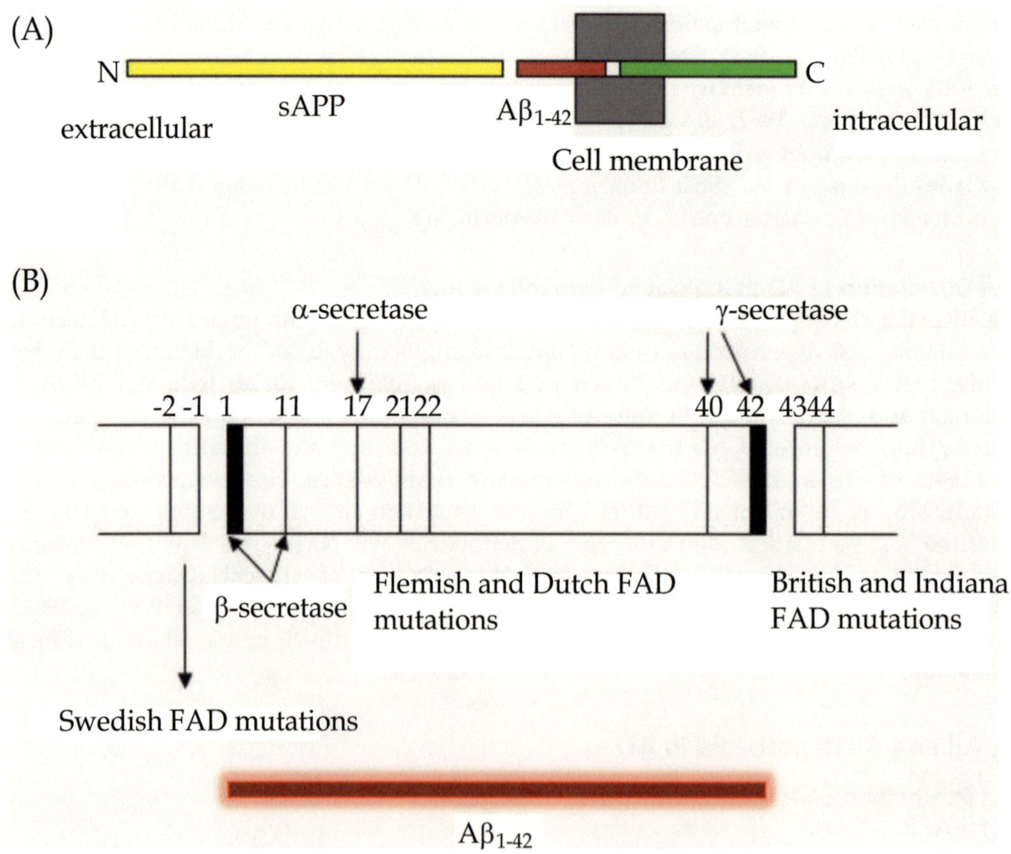

Fig. 1. Schematic diagram of APP and its cleavage. (A) Full-length APP is located in the cell membrane. (B) APP can be cleaved at α-, or β- and γ-secretase sites. FAD mutations are often at cleavage sites

outgrowth and extension, and probably in synaptic transmission and maintenance of axons (Yamaguchi et al., 1990; Yamaguchi et al., 1994). In addition, APP has been suggested to have neuroprotective function or neurotrophic roles (Mattson et al., 1993b). APP knockouts are fertile (Zheng et al., 1996). Neuroanatomical studies of APP knockout mouse brains show no significant differences relative to the wild-type control brains (Zheng et al., 1996). APP can be cleaved at the C terminal by α-secretase near the cell surface to generate a secreted fragment (Sinha and Lieberburg, 1999) (Figure 1B). The exact location of α-secretase activity is still unknown, although some data suggest that α-cleavage occurs mainly at trans-Golgi or plasma membrane (Kuentzel et al., 1993). One possible explanation for the uncertainty about the localization of α-secretase is that there may be more than one enzyme with the α-secretase activity. The candidates for α-secretase are two members of the family of disintegrin and metalloprotease ADAM: tumour necrosis factor-converting enzyme (TACE or ADAM-17) and ADAM-10. TACE can process pro-TNF, creating the extracellular TNF in a similar way to APP. The blockage or knockout of TACE can decrease the release of sAPP (Buxbaum et al., 1998). However, cells lacking TACE still retain part of α-secretase activity (Buxbaum et al., 1998). In addition to TACE, overexpression of ADAM-10 increases α-cleavage of APP (Lammich et al., 1999). A dominant negative form of ADAM-10 inhibits α-secretase activity, but does not totally abolish sAPP production (Lammich et al., 1999). ADAM-10 is inactive in the Golgi, while becomes activated at the plasma membrane (Lammich et al., 1999). Therefore, TACE and ADAM-10 may both contribute to α-cleavage.

In addition to α-secretase pathway, APP can also be cleaved by putative β- and γ-secretases to generate Aβ fragments containing 39-43 amino acids (Figure 1B). The majority of Aβ peptides is the 40 amino acid long $A\beta_{1\text{-}40}$, only 10% of the species are the 42 amino acid peptide $A\beta_{1\text{-}42}$. β-site APP cleaving enzyme (BACE or Asp2) has been suggested to be responsible for β-secretase activity. BACE is a member of pepsin family of aspartyl proteases (Vassar et al., 1999). BACE cleaves full-length APP at Asp1 (Vassar et al., 1999). The Swedish FAD mutation, which is known to enhance β-secretase cleavage, also promotes cleavage of APP at Asp1 by BACE (Vassar et al., 1999). BACE is co-localized with APP in many regions, especially in neurons. BACE also has a subcellular distribution similar to β-secretase (Vassar et al., 1999).

Recent studies suggest that γ-secretase may not be a single protein but rather mediated by a complex of a number of proteins. γ-secretase activity happens when APP is cleaved within the complex containing presenilin, APP binding proteins Nicastrin, Aph-1 and Pen-2 (Yu et al., 2000; Chen et al., 2001; Chung and Struhl, 2001; Satoh and Kuroda, 2001; Hu et al., 2002). There are two proposed β- and γ-secretase pathways. One is called the endosomal/lysosomal pathway. Secreted APP is endocytosed and delivered to endosomes and lysosomes where β- and γ-secretase cleavages occur. The other pathway suggests that Aβ generation occurs in the endoplasmic reticulum and Golgi-derived vesicles (Chyung et al., 1997; Sinha and Lieberburg, 1999). The γ-cleavage and the role of presenilins in this cleavage are discussed in details in the following section about presenilins.

Mutations in the APP gene identified 25 families of FAD worldwide (Chartier-Harlin et al., 1991a; Chartier-Harlin et al., 1991b) (Figure 1B). All these APP mutations are missense mutations. Double mutation Lys670Asn/Met671Leu ("Swedish" mutation), Ala693Gly ("Flemish" mutation), Glu693Gln ("Dutch" mutation) and Ile716Val (Czech et al., 2000) increase Aβ production, especially the generation of $A\beta_{1\text{-}42}$. The "Dutch" mutation is a point mutation within the Aβ peptide sequence and leads to a conformational change of Aβ, which increases the aggregation of Aβ peptides and forms fibrils (Levy et al., 1990; Wisniewski et al., 1997). The "Flemish" mutation is also located within Aβ sequence and alters γ-secretase activity leading to increased production of $A\beta_{1\text{-}42}$ (Haass et al., 1994). The "Arctic" mutation Glu693Gly does not increase Aβ production, but the amount of protofibrils of Aβ increases (Nilsberth et al., 2001). Besides the APP mutations leading to obligate AD phenotype, other evidence that APP is associated with AD comes from DS patients. DS patients have 3 copies of chromosome 21 leading to overexpression of APP. Almost all DS patients develop AD in their 30-40's (reviewed by (Lott and Head, 2001)). Two "APP-like" genes APLP1 amd APLP2 have been localized to human chromosome 19 and suggested to be a strong candidate for late onset FAD (Wasco et al., 1992).

4.1.2 Presenilin

Besides the APP gene, FAD is also associated with mutations in the presenilin (PS) genes (Deng et al., 1996a; Busciglio et al., 1997; Hartmann et al., 1997; Price and Sisodia, 1998; Grace et al., 2002; Grace and Busciglio, 2003). PSs are transmembrane proteins with 8 transmembrane domains, located mainly in the endoplasmic reticulum, Golgi, endoplasmic reticulum-Golgi intermediate structures, and synaptic terminals as detected by electron microscopy (Cook et al., 1996; Takashima et al., 1996; Culvenor et al., 1997; Huynh et al., 1997; Lah et al., 1997; McGeer et al., 1998; Tanimukai et al., 1999; Culvenor et al., 2000; Siman et al., 2001). The PS1 gene is located on human chromosome 14 and the PS2 gene is on chromosome 1 (Sherrington et al., 1996). In humans, both PS1 and PS2 are encoded by 12 exons (Hutton et al., 1996). PSs are highly expressed in human brain, especially in neurons, and in most peripheral tissues (Deng et al., 1996b; Sherrington et al., 1996). There is a strong sequence homology between PS1 and PS2 (Sherrington et al., 1996). PSs are highly conserved from Drosophila to human (Hong and Koo, 1997; Berezovska et al., 1999). While no PS homologues are found in yeast, a PS homologue is found in *Arabidopsis thaliana*, (Czech et al., 2000). PSs are not glycosylated, sulfated or acylated (De Strooper et al., 1997).

The physiological functions of PSs are widely studied. PS knockout studies show that PS1 is important for axial skeleton development. PS1 knockouts have severe defects in their bone and skeleton systems. Interestingly, the phenotype of PS1 knockouts is very similar to the Notch-1 knockouts, which indicates that PSs may play an important role in the Notch signaling pathway (Wong et al., 1997). In addition, the interaction between PSs and Notch is suggested by co-immunoprecipitation of endogenous Notch and PSs in cultured *Drosophila* cells (Ray et al., 1999). Notch is processed in the secretory pathway and cleaved at the Golgi. The two truncated subunits of Notch form a protein complex in the plasma membrane and act as a receptor. When Notch ligand binds to this receptor, one of the two subunits gets cleaved at the extracellular site near the membrane. Then, the intracellular fragment of the cleaved subunit is released into the cytosol. This fragment then translocates into the nucleus and acts as a part of a transcriptional factor complex. This complex can regulate, at the transcriptional level, Notch target genes (De Strooper et al., 1999). The studies of the PS knockouts and Notch function suggest that PSs may be the proteases responsible for Notch cleavage and regulating the trafficking of cleaved Notch to the cytosol (De Strooper et al., 1999). A similar scenario has been proposed for APP processing by PS (De Strooper et al., 1999).

The link between PS1 or PS2 with AD was found through genetic studies of FAD cases. PS1 mutation families have early onset of AD at around 50 years old, whereas PS2 mutation families develop AD symptoms between 40-80 years old (Rogaev et al., 1995). The majority of these PS mutations are missense mutations leading to amino acid change in the protein sequence. If an individual carries a PS mutation, the probability of developing early onset AD is higher than 95% (Annaert et al., 1999). PS mutations are likely to be a "gain of toxic function" resulting in the abnormal APP processing, probably as part of the "γ-secretase" complex that generates Aβ fragments. PS mutations increase Aβ, especially $A\beta_{1-42}$ production (Busciglio et al., 1997; Hartmann et al., 1997). PSs can interact with APP directly. This is supported by the fact that APP and PSs can be co-immunoprecipitated in transfected cells and interact in a yeast two-hybrid system (Waragai et al., 1997; Weidemann et al., 1997; Xia et al., 1998). Whether PSs act directly as the γ-secretase and how PSs cleave APP inside its transmembrane domain are still not clear yet. One model proposes that PSs regulate APP intracellular trafficking and lead APP to the subcellular compartments, most possibly, the endoplasmic reticulum, where γ-secretase cleavage happens (Davis et al., 1998). Two aspartic acid sites (D257, D385) on PS1 are likely to be critical for γ-secretase cleavage because mutations of these two sites significantly decrease γ-secretase cleavage (Tandon and Fraser, 2002). Since γ-secretase cleavage happens inside of the transmembrane domain of APP, it is suggested that the γ-secretase complex (PSs, Nicastrin, Aph-1 and Pen-2) form a pore structure on the membrane. APP is then located and stabilized in the middle of the pore by Nicastrin or Pen-2 (Yu et al., 2000; Chen et al., 2001; Chung and Struhl, 2001; Satoh and Kuroda, 2001; Hu et al., 2002).

4.2 Aβ involvement and Aβ hypothesis in AD

To date, the cause of AD is still not clear. Major pathological features of AD are intracellular NFTs composed of hyperphosphorylated tau, extracellular SPs containing Aβ peptides, and massive synaptic and neuronal loss. Accordingly, there are tau, Aβ and synaptic-neuronal loss hypotheses for the cause of AD. The amyloid hypothesis, on the other hand, emphasizes that increased Aβ production or failure of Aβ clearance induces gradual Aβ accumulation through life, resulting in the formation of amyloid plaques, which induces inflammatory responses and in turn induces synaptic damage, tangles, and then neuronal loss (Podlisny et al., 1987; Hardy and Higgins, 1992). The evidence supporting the amyloid hypothesis comes from studies showing that most of FAD mutations increase Aβ production (Czech et al., 2000). As mentioned in the Aβ section above, both extracellular and intracellular Aβ are toxic to cells. In addition, co-expression of mutant APP and mutant tau increase NFTs, but not SPs, suggesting that Aβ production and accumulation may be upstream to tau to induce tangle formation (Lewis et al., 2001). In addition, the evidence from Down's syndrome patients suggests that SP formation precedes NFT (Mann et al., 1989; Lemere et al., 1996). Furthermore, in a FAD mutation carrier who died from other disease unrelated to AD in middle life, autopsy showed that the load of amyloid deposition and SPs but not NFT (Smith et al., 2001), suggesting that SP formation may happen before NFT formation. However, tau mutants can cause fontotemporal dementia where lots of tangles, but not amyloid deposits, are found in the brain, suggesting that NFT and SP formation may be independent (Hutton et al., 1998; Poorkaj et al., 1998; Spillantini and Goedert, 1998). Therefore, from this point of view, it seems that Aβ accumulation is either preceding or independent of NFT formation. The Aβ deposition in the neural parenchyma occurs early in plaque formation, and this peptide species is the major component in the mature plaque (Price and Sisodia, 1998). Aβ production increases in the cells expressing FAD mutations (Price and Sisodia, 1998). These Aβ deposits may also act as a backbone for the subsequent deposits of other proteins, such as α_1-antichymotrypsin, apolipoprotein E (apoE) and J (Rogers et al., 1988).

The aggregations of Aβ are toxic to neurons and are thought to contribute to neuronal loss in AD development (Yankner, 1996). Since extracellular Aβ deposition is a major pathological hallmark of AD, considerable attention has been devoted to the Aβ cytotoxicity hypothesis, which argues that the extracellular Aβ (eAβ), especially $eA\beta_{1-42}$, induces neuronal death, therefore, is one of the primary causes of AD (Yankner et al., 1990; Roses, 1996; Scheuner et al., 1996; Sinha and Lieberburg, 1999; De Strooper and Annaert, 2000; Wang et al., 2001). The eAβ toxicity hypothesis is supported by the fact that fibrillar eAβ is toxic to various systems, including cell lines and primary cells in cultures (Yankner et al., 1990; Kowall et al., 1991; Pike et al., 1991; Busciglio et al., 1992, Busciglio, 1993 #189; Behl et al., 1994; Hoyer, 1994; Lorenzo and Yankner, 1994b; Price et al., 1995; Lorenzo and Yankner, 1996; Roher et al., 1996). Furthermore, levels of Aβ, especially $A\beta_{1-42}$, increase in the AD brains and in the serum or fibroblasts from the AD patients (reviewed by (Price and Sisodia, 1998)). Although the mechanism of eAβ cytotoxicity is still not fully understood, proposed eAβ toxicity mechanisms include: increasing vulnerability of cells to a secondary insult (Mattson et al., 1993a; Behl et al., 1994), changes in calcium influx (Ho et al., 2001), increasing oxidative stress (Behl et al., 1994), activation of inflammation and microglia (Eikelenboom et al., 2002; Gasic-Milenkovic et al., 2003), changes in tau phosphorylation (Ghribi et al., 2003), induction of apoptosis (Colurso et al., 2003; Hashimoto et al., 2003; Monsonego et al., 2003), induction of lysosomal protease activity and damaging membrane (Bahr and Bendiske, 2002; Bendiske and Bahr, 2003). Also, eAβ can interacts with receptors on the cell membrane, such as the p75 neurotrophin receptors, APP, receptors for advanced glycation endproducts (RAGE) (Loo et al., 1993; Yan et al., 1997; Yarr et al., 1997; Yaar et al., 2002).

Like many other amyloidogenous proteins, Aβ undergoes oligomerization and fibrillation under physiological situations (Zerovnik et al., 2011). The mechanisms of amyloid fibril formation have been suggested as "templating and nucleation models", "linear colloid-like assembly of spherical oligomers", and "domain-swapping" (Zerovnik et al., 2011). Recent studies have demonstrated that soluble Aβ oligomers have toxic role (Haass and Selkoe, 2007; Walsh and Selkoe, 2007). Aβ oligomers have been shown to induce cognitive defects when transferred into wild type murine brains (Podlisny et al., 1998; Walsh et al., 2000; Walsh et al., 2002b; Walsh et al., 2002a; Walsh et al., 2005b; Walsh et al., 2005a; Lesne et al., 2006; Townsend et al., 2006; Shankar et al., 2009). Soluble oligomers form trimers and tetramers that disrupt normal synaptic function (Salminen et al., 2008), precede synapse loss (Salminen et al., 2008). Aβ oligomers induce inhibited LTP and enhanced long-term depression (Malchiodi-Albedi et al., 2011). The mechanisms of Aβ oligomer toxicity have been suggested to be associated with calcium dysregulation (Malchiodi-Albedi et al., 2011), inflammation activation (Salminen et al., 2008), potassium efflux activation (Salminen et al., 2008) and interaction with membrane lipid rafts (Simons and Gerl, 2010) and microglia (Malchiodi-Albedi et al., 2011).

Several lines of evidence suggest that eAβ may not be the sole contributor to AD pathology. First, in AD patients, the severity of Aβ deposition correlates poorly with clinical dementia levels (Barcikowska et al., 1992). Second, in some AD animal models, Aβ accumulates and forms SPs in the absence of the other two AD pathological features, neuronal loss and NFTs (Price and Sisodia, 1998; Masliah et al., 2001a). Third, eAβ toxicity generally requires non-physiological micro molar levels of Aβ in the culture medium. Moreover, some groups have reported that eAβ is not toxic even at high micro molar concentration in rat PC12, human IMR32 cells and in monkey cerebral cortex (Busciglio et al., 1992; Podlisny et al., 1993; Gschwind and Huber, 1995). One of the best models to study human age-related diseases, human primary cultured neurons, is resistent to 10 μM of eAβ (Mattson et al., 1992; Paradis et al., 1996). A secondary insult, such as serum deprivation, is required for eAβ to induce cell death in human neurons (Paradis et al., 1996). Fourth, transgenic mice carrying FAD APP^{V717F} mutation show neuronal and synaptic loss before Aβ accumulation (Hsia et al., 1999). In addition, human neuronal cell death induced by serum deprivation increases eAβ production, suggesting that eAβ generation is a consequence instead of a cause of neuronal cell loss (LeBlanc et al., 1999). Interestingly, in human primary neurons, p75 neurotrophin receptors play a protective role against eAβ toxicity. Blocking p75 by anti-sense constructs or antibody significantly promotes eAβ toxicity (Zhang et al., 2003). In addition, in some AD animal models, Aβ accumulates to form SPs in the absence of two other AD pathological features, neuronal loss and NFT (Price and Sisodia, 1998; Masliah et al., 2001a). Furthermore, the number of SPs does not correlate with the degree of cognitive impairment. In some older people without dementia, lots of SPs are found in their brains.

Recently, findings implicating intracellular Aβ (iAβ) accumulation and toxicity in AD are attracting more and more attention. The accumulation of iAβ has been observed. First, $iAβ_{1-42}$ significantly accumulates in the pyramidal neurons of the hippocampus and the entorhinal cortex in mild cognitive impairment and AD patient brains (Chui et al., 1999; Gouras et al., 2000; D'Andrea et al., 2001; D'Andrea et al., 2002; Nagele et al., 2002; Tabira et al., 2002; Takahashi et al., 2002; Wang et al., 2002). Similar accumulations of $Aβ_{1-42}$ also occur in neurons of DS (Busciglio et al., 2002; Takahashi et al., 2002) and muscle cells of IBM individuals (Askanas et al., 1992; Sugarman et al., 2002), two degenerative disorders other than AD associated with amyloid deposition. Second, this $iAβ_{1-42}$ accumulation appears earlier than amyloid plaque formation (Gouras et al., 2000; D'Andrea et al., 2001; Tabira et al., 2002; Takahashi et al., 2002; Wang et al., 2002). Third, in the cell culture system, accumulation of $iAβ_{1-42}$ was reported (Yang et al., 1998; Greenfield et al., 1999). Fourth, in the transgenic animal models, iAβ accumulation precedes NFT formation in APP/PS1 double mutant mice (Wirths et al., 2001). In the APP mutant mice where synaptic loss happens before the presence of eAβ, iAβ was also reported (Li et al., 1996; Masliah et al., 1996; Hsia et al., 1999). Furthermore, using neuronal specific promoter NF-L, $Aβ_{1-42}$ expressed intracellularly in the neurons of transgenic mice induces dramatic cell loss (LaFerla et al., 1995). Microinjection of intracellular $Aβ_{1-42}$ into neurons induces dramatic cell death mediated through the activation of p53, Bax and caspase-6 (Zhang et al., 2002; Li et al., 2007). Intracellular $Aβ_{1-42}$ also causes electrophysiological property changes in primary human neurons (Hou et al., 2009). Androgen (Zhang et al., 2004), estrogen (Zhang et al., 2004), galanin (Cui et al., 2010) can protect against such toxicity.

Under physiological conditions, Aβ peptides are normally generated in the endoplasmic reticulum, Golgi or endosomal-lysosomal pathway, and secreted to the extracellular environment (Martin et al., 1995; Chyung et al., 1997; Tienari et al., 1997; Lee et al., 1998;

Greenfield et al., 1999). There are three possible pathways that may generate iAβ. One is that Aβ goes through endoplasmic reticulum-associated degradation (ERAD) pathway. When Aβ is made in the endoplasmic reticulum, the insoluble Aβ could be recognized as a misfolded protein and then reverse translocate from the endoplasmic reticulum to the cytosol. The misfolded proteins are then ubiquitinated and sent to proteasome for degradation (Werner et al., 1996; Greenfield et al., 1999; Friedlander et al., 2000; Ng et al., 2000; VanSlyke and Musil, 2002). It is possible that aging decreases proteasome activity (Merker et al., 2001), which leads to insufficient degradation and clearance of Aβ. The second possible way to generate iAβ is that Aβ fragments can be located in the endosome/lysosome transported from the trans-Golgi or through endocytosis. It has been suggested that Aβ can increase the membrane permeability of lysosome (Yang et al., 1998). Therefore, the Aβ within the endosome/lysosome can break the lysosome membrane and leak out of the vesicles. The third possible way is that there could be leakage happening along any of the secretory pathway. It is even possible that secreted Aβ passively diffuses into the cytosol through the plasma membrane or is actively uptaken by certain receptors on the plasma membrane.

5. Potential AD therapies based on Aβ hypothesis

5.1 Decreasing Aβ production

Aβ is generated from cleavage of APP by β- and γ-secretase (Vassar and Citron, 2000). β-secretase, a membrane-bound aspartic protease, is also called BACE, is most abundant in the brain (Vassar and Citron, 2000). BACE knockout mice apparently lack phenotype, which suggests that maybe inhibition of BACE in adult mice does not have side effect, and can be an excellent drug target for the cure of AD. However, there is a homologue of BACE, BACE2 (Vassar and Citron, 2000), which compensates the function of BACE. So, drugs which inhibit BACE, not BACE2, make sense in decreasing Aβ production. γ-secretase releases Aβ from APP. However, compared to β-secretase, γ-secretase is less understood. It is known that transmembrane proteins PS1 and PS2 (Strooper and Annaert, 2001), and nicastrin (Kopan and Goate, 2002) are required for the activity of γ-secretase. γ-secretase is involved in the cleavage of other integral membrane proteins including Notch (Strooper and Annaert, 2001), CD44 receptor (Okamoto et al., 2001). The mice die early in embryogenesis if γ-secretase is totally inhibited. Therefore, reasonable treatment with γ-secretase is partially inhibit γ-secretase, or inhibits the γ-secretase specifically cleaves APP to yield Aβ (Strooper and Annaert, 2001) (Figure 2).

Non-steroidal anti-inflammatory drugs (NSAIDs) are also candidates for AD drug target, because inflammation in AD is an important inducement for neuronal loss and it causes microglia activation, cytokines and complement components in the vicinity of the plaques (McGeer and McGeer, 1999; Akiyama et al., 2000). Clinic treatment of NSAIDs could specifically slow down the progression of AD (in t' Veld et al., 2001). NSAIDs target cyclooxygenases (COX) 1 and 2, while COX-2 inhibitors have little effects (McGeer, 2000). Recently, the study shows that the protective role of NSAIDs may be independent of their role in inflammation (Weggen et al., 2001). The production of Aβ in NSAIDs treated cells is apparently inhibited (De Strooper and Konig, 2001). But we still don't know how the NSAIDs specifically reduce the production of Aβ (Figure 2).

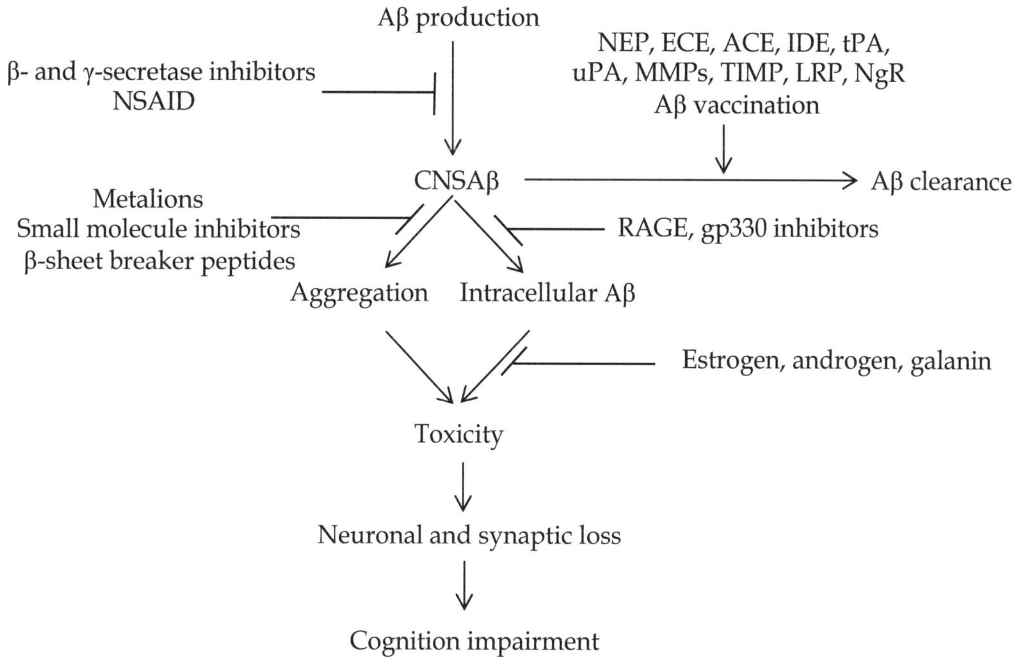

Fig. 2. Schematic diagram of Aβ production, clearance, aggregation and toxicity

5.2 Increasing Aβ clearance

5.2.1 Neprilysin (NEP)

Neprilysin, also called neutral endopeptidease (NEP), enkephalinase, CD10, or common acute lymphoblastic leukemia antigen (CALLA), is a zinc metallopeptidase with a zinc-binding motif (Turner and Tanzawa, 1997). NEP is a type II integral membrane protein with a short amino-terminal and localized at the cell membrane. NEP binds to many extracellular proteins or peptides, such as enkephalins, substance P, atrial natriuretic peptide, somatostatin, endothelin and insulin B chain. The physiological role of NEP is not fully understood yet. Studies suggest its possible implications in the regulation of natriuretic and vasodilator peptides in the kidney, the modulation of inflammatory response by neutrophils and the inactivation of mitogenic signaling in various cells (Turner et al., 2001). NEP is highly localized at the synapses (Schwartz et al., 1980) and colocalized with SP and Aβ (Sato et al., 1991). NEP can hydrolyze synthetic $A\beta_{1\text{-}40}$ *in vitro* (Howell et al., 1995) and synthetic $A\beta_{1\text{-}42}$ injected into rat hippocampus *in vivo* (Iwata et al., 2000). Mice with disrupted NEP gene show decreased ability of degrading exogenous $A\beta_{1\text{-}42}$ and endogenous $A\beta_{40/42}$ (Iwata et al., 2001). Endogenous Aβ accumulates in the hippocampus of this animal model which correlates with the severity of AD pathology (Iwata et al., 2001). Also, in human AD brain samples, NEP mRNA levels are low in the vulnerable areas, such as the hippocampus and the temporal cortex (Yasojima et al., 2001) (Figure 2).

Besides NEP, two other proteases related to NEP were also found to degrade Aβ. Endothelin-converting enzyme (ECE) hydrolyzes endogenous and synthetic Aβ in neuroblastoma cells and transfected CHO cells (Eckman et al., 2001). ECE can also degrade $A\beta_{1\text{-}40}$ and $A\beta_{1\text{-}42}$ into $A\beta_{1\text{-}16}$, $A\beta_{1\text{-}17}$ and $A\beta_{1\text{-}19}$ *in vitro* (Eckman et al., 2001). An intronic polymorphism of angiotensin converting enzyme (ACE) is found to be a possible susceptibility genetic factor (Narain et al., 2000). Purified ACE from human seminal fluid is able to degrade $A\beta_{1\text{-}40}$ and reduce Aβ fibrillogenesis and cytotoxicity (Hu et al., 2001) (Figure 2).

5.2.2 Insulin-degrading enzyme (IDE)

Insulin-degrading enzyme (IDE), also called insulysin and insulinase, is a neutral thiol metalloendopeptidase with an inverted zinc-binding site. IDE can hydrolyze multiple peptides, including amylin, and the APP intracellular domain in addition to Aβ (Duckworth et al., 1998; Selkoe, 2001). Purified nondenatured IDE migrates from 300kDa to 110kDa after denaturation, which indicates that native IDE exists as a mixture of dimers and tetramers (Authier et al., 1996; Duckworth et al., 1998). IDE is significantly activated in neutral pH and dimmers formation (Mirsky et al., 1949; Kurochkin, 2001; Song et al., 2003). IDE was found to be located to the ^{125}I-labeled synthetic Aβ in cytosol fractions from rat brain and liver (Kurochkin and Goto, 1994). Purified IDE effectively degrades Aβ *in vivo* and *in vitro* (McDermott and Gibson, 1997; Perez et al., 2000), proved by the transgenic APP mouse as well (Farris et al., 2003; Farris et al., 2004) (Figure 2).

5.2.3 Plasmin, tissue plasminogen activator (tPA), urokinase-type plaminogen activator (uPA), matrix metalloproteinases and endosomal/lysosomal proteases

Plasmin, a serin protease, can degrade many extracellular matrix components (Werb, 1997). Plasmin, tissue plasminogen activator (tPA), and urokinase-type plaminogen activator (uPA) all belong to the plasimin system (Henkin et al., 1991). Plasmin, the active serine protease, is generated from tPA expressed in neurons and uPA expressed in neurons and microglial cells by cleavage of plasminogen (Madani et al., 2003). It is reported that plasmin significantly decreases the neurotoxicity of Aβ aggregation by degrading Aβ, which has been proved by cell culture (Ledesma et al., 2000; Ledesma et al., 2003) (Figure 2).

Matrix metalloproteinases (MMPs) is a large family which can degrade and remodel extracellular matrix. MMPs have common propeptide and N-terminal catalytic domains (Yong et al., 1998). MMPs are activated by a proteolytic processing, regulated by tissue inhibitors of matrix metalloproteinases (TIMP), which can bind to the active or the inactive form of the MMPs (Brew et al., 2000). TIMP is found to co-localize with neuritic plaques and neurofibrillary tangles. Incubation of MMP-9 and synthetic Aβ1-40 can produce several products of degradation (Backstrom et al., 1996). The other MMPs can also performe this kind of cleavage (Figure 2).

Endosomal and lysosomal proteases can protect neuron cells by internalization of extracellular Aβ though a number of receptors such as lipoprotein receptor-related protein (LRP), receptor for advanced glycation and products (RAGE), gp330/megalin and P-glycoproein as indicated in the following text. In AD models, alterations occur to lysosomal, including the accumulation of lysosomes and lysosomal hydrolases, next to Aβ deposits (Ii et al., 1993; Cataldo et al., 1994). Cathepsin D protein level and activity are increased in aging brain, and the CSF of AD patients (Cataldo et al., 1995; Hoffman et al., 1998). It is reported that cathepsin D gene is associated with sporadic AD (Papassotiropoulos et al., 1999) (Figure 2).

5.2.4 Aβ vaccination

The active and passive immunizations have been examined in *in vitro* models and proven effective against Aβ pathology, cellular alterations and cognitive impairment in AD animal models (Schenk et al., 1999; Bard et al., 2000; Janus et al., 2000; Morgan et al., 2000; DeMattos et al., 2001; Lemere et al., 2001; DeMattos et al., 2002a; DeMattos et al., 2002b; Dodart et al., 2002; Matsuoka et al., 2003; Lemere et al., 2004; Hartman et al., 2005; Selkoe, 2007; Vasilevko et al., 2007; Yamada et al., 2009). After vaccination of Aβ, a transgenic mouse over expressing a mutant form of human APP is protected against amyloid plaque formation (Schenk et al., 1999). This vaccination not only protects Aβ aggregation, but also clears the amyloids in the brain of adult mice (Weiner et al., 2000). For vaccination, the antibody is directly injected by intraperitoneal immunization (Bard et al., 2000; DeMattos et al., 2001). The antibodies go across the blood-brain barrier, and probably trigger microglia to phagocytose Aβ. There is an alternative working mechanism: the antibodies make Aβ trapped in the plasma, which in turn reduce the extracellular concentration of Aβ (Janus et al., 2000; Morgan et al., 2000). Although the concentration of Aβ decreased after the vaccination, the cognitive function in these models is not apparently affected, which may due to the metabolism of Aβ; another problem for the vaccination is the clinical signs of inflammation in the CNS of several patients. According to Aβ vaccination, lower toxicity and higher immunogenicity (Nicolau et al., 2002) should be mainly considered (Figure 2).

5.2.5 Receptor mediated Aβ clearance

LRP and RAGE are both multi-ligand receptors binding to various ligands (Tanzi et al., 2004), trafficking Aβ across the blood-brain barrier (BBB) (Deane et al., 2004; Zlokovic, 2008). LRP1, a member of the low-density lipoprotein (LDL) receptor family, binds to various structurally unrelated ligands, apoE, APP, lactoferrin and Aβ included (Deane and Zlokovic, 2007). LRP1 antagonists (Shibata et al., 2000) or low expression level of LRP1 (Van Uden et al., 2002) apparently increase Aβ load (Deane et al., 2008; Marques et al., 2009). β-secretase cleaves the extracellular domain of LRP to produce soluble LRP, which can binds to free Aβ in the plasma in order to reduce the concentration of extracellular Aβ (Sagare et al., 2007). RAGE is a member of immunoglobulin super family, mediating the reentry of Aβ in to the brain through BBB. RAGE can bind to soluble Aβ at a nanomolar concentration (Deane et al., 2003), and this kind of interaction is indicated in injuries, imflammatory, and AD brains (Yan et al., 1996; Stern et al., 2002; Deane et al., 2003). In addition, Nogo-66 receptor (NgR) (Park and Strittmatter, 2007; Tang and Liou, 2007), gp330/megalin and P-glycoproein (Zlokovic, 1996; Lam et al., 2001) can also contribute to Aβ trafficking, with their respective role in transforming Aβ through BBB unknown (Figure 2).

Besides the clearance pathways mentioned above, one of the AD risk factor apoE ε4 allele can alter Aβ clearance (Castellano et al., 2011). In a mouse model of Aβ-amyloidosis expressing human apoE isoforms (PDAPP/TRE), the concentration and clearance of soluble Aβ in the brain interstitial fluid is reported to depend on the isoform type of apoE, especially in aged PDAPP/TRE mice (Castellano et al., 2011).

5.3 Preventing Aβ aggregation formation

Mental ions like Cu^{2+} and Zn^{2+} are found to reduce the aggregation and toxicity of Aβ (Atwood et al., 1998). Clioruinol, an antibiotic and Cu^{2+}/Zn^{2+} clelator that crosses the blood-brain barrier, can significantly decrease brain Aβ depositon in APP-transgenic mice after 9-week treatment (Cherny et al., 2001). In the progression of Aβ aggregation formation, a number of small molecules can interfere with the Aβ fibril *in vivo* or *in vitro,* such as rifampicin (Tomiyama et al., 1996), Congo red (Lorenzo and Yankner, 1994a), benzofuran

(Howlett et al., 1999), and Nicotine (Salomon et al., 1996) etc., with different principles as follows. Rifampicin prevents Aβ-induced oxidative damage as a free radical scavenger, because the nahpthohydroquinone and naphthoquinone structure protect the neuron cells (Tomiyama et al., 1996). Congo reds may inhibit the aggregation of Aβ through two sulfonate groups at a certain distance, which indicates the specific interaction of the negatively charged sulfonate moieties with Aβ (Pollack et al., 1995; Klunk et al., 1998). Just like a number of tetracyclic and carbazole-type compounds, benzofuran inhibits Aβ fibril formation, as a result of the inhibitory properties of these compounds (Howlett et al., 1999). Nicotine can prevent the conformational transition from α-helix to β-sheet (Salomon et al., 1996), and attenuate the neurotoxicity of Aβ through the nicotine receptor (Zamani et al., 1997). Nicotine also enhances the biosynthesis and secretion of transthyretin, which could bind to Aβ peptide to inhibit the formation of amyloid deposition (Tsuzuki et al., 2000). "β-sheet breaker peptides", another way to prevent Aβ aggregation formation, are two peptides with sequences complementary to Aβ, with additional proline residues, which inhibit the formation of β-sheet structures (Soto et al., 1996; Soto et al., 1998). The sequences of the "β sheet breaker peptides" are RDLPFFDVPID and LPFFD. According to the usage of peptides in the treatment of disease in the central nervous system, rapid proteolytic degradation in the plasma and cerebrospinal fluid, and low permeability across the blood-brain barrier should be taken into account (Poduslo et al., 1999) (Figure 2).

6. List of abbreviations

Aβ: amyloid β; ACE: angiotensin converting enzyme; AD: Alzheimer's disease; apoE: apolipoprotein E; APP: amyloid precursor protein; BACE: β-site APP cleaving enzyme; BBB: blood-brain barrier; CALLA: common acute lymphoblastic leukemia antigen; COX: cyclooxygenases; DS: Down's syndrome; eAβ: extracellular Aβ; ECE: endothelin-converting enzyme; ERAD: endoplasmic reticulum-associated degradation; FAD: familial AD; GABA: γ-aminobutyric acid; iAβ: intracellular Aβ; IDE: insulin-degrading enzyme; LRP: lipoprotein receptor-related protein; LTP: long-term potentiation; MMP: matrix metalloproteinases; NEP: neutral endopeptidease; NFT: neurofibrillary tangles; NgR: Nogo-66 receptor; NSAID: non-steroidal anti-inflammatory drug; PS: presenilin; RAGE: receptor for advanced glycation end products; SP: senile plaques; TACE: tumour necrosis factor-converting enzyme; TIMP: tissue inhibitors of matrix metalloproteinases; tPA: tissue plasminogen activator; uPA: urokinase-type plaminogen activator

7. Conclusions

Amyloid hypothesis stating that Aβ is the primary cause of AD has been proposed and examined in AD research field. However, many controversial issues still exist and further studies are needed to increase our understanding about AD development and progression. The therapeutics, which stem from the knowledge of basic research, may become another effective way to evaluate the theory itself.

8. Disclosure statement

All authors declare no actual or potential conflicts of interest including any financial, personal or other relationships with other people or organizations within three years of beginning the work submitted that could inappropriately influence (bias) their work.

9. Acknowledgements

This work was supported by the National Program of Basic Research sponsored by the Ministry of Science and Technology of China (2009CB941301), Peking University President Research Grant, Ministry of Education Recruiting Research Grant and Roche Research Grant.

10. References

Akiyama H et al. (2000) Inflammation and Alzheimer's disease. Neurobiol Aging 21:383-421.

Alorainy I (2000) Senile scleral plaques: CT. Neuroradiology 42:145-148.

Annaert WG, Levesque L, Craessaerts K, Dierinck I, Snellings G, Westaway D, George-Hyslop PS, Cordell B, Fraser P, De Strooper B (1999) Presenilin 1 controls gamma-secretase processing of amyloid precursor protein in pre-golgi compartments of hippocampal neurons. J Cell Biol 147:277-294.

Arnold SE, Hyman BT, Flory J, Damasio AR, van Hoesen GW (1991) The topographical and neuroanatomical distribution of neurofibrillary tangles and neuritic plaques in the cerebral cortex of patients with Alzheimer's disease. Cereb Cortex 1:103-116.

Ashe KH (2000) Synaptic structure and function in transgenic APP mice. Ann N Y Acad Sci 924:39-41.

Askanas V, Engel WK, Alvarez RB (1992) Light and electron microscopic localization of beta-amyloid protein in muscle biopsies of patients with inclusion-body myositis. Am J Pathol 141:31-36.

Atwood A, Choi J, Levin HL (1998) The application of a homologous recombination assay revealed amino acid residues in an LTR-retrotransposon that were critical for integration. J Virol 72:1324-1333.

Authier F, Posner BI, Bergeron JJ (1996) Insulin-degrading enzyme. Clin Invest Med 19:149-160.

Backstrom JR, Lim GP, Cullen MJ, Tokes ZA (1996) Matrix metalloproteinase-9 (MMP-9) is synthesized in neurons of the human hippocampus and is capable of degrading the amyloid-beta peptide (1-40). J Neurosci 16:7910-7919.

Bahr BA, Bendiske J (2002) The neuropathogenic contributions of lysosomal dysfunction. J Neurochem 83:481-489.

Baloyannis SJ, Manolidis SL, Manolidis LS (2000) Synaptic alterations in the vestibulocerebellar system in Alzheimer's disease--a Golgi and electron microscope study. Acta Otolaryngol 120:247-250.

Barcikowska M, Kujawa M, Wisniewski H (1992) beta-Amyloid deposits within the cerebellum of persons older than 80 years of age. Neuropatol Pol 30:285-293.

Bard F et al. (2000) Peripherally administered antibodies against amyloid beta-peptide enter the central nervous system and reduce pathology in a mouse model of Alzheimer disease. Nat Med 6:916-919.

Behl C, Davis J, Lesley R, Schubert D (1994) Hydrogen peroxide mediates amyloid b protein toxicity. Cell 77:817-827.

Bendiske J, Bahr BA (2003) Lysosomal activation is a compensatory response against protein accumulation and associated synaptopathogenesis--an approach for slowing Alzheimer disease? J Neuropathol Exp Neurol 62:451-463.

Berezovska O, Frosch M, McLean P, Knowles R, Koo E, Kang D, Shen J, Lu FM, Lux SE, Tonegawa S, Hyman BT (1999) The Alzheimer-related gene presenilin 1 facilitates notch 1 in primary mammalian neurons. Brain Res Mol Brain Res 69:273-280.

Boller F, Verny M, Hugonot-Diener L, Saxton J (2002) Clinical features and assessment of severe dementia. A review. Eur J Neurol 9:125-136.

Bondareff W, Mountjoy CQ, Roth M (1982) Loss of neurons of origin of the adrenergic projection to cerebral cortex (nucleus locus ceruleus) in senile dementia. Neurology 32:164-168.

Braak H, Braak E (1994) Pathology of Alzheimer's disease. In: Neurodegenerative Disease., pp 585-613. Philadelphia: Saunders.

Braak H, Braak E, Ohm T, Bohl J (1989) Alzheimer's disease: mismatch between amyloid plaques and neuritic plaques. Neurosci Lett 103:24-28.

Brew K, Dinakarpandian D, Nagase H (2000) Tissue inhibitors of metalloproteinases: evolution, structure and function. Biochim Biophys Acta 1477:267-283.

Busciglio J, Lorenzo A, Yankner BA (1992) Methodological variables in the assessment of beta amyloid neurotoxicity. Neurobiol Aging 13:609-612.

Busciglio J, Pelsman A, Wong C, Pigino G, Yuan M, Mori H, Yankner BA (2002) Altered metabolism of the amyloid beta precursor protein is associated with mitochondrial dysfunction in Down's syndrome. Neuron 33:677-688.

Busciglio J, Hartmann H, Lorenzo A, Wong C, Baumann K, Sommer B, Staufenbiel M, Yankner BA (1997) Neuronal localization of presenilin-1 and association with amyloid plaques and neurofibrillary tangles in Alzheimer's disease. J Neurosci 17:5101-5107.

Buxbaum JD, Liu KN, Luo Y, Slack JL, Stocking KL, Peschon JJ, Johnson RS, Castner BJ, Cerretti DP, Black RA (1998) Evidence that tumor necrosis factor alpha converting enzyme is involved in regulated alpha-secretase cleavage of the Alzheimer amyloid protein precursor. J Biol Chem 273:27765-27767.

Callahan LM, Vaules WA, Coleman PD (2002) Progressive reduction of synaptophysin message in single neurons in Alzheimer disease. J Neuropathol Exp Neurol 61:384-395.

Castellano JM, Kim J, Stewart FR, Jiang H, Demattos RB, Patterson BW, Fagan AM, Morris JC, Mawuenyega KG, Cruchaga C, Goate AM, Bales KR, Paul SM, Bateman RJ, Holtzman DM (2011) Human apoE Isoforms Differentially Regulate Brain Amyloid-{beta} Peptide Clearance. Sci Transl Med 3:89ra57.

Cataldo AM, Hamilton DJ, Nixon RA (1994) Lysosomal abnormalities in degenerating neurons link neuronal compromise to senile plaque development in Alzheimer disease. Brain Res 640:68-80.

Cataldo AM, Barnett JL, Berman SA, Li J, Quarless S, Bursztajn S, Lippa C, Nixon RA (1995) Gene expression and cellular content of cathepsin D in Alzheimer's disease brain: evidence for early up-regulation of the endosomal-lysosomal system. Neuron 14:671-680.

Chan SL, Furukawa K, Mattson MP (2002) Presenilins and APP in neuritic and synaptic plasticity: implications for the pathogenesis of Alzheimer's disease. Neuromolecular Med 2:167-196.

Chartier-Harlin MC, Crawford F, Hamandi K, Mullan M, Goate A, Hardy J, Backhovens H, Martin JJ, Broeckhoven CV (1991a) Screening for the beta-amyloid precursor protein mutation (APP717: Val----Ile) in extended pedigrees with early onset Alzheimer's disease. Neurosci Lett 129:134-135.

Chartier-Harlin MC, Crawford F, Houlden H, Warren A, Hughes D, Fidani L, Goate A, Rossor M, Roques P, Hardy J, et al. (1991b) Early-onset Alzheimer's disease caused by mutations at codon 717 of the beta-amyloid precursor protein gene. Nature 353:844-846.

Chen F, Yu G, Arawaka S, Nishimura M, Kawarai T, Yu H, Tandon A, Supala A, Song YQ, Rogaeva E, Milman P, Sato C, Yu C, Janus C, Lee J, Song L, Zhang L, Fraser PE, St George-Hyslop PH (2001) Nicastrin binds to membrane-tethered Notch. Nat Cell Biol 3:751-754.

Cherny RA, Atwood CS, Xilinas ME, Gray DN, Jones WD, McLean CA, Barnham KJ, Volitakis I, Fraser FW, Kim Y, Huang X, Goldstein LE, Moir RD, Lim JT, Beyreuther K, Zheng H, Tanzi RE, Masters CL, Bush AI (2001) Treatment with a copper-zinc chelator markedly and rapidly inhibits beta-amyloid accumulation in Alzheimer's disease transgenic mice. Neuron 30:665-676.

Chui DH, Tanahashi H, Ozawa K, Ikeda S, Checler F, Ueda O, Suzuki H, Araki W, Inoue H, Shirotani K, Takahashi K, Gallyas F, Tabira T (1999) Transgenic mice with Alzheimer presenilin 1 mutations show accelerated neurodegeneration without amyloid plaque formation. Nat Med 5:560-564.

Chung HM, Struhl G (2001) Nicastrin is required for Presenilin-mediated transmembrane cleavage in Drosophila. Nat Cell Biol 3:1129-1132.

Chyung AS, Greenberg BD, Cook DG, Doms RW, Lee VM (1997) Novel beta-secretase cleavage of beta-amyloid precursor protein in the endoplasmic reticulum/intermediate compartment of NT2N cells. J Cell Biol 138:671-680.

Colle MA, Duyckaerts C, Laquerriere A, Pradier L, Czech C, Checler F, Hauw JJ (2000) Laminar specific loss of isocortical presenilin 1 immunoreactivity in Alzheimer's disease. Correlations with the amyloid load and the density of tau-positive neurofibrillary tangles. Neuropathol Appl Neurobiol 26:117-123.

Colurso GJ, Nilson JE, Vervoort LG (2003) Quantitative assessment of DNA fragmentation and beta-amyloid deposition in insular cortex and midfrontal gyrus from patients with Alzheimer's disease. Life Sci 73:1795-1803.

Cook DG, Sung JC, Golde TE, Felsenstein KM, Wojczyk BS, Tanzi RE, Trojanowski JQ, Lee VM, Doms RW (1996) Expression and analysis of presenilin 1 in a human neuronal system: localization in cell bodies and dendrites. Proc Natl Acad Sci U S A 93:9223-9228.

Cork LC, Powers RE, Selkoe DJ, Davies P, Geyer JJ, Price DL (1988) Neurofibrillary tangles and senile plaques in aged bears. J Neuropathol Exp Neurol 47:629-641.

Cotman CW, Su JH (1996) Mechanism of neuronal death in Alzheimer's disease. Brain Pathol 6:493-506.

Cui J, Chen Q, Yue X, Jiang X, Gao GF, Yu LC, Zhang Y (2010) Galanin protects against intracellular amyloid toxicity in human primary neurons. J Alzheimers Dis 19:529-544.

Culvenor JG, Maher F, Evin G, Malchiodi-Albedi F, Cappai R, Underwood JR, Davis JB, Karran EH, Roberts GW, Beyreuther K, Masters CL (1997) Alzheimer's disease-associated presenilin 1 in neuronal cells: evidence for localization to the endoplasmic reticulum-Golgi intermediate compartment. J Neurosci Res 49:719-731.

Culvenor JG, Evin G, Cooney MA, Wardan H, Sharples RA, Maher F, Reed G, Diehlmann A, Weidemann A, Beyreuther K, Masters CL (2000) Presenilin 2 expression in neuronal cells: induction during differentiation of embryonic carcinoma cells. Exp Cell Res 255:192-206.

Cummings BJ, Satou T, Head E, Milgram NW, Cole GM, Savage MJ, Podlisny MB, Selkoe DJ, Siman R, Greenberg BD, Cotman CW (1996) Diffuse plaques contain C-terminal A beta 42 and not A beta 40: evidence from cats and dogs. Neurobiol Aging 17:653-659.

Czech C, Tremp G, Pradier L (2000) Presenilins and Alzheimer's disease: biological functions and pathogenic mechanisms. Prog Neurobiol 60:363-384.

D'Andrea MR, Nagele RG, Wang HY, Peterson PA, Lee DH (2001) Evidence that neurones accumulating amyloid can undergo lysis to form amyloid plaques in Alzheimer's disease. Histopathology 38:120-134.

D'Andrea MR, Nagele RG, Gumula NA, Reiser PA, Polkovitch DA, Hertzog BM, Andrade-Gordon P (2002) Lipofuscin and Abeta42 exhibit distinct distribution patterns in normal and Alzheimer's disease brains. Neurosci Lett 323:45-49.

Davies P, Maloney AJ (1976) Selective loss of central cholinergic neurons in Alzheimer's disease. Lancet 2:1403.

Davis JA, Naruse S, Chen H, Eckman C, Younkin S, Price DL, Borchelt DR, Sisodia SS, Wong PC (1998) An Alzheimer's disease-linked PS1 variant rescues the developmental abnormalities of PS1-deficient embryos. Neuron 20:603-609.

De Kosky ST, Scheff SW (1990) Synapse loss in frontal lobe biopsies in Alzheimer's disease: Correlation with cognitive severity. Ann Neurol 27:457-464.

De Strooper B, Annaert W (2000) Proteolytic processing and cell biological functions of the amyloid precursor protein. J Cell Sci 113:1857-1870.

De Strooper B, Konig G (2001) An inflammatory drug prospect. Nature 414:159-160.

De Strooper B, Beullens M, Contreras B, Levesque L, Craessaerts K, Cordell B, Moechars D, Bollen M, Fraser P, George-Hyslop PS, Van Leuven F (1997) Phosphorylation, subcellular localization, and membrane orientation of the Alzheimer's disease-associated presenilins. J Biol Chem 272:3590-3598.

De Strooper B, Annaert W, Cupers P, Saftig P, Craessaerts K, Mumm JS, Schroeter EH, Schrijvers V, Wolfe MS, Ray WJ, Goate A, Kopan R (1999) A presenilin-1-dependent gamma-secretase-like protease mediates release of Notch intracellular domain. Nature 398:518-522.

Deane R, Zlokovic BV (2007) Role of the blood-brain barrier in the pathogenesis of Alzheimer's disease. Curr Alzheimer Res 4:191-197.

Deane R, Sagare A, Zlokovic BV (2008) The role of the cell surface LRP and soluble LRP in blood-brain barrier Abeta clearance in Alzheimer's disease. Curr Pharm Des 14:1601-1605.

Deane R, Wu Z, Sagare A, Davis J, Du Yan S, Hamm K, Xu F, Parisi M, LaRue B, Hu HW, Spijkers P, Guo H, Song X, Lenting PJ, Van Nostrand WE, Zlokovic BV (2004) LRP/amyloid beta-peptide interaction mediates differential brain efflux of Abeta isoforms. Neuron 43:333-344.

Deane R et al. (2003) RAGE mediates amyloid-beta peptide transport across the blood-brain barrier and accumulation in brain. Nat Med 9:907-913.

Defigueiredo RJ, Cummings BJ, Mundkur PY, Cotman CW (1995) Color image analysis in neuroanatomical research: application to senile plaque subtype quantification in Alzheimer's disease. Neurobiol Aging 16:211-223.

DeMattos RB, Bales KR, Cummins DJ, Paul SM, Holtzman DM (2002a) Brain to plasma amyloid-beta efflux: a measure of brain amyloid burden in a mouse model of Alzheimer's disease. Science 295:2264-2267.

DeMattos RB, Bales KR, Cummins DJ, Dodart JC, Paul SM, Holtzman DM (2001) Peripheral anti-A beta antibody alters CNS and plasma A beta clearance and decreases brain A beta burden in a mouse model of Alzheimer's disease. Proc Natl Acad Sci U S A 98:8850-8855.

DeMattos RB, Bales KR, Parsadanian M, O'Dell MA, Foss EM, Paul SM, Holtzman DM (2002b) Plaque-associated disruption of CSF and plasma amyloid-beta (Abeta) equilibrium in a mouse model of Alzheimer's disease. J Neurochem 81:229-236.

Deng G, Pike CJ, Cotman CW (1996a) Alzheimer-associated presenilin-2 confers increased sensitivity to apoptosis in PC12 cells. FEBS Lett 397:50-54.

Deng G, Su JH, Cotman CW (1996b) Gene expression of Alzheimer-associated presenilin-2 in the frontal cortex of Alzheimer and aged control brain. FEBS Lett 394:17-20.

Dodart JC, Bales KR, Gannon KS, Greene SJ, DeMattos RB, Mathis C, DeLong CA, Wu S, Wu X, Holtzman DM, Paul SM (2002) Immunization reverses memory deficits without reducing brain Abeta burden in Alzheimer's disease model. Nat Neurosci 5:452-457.

Dodd PR (2002) Excited to death: different ways to lose your neurones. Biogerontology 3:51-56.

Duckworth WC, Bennett RG, Hamel FG (1998) Insulin degradation: progress and potential. Endocr Rev 19:608-624.

Eckman EA, Reed DK, Eckman CB (2001) Degradation of the Alzheimer's amyloid beta peptide by endothelin-converting enzyme. J Biol Chem 276:24540-24548.

Eikelenboom P, Bate C, Van Gool WA, Hoozemans JJ, Rozemuller JM, Veerhuis R, Williams A (2002) Neuroinflammation in Alzheimer's disease and prion disease. Glia 40:232-239.

Farris W, Mansourian S, Leissring MA, Eckman EA, Bertram L, Eckman CB, Tanzi RE, Selkoe DJ (2004) Partial loss-of-function mutations in insulin-degrading enzyme that induce diabetes also impair degradation of amyloid beta-protein. Am J Pathol 164:1425-1434.

Farris W, Mansourian S, Chang Y, Lindsley L, Eckman EA, Frosch MP, Eckman CB, Tanzi RE, Selkoe DJ, Guenette S (2003) Insulin-degrading enzyme regulates the levels of insulin, amyloid beta-protein, and the beta-amyloid precursor protein intracellular domain in vivo. Proc Natl Acad Sci U S A 100:4162-4167.

Francis PT, Webster MT, Chessell IP, Holmes C, Stratmann GC, Procter AW, Cross AJ, Green AR, Bowen DM (1993) Neurotransmitters and second messengers in aging and Alzheimer's disease. Ann N Y Acad Sci 695:19-26.

Friedlander R, Jarosch E, Urban J, Volkwein C, Sommer T (2000) A regulatory link between ER-associated protein degradation and the unfolded-protein response. Nat Cell Biol 2:379-384.

Garver TD, Harris KA, Lehman RA, Lee VM, Trojanowski JQ, Billingsley ML (1994) Tau phosphorylation in human, primate, and rat brain: evidence that a pool of tau is highly phosphorylated in vivo and is rapidly dephosphorylated in vitro. J Neurochem 63:2279-2287.

Gasic-Milenkovic J, Dukic-Stefanovic S, Deuther-Conrad W, Gartner U, Munch G (2003) beta-Amyloid peptide potentiates inflammatory responses induced by lipopolysaccharide, interferon -gamma and 'advanced glycation endproducts' in a murine microglia cell line. Eur J Neurosci 17:813-821.

Gearing M, Tigges J, Mori H, Mirra SS (1997) beta-Amyloid (A beta) deposition in the brains of aged orangutans. Neurobiol Aging 18:139-146.

Gearing M, Schneider JA, Robbins RS, Hollister RD, Mori H, Games D, Hyman BT, Mirra SS (1995) Regional variation in the distribution of apolipoprotein E and A beta in Alzheimer's disease. J Neuropathol Exp Neurol 54:833-841.

Geula C (1998) Abnormalities of neural circuitry in Alzheimer's disease: hippocampus and cortical cholinergic innervation. Neurology 51:S18-29; discussion S65-17.

Ghribi O, Herman MM, Savory J (2003) Lithium inhibits Abeta-induced stress in endoplasmic reticulum of rabbit hippocampus but does not prevent oxidative damage and tau phosphorylation. J Neurosci Res 71:853-862.

Glenner GG, Wong CW (1984) Alzheimer's disease: initial report of the purification and characterization of a novel cerebrovascular amyloid protein. biochem Biophys Res Comm 120:885-890.

Goate A, Chartier-Harlin MC, Mullan M, Brown J, Crawford F, Fidani L, Giuffra L, Haynes A, Irving N, James L, et al. (1991) Segregation of a missense mutation in the amyloid precursor protein gene with familial Alzheimer's disease. Nature 349:704-706.

Goedert M, Jakes R, Spillantini MG, Hasegawa M, Smith MJ, Crowther RA (1996) Assembly of microtubule-associated protein tau into Alzheimer-like filaments induced by sulphated glycosaminoglycans. Nature 383:550-553.

Gold M (2002) Tau therapeutics for Alzheimer's disease: the promise and the challenges. J Mol Neurosci 19:331-334.

Golde TE, Estus S, Younkin LH, Selkoe DJ, Younkin SG (1992) Processing of the amyloid protein precursor to potentially amyloidogenic derivatives. Science 255:728-730.

Gomez-Isla T, Price JL, McKeel DW, Jr., Morris JC, Growdon JH, Hyman BT (1996) Profound loss of layer II entorhinal cortex neurons occurs in very mild Alzheimer's disease. J Neurosci 16:4491-4500.

Gomez-Isla T, Growdon WB, McNamara M, Newell K, Gomez-Tortosa E, Hedley-Whyte ET, Hyman BT (1999) Clinicopathologic correlates in temporal cortex in dementia with Lewy bodies. Neurology 53:2003-2009.

Gomez-Isla T, Hollister R, West H, Mui S, Growdon JH, Petersen RC, Parisi JE, Hyman BT (1997) Neuronal loss correlates with but exceeds neurofibrillary tangles in Alzheimer's disease. Ann Neurol 41:17-24.

Gouras GK, Tsai J, Naslund J, Vincent B, Edgar M, Checler F, Greenfield JP, Haroutunian V, Buxbaum JD, Xu H, Greengard P, Relkin NR (2000) Intraneuronal Abeta42 accumulation in human brain. Am J Pathol 156:15-20.

Grace EA, Busciglio J (2003) Aberrant activation of focal adhesion proteins mediates fibrillar amyloid beta-induced neuronal dystrophy. J Neurosci 23:493-502.

Grace EA, Rabiner CA, Busciglio J (2002) Characterization of neuronal dystrophy induced by fibrillar amyloid beta: implications for Alzheimer's disease. Neuroscience 114:265-273.

Greenfield JP, Tsai J, Gouras GK, Hai B, Thinakaran G, Checler F, Sisodia SS, Greengard P, Xu H (1999) Endoplasmic reticulum and trans-Golgi network generate distinct populations of Alzheimer beta-amyloid peptides. Proc Natl Acad Sci U S A 96:742-747.

Gschwind M, Huber G (1995) Apoptotic cell death induced by beta-amyloid 1-42 peptide is cell type dependent. J Neurochem 65:292-300.

Haass C, Selkoe DJ (2007) Soluble protein oligomers in neurodegeneration: lessons from the Alzheimer's amyloid beta-peptide. Nat Rev Mol Cell Biol 8:101-112.

Haass C, Hung AY, Selkoe DJ, Teplow DB (1994) Mutations associated with a locus for familial Alzheimer's disease result in alternative processing of amyloid beta-protein precursor. J Biol Chem 269:17741-17748.

Haass C, Koo EH, Mellon A, Hung AY, Selkoe DJ (1992a) Targeting of cell-surface beta-amyloid precursor protein to lysosomes: alternative processing into amyloid-bearing fragments. Nature 357:500-503.

Haass C, Schlossmacher MG, Hung AY, Vigo-Pelfrey C, Mellon A, Ostaszewski BL, Lieberburg I, Koo EH, Schenk D, Teplow DB, et al. (1992b) Amyloid beta-peptide is produced by cultured cells during normal metabolism. Nature 359:322-325.

Hamos JE, DeGennaro LJ, Drachman DA (1989) Synaptic loss in Alzheimer's disease and other dementias. Neurology 39:355-361.

Hardy J (2003) The Relationship between Amyloid and Tau. J Mol Neurosci 20:203-206.

Hardy JA, Higgins GA (1992) Alzheimer's disease: the amyloid cascade hypothesis. Science 256:184-185.

Hartig W, Klein C, Brauer K, Schuppel KF, Arendt T, Bruckner G, Bigl V (2000) Abnormally phosphorylated protein tau in the cortex of aged individuals of various mammalian orders. Acta Neuropathol (Berl) 100:305-312.

Hartman RE, Izumi Y, Bales KR, Paul SM, Wozniak DF, Holtzman DM (2005) Treatment with an amyloid-beta antibody ameliorates plaque load, learning deficits, and hippocampal long-term potentiation in a mouse model of Alzheimer's disease. J Neurosci 25:6213-6220.

Hartmann H, Busciglio J, Baumann KH, Staufenbiel M, Yankner BA (1997) Developmental regulation of presenilin-1 processing in the brain suggests a role in neuronal differentiation. J Biol Chem 272:14505-14508.

Hashimoto Y, Niikura T, Chiba T, Tsukamoto E, Kadowaki H, Nishitoh H, Yamagishi Y, Ishizaka M, Yamada M, Nawa M, Terashita K, Aiso S, Ichijo H, Nishimoto I (2003) The Cytoplasmic Domain of Alzheimer's Amyloid-{beta} Protein Precursor Causes Sustained Apoptosis Signal-Regulating Kinase 1/c-Jun NH2-Terminal Kinase-Mediated Neurotoxic Signal via Dimerization. J Pharmacol Exp Ther 306:889-902.

Henkin J, Marcotte P, Yang HC (1991) The plasminogen-plasmin system. Prog Cardiovasc Dis 34:135-164.

Ho R, Ortiz D, Shea TB (2001) Amyloid-beta promotes calcium influx and neurodegeneration via stimulation of L voltage-sensitive calcium channels rather than NMDA channels in cultured neurons. J Alzheimers Dis 3:479-483.

Hoffman KB, Bi X, Pham JT, Lynch G (1998) Beta-amyloid increases cathepsin D levels in hippocampus. Neurosci Lett 250:75-78.

Hohmann GF, Wenk GL, Lowenstein P, Brown ME, Coyle JT (1987) Age-related recurrence of basal forebrain lesion-induced cholinergic deficits. Neurosci Lett 82:253-259.

Hong CS, Koo EH (1997) Isolation and characterization of Drosophila presenilin homolog. Neuroreport 8:665-668.

Hou JF, Cui J, Yu LC, Zhang Y (2009) Intracellular amyloid induces impairments on electrophysiological properties of cultured human neurons. Neurosci Lett 462:294-299.

Howell S, Nalbantoglu J, Crine P (1995) Neutral endopeptidase can hydrolyze beta-amyloid(1-40) but shows no effect on beta-amyloid precursor protein metabolism. Peptides 16:647-652.

Howlett DR, Perry AE, Godfrey F, Swatton JE, Jennings KH, Spitzfaden C, Wadsworth H, Wood SJ, Markwell RE (1999) Inhibition of fibril formation in beta-amyloid peptide by a novel series of benzofurans. Biochem J 340 (Pt 1):283-289.

Hoyer S (1994) Neurodegeneration, Alzheimer's disease, and beta-amyloid toxicity. Life Sci 55:1977-1983.

Hsia AY, Masliah E, McConlogue L, Yu GQ, Tatsuno G, Hu K, Kholodenko D, Malenka RC, Nicoll RA, Mucke L (1999) Plaque-independent disruption of neural circuits in Alzheimer's disease mouse models. Proc Natl Acad Sci U S A 96:3228-3233.

Hu J, Igarashi A, Kamata M, Nakagawa H (2001) Angiotensin-converting enzyme degrades Alzheimer amyloid beta-peptide (A beta); retards A beta aggregation, deposition, fibril formation; and inhibits cytotoxicity. J Biol Chem 276:47863-47868.

Hu Y, Ye Y, Fortini ME (2002) Nicastrin is required for gamma-secretase cleavage of the Drosophila Notch receptor. Dev Cell 2:69-78.

Hutton M et al. (1996) Complete analysis of the presenilin 1 gene in early onset Alzheimer's disease. Neuroreport 7:801-805.

Hutton M et al. (1998) Association of missense and 5'-splice-site mutations in tau with the inherited dementia FTDP-17. Nature 393:702-705.

Huynh DP, Vinters HV, Ho DH, Ho VV, Pulst SM (1997) Neuronal expression and intracellular localization of presenilins in normal and Alzheimer disease brains. J Neuropathol Exp Neurol 56:1009-1017.

Ii K, Ito H, Kominami E, Hirano A (1993) Abnormal distribution of cathepsin proteinases and endogenous inhibitors (cystatins) in the hippocampus of patients with Alzheimer's disease, parkinsonism-dementia complex on Guam, and senile dementia and in the aged. Virchows Arch A Pathol Anat Histopathol 423:185-194.

in t' Veld BA, Ruitenberg A, Hofman A, Launer LJ, van Duijn CM, Stijnen T, Breteler MM, Stricker BH (2001) Nonsteroidal antiinflammatory drugs and the risk of Alzheimer's disease. N Engl J Med 345:1515-1521.

Iwata N, Tsubuki S, Takaki Y, Shirotani K, Lu B, Gerard NP, Gerard C, Hama E, Lee HJ, Saido TC (2001) Metabolic regulation of brain Abeta by neprilysin. Science 292:1550-1552.

Iwata N, Tsubuki S, Takaki Y, Watanabe K, Sekiguchi M, Hosoki E, Kawashima-Morishima M, Lee HJ, Hama E, Sekine-Aizawa Y, Saido TC (2000) Identification of the major Abeta1-42-degrading catabolic pathway in brain parenchyma: suppression leads to biochemical and pathological deposition. Nat Med 6:143-150.

Janus C, Pearson J, McLaurin J, Mathews PM, Jiang Y, Schmidt SD, Chishti MA, Horne P, Heslin D, French J, Mount HT, Nixon RA, Mercken M, Bergeron C, Fraser PE, St George-Hyslop P, Westaway D (2000) A beta peptide immunization reduces behavioural impairment and plaques in a model of Alzheimer's disease. Nature 408:979-982.

Jellinger K (2002a) Prevalence of Alzheimer's disease in very elderly people: a prospective neuropathological study. Neurology 58:671-672; author reply 671-672.

Jellinger KA (2002b) Vascular-ischemic dementia: an update. J Neural Transm Suppl:1-23.

Jellinger KA (2002c) Alzheimer disease and cerebrovascular pathology: an update. J Neural Transm 109:813-836.

Jellinger KA, Attems J (2003) Incidence of cerebrovascular lesions in Alzheimer's disease: a postmortem study. Acta Neuropathol (Berl) 105:14-17.

Jucker M, Walker LC, Kuo H, Tian M, Ingram DK (1994) Age-related fibrillar deposits in brains of C57BL/6 mice. A review of localization, staining characteristics, and strain specificity. Mol Neurobiol 9:125-133.

Kang J, Muller-Hill B (1990) Differential splicing of Alzheimer's disease amyloid A4 precursor RNA in rat tissue: PreA4695 mRNA is predominantly produced in rat and human brain. BBRC 166:1192-1200.

Kang J, Lemaire HG, Unterbeck A, Salbaum JM, Masters CL, Grzeschik KH, Multhaup G, Beyreuther K, Muller-Hill B (1987) The precursor of Alzheimer's disease amyloid A4 protein resembles a cell-surface receptor. Nature 325:733-736.

Kitaguchi N, Takahashi Y, Tokushima Y, Shiojiri S, Ito H (1988) Novel precursor of Alzheimer's disease amyloid protein shows protease inhibitory activity. Nature 331:530-532.

Klunk WE, Debnath ML, Koros AM, Pettegrew JW (1998) Chrysamine-G, a lipophilic analogue of Congo red, inhibits A beta-induced toxicity in PC12 cells. Life Sci 63:1807-1814.

Koo EH, Sisodia SS, Archer DR, Martin LJ, Weidemann A, Beyreuther K, Fischer P, Masters CL, Price DL (1990) Precursor of amyloid protein in Alzheimer disease undergoes fast anterograde axonal transport. Proc Natl Acad USA 87:1561-1565.

Kopan R, Goate A (2002) Aph-2/Nicastrin: an essential component of gamma-secretase and regulator of Notch signaling and Presenilin localization. Neuron 33:321-324.

Kowall NW, Beal MF, Busciglio J, Duffy LK, Yankner BA (1991) An in vivo model for the neurodegenerative effects of beta amyloid and protection by substance P. Proc Natl Acad Sci U S A 88:7247-7251.

Kuentzel SL, Ali SM, Altman RA, Greenberg BD, Raub TJ (1993) The Alzheimer beta-amyloid protein precursor/protease nexin-II is cleaved by secretase in a trans-Golgi secretory compartment in human neuroglioma cells. Biochem J 295:367-378.

Kurochkin IV (2001) Insulin degrading enzyme: embarking on amyloid destruction. Trends Biochem Sci 26:421-425.

Kurochkin IV, Goto S (1994) Alzheimer's beta-amyloid peptide specifically interacts with and is degraded by insulin degrading enzyme. FEBS Lett 345:33-37.

LaFerla FM, Tinkle BT, Bieberich CJ, Haudenschild CC, Jay G (1995) The Alzheimer's A beta peptide induces neurodegeneration and apoptotic cell death in transgenic mice. Nat Genet 9:21-30.

Lah JJ, Heilman CJ, Nash NR, Rees HD, Yi H, Counts SE, Levey AI (1997) Light and electron microscopic localization of presenilin-1 in primate brain. J Neurosci 17:1971-1980.

Lai A, Sisodia SS, Trowbridge IS (1995) Characterization of sorting signals in the beta-amyloid precursor protein cytoplasmic domain. J Biol Chem 270:3565-3573.

Lam FC, Liu R, Lu P, Shapiro AB, Renoir JM, Sharom FJ, Reiner PB (2001) beta-Amyloid efflux mediated by p-glycoprotein. J Neurochem 76:1121-1128.

Lammich S, Kojro E, Postina R, Gilbert S, Pfeiffer R, Jasionowski M, Haass C, Fahrenholz F (1999) Constitutive and regulated alpha-secretase cleavage of Alzheimer's amyloid precursor protein by a disintegrin metalloprotease. Proc Natl Acad Sci U S A 96:3922-3927.

Larson J, Lynch G, Games D, Seubert P (1999) Alterations in synaptic transmission and long-term potentiation in hippocampal slices from young and aged PDAPP mice. Brain Res 840:23-35.

Lassmann H, Bancher C, Breitschopf H, Wegiel J, Bobinski M (1995) Cell death in Alzheimer's disease evaluated by DNA fragmentation in situ. Acta Neuropathol 89:35-41.

LeBlanc A, Liu H, Goodyer C, Bergeron C, Hammond J (1999) Caspase-6 role in apoptosis of human neurons, amyloidogenesis, and Alzheimer's disease. J Biol Chem 274:23426-23436.

LeBlanc AC, Chen HY, Autilio-Gambetti L, Gambetti P (1991) Differential APP gene expression in rat cerebral cortex, meninges, and primary astroglial, microglial and neuronal cultures. FEBS Lett 292:171-178.

Ledesma MD, Da Silva JS, Crassaerts K, Delacourte A, De Strooper B, Dotti CG (2000) Brain plasmin enhances APP alpha-cleavage and Abeta degradation and is reduced in Alzheimer's disease brains. EMBO Rep 1:530-535.

Ledesma MD, Abad-Rodriguez J, Galvan C, Biondi E, Navarro P, Delacourte A, Dingwall C, Dotti CG (2003) Raft disorganization leads to reduced plasmin activity in Alzheimer's disease brains. EMBO Rep 4:1190-1196.

Lee SJ, Liyanage U, Bickel PE, Xia W, Lansbury PT, Jr., Kosik KS (1998) A detergent-insoluble membrane compartment contains A beta in vivo. Nat Med 4:730-734.

Lee VMY, Balin BJ, Otvos LJ, Trojanowski JQ (1991) A68: a major subunit of paired helical filaments and derivatized forms of normal tau. Science 251:675-678.

Lemere CA, Maron R, Selkoe DJ, Weiner HL (2001) Nasal vaccination with beta-amyloid peptide for the treatment of Alzheimer's disease. DNA Cell Biol 20:705-711.

Lemere CA, Beierschmitt A, Iglesias M, Spooner ET, Bloom JK, Leverone JF, Zheng JB, Seabrook TJ, Louard D, Li D, Selkoe DJ, Palmour RM, Ervin FR (2004) Alzheimer's disease abeta vaccine reduces central nervous system abeta levels in a non-human primate, the Caribbean vervet. Am J Pathol 165:283-297.

Lemere CA, Lopera F, Kosik KS, Lendon CL, Ossa J, Saido TC, Yamaguchi H, Ruiz A, Martinez A, Madrigal L, Hincapie L, Arango JC, Anthony DC, Koo EH, Goate AM, Selkoe DJ (1996) The E280A presenilin 1 Alzheimer mutation produces increased A beta 42 deposition and severe cerebellar pathology. Nat Med 2:1146-1150.

Lesne S, Koh MT, Kotilinek L, Kayed R, Glabe CG, Yang A, Gallagher M, Ashe KH (2006) A specific amyloid-beta protein assembly in the brain impairs memory. Nature 440:352-357.

Levy E, Carman MD, Fernandez-Madrid IJ, Power MD, Lieberburg I, van Duinen SG, Bots GT, Luyendijk W, Frangione B (1990) Mutation of the Alzheimer's disease amyloid gene in hereditary cerebral hemorrhage, Dutch type. Science 248:1124-1126.

Lewis J, Dickson DW, Lin WL, Chisholm L, Corral A, Jones G, Yen SH, Sahara N, Skipper L, Yager D, Eckman C, Hardy J, Hutton M, McGowan E (2001) Enhanced neurofibrillary degeneration in transgenic mice expressing mutant tau and APP. Science 293:1487-1491.

Li M, Chen L, Lee DH, Yu LC, Zhang Y (2007) The role of intracellular amyloid beta in Alzheimer's disease. Prog Neurobiol 83:131-139.

Li WP, Chan WY, Lai HW, Yew DT (1997) Terminal dUTP nick end labeling (TUNEL) positive cells in the different regions of the brain in normal aging and Alzheimer patients. J Mol Neurosci 8:75-82.

Li YP, Bushnell AF, Lee CM, Perlmutter LS, Wong SK (1996) Beta-amyloid induces apoptosis in human-derived neurotypic SH-SY5Y cells. Brain Res 738:196-204.

Lippa CF, Hamos JE, Pulaski-Salo D, DeGennaro LJ, Drachman DA (1992) Alzheimer's disease and aging: effects on perforant pathway perikarya and synapses. Neurobiol Aging 13:405-411.

Loo DT, Copani A, Pike CJ, Whitemore ER, Walencewica Aj, Cotman CW (1993) Apoptosis is induced by beta-amyloid in cultured central nervous system neurons. Proc Natl Acad Sci USA 90:7951-7955.

Lorenzo A, Yankner BA (1994a) Beta-amyloid neurotoxicity requires fibril formation and is inhibited by congo red. Proc Natl Acad Sci U S A 91:12243-12247.

Lorenzo A, Yankner BA (1994b) Beta-amyloid neurotoxicity requires fibril formation and is inhibited by congo red. Proc Natl Acad Sci U S A 91:12243-12247.

Lorenzo A, Yankner BA (1996) Amyloid fibril toxicity in Alzheimer's disease and diabetes. Ann N Y Acad Sci 777:89-95.

Lott IT, Head E (2001) Down syndrome and Alzheimer's disease: a link between development and aging. Ment Retard Dev Disabil Res Rev 7:172-178.

Madani R, Nef S, Vassalli JD (2003) Emotions are building up in the field of extracellular proteolysis. Trends Mol Med 9:183-185.

Malchiodi-Albedi F, Paradisi S, Matteucci A, Frank C, Diociaiuti M (2011) Amyloid oligomer neurotoxicity, calcium dysregulation, and lipid rafts. Int J Alzheimers Dis 2011:906964.

Mann DM, Brown A, Wilks DP, Davies CA (1989) Immunocytochemical and lectin histochemical studies of plaques and tangles in Down's syndrome patients at different ages. Prog Clin Biol Res 317:849-856.

Mann DMA, Yates PO, Marcynuik B (1985) Some morphometric observations on the cerebral cortex and hippocampus in presenile Alzheimer's disease, senile dementia of Alzheimer's type and Down's syndrome in middle age. J Neurol Sci 69:139-159.

Marques MA, Kulstad JJ, Savard CE, Green PS, Lee SP, Craft S, Watson GS, Cook DG (2009) Peripheral amyloid-beta levels regulate amyloid-beta clearance from the central nervous system. J Alzheimers Dis 16:325-329.

Martin BL, Schrader-Fischer G, Busciglio J, Duke M, Paganetti P, Yankner BA (1995) Intracellular accumulation of beta-amyloid in cells expressing the Swedish mutant amyloid precursor protein. J Biol Chem 270:26727-26730.

Masliah E (2001) Recent advances in the understanding of the role of synaptic proteins in Alzheimer's Disease and other neurodegenerative disorders. J Alzheimers Dis 3:121-129.

Masliah E, Terry RD, DeTeresa RM, Hansen LA (1989) Immunohistochemical quantification of the synapse-related protein synaptophysin in Alzheimer disease. Neurosci Lett 103:234-239.

Masliah E, Sisk A, Mallory M, Mucke L, Schenk D, Games D (1996) Comparison of neurodegenerative pathology in transgenic mice overexpressing V717F beta-amyloid precursor protein and Alzheimer's disease. J Neurosci 16:5795-5811.

Masliah E, Rockenstein E, Veinbergs I, Sagara Y, Mallory M, Hashimoto M, Mucke L (2001a) beta-amyloid peptides enhance alpha-synuclein accumulation and neuronal deficits in a transgenic mouse model linking Alzheimer's disease and Parkinson's disease. Proc Natl Acad Sci U S A 98:12245-12250.

Masliah E, Mallory M, Alford M, DeTeresa R, Hansen LA, McKeel DW, Jr., Morris JC (2001b) Altered expression of synaptic proteins occurs early during progression of Alzheimer's disease. Neurology 56:127-129.

Masters CL, Simms G, Weinman NA, Multhaup G, McDonald BL, Beyreuther K (1985) Amyloid plaque core protein in Alzheimer disease and Down syndrome. Proc Natl Acad Sci USA 82:4245-4249.

Matsuoka Y, Saito M, LaFrancois J, Gaynor K, Olm V, Wang L, Casey E, Lu Y, Shiratori C, Lemere C, Duff K (2003) Novel therapeutic approach for the treatment of Alzheimer's disease by peripheral administration of agents with an affinity to beta-amyloid. J Neurosci 23:29-33.

Mattson MP, Cheng B, Davis D, Bryant K, Lieberburg I, Rydel RE (1992) beta-Amyloid peptides destabilize calcium homeostasis and render human cortical neurons vulnerable to excitotoxicity. J Neurosci 12:376-389.

Mattson MP, Barger SW, Cheng B, Lieberburg I, Smith-Swintosky VL, Rydel RE (1993a) beta-Amyloid precursor protein metabolites and loss of neuronal Ca2+ homeostasis in Alzheimer's disease. Trends Neurosci 16:409-414.

Mattson MP, Cheng B, Culwell AR, Esch FS, Lieberburg I, Rydel RE (1993b) Evidence for excitoprotective and intraneuronal calcium-regulating roles for secreted forms of the beta-amyloid precursor protein. Neuron 10:243-254.

McDermott JR, Gibson AM (1997) Degradation of Alzheimer's beta-amyloid protein by human and rat brain peptidases: involvement of insulin-degrading enzyme. Neurochem Res 22:49-56.

McGeer EG, McGeer PL (1999) Brain inflammation in Alzheimer disease and the therapeutic implications. Curr Pharm Des 5:821-836.

McGeer PL (2000) Cyclo-oxygenase-2 inhibitors: rationale and therapeutic potential for Alzheimer's disease. Drugs Aging 17:1-11.

McGeer PL, Kawamata T, McGeer EG (1998) Localization and possible functions of presenilins in brain. Rev Neurosci 9:1-15.

McKhann G, Drachman D, Folstein M, Katzman R, Price DL, Stadlan EM (1984) Clinical diagnosis of Alzheimer's disease: report of the NINCDS-ADRDA Work Group under the auspices of Department of Health and Human Services Task Force on Alzheimer's disease. Neurology 34:939-944.

Merker K, Stolzing A, Grune T (2001) Proteolysis, caloric restriction and aging. Mech Ageing Dev 122:595-615.

Mesulam MM (1986) Alzheimer plaques and cortical cholinergic innervation. Neuroscience 17:275-276.

Mesulam MM, Geula C (1988) Acetychollinesterase-rich pyramidal neurons in the human neocortex and hippocampus: absence at birth, development during the life span, and dissolution in Alzheimer's disease. Ann Neurol 24:765-773.

Michaelis ML, Dobrowsky RT, Li G (2002) Tau neurofibrillary pathology and microtubule stability. J Mol Neurosci 19:289-293.

Mirsky IA, Kaplan S, Broh-Kahn RH (1949) Persinogen excretion (uropepsin as an index of the influence of various life situations on gastric secretion. Res Publ Assoc Res Nerv Ment Dis 29:628-646.

Monsonego A, Imitola J, Zota V, Oida T, Weiner HL (2003) Microglia-Mediated Nitric Oxide Cytotoxicity of T Cells Following Amyloid beta-Peptide Presentation to Th1 Cells. J Immunol 171:2216-2224.

Morgan D, Diamond DM, Gottschall PE, Ugen KE, Dickey C, Hardy J, Duff K, Jantzen P, DiCarlo G, Wilcock D, Connor K, Hatcher J, Hope C, Gordon M, Arendash GW (2000) A beta peptide vaccination prevents memory loss in an animal model of Alzheimer's disease. Nature 408:982-985.

Mori H, Takio k, Ogawara M, Selkie D (1992) Mass spectrometry of purified amyloid b protein in Alzheimer's disease. J Biol Chem 267:17082-17086.

Morris JC, McKeel DWJ, Storandt M, Rubin EH, Price JL, Grant EA, Ball MJ, Berg L (1991) Very mild Alzheimer's disease: informant-based clinical, psychometric, and pathologic distinction from normal aging. Neurology 41:469-478.

Nagele RG, D'Andrea MR, Anderson WJ, Wang HY (2002) Intracellular accumulation of beta-amyloid (1-42) in neurons is facilitated by the alpha7 nicotinic acetylcholine receptor in Alzheimer's disease. Neuroscience 110:199-211.

Narain Y, Yip A, Murphy T, Brayne C, Easton D, Evans JG, Xuereb J, Cairns N, Esiri MM, Furlong RA, Rubinsztein DC (2000) The ACE gene and Alzheimer's disease susceptibility. J Med Genet 37:695-697.

Ng DT, Spear ED, Walter P (2000) The unfolded protein response regulates multiple aspects of secretory and membrane protein biogenesis and endoplasmic reticulum quality control. J Cell Biol 150:77-88.
Nicolau C, Greferath R, Balaban TS, Lazarte JE, Hopkins RJ (2002) A liposome-based therapeutic vaccine against beta -amyloid plaques on the pancreas of transgenic NORBA mice. Proc Natl Acad Sci U S A 99:2332-2337.
Nilsberth C, Westlind-Danielsson A, Eckman CB, Condron MM, Axelman K, Forsell C, Stenh C, Luthman J, Teplow DB, Younkin SG, Naslund J, Lannfelt L (2001) The 'Arctic' APP mutation (E693G) causes Alzheimer's disease by enhanced Abeta protofibril formation. Nat Neurosci 4:887-893.
Okamoto I, Kawano Y, Murakami D, Sasayama T, Araki N, Miki T, Wong AJ, Saya H (2001) Proteolytic release of CD44 intracellular domain and its role in the CD44 signaling pathway. J Cell Biol 155:755-762.
Papassotiropoulos A, Bagli M, Feder O, Jessen F, Maier W, Rao ML, Ludwig M, Schwab SG, Heun R (1999) Genetic polymorphism of cathepsin D is strongly associated with the risk for developing sporadic Alzheimer's disease. Neurosci Lett 262:171-174.
Paradis E, Douillard H, Koutroumanis M, Goodyer C, LeBlanc A (1996) Amyloid beta peptide of Alzheimer's disease downregulates Bcl-2 and upregulates bax expression in human neurons. J Neurosci 16:7533-7539.
Park JH, Strittmatter SM (2007) Nogo receptor interacts with brain APP and Abeta to reduce pathologic changes in Alzheimer's transgenic mice. Curr Alzheimer Res 4:568-570.
Pearson RC, Powell TP (1987) Anterograde vs. retrograde degeneration of the nucleus basalis medialis in Alzheimer's disease. J Neural Transm Suppl 24:139-146.
Perez A, Morelli L, Cresto JC, Castano EM (2000) Degradation of soluble amyloid beta-peptides 1-40, 1-42, and the Dutch variant 1-40Q by insulin degrading enzyme from Alzheimer disease and control brains. Neurochem Res 25:247-255.
Pike CJ, Walencewicz AJ, Glabe CG, Cotman CW (1991) In vitro aging of beta-amyloid protein causes peptide aggregation and neurotoxicity. Brain Res 563:311-314.
Podlisny MB, Lee G, Selkoe DJ (1987) Gene dosage of the amyloid beta precursor protein in Alzheimer's disease. Science 238:669-671.
Podlisny MB, Stephenson DT, Frosch MP, Tolan DR, Lieberburg I, Clemens JA, Selkoe DJ (1993) Microinjection of synthetic amyloid beta-protein in monkey cerebral cortex fails to produce acute neurotoxicity. Am J Pathol 142:17-24.
Podlisny MB, Walsh DM, Amarante P, Ostaszewski BL, Stimson ER, Maggio JE, Teplow DB, Selkoe DJ (1998) Oligomerization of endogenous and synthetic amyloid beta-protein at nanomolar levels in cell culture and stabilization of monomer by Congo red. Biochemistry 37:3602-3611.
Poduslo JF, Curran GL, Kumar A, Frangione B, Soto C (1999) Beta-sheet breaker peptide inhibitor of Alzheimer's amyloidogenesis with increased blood-brain barrier permeability and resistance to proteolytic degradation in plasma. J Neurobiol 39:371-382.
Pollack SJ, Sadler, II, Hawtin SR, Tailor VJ, Shearman MS (1995) Sulfonated dyes attenuate the toxic effects of beta-amyloid in a structure-specific fashion. Neurosci Lett 197:211-214.
Ponte P, Gonzalez-Dewhittt P, Schilling J, Miller J, Hsu D, Greenberg B, Davis K, Wallace W, Lieberburg I, Fuller F (1988) A new A4 amyloid mRNA contains a domain homologous to serine proteinase inhibitors. Nature 331:525-527.

Poorkaj P, Bird TD, Wijsman E, Nemens E, Garruto RM, Anderson L, Andreadis A, Wiederholt WC, Raskind M, Schellenberg GD (1998) Tau is a candidate gene for chromosome 17 frontotemporal dementia. Ann Neurol 43:815-825.

Price DL, Sisodia SS (1998) Mutant genes in familial Alzheimer's disease and transgenic models. Annu Reve Neurosci 21:479-505.

Price DL, Sisodia SS, Gandy SE (1995) Amyloid beta amyloidosis in Alzheimer's disease. Curr Opin Neurol 8:268-274.

Price JL, McKeel DW, Jr., Morris JC (2001) Synaptic loss and pathological change in older adults--aging versus disease? Neurobiol Aging 22:351-352.

Ray WJ, Yao M, Nowotny P, Mumm J, Zhang W, Wu JY, Kopan R, Goate AM (1999) Evidence for a physical interaction between presenilin and Notch. Proc Natl Acad Sci U S A 96:3263-3268.

Roder H (2003) Prospect of therapeutic approaches to tauopathies. J Mol Neurosci 20:195-202.

Rogaev EI, Sherrington R, Rogaeva EA, Levesque G, Ikeda M, Liang Y, Chi H, Lin C, Holman K, Tsuda T, et al. (1995) Familial Alzheimer's disease in kindreds with missense mutations in a gene on chromosome 1 related to the Alzheimer's disease type 3 gene. Nature 376:775-778.

Rogers J, Luber-Narod J, Styren SD, Civin WH (1988) Expression of immune system-associated antigens by cells of the human central nervous system: relationship to the pathology of Alzheimer's disease. Neurobiol Aging 9:339-349.

Roher A, Lowenson J, Clarke S, Woods S, Cotter R, Gowing E, Ball MJ (1993) beta-Amyloid-(1-42) is a major component of cerebrovascular amyloid deposits: implications for the pathology of Alzheimer's disease. Proc Natl Acad Sci USA 90:10836-10840.

Roher AE, Chaney MO, Kuo YM, Webster SD, Stine WB, Haverkamp LJ, Woods AS, Cotter RJ, Tuohy JM, Krafft GA, Bonnell BS, Emmerling MR (1996) Morphology and toxicity of Abeta-(1-42) dimer derived from neuritic and vascular amyloid deposits of Alzheimer's disease. J Biol Chem 271:20631-20635.

Roses AD (1996) The Alzheimer diseases. Curr Opin Neurobiol 6:644-650.

Sagare A, Deane R, Bell RD, Johnson B, Hamm K, Pendu R, Marky A, Lenting PJ, Wu Z, Zarcone T, Goate A, Mayo K, Perlmutter D, Coma M, Zhong Z, Zlokovic BV (2007) Clearance of amyloid-beta by circulating lipoprotein receptors. Nat Med 13:1029-1031.

Salminen A, Ojala J, Suuronen T, Kaarniranta K, Kauppinen A (2008) Amyloid-beta oligomers set fire to inflammasomes and induce Alzheimer's pathology. J Cell Mol Med 12:2255-2262.

Salomon AR, Marcinowski KJ, Friedland RP, Zagorski MG (1996) Nicotine inhibits amyloid formation by the beta-peptide. Biochemistry 35:13568-13578.

Samuel W, Masliah E, Hill LR, Butters N, Terry R (1994) Hippocampal connectivity and Alzheimer's dementia: effects of synapse loss and tangle frequency in a two-component model. Neurology 44:2081-2088.

Sato M, Ikeda K, Haga S, Allsop D, Ishii T (1991) A monoclonal antibody to common acute lymphoblastic leukemia antigen (neutral endopeptidase) immunostains senile plaques in the brains of patients with Alzheimer's disease. Neurosci Lett 121:271-273.

Satoh J, Kuroda Y (2001) Nicastrin, a key regulator of presenilin function, is expressed constitutively in human neural cell lines. Neuropathology 21:115-122.

Scheff SW, Price DA (2001) Alzheimer's disease-related synapse loss in the cingulate cortex. J Alzheimers Dis 3:495-505.
Scheff SW, Price DA, Sparks DL (2001) Quantitative assessment of possible age-related change in synaptic numbers in the human frontal cortex. Neurobiol Aging 22:355-365.
Schenk D et al. (1999) Immunization with amyloid-beta attenuates Alzheimer-disease-like pathology in the PDAPP mouse. Nature 400:173-177.
Scheuner D et al. (1996) Secreted amyloid beta-protein similar to that in the senile plaques of Alzheimer's disease is increased in vivo by the presenilin 1 and 2 and APP mutations linked to familial Alzheimer's disease. Nat Med 2:864-870.
Schwartz JC, de la Baume S, Malfroy B, Patey G, Perdrisot R, Swerts JP, Fournie-Zaluski MC, Gacel G, Roques BP (1980) "Enkephalinase", a newly characterised dipeptidyl carboxypeptidase: properties and possible role in enkephalinergic transmission. Int J Neurol 14:195-204.
Selkoe DJ (2001) Clearing the brain's amyloid cobwebs. Neuron 32:177-180.
Selkoe DJ (2002) Alzheimer's disease is a synaptic failure. Science 298:789-791.
Selkoe DJ (2007) Developing preventive therapies for chronic diseases: lessons learned from Alzheimer's disease. Nutr Rev 65:S239-243.
Shankar GM, Leissring MA, Adame A, Sun X, Spooner E, Masliah E, Selkoe DJ, Lemere CA, Walsh DM (2009) Biochemical and immunohistochemical analysis of an Alzheimer's disease mouse model reveals the presence of multiple cerebral Abeta assembly forms throughout life. Neurobiol Dis 36:293-302.
Sherrington R et al. (1996) Alzheimer's disease associated with mutations in presenilin 2 is rare and variably penetrant. Hum Mol Genet 5:985-988.
Shibata M, Yamada S, Kumar SR, Calero M, Bading J, Frangione B, Holtzman DM, Miller CA, Strickland DK, Ghiso J, Zlokovic BV (2000) Clearance of Alzheimer's amyloid-ss(1-40) peptide from brain by LDL receptor-related protein-1 at the blood-brain barrier. J Clin Invest 106:1489-1499.
Siman R, Flood DG, Thinakaran G, Neumar RW (2001) Endoplasmic reticulum stress-induced cysteine protease activation in cortical neurons: effect of an Alzheimer's disease-linked presenilin-1 knock-in mutation. J Biol Chem 276:44736-44743.
Simons K, Gerl MJ (2010) Revitalizing membrane rafts: new tools and insights. Nat Rev Mol Cell Biol 11:688-699.
Sinha S, Lieberburg I (1999) Cellular mechanisms of beta-amyloid production and secretion. Proc Natl Acad Sci USA 96:11049-11053.
Sisodia SS, Koo EH, Hoffman PN, Perry G, Price DL (1993) Identification and transport of full-length amyloid precursor proteins in rat peripheral nervous system. J Neurosci 13:3136-3142.
Smale G, Nichols NR, Brady DR, Finch CE, Horton WEJ (1995) Evidence for apoptotic cell death in Alzheimer's disease. Exp Neurol 133:225-230.
Smith MJ, Kwok JB, McLean CA, Kril JJ, Broe GA, Nicholson GA, Cappai R, Hallupp M, Cotton RG, Masters CL, Schofield PR, Brooks WS (2001) Variable phenotype of Alzheimer's disease with spastic paraparesis. Ann Neurol 49:125-129.
Song ES, Juliano MA, Juliano L, Hersh LB (2003) Substrate activation of insulin-degrading enzyme (insulysin). A potential target for drug development. J Biol Chem 278:49789-49794.

Soto C, Kindy MS, Baumann M, Frangione B (1996) Inhibition of Alzheimer's amyloidosis by peptides that prevent beta-sheet conformation. Biochem Biophys Res Commun 226:672-680.

Soto C, Sigurdsson EM, Morelli L, Kumar RA, Castano EM, Frangione B (1998) Beta-sheet breaker peptides inhibit fibrillogenesis in a rat brain model of amyloidosis: implications for Alzheimer's therapy. Nat Med 4:822-826.

Spillantini MG, Goedert M (1998) Tau protein pathology in neurodegenerative diseases. Trends Neurosci 21:428-433.

Stephan A, Laroche S, Davis S (2001) Generation of aggregated beta-amyloid in the rat hippocampus impairs synaptic transmission and plasticity and causes memory deficits. J Neurosci 21:5703-5714.

Stern DM, Yan SD, Yan SF, Schmidt AM (2002) Receptor for advanced glycation endproducts (RAGE) and the complications of diabetes. Ageing Res Rev 1:1-15.

Strooper BD, Annaert W (2001) Presenilins and the intramembrane proteolysis of proteins: facts and fiction. Nat Cell Biol 3:E221-225.

Struble RG, Kitt CA, Walker LC, Cork LC, Price DL (1984) Somatostatinergic neurites in senile plaques of aged non-human primates. Brain Res 324:394-396.

Struble RG, Lehmann J, Mitchell SJ, McKinney M, Price DL, Coyle JT, DeLong MR (1986) Basal forebrain neurons provide major cholinergic innervation of primate neocortex. Neurosci Lett 66:215-220.

Su JH, Deng G, Cotman CW (1997) Bax protein expression is increased in Alzheimer's brain: correlations with DNA damage, Bcl-2 expression, and brain pathology. J Neuropathol Exp Neurol 56:86-93.

Sugarman MC, Yamasaki TR, Oddo S, Echegoyen JC, Murphy MP, Golde TE, Jannatipour M, Leissring MA, LaFerla FM (2002) Inclusion body myositis-like phenotype induced by transgenic overexpression of beta APP in skeletal muscle. Proc Natl Acad Sci U S A 99:6334-6339.

Tabira T, Chui DH, Kuroda S (2002) Significance of intracellular Abeta42 accumulation in Alzheimer's disease. Front Biosci 7:a44-49.

Takahashi RH, Milner TA, Li F, Nam EE, Edgar MA, Yamaguchi H, Beal MF, Xu H, Greengard P, Gouras GK (2002) Intraneuronal Alzheimer abeta42 accumulates in multivesicular bodies and is associated with synaptic pathology. Am J Pathol 161:1869-1879.

Takashima A, Sato M, Mercken M, Tanaka S, Kondo S, Honda T, Sato K, Murayama M, Noguchi K, Nakazato Y, Takahashi H (1996) Localization of Alzheimer-associated presenilin 1 in transfected COS-7 cells. Biochem Biophys Res Commun 227:423-426.

Tandon A, Fraser P (2002) The presenilins. Genome Biol 3:reviews3014.

Tang BL, Liou YC (2007) Novel modulators of amyloid-beta precursor protein processing. J Neurochem 100:314-323.

Tanimukai H, Sato K, Kudo T, Kashiwagi Y, Tohyama M, Takeda M (1999) Regional distribution of presenilin-1 messenger RNA in the embryonic rat brain: comparison with beta-amyloid precursor protein messenger RNA localization. Neuroscience 90:27-39.

Tanzi RE, Moir RD, Wagner SL (2004) Clearance of Alzheimer's Abeta peptide: The many roads to perdition. Neuron 43:605-608.

Tekirian TL, Cole GM, Russell MJ, Yang F, Wekstein DR, Patel E, Snowdon DA, Markesbery WR, Geddes JW (1996) Carboxy terminal of beta-amyloid deposits in aged human, canine, and polar bear brains. Neurobiol Aging 17:249-257.

Terry RD (2000) Cell death or synaptic loss in Alzheimer disease. J Neuropathol Exp Neurol 59:1118-1119.

Terry RD, Masliah E, Salmon DP (1991) Physical basis of cognitive alterations in Alzheimer's disease: Synaptic loss is a major correlate of cognitive impairment. Ann Neurol 30:572-580.

Tienari PJ, Ida N, Ikonen E, Simons M, Weidemann A, Multhaup G, Masters CL, Dotti CG, Beyreuther K (1997) Intracellular and secreted Alzheimer beta-amyloid species are generated by distinct mechanisms in cultured hippocampal neurons. Proc Natl Acad Sci U S A 94:4125-4130.

Tomiyama T, Shoji A, Kataoka K, Suwa Y, Asano S, Kaneko H, Endo N (1996) Inhibition of amyloid beta protein aggregation and neurotoxicity by rifampicin. Its possible function as a hydroxyl radical scavenger. J Biol Chem 271:6839-6844.

Townsend M, Cleary JP, Mehta T, Hofmeister J, Lesne S, O'Hare E, Walsh DM, Selkoe DJ (2006) Orally available compound prevents deficits in memory caused by the Alzheimer amyloid-beta oligomers. Ann Neurol 60:668-676.

Troncoso JC, Sukhov RR, Kawas CH, Koliatsos VE (1996) In situ labeling of dying cortical neurons in normal aging and in Alzheimer's disease: correlations with senile plaques and disease progression. J Nuropathol Exp Neurol 55:1134-1142.

Tseng BP, Esler WP, Clish CB, Stimson ER, Ghilardi JR, Vinters HV, Mantyh PW, Lee JP, Maggio JE (1999) Deposition of monomeric, not oligomeric, Abeta mediates growth of Alzheimer's disease amyloid plaques in human brain preparations. Biochemistry 38:10424-10431.

Tsuzuki K, Fukatsu R, Yamaguchi H, Tateno M, Imai K, Fujii N, Yamauchi T (2000) Transthyretin binds amyloid beta peptides, Abeta1-42 and Abeta1-40 to form complex in the autopsied human kidney - possible role of transthyretin for abeta sequestration. Neurosci Lett 281:171-174.

Turner AJ, Tanzawa K (1997) Mammalian membrane metallopeptidases: NEP, ECE, KELL, and PEX. FASEB J 11:355-364.

Turner AJ, Isaac RE, Coates D (2001) The neprilysin (NEP) family of zinc metalloendopeptidases: genomics and function. Bioessays 23:261-269.

Urbanc B, Cruz L, Buldyrev SV, Havlin S, Irizarry MC, Stanley HE, Hyman BT (1999) Dynamics of plaque formation in Alzheimer's disease. Biophys J 76:1330-1334.

Van Uden E, Mallory M, Veinbergs I, Alford M, Rockenstein E, Masliah E (2002) Increased extracellular amyloid deposition and neurodegeneration in human amyloid precursor protein transgenic mice deficient in receptor-associated protein. J Neurosci 22:9298-9304.

VanSlyke JK, Musil LS (2002) Dislocation and degradation from the ER are regulated by cytosolic stress. J Cell Biol 157:381-394.

Vasilevko V, Xu F, Previti ML, Van Nostrand WE, Cribbs DH (2007) Experimental investigation of antibody-mediated clearance mechanisms of amyloid-beta in CNS of Tg-SwDI transgenic mice. J Neurosci 27:13376-13383.

Vassar R, Citron M (2000) Abeta-generating enzymes: recent advances in beta- and gamma-secretase research. Neuron 27:419-422.

Vassar R et al. (1999) Beta-secretase cleavage of Alzheimer's amyloid precursor protein by the transmembrane aspartic protease BACE. Science 286:735-741.

Walsh DM, Selkoe DJ (2007) A beta oligomers - a decade of discovery. J Neurochem 101:1172-1184.

Walsh DM, Tseng BP, Rydel RE, Podlisny MB, Selkoe DJ (2000) The oligomerization of amyloid beta-protein begins intracellularly in cells derived from human brain. Biochemistry 39:10831-10839.

Walsh DM, Klyubin I, Fadeeva JV, Rowan MJ, Selkoe DJ (2002a) Amyloid-beta oligomers: their production, toxicity and therapeutic inhibition. Biochem Soc Trans 30:552-557.

Walsh DM, Klyubin I, Fadeeva JV, Cullen WK, Anwyl R, Wolfe MS, Rowan MJ, Selkoe DJ (2002b) Naturally secreted oligomers of amyloid beta protein potently inhibit hippocampal long-term potentiation in vivo. Nature 416:535-539.

Walsh DM, Townsend M, Podlisny MB, Shankar GM, Fadeeva JV, El Agnaf O, Hartley DM, Selkoe DJ (2005a) Certain inhibitors of synthetic amyloid beta-peptide (Abeta) fibrillogenesis block oligomerization of natural Abeta and thereby rescue long-term potentiation. J Neurosci 25:2455-2462.

Walsh DM, Klyubin I, Shankar GM, Townsend M, Fadeeva JV, Betts V, Podlisny MB, Cleary JP, Ashe KH, Rowan MJ, Selkoe DJ (2005b) The role of cell-derived oligomers of Abeta in Alzheimer's disease and avenues for therapeutic intervention. Biochem Soc Trans 33:1087-1090.

Wang HY, D'Andrea MR, Nagele RG (2002) Cerebellar diffuse amyloid plaques are derived from dendritic Abeta42 accumulations in Purkinje cells. Neurobiol Aging 23:213-223.

Wang SS, Rymer DL, Good TA (2001) Reduction in cholesterol and sialic acid content protects cells from the toxic effects of beta-amyloid peptides. J Biol Chem 276:42027-42034.

Waragai M, Imafuku I, Takeuchi S, Kanazawa I, Oyama F, Udagawa Y, Kawabata M, Okazawa H (1997) Presenilin 1 binds to amyloid precursor protein directly. Biochem Biophys Res Commun 239:480-482.

Wasco W, Bupp K, Magendantz M, Gusella JF, Tanzi RE, Solomon F (1992) Identification of a mouse brain cDNA that encodes a protein related to the Alzheimer disease-associated amyloid beta protein precursor. Proc Natl Acad Sci U S A 89:10758-10762.

Weggen S, Eriksen JL, Das P, Sagi SA, Wang R, Pietrzik CU, Findlay KA, Smith TE, Murphy MP, Bulter T, Kang DE, Marquez-Sterling N, Golde TE, Koo EH (2001) A subset of NSAIDs lower amyloidogenic Abeta42 independently of cyclooxygenase activity. Nature 414:212-216.

Weidemann A, Paliga K, Durrwang U, Czech C, Evin G, Masters CL, Beyreuther K (1997) Formation of stable complexes between two Alzheimer's disease gene products: presenilin-2 and beta-amyloid precursor protein. Nat Med 3:328-332.

Weiner HL, Lemere CA, Maron R, Spooner ET, Grenfell TJ, Mori C, Issazadeh S, Hancock WW, Selkoe DJ (2000) Nasal administration of amyloid-beta peptide decreases cerebral amyloid burden in a mouse model of Alzheimer's disease. Ann Neurol 48:567-579.

Weinstock M (1997) Possible role of the cholinergic system and disease models. J Neural Transm Suppl 49:93-102.

Werb Z (1997) ECM and cell surface proteolysis: regulating cellular ecology. Cell 91:439-442.

Werner ED, Brodsky JL, McCracken AA (1996) Proteasome-dependent endoplasmic reticulum-associated protein degradation: an unconventional route to a familiar fate. Proc Natl Acad Sci U S A 93:13797-13801.

West MJ, Coleman PS, Flood DG, Troncoso JC (1994) Differences in the pattern of hippocampal neuronal loss in normal aging and Alzheimer's disease. Lancet 344:769-772.

Whitehouse PJ, Price DL, Clark AW, Coyle JT, DeLong MR (1981) Alzheimer disease: evidence for selective loss of cholinergic neurons in the nucleus basalis. Ann Neurol 10:122-126.

Whitehouse PJ, Price DL, Struble RG, Clark AW, Coyle JT, Delon MR (1982) Alzheimer's disease and senile dementia: loss of neurons in the basal forebrain. Science 215:1237-1239.

Wirths O, Multhaup G, Czech C, Blanchard V, Moussaoui S, Tremp G, Pradier L, Beyreuther K, Bayer TA (2001) Intraneuronal Abeta accumulation precedes plaque formation in beta-amyloid precursor protein and presenilin-1 double-transgenic mice. Neurosci Lett 306:116-120.

Wisniewski T, Ghiso J, Frangione B (1997) Biology of A beta amyloid in Alzheimer's disease. Neurobiol Dis 4:313-328.

Wong PC, Zheng H, Chen H, Becher MW, Sirinathsinghji DJ, Trumbauer ME, Chen HY, Price DL, Van der Ploeg LH, Sisodia SS (1997) Presenilin 1 is required for Notch1 and DII1 expression in the paraxial mesoderm. Nature 387:288-292.

Xia W, Zhang J, Ostaszewski BL, Kimberly WT, Seubert P, Koo EH, Shen J, Selkoe DJ (1998) Presenilin 1 regulates the processing of beta-amyloid precursor protein C-terminal fragments and the generation of amyloid beta-protein in endoplasmic reticulum and Golgi. Biochemistry 37:16465-16471.

Yaar M, Zhai S, Fine RE, Eisenhauer PB, Arble BL, Stewart KB, Gilchrest BA (2002) Amyloid beta binds trimers as well as monomers of the 75-kDa neurotrophin receptor and activates receptor signaling. J Biol Chem 277:7720-7725.

Yamada K, Yabuki C, Seubert P, Schenk D, Hori Y, Ohtsuki S, Terasaki T, Hashimoto T, Iwatsubo T (2009) Abeta immunotherapy: intracerebral sequestration of Abeta by an anti-Abeta monoclonal antibody 266 with high affinity to soluble Abeta. J Neurosci 29:11393-11398.

Yamada T, Sasaki H, Dohura K, Goto I, Sadadi Y (1989) Structure and expressionof the alternatively-spliced forms of mRNA for the mouse homolog of Alzheimer's disease amyloid beta protein precursor. Biochem Biophys Res Comm 158:906-912.

Yamaguchi H, Yamazaki T, Kawarabayashi T, Sun X, Sakai Y, Hirai S (1994) Localization of Alzheimer amyloid beta protein precursor and its relation to senile plaque amyloid. Gerontology 40:65-70.

Yamaguchi H, Ishiguro K, Shoji M, Yamazaki T, Nakazato Y, Ihara Y, Hirai S (1990) Amyloid beta/A4 protein precursor is bound to neurofibrillary tangles in Alzheimer-type dementia. Brain Res 537:318-322.

Yan SD, Chen X, Fu J, Chen M, Zhu H, Roher A, Slattery T, Zhao L, Nagashima M, Morser J, Migheli A, Nawroth P, Stern D, Schmidt AM (1996) RAGE and amyloid-beta peptide neurotoxicity in Alzheimer's disease. Nature 382:685-691.

Yan SD, Fu J, Soto C, Chen X, Zhu H, Al-Mohanna F, Collison K, Zhu A, Stern E, Saido T, Tohyama M, Ogawa S, Roher A, Stern D (1997) An intracellular protein that binds amyloid-beta peptide and mediates neurotoxicity in Alzheimer's disease. Nature 389:689-695.

Yang AJ, Chandswangbhuvana D, Margol L, Glabe CG (1998) Loss of endosomal/lysosomal membrane impermeability is an early event in amyloid Abeta1-42 pathogenesis. J Neurosci Res 52:691-698.

Yankner BA (1996) Mechanisms of neuronal degeneration in Alzheimer's disease. Neuron 16:921-932.

Yankner BA, Caceres A, Duffy LK (1990) Nerve growth factor potentiates the neurotoxicity of beta amyloid. Proc Natl Acad Sci U S A 87:9020-9023.

Yao PJ, Morsch R, Callahan LM, Coleman PD (1999) Changes in synaptic expression of clathrin assembly protein AP180 in Alzheimer's disease analysed by immunohistochemistry. Neuroscience 94:389-394.

Yarr M, Zhai S, Pilch PF, Doyle SM, Eisenhauer PB, Fine RE, Gilchrest BA (1997) Binding of beta-amyloid to the p75 neurotrophin receptor induces apoptosis. A possible mechanism for Alzheimer's disease. J Clin Invest 100:2333-2340.

Yasojima K, Akiyama H, McGeer EG, McGeer PL (2001) Reduced neprilysin in high plaque areas of Alzheimer brain: a possible relationship to deficient degradation of beta-amyloid peptide. Neurosci Lett 297:97-100.

Yong VW, Krekoski CA, Forsyth PA, Bell R, Edwards DR (1998) Matrix metalloproteinases and diseases of the CNS. Trends Neurosci 21:75-80.

Yu G et al. (2000) Nicastrin modulates presenilin-mediated notch/glp-1 signal transduction and betaAPP processing. Nature 407:48-54.

Zamani MR, Allen YS, Owen GP, Gray JA (1997) Nicotine modulates the neurotoxic effect of beta-amyloid protein(25-35)) in hippocampal cultures. Neuroreport 8:513-517.

Zerovnik E, Stoka V, Mirtic A, Guncar G, Grdadolnik J, Staniforth RA, Turk D, Turk V (2011) Mechanisms of amyloid fibril formation - focus on domain-swapping. FEBS J 278:2263-2282.

Zhang Y, McLaughlin R, Goodyer C, LeBlanc A (2002) Selective cytotoxicity of intracellular amyloid beta peptide1-42 through p53 and Bax in cultured primary human neurons. J Cell Biol 156:519-529.

Zhang Y, Champagne N, Beitel LK, Goodyer CG, Trifiro M, LeBlanc A (2004) Estrogen and androgen protection of human neurons against intracellular amyloid beta1-42 toxicity through heat shock protein 70. J Neurosci 24:5315-5321.

Zhang Y, Hong Y, Bounhar Y, Blacker M, Roucou X, Tounekti O, Vereker E, Bowers WJ, Federoff HJ, Goodyer CG, LeBlanc A (2003) p75 neurotrophin receptor protects primary cultures of human neurons against extracellular amyloid beta peptide cytotoxicity. J Neurosci 23:7385-7394.

Zheng H, Jiang M, Trumbauer ME, Hopkins R, Sirinathsinghji DJ, Stevens KA, Conner MW, Slunt HH, Sisodia SS, Chen HY, Van der Ploeg LH (1996) Mice deficient for the amyloid precursor protein gene. Ann N Y Acad Sci 777:421-426.

Zlokovic BV (1996) Cerebrovascular transport of Alzheimer's amyloid beta and apolipoproteins J and E: possible anti-amyloidogenic role of the blood-brain barrier. Life Sci 59:1483-1497.

Zlokovic BV (2008) New therapeutic targets in the neurovascular pathway in Alzheimer's disease. Neurotherapeutics 5:409-414.

4

Structure-Toxicity Relationships of Amyloid Peptide Oligomers

Patrick Walsh and Simon Sharpe
The Hospital for Sick Children, and the University of Toronto
Canada

1. Introduction

The accumulation of misfolded proteins as insoluble, fibrillar aggregates is characteristic of several degenerative diseases. Examples include the proteins involved in amyloid diseases such as Alzheimer's disease (Aβ) (Glenner and Wong 1984), type II diabetes (amylin) (Cooper et al. 1987) and Parkinson's disease (α-synuclein) (Spillantini et al. 1997), as well as the mammalian prion diseases (PrP) (Prusiner 1982). While infectivity and onset differ between amyloid and prion diseases, recent evidence suggests that soluble protein oligomers, rather than fibrils, are the cytotoxic species in each case (Lambert et al. 1998; Bucciantini et al. 2002; Kayed et al. 2003; Walsh and Selkoe 2004; Silveira et al. 2005; Baglioni et al. 2006; Simoneau et al. 2007). It has been suggested that these non-fibrillar assemblies may be a common element of all amyloid diseases, and non-fibrillar oligomers formed by several amyloid proteins have been identified *in vivo* or produced *in vitro.* Regardless of protein sequence, these oligomers share several key features, including reactivity to structural antibodies, the ability to permeabilize model membranes, and cytotoxicity to cultured neurons. However, despite their potential importance in the pathogenesis of amyloid diseases, the details of the molecular structure of these non-fibrillar oligomers are only now beginning to emerge, as is their relationship to mature fibrils, and to the onset of disease.

The mechanism or mechanisms through which these oligomeric species induce cell death and contribute to the pathology of amyloid diseases remain a matter of some debate. Current hypotheses include a physical disruption of cellular membranes, formation of amyloid pores or channels, induction of oxidative stress, or interactions with receptor proteins on the cell surface leading to either altered protein function, or the initiation of a signaling event. Defining the link between the structure of misfolded protein aggregates and the concurrent gain of a toxic functionality is inhibited by the inherent difficulties of studying aggregative proteins, and is further complicated by the ability of amyloid proteins and peptides to form several distinct types of oligomers and fibrils, which often exist as heterogeneous mixtures. Each species of aggregate may exhibit varied biological activity, different local structure or gross morphology and typically contains different numbers of monomers per assembly. Despite these challenges, there has been significant recent progress in obtaining high-resolution structural details of amyloid fibrils and non-fibrillar oligomers, and in defining their biological mode of action. In this chapter, we review the current knowledge of the structure-toxicity relationship of non-fibrillar amyloid oligomers.

2. Amyloid fibrils

2.1 Overview of amyloid fibril structure

As the final stage in the assembly pathway for misfolded amyloid proteins, accumulation of fibrils has long been seen as the hallmark of amyloid diseases. Since they were the only readily detectable amyloid assembly present in disease tissue, early work suggested that fibrils were likely to be the mediators of cell death and disease progression. In addition, preparation of stable mature amyloid fibrils has generally been more accessible than the potentially transient non-fibrillar oligomers, facilitating biophysical and structural analysis. With recent advances in methodology and instrumentation, high-resolution structural details have been reported for amyloid fibrils formed by several proteins and peptides, based on data from crystallographic and solid state (nuclear magnetic resonance) NMR studies (Petkova et al. 2002; Jaroniec et al. 2004; Sawaya et al. 2007; Lee et al. 2008; 2009). While the details of each structure differ, based on sequence and solution conditions used for assembly, these studies have confirmed the presence of a cross-β architecture within the core of all amyloid fibrils studied to date. This structural motif is characterized by having protein or peptide strands form extended β-sheets running perpendicular to the long axis of the filament, and was initially identified from x-ray fiber diffraction studies of amyloid fibrils (Eanes and Glenner 1968; Geddes et al. 1968; Jahn et al. 2009). The cross-β diffraction pattern contains intense reflections at 4.7-4.8 Å (meridional) and 10 Å (equatorial) due to the characteristic spacing between β-strands along the long axis and between the perpendicularly stacked β-sheets, respectively.

In general, the core of most amyloid fibrils is considered to contain a dehydrated interface between adjacent β-sheets. This is typically considered to result from packing of hydrophobic residues in a water-excluded core, giving rise to one of 8 possible steric zipper arrangements, as first proposed by Sawaya *et al.* (Sawaya et al. 2007) (Figure 1A). These permutations arise from the fact that there are 2 possible types of β-sheet (parallel or antiparallel), 2 stacking possibilities (parallel or anti-parallel) and 2 surfaces for inter-sheet packing (face-to-face or face-to-back). The presence of steric zipper motifs was initially observed in X-ray structures of fibril-like crystals formed by short amyloidogenic peptides (Sawaya et al. 2007), and a subset of these classes of intersheet packing have been observed in solid-state NMR structures of amyloid fibrils (Nielsen et al. 2009). It is important to note, however, that recent NMR studies have revealed some possible structural differences between the crystalline and fibrillar forms of the GNNQQNY peptide derived from the yeast prion Sup35 (van der Wel et al. 2007), such that more structures of amyloid fibrils are required to confirm the crystallographic data.

Additional complexity in fibril structure comes from quaternary interactions in which protofilaments containing a basic building block (for example a filament formed by extended arrangement of a pair of stacked β-sheets) are bundled or twisted together to form the mature amyloid fibril. It is clear from electron microscopy studies of fibrils formed by numerous amyloid peptides that significant heterogeneity can exist between fibrils formed by the same peptide (Fandrich et al. 2009). This can be rationalized as variations in the interchain, intersheet, and interprotofilament packing, as well as conformational heterogeneity between peptide chains. The heterogeneous nature of many fibril preparations has been supported by solid state NMR for Aβ(1-40) (Petkova et al. 2005), α-synuclein (Heise et al. 2005), GNQQNY fibrils (van der Wel et al.), and amylin (Madine et al. 2008).

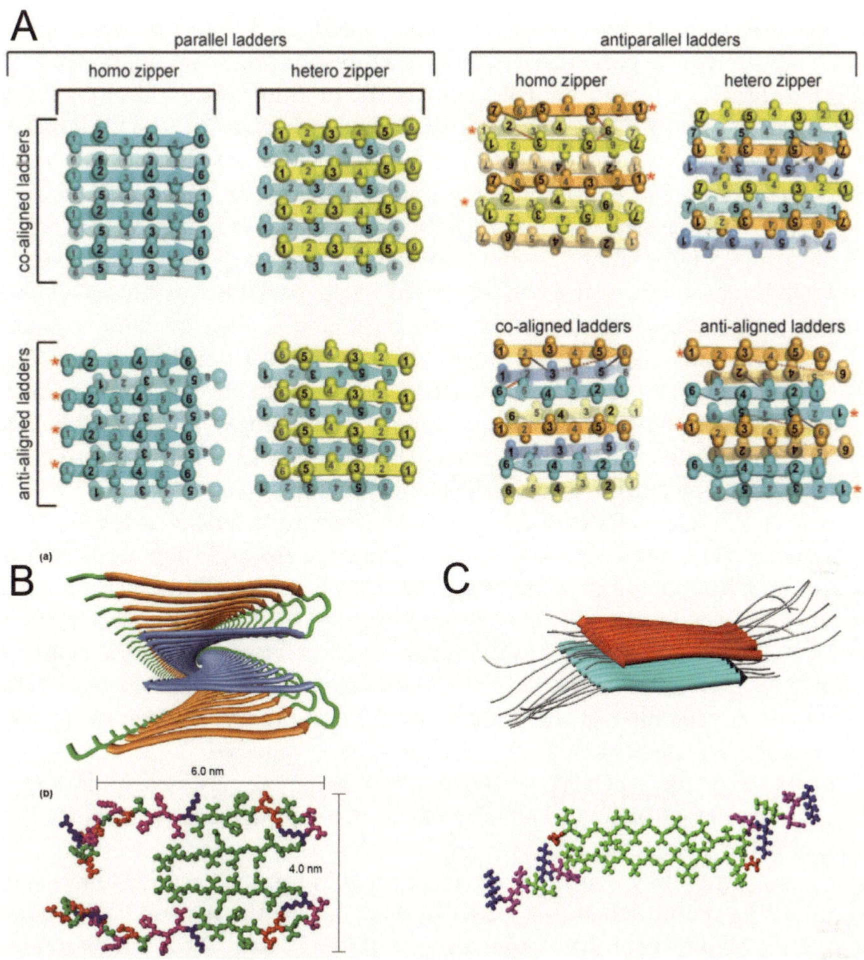

Fig. 1. Stuctural models for amyloid fibrils. (A) Possible arrangements of beta-strands in an amyloid fibril. Eight permutations exist, four containing parallel β-sheets and four containing anti-parallel β-sheets, each with the possibility of parallel or antiparallel stacking of the two sheets, which may align in a face-to-face or face-to-back manner. In each case, the interface between the sheets forms a so-called steric zipper, with opposing side chains interdigitating to exclude water. Reprinted with permission from Nielsen *et al.*, 2009. Copyright 2009 Angewandte Chimie. (B) Structural model for Aβ(1-40) fibrils, as determined by solid state NMR. This structure contains a class 1 steric zipper with parallel β-sheets stacked in a face-to-face antiparallel arrangement. The upper image shows the backbone of several monomers, arranged with the fibril axis extending into the page, while the lower image focuses on a representative pair of peptides, showing the interdigitation of sidechains within the hydrophobic core, as well as depicting quaternary contacts between adjacent protofilaments. Reprinted with permission from Petkova *et al.*, 2002. Copyright 2002 Proceedings of the National Acadamy of Science of the United States. (C) Structural model for amyloid fibrils formed by PrP(106-126), determined using solid state NMR. The peptide strands are arranged in a class 1 steric zipper motif with a salt bridge between K110 and the carboxylate of the C-terminus. The overall structural effect is similar to a single layer of the Aβ structure. Reprinted with permission from Walsh *et al.*, 2009. Copyright 2009 Structure

Probably the best characterized fibril structures are those formed by fragments of the Alzheimer's Aβ protein. In particular, several structures for fibrils formed by Aβ(1-40) have been reported, based primarily on solid state NMR or transmission electron microscopy (TEM) (Chan 2011; Tycko 2011; Petkova et al. 2002; Sachse et al. 2008). The fibril morphology and subunit peptide structure in each case is dependent on the incubation conditions during *in vitro* fibrillization, and can exhibit significant heterogeneity in both TEM and NMR experiments. An example structure for Aβ(1-40) fibrils is shown in Figure 1B. Each peptide adopts a β-turn-β conformation, forming parallel in-register β-sheets with neighboring peptides down the long axis of the fibril. The two sheets pack into an internal class 1 steric zipper motif within the protofilament. In this structural model, quaternary interactions between two protofilaments were determined using intermolecular dipolar couplings from solid state NMR, giving rise to the depicted structure for the mature fibril. These quaternary interactions vary between fibrils with different morphology, such as the three-fold symmetric fibrils reported by Paravastu *et al.*, (Paravastu et al. 2006) or those studied by cryoelectron microscopy (Sachse et al. 2008; Schmidt et al. 2009).

By contrast, only a single well-defined structure has been reported so far for protofilaments formed by the far more neurotoxic and more aggregative Aβ(1-42) peptide, which is a less abundant form of Aβ, but which correlated more closely with pathogenesis (Burdick et al. 1992; Jarrett et al. 1993; Luhrs et al. 2005; Kumar-Singh et al. 2006). This structure is similar to that of Aβ(1-40), but rather than intramolecular contacts forming the steric zipper, the top strand from one monomer makes side chain contacts with the bottom strand from an adjacent monomer. Modeling of the mature fibril based on cryoelectron microscopy and hydrogen/deuterium exchange measurements has suggested a distinctly different quaternary assembly for Aβ(1-42) fibrils, but the potential relationship between these structures and the varied biological activity of the two Aβ peptides remains (Miller et al.; Olofsson et al. 2007; Zhang et al. 2009).

Numerous solid state NMR structures of small amyloid-forming peptides have now been reported, including short fragments of Aβ (Balbach et al. 2000; Tycko and Ishii 2003), amylin (Luca et al. 2007; Madine et al. 2008), transthyretin (Jaroniec et al. 2002; Jaroniec et al. 2004), calcitonin (Naito et al. 2004) and neurotoxic fragments of PrP (Cheng et al. 2011; Lee et al. 2008; 2009). As shown for PrP(106-126) fibrils in Figure 1C, most of these structures reflect similar architecture as observed for Aβ, parallel β-sheets and a class 1 steric zipper packing. Some short peptides display alternate packing arrangements in the fibrils, such as the antiparallel β-sheets formed by Aβ(16-22) (Balbach et al. 2000) or the antiparallel heterozipper arrangement of amylin(20-29) fibrils (Nielsen et al. 2009). Longer amyloid proteins have remained more challenging. For example, initial studies of full-length α-synuclein by hydrogen—deuterium exchange and solid state NMR have allowed identification of secondary structure elements and delineation of the fibril core, but a high-resolution fibril structure is lacking (Heise et al. 2005; Vilar et al. 2008).

2.2 Prion fibrils

The prion protein (PrP) is the major causative agent of neurodegenerative prion diseases, such as scrapie in sheep, BSE in cattle, and CJD among others in humans. The protein converts from a monomeric, primarily helical cellular form (PrP^{C}), to an infectious, oligomeric, scrapie form (PrP^{Sc}), with increased β-structure. In addition, there are several known fungal prion proteins, unrelated to PrP in amino acid sequence, but sharing the ability to adopt a fibrillar, infectious, β-sheet rich structure. While sharing some common structural elements with fibrils formed by amyloid proteins, some striking differences have been observed. For example, the fungal Het-S prion protein structure solved by solid state NMR contains a β-solenoid structure with two protein molecules per "rung" of the solenoid ladder, rather than the cross-β packing typical of amyloid (Figure 2) (Wasmer et al. 2008). By contrast, amyloid fibrils formed by PrP *in vitro* were shown by electron paramagnetic resonance (EPR) to contain amyloid-like in-register parallel beta-sheet structure (Cobb et al. 2007) (Figure 2), similar to the yeast prion proteins Ure2 (Baxa et al. 2007) and Sup35 (Shewmaker et al. 2006). Interestingly, it has been shown through electron crystallography, X-ray fibre diffraction, and molecular dynamics simulations that the infectious PrP^{Sc} form of PrP from infected brains likely differs from *in vitro* fibrils and may contain a β-helix or β-solenoid structure (Govaerts et al. 2004), similar to Het-S.

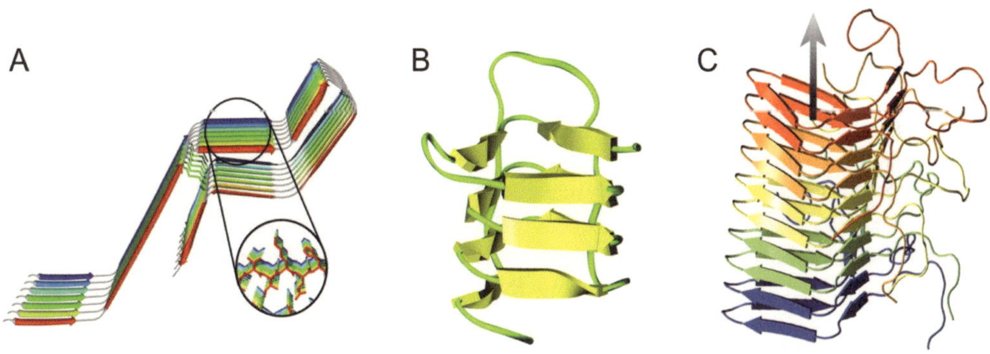

Fig. 2. Structures formed by prion proteins from human and yeast systems. (A) Structure of amyloid fibrils formed by PrP, showing parallel in-register β-sheets. The structure is also stabilized by a disulphide bond. Reprinted with permission from Cobb *et al.*, 2007. Copyright 2007 Proceedings of the National Acadamy of Science of the United States. (B) β-helical structure formed by human PrP taken from infectious material. Reprinted with permission from Govaerts *et al.*, 2004. Copyright 2004 Proceedings of the National Acadamy of Science of the United States. (C) The Het-S prion structure from solid state NMR showing residues 218-289 in a β-solenoid. Reprinted with permission from Wasmer *et al.*, 2008. Copyright 2008 Science

3. Non-fibrillar amyloid oligomers

3.1 Overview

While a wealth of structural information is becoming available for the fibrillar forms of many model and disease related amyloid proteins and peptides, relatively little is known about the molecular structure of non-fibrillar oligomers formed by the same polypeptides. Structural characterization has been made particularly challenging by the transient nature of many of these assemblies, which are widely considered to form as intermediates along the amyloid misfolding pathway. Thus, the difficulty of obtaining highly pure samples of non-fibrillar oligomers which are sufficiently long-lived for biophysical studies has significantly slowed progress in this field. A number of studies have used small molecules, including detergents or lipids, to trap or stabilize oligomeric states of amyloid proteins (Laurents et al. 2005; Yu et al. 2009), but this approach risks formation of off-pathway or non-productive assemblies, rather than the on-pathway intermediates likely to play a role in amyloid disease (Kayed et al. 2003).

Despite these challenges, however, a number of low-resolution studies have been reported, using TEM, atomic force microscopy (AFM), hydrogen/deuterium exchange, and fluorescence spectroscopy-based approaches (Huang et al. 2000; Williams et al. 2005; Losic et al. 2006; Ono et al. 2009). Microscopy and size exclusion chromatography have shown that, similar to amyloid fibrils, there are a wide range of non-fibrillar oligomers that can be categorized based on their size (ranging from dimers of Aβ(1-40) to large globular assemblies containing hundreds of peptide monomers) or morphology (Haass and Selkoe 2007; Walsh and Selkoe 2007). In terms of the latter, most oligomers reported have either exhibited a roughly globular appearance by AFM and TEM, or have been annular in nature - exhibiting a pore or ring shaped structure (Janson et al. 1999; Conway et al. 2000; Lashuel et al. 2002). These two morphologies appear to exhibit different degrees of biological activity, with spherical oligomers, but not annular oligomers, increasing membrane conductance and inducing apoptosis in cell culture (Kayed et al. 2009). The large (3-10 nm diameter), spherical oligomers formed by several amyloid proteins have been shown to bind to a single conformational antibody, suggesting that a common structural motif exists in these assemblies, despite having no sequence similarity. Antibody binding was also shown to inhibit the inherent cytotoxicity of these large amyloid oligomers (Figure 3). Likewise, annular oligomers formed by Aβ(1-42), amylin and α-synuclein are all recognized by an antibody that does not bind to monomeric or fibrillar material, and that shows only weak binding to spherical oligomers, indicating that these contain distinct structural elements from the other assemblies (Kayed et al. 2009).

More recently, solid state NMR has been successfully used to obtain high-resolution structural details of non-fibrillar oligomers formed by Aβ (Chimon and Ishii 2005; Chimon et al. 2007), PrP(106-126) (Walsh et al. 2009; Walsh et al. 2010), and α-synuclein (Kim et al. 2009), and solution NMR has been used to investigate the structure of small detergent stabilized oligomers of Aβ(1-42) (Yu et al. 2009). Advances in computational infrastructure and methodologies have also led to an increased use of molecular dynamics simulations to investigate the structure and assembly of non-fibrillar amyloid oligomers.

3.2 Aβ oligomers

The non-fibrillar oligomers formed by Aβ(1-40) and Aβ(1-42) have been implicated as the main toxic species associated with Alzheimer's disease, and as such have been the focus of the majority of studies on amyloid oligomers reported to date. Structural characterization has been impeded by the wide spectrum of oligomeric states that can be adopted by these peptides along their aggregation pathways. As indicated above, species ranging in size from dimers to oligomers containing hundreds of peptides have been reported, both *in vitro*, and in material isolated from the brains of Alzheimer's patients (Haass and Selkoe 2007; Walsh and Selkoe 2007).

The larger oligomers can also be subdivided into spherical, so-called pre-fibrillar oligomers and ring-shaped annular oligomers, each with different antibody reactivity. From a high-resolution standpoint, most experimental progress has been made in defining the molecular structures of small and large pre-fibrillar oligomers formed by Aβ, although numerous molecular dynamics simulations have been carried out on membrane-bound amyloid channels or pores that closely resemble the overall morphology of annular protofibrils as

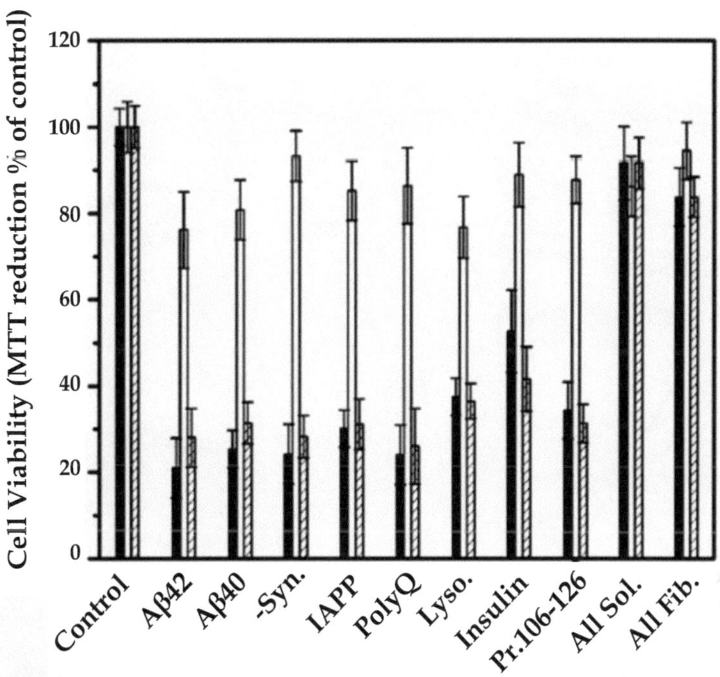

Fig. 3. Amyloid oligomers are toxic and share a common structural element. A graph showing the viability of neuroblastoma SH-SY5Y cells, monitored by the 3-(4,5-dimethyl-2-thiazoyl)-2,5-diphenyltetrasodium bromide (MTT) reduction assay, as a function of treatment with preparations of several amyloid proteins. The toxicity of non-fibrillar oligomers formed by each peptide is shown to significantly decrease cell survival (black bars) relative to the control, soluble (presumed monomeric) peptide and mature amyloid fibrils. In each case, the effects of the oligomers on cell survival are attenuated by the addition of an amyloid oligomer specific antibody (A11, white bars). Non-specific IgG is shown in hatched bars, and exerts no effect on the system. Reprinted with permission from Kayed *et al.*, 2003. Copyright 2003 Science

seen in TEM and AFM images (Jang et al. 2007; Zheng et al. 2008). These annular oligomers are 8-20 nm in diameter by TEM and AFM, and like the spherical oligomers, circular dichroism (CD) spectroscopy shows that they contain high levels of β-sheet (Kayed et al. 2008). The anti-annular oligomer antibodies also bind to the β-barrel pores formed by the bacterial toxin α-hemolysin, such that they may share the same general architecture (Kayed et al. 2009). Interestingly, preformed annular oligomers did not permeabilize membranes, instead converting to prefibrillar oligomers upon interaction with membranes. This may suggest that any pore like structure formed by Aβ would need to assemble within the membrane, rather than acting through insertion of a preformed assembly.

In the pre-fibrillar oligomers, the structural data that has emerged from recent studies suggests that even at the earliest stages of aggregation they share common features with the fibrillar forms of Aβ. For example, Yu et al., used 0.05% SDS to stabilize very small pre-globulomers and globulomers of Aβ(1-42), with molecular weights of 16 and 64 kDa respectively (Yu et al. 2009). These were assumed to represent very early points in the amyloid aggregation pathway, and structural studies were conducted using solution NMR.

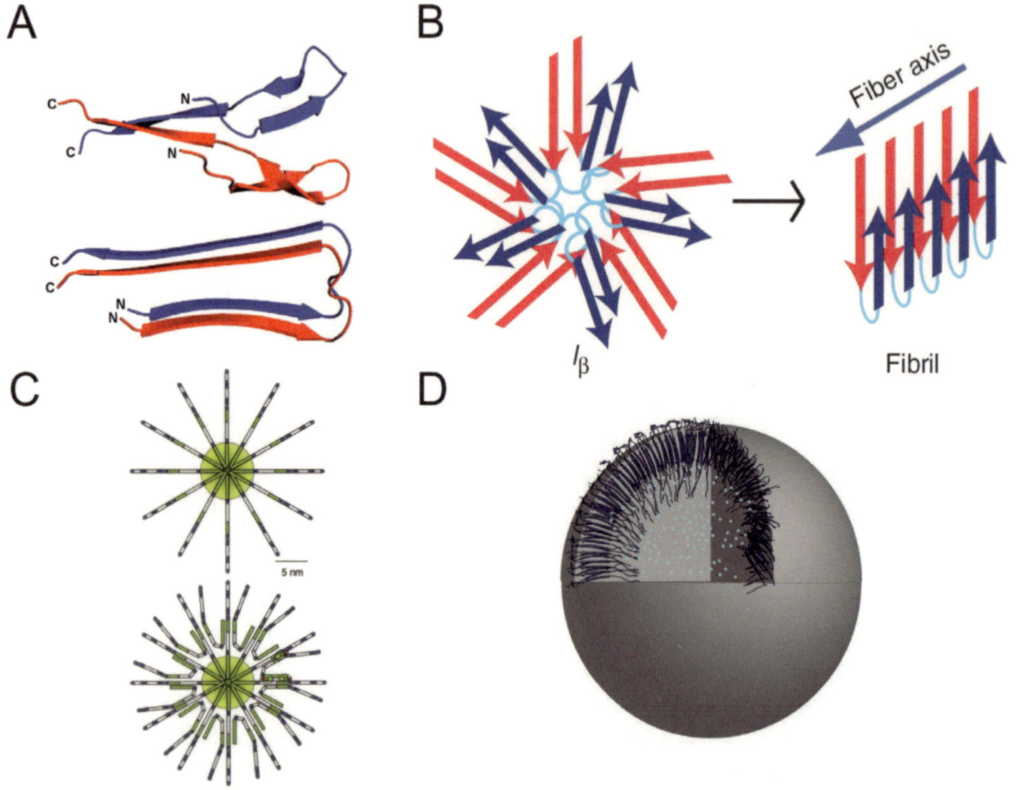

Fig. 4. Structures of non-fibrillar amyloid oligomers. (A) Pre-globulomer(top) and globulomer (bottom) structures formed by Aβ(1-42) are shown. Both structures show similarities to the basic Aβ(1-40) fibril subunit shown in Figure 1B. Reprinted with permission from Yu *et al.*, 2009. Copyright 2009 The American Chemical Society. (B) Structural model of large spherical Aβ(1-40) oligomers obtained using solid state NMR. Reprinted with permission from Chimon *et al.*, 2008. Copyright 2008 Nature Publishing Group. (C) A structural model of large, DSS stabilized Aβ(1-40) oligomers shown as extended micelle-like structures, approximately 35nm in diameter. Significant structural similarity with the solid state NMR derived model shown in (B) is evident. Reprinted with permission from Laurents *et al.*, 2005. Copyright 2005 Journal of Biological Chemistry. (D) A structural model for non-fibrillar PrP(106-126) oligomers, obtained from solid state NMR, showing similar contacts to those seen in fibrils formed by the same peptide (Figure 1C). The basic subunit is a parallel beta sheet stacked two high to form a class 1 steric zipper which are arranged in a micelle-like formation. Reprinted with permission from Walsh *et al.*, 2010. Copyright 2010 The American Chemical Society

The intra-chain and inter-chain contacts in these oligomers are share similarities with the Aβ (1-40) and Aβ(1-42) fibril structures reported to date. Both contain similar secondary structure elements with the fibrillar form, and contain intermolecular contacts reminiscent of the fibrils, although in the small oligomers, the N-terminal strand folds back on itself, rather than participating in intermolecular β-sheet formation (Figure 4A). In a similar vein, DSS was used to stabilize very large (764 kDa) Aβ(1-40) oligomers, and subsequent structural analysis suggested the presence of micelle-like assemblies containing a radial arrangement of Aβ monomers in an extended β-sheet conformation (Figure 4C) (Laurents et al. 2005). The nature of intermolecular or intramolecular β-sheets was not determined in this study, so it is difficult to relate the resulting models to the fibrillar form of the protein.

For both of the aforementioned studies, it is important to note that the effect of detergents and other small molecules on the structure and assembly of amyloid peptides remains unclear. Addition of cofactors may lead to formation or stabilization of otherwise unpopulated structures. Recent studies of on-pathway prefibrillar oligomers of Aβ(1-40) and Aβ(1-42) have circumvented this requirement by using either gel filtration and lyophilization (Chimon and Ishii 2005; Chimon et al. 2007) or careful modulation of solution salt and pH conditions to trap non-fibrillar oligomers for structural studies (Ahmed et al. 2010).

Solid state NMR of large (15-35nm) spherical oligomers of Aβ(1-40) prepared by freeze-trapping revealed fibril-like secondary and quaternary structures, leading to a model in which the location and intermolecular assembly of β-sheets is shared between the two forms (Chimon et al. 2007). A schematic for the proposed architecture of these oligomers is shown in Figure 4B, along with a model of the Aβ(1-40) protofilament structure determined by Petkova *et al.* (Petkova et al. 2002). This micelle-like arrangement is reminiscent of that proposed for DSS-stabilized oligomers (Figure 4C), potentially validating the use of small molecules to trap transient amyloid oligomers. These large oligomers were shown to exhibit neurotoxicity, and based on their transient nature can be assumed to lie on the fibril assembly pathway.

Ahmed *et al.* have used altered solution conditions to trap discoidal pentamers and decamers of Aβ(1-42) with potent neurotoxicity (Ahmed et al. 2010). When incubated at 37°C for several hours, these oligomers convert to amyloid fibrils, suggesting that they are productive intermediates on the assembly pathway. In contrast to the large Aβ(1-40) oligomers studies by Chimon *et al.* (2007), Fourier-transform infrared (FTIR) spectroscopy and solid-state NMR studies of these small oligomers indicated the presence of significantly increased disorder and solvent accessibility relative to fibrils of Aβ(1-42), and showed that the oligomers lack the in-register parallel β-sheet architecture of the fibrillar form. The oligomeric peptides do, however contain the same β-loop-β secondary and tertiary fold observed in Aβ(1-42) and Aβ(1-40) fibrils. This is supported by molecular dynamics and hydrogen-deuterium exchange studies from several other groups, and leads to an overall picture in which Aβ peptides adopt a β-loop-β structure as a common element of all oligomeric states, with intermolecular contacts and solvent accessibility varying between different types of oligomers. MD and H/D exchange studies support these conclusions, leading to the general concept that early intermediates formed during Aβ assembly may be more solvent accessible and potentially more labile, and that conformational flexibility is likely to play an important role in their biological activity (Pan et al. 2011; Yu et al. 2010; Yu and Zheng 2011; Cheon et al. 2007; Zhang et al. 2009).

3.3 PrP(106-126) oligomers

The PrP derived peptide PrP(106-126) poses an interesting structure-toxicity relationship. Evidence has been presented both in favour of, and against, a dependence of PrP(106-126) toxicity on expression of cell-surface full length PrP (Brown 1998). However, it has also been shown that this PrP derived peptide is able to form both amyloid fibrils and cytotoxic oligomers, making it a useful model for studying the structural and mechanistic details of non-fibrillar amyloid oligomers (Forloni et al. 1993; Selvaggini et al. 1993; Jobling et al. 1999;

Salmona et al. 1999). For example, in studies by Kayed *et al.*, non-fibrillar oligomers of PrP(106-126) were shown to form large (10-20nm diameter) spherical oligomers with similar morphology to Aβ, amylin, and several other amyloid proteins (Kayed et al. 2003). These oligomers cause increase membrane conductance and were cytotoxic to neuronal cell cultures, and have also been shown to disrupt model-membranes in a concentration dependent manner, as revealed by a liposome dye-release assay (Kayed et al. 2004; Walsh et al. 2009). Utilizing solid state NMR, a structural model was developed for these non-fibrillar oligomers (Figure 4D) (Walsh et al. 2010). Similar to the Aβ(1-40) oligomers reported by Ishii *et al.* (Chimon et al. 2007), large PrP(106-126) oligomers contain fibril-like secondary structure and intermolecular contacts, suggesting that they are composed of small fibril-like segments arranged in a micelle-like assembly. This is an interesting observation considering that these oligomers do not bind thioflavin-T, unlike the amyloid fibrils formed by PrP(106-126), implying that the oligomers either lack the extended cross-β structure required for dye-binding, or that the binding site for the dye is occluded in the oligomer structure.

3.4 α-synuclein oligomers

In the case of α-synuclein, despite its innate lipid binding ability, it is the aggregated state that is considered to gain cytotoxic function, likely acting through membrane permeabilization (Haass and Selkoe 2007). Strong evidence has been presented to suggest that oligomers lying on misfolding pathway leading to amyloid fibril formation are the most cytotoxic species formed by this protein (Lashuel et al. 2002). These oligomers were found to share common structural elements with other amyloid oligomers as seen by A11 antibody binding (Kayed et al. 2007), and the presence of extensive β-sheet secondary structure in baicalin stabilized oligomers has been confirmed through FTIR and CD spectroscopy (Zhu et al. 2004; Hong et al. 2008). A recent study combined biophysical analysis with solution and solid state NMR to more closely investigate the structure and membrane interaction of non-fibrillar α-synuclein oligomers (Kim et al. 2009). Through solid state NMR it was shown that the pore forming contained β-sheet secondary structure but that there were significant differences between the structures of the monomeric, oligomeric and fibrillar states of this protein - contrasting with the studies of Aβ and PrP(106-126) oligomers referenced above.

3.5 Other amyloid oligomers and common structural elements

While several other amyloid proteins and peptides, including amylin and polyglutamine, have been shown to form neurotoxic, non-fibrillar oligomers, there is currently no high-resolution structural information available on these systems. It is known that at least one oligomeric state populated by each peptide is morphologically similar to that observed for spherical aggregates of Aβ, PrP(106-126), and α-synuclein. These oligomers also cause increased membrane permeability (Kayed et al. 2004; Demuro et al. 2005), and furthermore share the common structural element that allows recognition by the A11 anti-oligomer antibody developed by Kayed *et al.* (Kayed et al. 2003).

In the case of the mammalian prion protein, non-fibrillar oligomers of various sizes have been identified and shown to be neurotoxic (Baskakov et al. 2002; Sokolowski et al. 2003; Silveira et al. 2005; Simoneau et al. 2007). Small oligomers (composed of < 30 monomers) of PrP purified from the brains of infected animals have been shown to be the most infectious and toxic form of the protein, echoing the biological activity of amyloid oligomers (Silveira et al. 2005). PrP oligomers have been shown to contain a predominantly β-sheet secondary structure by FTIR spectroscopy and CD, but no detailed structural information has been reported (Baskakov et al. 2001; Sokolowski et al. 2003). Of particular interest, the population of a β-sheet rich octamer formed during the misfolding of PrP has been shown to correlate with the susceptibility of different mammals to prion disease, further highlighting the role of oligomeric species in pathogenesis (Khan et al. 2010).

3.6 Where do non-fibrillar oligomers fit into the misfolding pathways of amyloid proteins?

The relationship between the formation of non-fibrillar oligomers and the misfolding pathway leading to amyloid fibril formation has not been definitively determined. While there have been conflicting reports (Necula et al. 2007), most evidence points to the spherical, cytotoxic oligomers existing as on-pathway intermediates. In particular, various prefibrillar oligomers of Aβ have been shown to be transient, disappearing as they reorganize into mature fibrils (Chimon and Ishii 2005). Similarly, pore forming oligomers of α-synuclein are considered to be on-pathway for fibrillization (Kim et al. 2009). From a mechanistic standpoint, the structural data on prefibrillar oligomers suggests early adoption of an extended β-structure, followed by formation of tertiary and quaternary contacts as the oligomers increase in size. The precise steps involved in the transition from discoidal or spherical oligomers to an extended amyloid fibril have not been determined, but likely involve an increase in the tightness of lateral associations between strands, with optimized hydrophobic packing and hydrogen bond formation driving the final steps of assembly. Taken together, the transient nature and fibril-like structure show that these entities exist on the aggregation pathway toward fibril. As described above, annular oligomers do not appear to exist as productive intermediates, but may instead represent off-pathway assembly. In the case of Aβ, it has been shown that in the presence of lipid membranes, prefibrillar oligomers are capable of rearranging to form annular oligomers, suggesting that in this case they may represent an alternate end-stage of the misfolding pathway (Kayed et al. 2009). This may also present a possible mechanism for formation of membrane-disrupting entities from the on-pathway non fibrillar oligomers, as discussed below.

4. Non-fibrillar amyloid oligomers as the cytotoxic agents in amyloid disease

While early studies focused on the amyloid fibrils or plaques as the causative agents of neurotoxicity in Alzheimer's disease, more recently it has become evident that small non-fibrillar oligomers correlate much more closely with loss of neuronal function and neurodegenerative disease progression (Kayed et al. 2003; Haass and Selkoe 2007; Walsh and Selkoe 2007). This finding has been echoed for non-fibrillar oligomers formed by a broad array of disease related and non-disease related amyloid proteins (Baglioni et al. 2006). Given the potential for some amyloid oligomers to have similar structural properties, regardless of amino acid sequence, it is possible that many of these may act via a similar toxic mechanism. The conformations accessible to aggregative proteins may create interactions with components of the cellular ion transport system or may allow them to form channels or pores in cell membranes (Lin et al. 2001; Kayed et al. 2004; Demuro et al. 2005). This may represent a general mechanism through which cytotoxic effects are exerted during the early stages of protein aggregation. Supporting this hypothesis, soluble amyloid oligomers with spherical morphology, induce vesicle leakage, and are toxic to cultured cells, possibly through disruption of calcium homeostasis (Thellung et al. 2000; Demuro et al. 2005; Ferreiro et al. 2008).

Alternatively, hydrophobic, misfolded proteins are likely to have a high propensity to associate with membranes, and membrane binding of many amyloid peptides has been described extensively (McLaurin and Chakrabartty 1996; Yip et al. 2002; Kayed et al. 2004). Once bound to the membrane surface, or inserted into the bilayer, non-fibrillar oligomers would have the potential to rearrange into channels, pores, or non-specific aggregates at the membrane surface. Any of these mechanisms are likely to cause membrane destabilization and cell death, and it has recently been demonstrated for Aβ oligomers that increased membrane conductance can occur in the absence of channel formation (Sokolov et al. 2006). Physical disruption such as the introduction of membrane defects, possibly through insertion of oligomers, or through membrane-catalyzed fibril formation, would also be sufficient to induce leakage of cell contents and ultimately lead to cell death (McLaurin and Chakrabartty 1997; Yip et al. 2002).

While the oligomer fold is distinct from that of fibrils, as determined by differential antibody reactivity, a common theme emerging from structural studies of non-fibrillar amyloid oligomers is the presence of local fibril-like structure. While it does not speak to the actual mechanism through which toxicity is exerted, this observation may suggest that small fibril-like assemblies are the key element required for cytotoxicity. A similar phenomenon has been reported by Xue *et al.* (Xue et al. 2009), who demonstrated that fragmentation of mature amyloid fibrils formed by α-synuclein, β2-microglobulin and lysozyme leads to an increase in membrane disruption and cytotoxicity (Figure 5). Likewise amyloid fibrils formed by hexapeptides gained cytotoxicity towards primary neuronal cell culture after physical disruption (Pastor et al. 2008). In both studies, it is likely that the increase in active ends allows improved interactions with cellular targets - membranes or other cell surface molecules, where they are able to rearrange to form active, toxic entities. Oligomeric species, which are known to be more conformationally flexible and less stable than their fibrillar counterparts, may act through a similar mechanism, carrying active fibril-like segments to the site of toxic activity.

4.1 Aβ toxicity

As with molecular structure, the link between oligomerization of an amyloid protein and disease progression has been explored in detail for Aβ. Several lines of evidence support a role for oligomers as the toxic entity in Alzheimer's patients. Anti-oligomer antibodies stain diffuse amyloid in human brains, showing that soluble oligomers with similar structural properties as those formed *in vitro* exist *in vivo* (Kayed et al. 2007). In addition, both injection of *in vitro* formed oligomers into brain tissue, and reinjection of small soluble Aβ oligomers isolated from diseased animals are able to induce loss of synaptic function and neuronal death (Walsh and Selkoe 2004; Cleary et al. 2005; Haass and Selkoe 2007; Walsh and Selkoe 2007). This experiment has also been performed for non-disease causing amyloid proteins, supporting a role for other amyloid oligomers as *in vivo* cytotoxins (Baglioni et al. 2006).

Aβ oligomer toxicity *in vitro* has been attributed to several distinct mechanisms, including but not limited to, membrane disruption and the direct formation of ion channels. Certainly there have been numerous reports of increased membrane conductance or leakage in the presence of Aβ oligomers ranging from small globulomers to large prefibrillar assemblies (Chimon and Ishii 2005; Yu et al. 2009), with some evidence presented to support formation of discrete ion channels of pores (Arispe 2004; Quist et al. 2005). A lot of attention has been focused on the latter, and several molecular modeling studies have proposed models for the structure of a putative pore or channel – typically a picket-fence arrangement of monomers adopting the β-loop-β structure from the fibril structures (Jang et al. 2007). Alternatively, alteration of the mechanical properties of the membrane could lead to increased conductance as observed by Sokolov *et al.* (Sokolov et al. 2006), although the structural basis for this is unclear.

Several very specific proposals for Aβ oligomer toxicity have been proposed as alternatives to membrane disruption. As a group these invoke interactions with specific cell-surface targets, with subsequent alteration of normal protein activity leading to loss of neuronal function and possibly to cell death (Verdier et al. 2004; Yankner and Lu 2009). While too numerous to describe in detail here, proposed interaction partners for Aβ have included the serpin-enzyme complex receptor (SEC-R) and the insulin receptor, both of which are capable of binding to monomeric Aβ, although the physiological effects are unclear (Verdier and Penke 2004). Fibrillar Aβ, on the other hand has been shown to bind a wide array of cell-surface proteins, including the receptor for advanced glycation end products (RAGE) complex and the amyloid precursor protein (Verdier and Penke 2004), leading in some cases in increased radical formation and oxidative stress. Similarly, binding to the α-7 nicotinic receptor can mediate N-methyl-D-aspartate (NMDA) receptor activity, with broad effects on cellular metabolism (Snyder et al. 2005). Any or all of these effects may play a role in loss of synaptic function, leading to symptomatic Alzheimer's disease. Other proposed interactions, such as dysregulation of calcium channels, may be confounded by membrane disruption effects, making them harder to confirm.

Less is known about potential interactions of soluble oligomers with cell surface receptor molecules, although similar targets to the fibrillar material have been proposed. An intriguing possibility arises from recent reports that oligomeric Aβ binds to the unstructured N-terminus of cellular PrP, with initial reports suggesting that the toxic effects of small Aβ oligomers may be mediated by this interaction (Lauren et al. 2009). If true, such an association may lead to an alteration of the as yet unidentified signaling functions of PrP, or may allow PrP to act as carrier for internalization of oligomeric Aβ. In this model, once inside the cell, the prefibrillar oligomers would exert loss of function effects on internal cellular components through mechanisms not yet identified. While this observation may provide a tantalizing link between two neurodegenerative disorders, more work need to be done to confirm the specificity of the interaction, and to define the potential role played by PrP.

It is important to note that since Aβ exists *in vitro* and *in vivo* as a continuum of different oligomeric states, none of which are particularly stable, it is difficult to distinguish biological effects induced by one specific type of non-fibrillar oligomer. Therefore, it is entirely feasible that Aβ has significantly different physiological effects when in different oligomeric forms. Thus, it is difficult to exclude any of the putative mechanisms for involvement of Aβ oligomers in progression of amyloid disease without further study.

4.2 PrP(106-126) toxicity

There have been conflicting reports on the toxicity of PrP(106-126) largely due to confounding effects of its ability to form amyloid oligomers as well as potentially playing a role in conversion of full-length PrP to the infectious PrP^{Sc} form (Gu et al. 2002). PrP(106-126) has been shown to be toxic in a number of different ways. Reports initially characterized PrP(106-126) as requiring full-length PrP for toxicity in cerebral endothelial cells (Deli et al. 2000). There is also significant evidence for PrP-independent cytotoxicity,

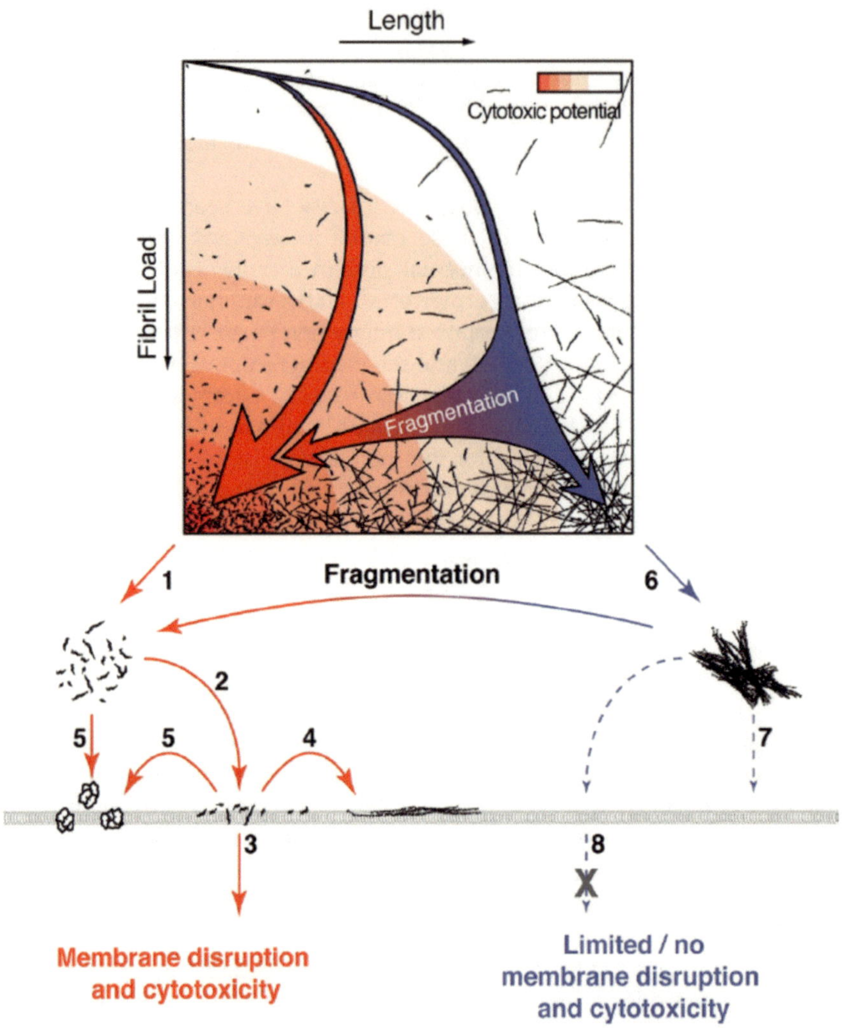

Fig. 5. The relationship between amyloid fibril length and toxicity. As the concentration of small fragments increases, increased membrane disruption and cellular toxicity are observed. As the fragments become smaller, it is proposed that they will be increasingly toxic to the cell. Reprinted with permission from Xue *et al.*, 2009. Copyright 2009 The American Chemical Society

but it is important to note that in most studies of PrP(106-126), the aggregation state of the peptide was not clearly defined, so the activity of prefibrillar oligomers is implicit rather than explicit in the results. PrP(106-126) has been shown to interact with L-type voltage sensitive calcium channels, causing apoptosis (Florio et al. 1998; Silei et al. 1999; Thellung et al. 2000). It has also been demonstrated that this peptide causes the activation of the JNK-c-Jun pathway, leading to apoptosis shortly after peptide treatment (Carimalo et al. 2005).

There have been several reports of direct membrane destabilization by PrP(106-126), including the formation of ion channels (Lin et al. 1997), or alterations in membrane viscosity (Salmona et al. 1997). More recent work using well-defined prefibrillar oligomers of PrP(106-126) have shown that it causes permeabilization of model membranes (Kayed et al. 2004; Walsh et al. 2009) and induces cytotoxicity in neuroblastoma cell cultures (Kayed et al. 2003). It is well known that PrP(106-126) interacts with phospholipid membranes even as a monomeric peptide, with lipid composition playing a role both in interaction and post-binding events. For example, PrP(106-126) has been shown to cause the aggregation of liposomes containing the ganglioside GM1 (Kurganov et al. 2004). While there is no direct link to the disruption of calcium channels or activation of the JNK-c-jun pathway, current evidence supports direct membrane interaction and disruption as a mechanism for PrP(106-126) cytotoxicity - at least in the absence of cell surface PrP. While unlikely in the face of recent studies for Aβ oligomers that show that structural alterations of the membrane are sufficient to increase conductance without requiring channels, rearrangement of the protein in the membrane to form discrete pores or channels cannot be ruled out (Eliezer 2006; Sokolov et al. 2006).

In terms of the structure-function relationship of PrP(106-126) oligomers, the similarities between the peptide subunits within the oligomeric and fibrillar forms of this protein are reminiscent of the large oligomers of Aβ(1-40) described by Chimon *et al.* (Chimon et al. 2007). Similar to one of the hypotheses proposed for Aβ, the insertion of small fibril fragments into the membrane may directly disrupt the membrane, nucleate the assembly of membrane-disruptive amyloid fibrils, or potentially rearrange into a toroidal or barrel stave type pore. In either case, the structural data supports the possibility of a common mechanism of action linking large spherical oligomers of Aβ and PrP(106-126).

4.3 α-synuclein toxicity

The toxicity associated with α-synuclein appears to be slightly different than other amyloid systems. To start with, α-synuclein is significantly larger (140 amino acids) than Aβ (40 or 42 residues), amylin (37 residues), or many other amyloidogenic proteins. Additionally, in its native state α-synuclein is intrinsically disordered, gaining α-helical structure upon binding to phospholipid membranes (Weinreb et al. 1996; Eliezer et al. 2001; Ulmer et al. 2005). In Parkinson's disease, α-synuclein forms β-sheet rich aggregates, culminating in the formation of amyloid fibrils (Lashuel et al. 2002; Lashuel et al. 2002). Not surprisingly, given its innate propensity to interact with membranes, the cytotoxic oligomers of α-synuclein have been shown to physically alter the conductance of planar bilayer membranes, presumably through the formation of pores (Kim et al. 2009). Multiple conductance levels were observed upon addition of these spherical, 15-30 nm diameter oligomers to lipid bilayers. The conductance profiles were similar to those observed for bee-venom mellitin, further supporting the formation of amyloid pores by these oligomers. Intriguingly, these pore-forming α-synuclein oligomers were recognized by the A11 antibody, which is specific for prefibrillar oligomers, suggesting that there are some common structural features shared with other amyloid oligomers, and providing an additional argument in favor of direct membrane disruption by prefibrillar oligomers.

5. Conclusion

It is clear that despite significant advances in the past decade, the link between accumulation of amyloidogenic proteins as β-sheet rich oligomers and disease pathogenesis remains somewhat unclear. In particular, the mechanism or mechanisms through which various non-fibrillar oligomers are capable of inducing cell death remain to be unambiguously determined. This is inextricably linked to questions of disease relevance - do all of the oligomers observed *in vitro* play a role in cell death during amyloidosis, and do they act through the same mechanisms? While the concept of a common mechanism of amyloid toxicity is attractive, given the broad range of cellular and tissue level effects reported to date, it may represent an oversimplification of a complex system.

Certainly it is possible that despite some common structural motifs and a shared ability to physically disrupt membranes, different oligomeric species formed by different amyloid proteins may exert a range of activities, all leading to the same effective endpoint - cell death and degenerative disease progression. Additional questions surround the fibril-like structures observed in most toxic amyloid oligomers described to date. Does this relate to studies showing that fragmentation of amyloid fibrils can create cytotoxic, membrane disrupting species, or are these fibril fragments acting via distinct pathways from prefibrillar oligomers? Ongoing efforts in structure determination of oligomers formed by different amyloid proteins, and in defining the molecular mechanisms for their cytotoxicity, will be required in order to address these important questions and to elucidate the link between structure and toxic function.

6. References

Ahmed, M., Davis, J., Aucoin, D., Sato, T., Ahuja, S., Aimoto, S., Elliott, J. I., Van Nostrand, W. E. and Smith, S. O. (2010). Structural conversion of neurotoxic amyloid-beta(1-42) oligomers to fibrils. *Nature Structural and Molecular Biology,* Vol. 17, No. 5, (May 2010), pp. 561-7, ISSN 1545-9985.

Arispe, N. (2004). Architecture of the Alzheimer's A beta P ion channel pore. *Journal of Membrane Biology,* Vol. 197, No. 1, (Jan 2004), pp. 33-48, ISSN 0022-2631.

Baglioni, S., Casamenti, F., Bucciantini, M., Luheshi, L. M., Taddei, N., Chiti, F., Dobson, C. M. and Stefani, M. (2006). Prefibrillar amyloid aggregates could be generic toxins in higher organisms. *Journal of Neuroscience,* Vol. 26, No. 31, (Aug 2006), pp. 8160-7, ISSN 1529-2401.

Balbach, J. J., Ishii, Y., Antzutkin, O. N., Leapman, R. D., Rizzo, N. W., Dyda, F., Reed, J. and Tycko, R. (2000). Amyloid fibril formation by A beta 16-22, a seven-residue fragment of the Alzheimer's beta-amyloid peptide, and structural characterization by solid state NMR. *Biochemistry,* Vol. 39, No. 45, (Nov 2000), pp. 13748-59, ISSN 0006-2960.

Baskakov, I. V., Legname, G., Baldwin, M. A., Prusiner, S. B. and Cohen, F. E. (2002). Pathway complexity of prion protein assembly into amyloid. *Journal of Biological Chemistry,* Vol. 277, No. 24, (Jun 2002), pp. 21140-8, ISSN 0021-9258.

Baskakov, I. V., Legname, G., Prusiner, S. B. and Cohen, F. E. (2001). Folding of prion protein to its native alpha-helical conformation is under kinetic control. *Journal of Biological Chemistry,* Vol. 276, No. 23, (Jun 2001), pp. 19687-90, ISSN 0021-9258.

Baxa, U., Wickner, R. B., Steven, A. C., Anderson, D. E., Marekov, L. N., Yau, W. M. and Tycko, R. (2007). Characterization of beta-sheet structure in Ure2p1-89 yeast prion fibrils by solid-state nuclear magnetic resonance. *Biochemistry,* Vol. 46, No. 45, (Nov 2007), pp. 13149-13162, ISSN 0006-2960.

Brown, D. R. (1998). Prion protein-overexpressing cells show altered response to a neurotoxic prion protein peptide. *Journal of Neuroscience Research,* Vol. 54, No. 3, (Nov 1998), pp. 331-40, ISSN 0360-4012.

Bucciantini, M., Giannoni, E., Chiti, F., Baroni, F., Formigli, L., Zurdo, J., Taddei, N., Ramponi, G., Dobson, C. M. and Stefani, M. (2002). Inherent toxicity of aggregates implies a common mechanism for protein misfolding diseases. *Nature,* Vol. 416, No. 6880, (Apr 2002), pp. 507-11, ISSN 0028-0836.

Burdick, D., Soreghan, B., Kwon, M., Kosmoski, J., Knauer, M., Henschen, A., Yates, J., Cotman, C. and Glabe, C. (1992). Assembly and aggregation properties of synthetic Alzheimer's A4/beta amyloid peptide analogs. *Journal of Biological Chemistry,* Vol. 267, No. 1, (Jan 1992), pp. 546-54, ISSN 0021-9258.

Carimalo, J., Cronier, S., Petit, G., Peyrin, J. M., Boukhtouche, F., Arbez, N., Lemaigre-Dubreuil, Y., Brugg, B. and Miquel, M. C. (2005). Activation of the JNK-c-Jun pathway during the early phase of neuronal apoptosis induced by PrP106-126 and prion infection. *European Journal of Neuroscience,* Vol. 21, No. 9, (May 2005), pp. 2311-9, ISSN 0953-816X.

Chan, J. C. Solid-State NMR Techniques for the Structural Determination of Amyloid Fibrils. *Topics in Current Chemistry,* Vol. 2011, (Jun pp. 1, ISSN 0340-1022.

Cheng, H. M., Tsai, T. W., Huang, W. Y., Lee, H. K., Lian, H. Y., Chou, F. C., Mou, Y. and Chan, J. C. (2011). Steric Zipper Formed by Hydrophobic Peptide Fragment of Syrian Hamster Prion Protein. *Biochemistry,* Vol. 50, No. 32, (Aug 2011), pp. 13, ISSN 1520-4995.

Cheon, M., Chang, I., Mohanty, S., Luheshi, L. M., Dobson, C. M., Vendruscolo, M. and Favrin, G. (2007). Structural reorganisation and potential toxicity of oligomeric species formed during the assembly of amyloid fibrils. *PLoS Computational Biology,* Vol. 3, No. 9, (Sep 2007), pp. 1727-38, ISSN 1553-7358.

Chimon, S. and Ishii, Y. (2005). Capturing intermediate structures of Alzheimer's beta-amyloid, Abeta(1-40), by solid-state NMR spectroscopy. *Journal of the American Chemical Society,* Vol. 127, No. 39, (Oct 2005), pp. 13472-3, ISSN 0002-7863.

Chimon, S., Shaibat, M. A., Jones, C. R., Calero, D. C., Aizezi, B. and Ishii, Y. (2007). Evidence of fibril-like beta-sheet structures in a neurotoxic amyloid intermediate of Alzheimer's beta-amyloid. *Nature Structural and Molecular Biology,* Vol. 14, No. 12, (Dec 2007), pp. 1157-1164, ISSN 1545-9985.

Cleary, J. P., Walsh, D. M., Hofmeister, J. J., Shankar, G. M., Kuskowski, M. A., Selkoe, D. J. and Ashe, K. H. (2005). Natural oligomers of the amyloid-beta protein specifically disrupt cognitive function. *Nature Neuroscience,* Vol. 8, No. 1, (Jan 2005), pp. 79-84, ISSN 1097-6256.

Cobb, N. J., Sonnichsen, F. D., McHaourab, H. and Surewicz, W. K. (2007). Molecular architecture of human prion protein amyloid: a parallel, in-register beta-structure. *Proceedings of the National Academy of Sciences of the United States of America,* Vol. 104, No. 48, (Nov 2007), pp. 18946-51, ISSN 1091-6490.

Conway, K. A., Harper, J. D. and Lansbury, P. T., Jr. (2000). Fibrils formed in vitro from alpha-synuclein and two mutant forms linked to Parkinson's disease are typical amyloid. *Biochemistry,* Vol. 39, No. 10, (Mar 2000), pp. 2552-63, ISSN 0006-2960.

Cooper, G. J., Willis, A. C., Clark, A., Turner, R. C., Sim, R. B. and Reid, K. B. (1987). Purification and characterization of a peptide from amyloid-rich pancreases of type

2 diabetic patients. *Proceedings of the National Academy of Sciences of the United States of America,* Vol. 84, No. 23, (Dec 1987), pp. 8628-32, ISSN 0027-8424.

Deli, M. A., Sakaguchi, S., Nakaoke, R., Abraham, C. S., Takahata, H., Kopacek, J., Shigematsu, K., Katamine, S. and Niwa, M. (2000). PrP fragment 106-126 is toxic to cerebral endothelial cells expressing PrP(C). *Neuroreport,* Vol. 11, No. 17, (Nov 2000), pp. 3931-6, ISSN 0959-4965.

Demuro, A., Mina, E., Kayed, R., Milton, S. C., Parker, I. and Glabe, C. G. (2005). Calcium dysregulation and membrane disruption as a ubiquitous neurotoxic mechanism of soluble amyloid oligomers. *Journal of Biological Chemistry,* Vol. 280, No. 17, (Apr 2005), pp. 17294-300, ISSN 0021-9258.

Eanes, E. D. and Glenner, G. G. (1968). X-ray diffraction studies on amyloid filaments. *Journal of Histochemistry & Cytochemistry,* Vol. 16, No. 11, (Nov 1968), pp. 673-7, ISSN 0022-1554.

Eliezer, D. (2006). Amyloid ion channels: a porous argument or a thin excuse? *The Journal of General Physiology,* Vol. 128, No. 6, (Dec 2006), pp. 631-3, ISSN 0022-1295.

Eliezer, D., Kutluay, E., Bussell, R., Jr. and Browne, G. (2001). Conformational properties of alpha-synuclein in its free and lipid-associated states. *Journal of Molecular Biology,* Vol. 307, No. 4, (Apr 2001), pp. 1061-73, ISSN 0022-2836.

Fandrich, M., Meinhardt, J. and Grigorieff, N. (2009). Structural polymorphism of Alzheimer Abeta and other amyloid fibrils. *Prion,* Vol. 3, No. 2, (Apr 2009), pp. 89-93, ISSN 1933-6896.

Ferreiro, E., Oliveira, C. R. and Pereira, C. M. (2008). The release of calcium from the endoplasmic reticulum induced by amyloid-beta and prion peptides activates the mitochondrial apoptotic pathway. *Neurobiology of Disease,* Vol. 30, No. 3, (Jun 2008), pp. 331-42, ISSN 1095-953X.

Florio, T., Thellung, S., Amico, C., Robello, M., Salmona, M., Bugiani, O., Tagliavini, F., Forloni, G. and Schettini, G. (1998). Prion protein fragment 106-126 induces apoptotic cell death and impairment of L-type voltage-sensitive calcium channel activity in the GH3 cell line. *Journal of Neuroscience Research,* Vol. 54, No. 3, (Nov 1998), pp. 341-52, ISSN 0360-4012.

Forloni, G., Angeretti, N., Chiesa, R., Monzani, E., Salmona, M., Bugiani, O. and Tagliavini, F. (1993). Neurotoxicity of a prion protein fragment. *Nature,* Vol. 362, No. 6420, (Apr 1993), pp. 543-6, ISSN 0028-0836.

Geddes, A. J., Parker, K. D., Atkins, E. D. and Beighton, E. (1968). "Cross-beta" conformation in proteins. *Journal of Molecular Biology,* Vol. 32, No. 2, (Mar 1968), pp. 343-58, ISSN 0022-2836.

Glenner, G. G. and Wong, C. W. (1984). Alzheimer's disease: initial report of the purification and characterization of a novel cerebrovascular amyloid protein. *Biochemical and Biophysical Research Communications,* Vol. 120, No. 3, (May 1984), pp. 885-90, ISSN 0006-291X.

Govaerts, C., Wille, H., Prusiner, S. B. and Cohen, F. E. (2004). Evidence for assembly of prions with left-handed beta-helices into trimers. *Proceedings of the National Academy of Sciences of the United States of America,* Vol. 101, No. 22, (Jun 2004), pp. 8342-7, ISSN 0027-8424.

Gu, Y., Fujioka, H., Mishra, R. S., Li, R. and Singh, N. (2002). Prion peptide 106-126 modulates the aggregation of cellular prion protein and induces the synthesis of potentially neurotoxic transmembrane PrP. *Journal of Biological Chemistry,* Vol. 277, No. 3, (Jan 2002), pp. 2275-86, ISSN 0021-9258.

Haass, C. and Selkoe, D. J. (2007). Soluble protein oligomers in neurodegeneration: lessons from the Alzheimer's amyloid beta-peptide. *Nature Reviews Molecular Cell Biology,* Vol. 8, No. 2, (Feb 2007), pp. 101-12, ISSN 1471-0072.

Heise, H., Hoyer, W., Becker, S., Andronesi, O. C., Riedel, D. and Baldus, M. (2005). Molecular-level secondary structure, polymorphism, and dynamics of full-length alpha-synuclein fibrils studied by solid-state NMR. *Proceedings of the National Academy of Sciences of the United States of America,* Vol. 102, No. 44, (Nov 2005), pp. 15871-6, ISSN 0027-8424.

Hong, D. P., Fink, A. L. and Uversky, V. N. (2008). Structural characteristics of alpha-synuclein oligomers stabilized by the flavonoid baicalein. *Journal of Molecular Biology,* Vol. 383, No. 1, (Oct 2008), pp. 214-23, ISSN 1089-8638.

Huang, T. H., Yang, D. S., Plaskos, N. P., Go, S., Yip, C. M., Fraser, P. E. and Chakrabartty, A. (2000). Structural studies of soluble oligomers of the Alzheimer beta-amyloid peptide. *Journal of Molecular Biology,* Vol. 297, No. 1, (Mar 2000), pp. 73-87, ISSN 0022-2836.

Jahn, T. R., Makin, O. S., Morris, K. L., Marshall, K. E., Tian, P., Sikorski, P. and Serpell, L. C. (2009). The common architecture of cross-beta amyloid. *Journal of Molecular Biology,* Vol. 395, No. 4, (Jan 2009), pp. 717-27, ISSN 1089-8638.

Jang, H., Zheng, J. and Nussinov, R. (2007). Models of beta-amyloid ion channels in the membrane suggest that channel formation in the bilayer is a dynamic process. *Biophysical Journal,* Vol. 93, No. 6, (Sep 2007), pp. 1938-49, ISSN 0006-3495.

Janson, J., Ashley, R. H., Harrison, D., McIntyre, S. and Butler, P. C. (1999). The mechanism of islet amyloid polypeptide toxicity is membrane disruption by intermediate-sized toxic amyloid particles. *Diabetes,* Vol. 48, No. 3, (Mar 1999), pp. 491-8, ISSN 0012-1797.

Jaroniec, C. P., MacPhee, C. E., Astrof, N. S., Dobson, C. M. and Griffin, R. G. (2002). Molecular conformation of a peptide fragment of transthyretin in an amyloid fibril. *Proceedings of the National Academy of Sciences of the United States of America,* Vol. 99, No. 26, (Dec 2002), pp. 16748-53, ISSN 0027-8424.

Jaroniec, C. P., MacPhee, C. E., Bajaj, V. S., McMahon, M. T., Dobson, C. M. and Griffin, R. G. (2004). High-resolution molecular structure of a peptide in an amyloid fibril determined by magic angle spinning NMR spectroscopy. *Proceedings of the National Academy of Sciences of the United States of America,* Vol. 101, No. 3, (Jan 2004), pp. 711-6, ISSN 0027-8424.

Jarrett, J. T., Berger, E. P. and Lansbury, P. T., Jr. (1993). The carboxy terminus of the beta amyloid protein is critical for the seeding of amyloid formation: implications for the pathogenesis of Alzheimer's disease. *Biochemistry,* Vol. 32, No. 18, (May 1993), pp. 4693-7, ISSN 0006-2960.

Jobling, M. F., Stewart, L. R., White, A. R., McLean, C., Friedhuber, A., Maher, F., Beyreuther, K., Masters, C. L., Barrow, C. J., Collins, S. J. and Cappai, R. (1999). The hydrophobic core sequence modulates the neurotoxic and secondary structure properties of the prion peptide 106-126. *Journal of Neurochemistry,* Vol. 73, No. 4, (Oct 1999), pp. 1557-1565, ISSN 0022-3042.

Kayed, R., Head, E., Sarsoza, F., Saing, T., Cotman, C. W., Necula, M., Margol, L., Wu, J., Breydo, L., Thompson, J. L., Rasool, S., Gurlo, T., Butler, P. and Glabe, C. G. (2007). Fibril specific, conformation dependent antibodies recognize a generic epitope common to amyloid fibrils and fibrillar oligomers that is absent in prefibrillar oligomers. *Molecular Neurodegeneration,* Vol. 2, No. 2, (Sept 2007), pp. 18, ISSN 1750-1326.

Kayed, R., Head, E., Thompson, J. L., McIntire, T. M., Milton, S. C., Cotman, C. W. and Glabe, C. G. (2003). Common structure of soluble amyloid oligomers implies common mechanism of pathogenesis. *Science,* Vol. 300, No. 5618, (Apr 2003), pp. 486-9, ISSN 1095-9203.

Kayed, R., Pensalfini, A., Margol, L., Sokolov, Y., Sarsoza, F., Head, E., Hall, J. and Glabe, C. (2009). Annular protofibrils are a structurally and functionally distinct type of amyloid oligomer. *Journal of Biological Chemistry,* Vol. 284, No. 7, (Feb 2009), pp. 4230-7, ISSN 0021-9258.

Kayed, R., Sokolov, Y., Edmonds, B., McIntire, T. M., Milton, S. C., Hall, J. E. and Glabe, C. G. (2004). Permeabilization of lipid bilayers is a common conformation-dependent activity of soluble amyloid oligomers in protein misfolding diseases. *Journal of Biological Chemistry,* Vol. 279, No. 45, (Nov 2004), pp. 46363-6, ISSN 0021-9258.

Khan, M. Q., Sweeting, B., Mulligan, V. K., Arslan, P. E., Cashman, N. R., Pai, E. F. and Chakrabartty, A. (2010). Prion disease susceptibility is affected by beta-structure folding propensity and local side-chain interactions in PrP. *Proceedings of the National Academy of Sciences of the United States of America,* Vol. 107, No. 46, (Nov 2010), pp. 19808-13, ISSN 1091-6490.

Kim, H. Y., Cho, M. K., Kumar, A., Maier, E., Siebenhaar, C., Becker, S., Fernandez, C. O., Lashuel, H. A., Benz, R., Lange, A. and Zweckstetter, M. (2009). Structural Properties of Pore-Forming Oligomers of alpha-Synuclein. *Journal of the American Chemical Society,* Vol. 4, (Nov 2009), pp. 4, ISSN 1520-5126.

Kumar-Singh, S., Theuns, J., Van Broeck, B., Pirici, D., Vennekens, K., Corsmit, E., Cruts, M., Dermaut, B., Wang, R. and Van Broeckhoven, C. (2006). Mean age-of-onset of familial alzheimer disease caused by presenilin mutations correlates with both increased Abeta42 and decreased Abeta40. *Human Mutation,* Vol. 27, No. 7, (Jul 2006), pp. 686-95, ISSN 1098-1004.

Kurganov, B., Doh, M. and Arispe, N. (2004). Aggregation of liposomes induced by the toxic peptides Alzheimer's Abs, human amylin and prion(106-126): facilitation by membrane-bound G_{M1} ganglioside. *Peptides,* Vol. 25, No. 2, 2004), pp. 217-232, ISSN 0196-9781.

Lambert, M. P., Barlow, A. K., Chromy, B. A., Edwards, C., Freed, R., Liosatos, M., Morgan, T. E., Rozovsky, I., Trommer, B., Viola, K. L., Wals, P., Zhang, C., Finch, C. E., Krafft, G. A. and Klein, W. L. (1998). Diffusible, nonfibrillar ligands derived from Abeta1-42 are potent central nervous system neurotoxins. *Proceedings of the National Academy of Sciences of the United States of America,* Vol. 95, No. 11, (May 26 1998), pp. 6448-53, ISSN 0027-8424.

Lashuel, H. A., Hartley, D., Petre, B. M., Walz, T. and Lansbury, P. T., Jr. (2002). Neurodegenerative disease: amyloid pores from pathogenic mutations. *Nature,* Vol. 418, No. 6895, (Jul 2002), pp. 291, ISSN 0028-0836.

Lashuel, H. A., Petre, B. M., Wall, J., Simon, M., Nowak, R. J., Walz, T. and Lansbury, P. T., Jr. (2002). Alpha-synuclein, especially the Parkinson's disease-associated mutants, forms pore-like annular and tubular protofibrils. *Journal of Molecular Biology,* Vol. 322, No. 5, (Oct 2002), pp. 1089-102, ISSN 0022-2836.

Lauren, J., Gimbel, D. A., Nygaard, H. B., Gilbert, J. W. and Strittmatter, S. M. (2009). Cellular prion protein mediates impairment of synaptic plasticity by amyloid-beta oligomers. *Nature,* Vol. 457, No. 7233, (Feb 2009), pp. 1128-32, ISSN 1476-4687.

Laurents, D. V., Gorman, P. M., Guo, M., Rico, M., Chakrabartty, A. and Bruix, M. (2005). Alzheimer's Abeta40 studied by NMR at low pH reveals that sodium 4,4-dimethyl-4-silapentane-1-sulfonate (DSS) binds and promotes beta-ball oligomerization. *Journal of Biological Chemistry,* Vol. 280, No. 5, (Feb 2005), pp. 3675-85, ISSN 0021-9258.

Lee, S. W., Mou, Y., Lin, S. Y., Chou, F. C., Tseng, W. H., Chen, C. H., Lu, C. Y., Yu, S. S. and Chan, J. C. (2008). Steric zipper of the amyloid fibrils formed by residues 109-122 of the Syrian hamster prion protein. *Journal of Molecular Biology,* Vol. 378, No. 5, (May 2008), pp. 1142-54, ISSN 1089-8638.

Lin, H., Bhatia, R. and Lal, R. (2001). Amyloid beta protein forms ion channels: implications for Alzheimer's disease pathophysiology. *FASEB Journal,* Vol. 15, No. 13, (Nov 2001), pp. 2433-44, ISSN 1530-6860.

Lin, M. C., Mirzabekov, T. and Kagan, B. L. (1997). Channel formation by a neurotoxic prion protein fragment. *Journal of Biological Chemistry,* Vol. 272, No. 1, (Jan 1997), pp. 44-7, ISSN 0021-9258.

Losic, D., Martin, L. L., Mechler, A., Aguilar, M. I. and Small, D. H. (2006). High resolution scanning tunnelling microscopy of the beta-amyloid protein (Abeta1-40) of Alzheimer's disease suggests a novel mechanism of oligomer assembly. *Journal of Structural Biology,* Vol. 155, No. 1, (Jul 2006), pp. 104-10, ISSN 1047-8477.

Luca, S., Yau, W. M., Leapman, R. and Tycko, R. (2007). Peptide conformation and supramolecular organization in amylin fibrils: constraints from solid-state NMR. *Biochemistry,* Vol. 46, No. 47, (Nov 2007), pp. 13505-22, ISSN 0006-2960.

Luhrs, T., Ritter, C., Adrian, M., Riek-Loher, D., Bohrmann, B., Dobeli, H., Schubert, D. and Riek, R. (2005). 3D structure of Alzheimer's amyloid-beta(1-42) fibrils. *Proceedings of the National Academy of Sciences of the United States of America,* Vol. 102, No. 48, (Nov 2005), pp. 17342-7, ISSN 0027-8424.

Madine, J., Jack, E., Stockley, P. G., Radford, S. E., Serpell, L. C. and Middleton, D. A. (2008). Structural insights into the polymorphism of amyloid-like fibrils formed by region 20-29 of amylin revealed by solid-state NMR and X-ray fiber diffraction. *Journal of the American Chemical Society,* Vol. 130, No. 45, (Nov 2008), pp. 14990-5001, ISSN 1520-5126.

McLaurin, J. and Chakrabartty, A. (1996). Membrane disruption by Alzheimer beta-amyloid peptides mediated through specific binding to either phospholipids or gangliosides. Implications for neurotoxicity. *Journal of Biological Chemistry,* Vol. 271, No. 43, (Oct 1996), pp. 26482-9, ISSN 0021-9258.

McLaurin, J. and Chakrabartty, A. (1997). Characterization of the interactions of Alzheimer beta-amyloid peptides with phospholipid membranes. *European Journal of Biochemistry,* Vol. 245, No. 2, (Apr 1997), pp. 355-63, ISSN 0014-2956.

Miller, Y., Ma, B., Tsai, C. J. and Nussinov, R. Hollow core of Alzheimer's Abeta42 amyloid observed by cryoEM is relevant at physiological pH. *Proceedings of the National Academy of Sciences of the United States of America,* Vol. 107, No. 32, (Aug pp. 14128-33, ISSN 1091-6490.

Naito, A., Kamihira, M., Inoue, R. and Saito, H. (2004). Structural diversity of amyloid fibril formed in human calcitonin as revealed by site-directed 13C solid-state NMR spectroscopy. *Magnetic Resonance in Chemistry,* Vol. 42, No. 2, (Feb 2004), pp. 247-57, ISSN 0749-1581.

Necula, M., Kayed, R., Milton, S. and Glabe, C. G. (2007). Small molecule inhibitors of aggregation indicate that amyloid beta oligomerization and fibrillization pathways are independent and distinct. *Journal of Biological Chemistry,* Vol. 282, No. 14, (Apr 2007), pp. 10311-24, ISSN 0021-9258.

Nielsen, J. T., Bjerring, M., Jeppesen, M. D., Pedersen, R. O., Pedersen, J. M., Hein, K. L., Vosegaard, T., Skrydstrup, T., Otzen, D. E. and Nielsen, N. C. (2009). Unique identification of supramolecular structures in amyloid fibrils by solid-state NMR spectroscopy. *Angewandte Chemie International Edition,* Vol. 48, No. 12, (Mar 2009), pp. 2118-21, ISSN 1521-3773.

Olofsson, A., Lindhagen-Persson, M., Sauer-Eriksson, A. E. and Ohman, A. (2007). Amide solvent protection analysis demonstrates that amyloid-beta(1-40) and amyloid-beta(1-42) form different fibrillar structures under identical conditions. *Biochemical Journal,* Vol. 404, No. 1, (May 2007), pp. 63-70, ISSN 1470-8728.

Ono, K., Condron, M. M. and Teplow, D. B. (2009). Structure-neurotoxicity relationships of amyloid beta-protein oligomers. *Proceedings of the National Academy of Sciences of the United States of America,* Vol. 106, No. 35, (Sep 2009), pp. 14745-50, ISSN 1091-6490.

Pan, J., Han, J., Borchers, C. H. and Konermann, L. (2011). Conformer-specific hydrogen exchange analysis of abeta(1-42) oligomers by top-down electron capture dissociation mass spectrometry. *Analytical Chemistry,* Vol. 83, No. 13, (Jul 2011), pp. 5386-93, ISSN 1520-6882.

Paravastu, A. K., Petkova, A. T. and Tycko, R. (2006). Polymorphic fibril formation by residues 10-40 of the Alzheimer's beta-amyloid peptide. *Biophysical Journal,* Vol. 90, No. 12, (Jun 2006), pp. 4618-29, ISSN 0006-3495.

Pastor, M. T., Kummerer, N., Schubert, V., Esteras-Chopo, A., Dotti, C. G., Lopez de la Paz, M. and Serrano, L. (2008). Amyloid toxicity is independent of polypeptide sequence, length and chirality. *Journal of Molecular Biology,* Vol. 375, No. 3, (Jan 2008), pp. 695-707, ISSN 1089-8638.

Petkova, A. T., Ishii, Y., Balbach, J. J., Antzutkin, O. N., Leapman, R. D., Delaglio, F. and Tycko, R. (2002). A structural model for Alzheimer's beta -amyloid fibrils based on experimental constraints from solid state NMR. *Proceedings of the National Academy of Sciences of the United States of America,* Vol. 99, No. 26, (Dec 2002), pp. 16742-7, ISSN 0027-8424.

Petkova, A. T., Leapman, R. D., Guo, Z., Yau, W. M., Mattson, M. P. and Tycko, R. (2005). Self-propagating, molecular-level polymorphism in Alzheimer's beta-amyloid fibrils. *Science,* Vol. 307, No. 5707, (Jan 2005), pp. 262-5, ISSN 1095-9203.

Prusiner, S. B. (1982). Novel proteinaceous infectious particles cause scrapie. *Science,* Vol. 216, No. 4542, (Apr 1982), pp. 136-44, ISSN 0036-8075.

Quist, A., Doudevski, I., Lin, H., Azimova, R., Ng, D., Frangione, B., Kagan, B., Ghiso, J. and Lal, R. (2005). Amyloid ion channels: a common structural link for protein-misfolding disease. *Proceedings of the National Academy of Sciences of the United States of America,* Vol. 102, No. 30, (Jul 2005), pp. 10427-32, ISSN 0027-8424.

Sachse, C., Fandrich, M. and Grigorieff, N. (2008). Paired beta-sheet structure of an Abeta(1-40) amyloid fibril revealed by electron microscopy. *Proceedings of the National Academy of Sciences of the United States of America,* Vol. 105, No. 21, (May 2008), pp. 7462-6, ISSN 1091-6490.

Salmona, M., Forloni, G., Diomede, L., Algeri, M., De Gioia, L., Angeretti, N., Giaccone, G., Tagliavini, F. and Bugiani, O. (1997). A neurotoxic and gliotrophic fragment of the prion protein increases plasma membrane microviscosity. *Neurobiology of Disease,* Vol. 4, No. 1, 1997), pp. 47-57, ISSN 0969-9961.

Salmona, M., Malesani, P., DeGioia, L., Gorla, S., Bruschi, M., Molinari, A., Della Vedova, F., Pedrotti, B., Marrari, M. A., Awan, T., Bugiani, O., Forloni, G. and Tagliavini, F. (1999). Molecular determinants of the physicochemical properties of a critical prion protein region comprising residues 106-126. *Biochemical Journal,* Vol. 342, (Aug 1999), pp. 207-214, ISSN 0264-6021.

Sawaya, M. R., Sambashivan, S., Nelson, R., Ivanova, M. I., Sievers, S. A., Apostol, M. I., Thompson, M. J., Balbirnie, M., Wiltzius, J. J., McFarlane, H. T., Madsen, A. O., Riekel, C. and Eisenberg, D. (2007). Atomic structures of amyloid cross-beta spines reveal varied steric zippers. *Nature,* Vol. 447, No. 7143, (May 2007), pp. 453-7, ISSN 1476-4687.

Schmidt, M., Sachse, C., Richter, W., Xu, C., Fandrich, M. and Grigorieff, N. (2009). Comparison of Alzheimer Abeta(1-40) and Abeta(1-42) amyloid fibrils reveals similar protofilament structures. *Proceedings of the National Academy of Sciences of the United States of America,* Vol. 106, No. 47, (Nov 2009), pp. 19813-8, ISSN 1091-6490.

Selvaggini, C., De Gioia, L., Cantu, L., Ghibaudi, E., Diomede, L., Passerini, F., Forloni, G., Bugiani, O., Tagliavini, F. and Salmona, M. (1993). Molecular characteristics of a protease-resistant, amyloidogenic and neurotoxic peptide homologous to residues 106-126 of the prion protein. *Biochemical and Biophysical Research Communications,* Vol. 194, No. 3, (Aug 1993), pp. 1380-6, ISSN 0006-291X.

Shewmaker, F., Wickner, R. B. and Tycko, R. (2006). Amyloid of the prion domain of Sup35p has an in-register parallel beta-sheet structure. *Proceedings of the National Academy of Sciences of the United States of America,* Vol. 103, No. 52, (Dec 2006), pp. 19754-9, ISSN 0027-8424.

Silei, V., Fabrizi, C., Venturini, G., Salmona, M., Bugiani, O., Tagliavini, F. and Lauro, G. M. (1999). Activation of microglial cells by PrP and beta-amyloid fragments raises intracellular calcium through L-type voltage sensitive calcium channels. *Brain Research,* Vol. 818, No. 1, 1999), pp. 168-170, ISSN 0006-8993.

Silveira, J. R., Raymond, G. J., Hughson, A. G., Race, R. E., Sim, V. L., Hayes, S. F. and Caughey, B. (2005). The most infectious prion protein particles. *Nature,* Vol. 437, No. 7056, (Sep 2005), pp. 257-61, ISSN 1476-4687.

Simoneau, S., Rezaei, H., Sales, N., Kaiser-Schulz, G., Lefebvre-Roque, M., Vidal, C., Fournier, J. G., Comte, J., Wopfner, F., Grosclaude, J., Schatzl, H. and Lasmezas, C. I. (2007). In vitro and in vivo neurotoxicity of prion protein oligomers. *PLoS Pathogens,* Vol. 3, No. 8, (Aug 2007), pp. e125, ISSN 1553-7374.

Snyder, E. M., Nong, Y., Almeida, C. G., Paul, S., Moran, T., Choi, E. Y., Nairn, A. C., Salter, M. W., Lombroso, P. J., Gouras, G. K. and Greengard, P. (2005). Regulation of NMDA receptor trafficking by amyloid-beta. *Nature Neuroscience,* Vol. 8, No. 8, (Aug 2005), pp. 1051-8, ISSN 1097-6256.

Sokolov, Y., Kozak, J. A., Kayed, R., Chanturiya, A., Glabe, C. and Hall, J. E. (2006). Soluble amyloid oligomers increase bilayer conductance by altering dielectric structure. *Journal of General Physiology,* Vol. 128, No. 6, (Dec 2006), pp. 637-47, ISSN 0022-1295.

Sokolowski, F., Modler, A. J., Masuch, R., Zirwer, D., Baier, M., Lutsch, G., Moss, D. A., Gast, K. and Naumann, D. (2003). Formation of critical oligomers is a key event during conformational transition of recombinant syrian hamster prion protein. *Journal of Biological Chemistry,* Vol. 278, No. 42, (Oct 2003), pp. 40481-92, ISSN 0021-9258.

Spillantini, M. G., Schmidt, M. L., Lee, V. M., Trojanowski, J. Q., Jakes, R. and Goedert, M. (1997). Alpha-synuclein in Lewy bodies. *Nature,* Vol. 388, No. 6645, (Aug 1997), pp. 839-40, ISSN 0028-0836.

Thellung, S., Florio, T., Villa, V., Corsaro, A., Arena, S., Amico, C., Robello, M., Salmona, M., Forloni, G., Bugiani, O., Tagliavini, F. and Schettini, G. (2000). Apoptotic cell death and impairment of L-type voltage-sensitive calcium channel activity in rat cerebellar granule cells treated with the prion protein fragment 106-126. *Neurobiology of Disease,* Vol. 7, No. 4, (Aug 2000), pp. 299-309, ISSN 0969-9961.

Tycko, R. (2011). Solid-state NMR studies of amyloid fibril structure. *Annu Rev Phys Chem,* Vol. 62, (May 2011), pp. 279-99, ISSN 0066-426X.

Tycko, R. and Ishii, Y. (2003). Constraints on supramolecular structure in amyloid fibrils from two-dimensional solid-state NMR spectroscopy with uniform isotopic labeling. *Journal of the American Chemical Society,* Vol. 125, No. 22, (Jun 2003), pp. 6606-7, ISSN 0002-7863.

Ulmer, T. S., Bax, A., Cole, N. B. and Nussbaum, R. L. (2005). Structure and dynamics of micelle-bound human alpha-synuclein. *Journal of Biological Chemistry,* Vol. 280, No. 10, (Mar 2005), pp. 9595-603, ISSN 0021-9258.

van der Wel, P. C., Lewandowski, J. R. and Griffin, R. G. (2007). Solid-state NMR study of amyloid nanocrystals and fibrils formed by the peptide GNNQQNY from yeast prion protein Sup35p. *Journal of the American Chemical Society,* Vol. 129, No. 16, (Apr 2007), pp. 5117-30, ISSN 0002-7863.

van der Wel, P. C., Lewandowski, J. R. and Griffin, R. G. (2007). Structural characterization of GNNQQNY amyloid fibrils by magic angle spinning NMR. *Biochemistry,* Vol. 49, No. 44, (Nov 2007), pp. 9457-69, ISSN 1520-4995.

Verdier, Y. and Penke, B. (2004). Binding sites of amyloid beta-peptide in cell plasma membrane and implications for Alzheimer's disease. *Current Protein & Peptide Science,* Vol. 5, No. 1, (Feb 2004), pp. 19-31, ISSN 1389-2037.

Verdier, Y., Zarandi, M. and Penke, B. (2004). Amyloid beta-peptide interactions with neuronal and glial cell plasma membrane: binding sites and implications for Alzheimer's disease. *Journal of Peptide Science,* Vol. 10, No. 5, (May 2004), pp. 229-48, ISSN 1075-2617.

Vilar, M., Chou, H. T., Luhrs, T., Maji, S. K., Riek-Loher, D., Verel, R., Manning, G., Stahlberg, H. and Riek, R. (2008). The fold of alpha-synuclein fibrils. *Proceedings of the National Academy of Sciences of the United States of America,* Vol. 105, No. 25, (Jun 2008), pp. 8637-42, ISSN 1091-6490.

Walsh, D. M. and Selkoe, D. J. (2004). Oligomers on the brain: the emerging role of soluble protein aggregates in neurodegeneration. *Protein & Peptide Letters,* Vol. 11, No. 3, (Jun 2004), pp. 213-28, ISSN 0929-8665.

Walsh, D. M. and Selkoe, D. J. (2007). A beta oligomers - a decade of discovery. *Journal of Neurochemistry,* Vol. 101, No. 5, (Jun 2007), pp. 1172-84, ISSN 0022-3042.

Walsh, P., Neudecker, P. and Sharpe, S. (2010). Structural Properties and Dynamic Behavior of Nonfibrillar Oligomers Formed by PrP(106-126). *Journal of the American Chemical Society,* Vol. 132, No. 22, (Jun 2010), pp. 7684-7695, ISSN 0002-7863.

Walsh, P., Simonetti, K. and Sharpe, S. (2009). Core structure of amyloid fibrils formed by residues 106-126 of the human prion protein. *Structure,* Vol. 17, No. 3, (Mar 2009), pp. 417-426, ISSN 0969-2126 (Print).

Walsh, P., Yau, J., Simonetti, K. and Sharpe, S. (2009). Morphology and Secondary Structure of Stable β-Oligomers Formed by Amyloid Peptide PrP(106-126). *Biochemistry,* Vol. 48, No. 25, (Jun 2009), pp. 5779-5781, ISSN 0969-2126.

Wasmer, C., Lange, A., Van Melckebeke, H., Siemer, A. B., Riek, R. and Meier, B. H. (2008). Amyloid fibrils of the HET-s(218-289) prion form a beta solenoid with a triangular hydrophobic core. *Science,* Vol. 319, No. 5869, (Mar 2008), pp. 1523-6, ISSN 1095-9203.

Weinreb, P. H., Zhen, W., Poon, A. W., Conway, K. A. and Lansbury, P. T., Jr. (1996). NACP, a protein implicated in Alzheimer's disease and learning, is natively unfolded. *Biochemistry,* Vol. 35, No. 43, (Oct 1996), pp. 13709-15, ISSN 0006-2960.

Williams, A. D., Sega, M., Chen, M., Kheterpal, I., Geva, M., Berthelier, V., Kaleta, D. T., Cook, K. D. and Wetzel, R. (2005). Structural properties of Abeta protofibrils stabilized by a small molecule. *Proceedings of the National Academy of Sciences of the United States of America,* Vol. 102, No. 20, (May 2005), pp. 7115-20, ISSN 0027-8424.

Xue, W. F., Hellewell, A. L., Gosal, W. S., Homans, S. W., Hewitt, E. W. and Radford, S. E. (2009). Fibril fragmentation enhances amyloid cytotoxicity. *Journal of Biological Chemistry,* Vol. 284, No. 49, (Dec 2009), pp. 34272-82, ISSN 1083-351X.

Yankner, B. A. and Lu, T. (2009). Amyloid beta-protein toxicity and the pathogenesis of Alzheimer disease. *Journal of Biological Chemistry,* Vol. 284, No. 8, (Feb 2009), pp. 4755-9, ISSN 0021-9258.

Yip, C. M., Darabie, A. A. and McLaurin, J. (2002). Abeta42-peptide assembly on lipid bilayers. *Journal of Molecular Biology,* Vol. 318, No. 1, (Apr 2002), pp. 97-107, ISSN 0022-2836.

Yu, L., Edalji, R., Harlan, J. E., Holzman, T. F., Lopez, A. P., Labkovsky, B., Hillen, H., Barghorn, S., Ebert, U., Richardson, P. L., Miesbauer, L., Solomon, L., Bartley, D., Walter, K., Johnson, R. W., Hajduk, P. J. and Olejniczak, E. T. (2009). Structural Characterization of a Soluble Amyloid beta-Peptide Oligomer. *Biochemistry,* Vol. 48, No. 9, (Feb 2009), pp. 1870-1877, ISSN 1520-4995.

Yu, X., Wang, Q. and Zheng, J. (2010). Structural determination of Abeta25-35 micelles by molecular dynamics simulations. *Biophysical Journal,* Vol. 99, No. 2, (Jul 2010), pp. 666-74, ISSN 1542-0086.

Yu, X. and Zheng, J. (2011). Polymorphic Structures of Alzheimer's beta-Amyloid Globulomers. *PLoS One,* Vol. 6, No. 6, (Jun 2011), pp. e20575, ISSN 1932-6203.

Zhang, A., Qi, W., Good, T. A. and Fernandez, E. J. (2009). Structural differences between Abeta(1-40) intermediate oligomers and fibrils elucidated by proteolytic fragmentation and hydrogen/deuterium exchange. *Biophysical Journal,* Vol. 96, No. 3, (Feb 2009), pp. 1091-104, ISSN 1542-0086.

Zhang, R., Hu, X., Khant, H., Ludtke, S. J., Chiu, W., Schmid, M. F., Frieden, C. and Lee, J. M. (2009). Interprotofilament interactions between Alzheimer's Abeta1-42 peptides in amyloid fibrils revealed by cryoEM. *Proceedings of the National Academy of Sciences of the United States of America,* Vol. 106, No. 12, (Mar 2009), pp. 4653-8, ISSN 1091-6490.

Zheng, J., Jang, H., Ma, B. and Nussinov, R. (2008). Annular structures as intermediates in fibril formation of Alzheimer Abeta17-42. *Journal of Physical Chemistry B,* Vol. 112, No. 22, (Jun 2008), pp. 6856-65, ISSN 1520-6106.

Zhu, M., Rajamani, S., Kaylor, J., Han, S., Zhou, F. and Fink, A. L. (2004). The flavonoid baicalein inhibits fibrillation of alpha-synuclein and disaggregates existing fibrils. *Journal of Biological Chemistry,* Vol. 279, No. 26, (Jun 2004), pp. 26846-57, ISSN 0021-9258.

5

Disruption of Calcium Homeostasis in Alzheimer's Disease: Role of Channel Formation by β Amyloid Protein

Masahiro Kawahara[1], Hironari Koyama[1], Susumu Ohkawara[1] and Midori Negishi-Kato[2]
[1]*Department of Analytical Chemistry, School of Pharmaceutical Sciences, Kyushu University of Health and Welfare,*
[2]*Institute of Industrial Science (IIS), The University of Tokyo, Japan*

1. Introduction

Alzheimer's disease (AD) is a severe senile type of dementia that affects a large number of elderly people. It is estimated that 5.4 million people in the worldwide are affected by this disease in 2011 and this number continues to grow yearly. AD is characterized by profound memory loss and severe cognitive decline. The pathological hallmarks of AD are the presence of numerous extracellular deposits termed senile plaques and intraneuronal neurofibrillary tangles (NFTs) (Selkoe, 1991). The selective loss of synapses and neurons is observed in the brain of patients, and this decrease in the number of synapses is strongly correlated with memory impairment (Terry et al., 1991). The major component of NFTs is the phosphorylated tau protein, while β-amyloid protein (AβP) is the major component of senile plaques.

Although the pathological cause of AD has not yet strictly been elucidated, numerous biochemical, toxicological, cell biological, and genetic studies have supported the "amyloid cascade hypothesis", which suggests that the neurotoxicity and synaptotoxicity (synaptic degeneration) caused by AβP play a central role in AD (Hardy & selkoe, 2002). Moreover, oligomerization and conformational changes in AβP are important for its neurodegenerative capacity.

There is considerable interest regarding the mechanism by which AβPs cause neurodegeneration. AβPs reportedly cause numerous adverse effects on neuronal survival, e.g., reactive oxygen species (ROS) production, cytokine induction, endoplasmic reticulum (ER) stresses induction, and the abnormal increase in intracellular Ca^{2+} levels ($[Ca^{2+}]_i$) (Small et al., 2001). These adverse effects are complex and may be interwoven. Among them, the disruption of Ca^{2+} homeostasis could be the primary event in the pathogenesis of AD, since Ca^{2+} ions play critical roles in the function and structure of neurons and other cells. Increasing evidence suggests the implications of Ca^{2+} dyshomeostasis in the pathogenesis of AD (Green and LaFerla, 2008; Demuro et al., 2010).

Several possible mechanisms account for AβP-induced Ca^{2+} dyshomeostasis, e.g., its interaction with endogenous Ca^{2+}-permeable ion channels, disruption of membrane integrity, and the formation of Ca^{2+} permeable channels (pores) by the direct incorporation of AβP into membranes. Here, we focus on the 'amyloid channel hypothesis' (Arispe et al., 2007; Lin et al. 2001; Kawahara, 2011b), namely, that the direct incorporation of AβPs and the subsequent imbalances of Ca^{2+} and other ions through amyloid channels may be the primary event in AßP neurotoxicity.
In this chapter, we review the current understanding of the link between Ca^{2+} homeostasis and AD pathogenesis based on the amyloid channel hypothesis the characteristics of AβP-induced neurotoxicity and synaptotoxicity caused by Ca^{2+} dyshomeostasis *via* amyloid channels. We also discuss the possible development of new drugs for the treatment and prevention of AD by attenuating amyloid channels and inhibiting AβP-induced Ca^{2+} dyshomeostasis.

2. Amyloid cascade hypothesis

AβP is a small peptide with 39–43 amino acid residues. It is derived from the proteolytic cleavage of a large precursor protein (amyloid precursor protein; APP) by the cleavage of its N-terminal by β-secretase (BACE), followed by the intra-membrane cleavage of its C-terminal by γ-secretase. There are several species of AβP, such as AβP(1–40), the first 40 amino acid residues, or AβP(1–42), which are generated by the different cleavage processes in its C-terminal domain. Genetic studies of early-onset cases of familial AD indicated that APP mutations and the consequent changes in AβP metabolism are associated with AD (Goate et al., 1991). Moreover, mutations in the presenilin genes also account for the majority of cases of early-onset familial AD (Sherrington et al., 1995). Presenilins have been identified as one of γ -secretase proteins, and their mutations also influence the production of AβP and its neurotoxicity (Selkoe and Wolfe, 2007).
Yankner *et al.* reported that AβP(1–40) caused the death of cultured rat hippocampal neurons and the neurodegeneration in the brains of experimental animals (Yankner et al., 1991). A smaller fragment of AβP (AβP (25–35)) or a longer variant (AβP (1–42)) were also reported to cause neuronal death. AβP is a hydrophobic peptide with an intrinsic tendency to self-assemble to form sodium dodecyl sulfate (SDS)-stable oligomers. In an aqueous solution, freshly prepared and dissolved AβP exists as a monomeric protein with a random coil structure. However, following incubation at 37°C for several days (*aging*), AβPs form aggregates (oligomers) with β-pleated sheet structures, and finally form insoluble aggregates, termed amyloid fibrils (Fig. 1). Pike et al. revealed that *aged* AβP(1–40) peptides were considerably more toxic to cultured neurons than *fresh* (freshly prepared just before the experiment) AβP(1–40) (Pike et al, 1991). The ß-sheet content of AßP solutions, as determined by circular dichroism (CD) spectroscopy, correlates with its neurotoxicity (Simmons et al., 1994). Jarrett and Lansbury demonstrated that the longer peptide variant, AβP(1–42), polymerizes much quicker than AβP(1–40) (Jarrett and Lansbury, 1993). AβP(1–42) enhances the aggregation of AβP(1–40) and functions as a "seed" for amyloid fibrils. AβP (1–42) is more abundant in the brains of AD patients than in age-matched controls. The point mutations of APP are located near the γ-secretase cleavage-site and influences the ratio of AβP(1–40) and AβP(1–42). Mutations of APP and the presenilin genes increase the production of AβP (1–42) in the transfected cell lines.

Recent studies on the identified AβP species further strengthened and refined the amyloid cascade hypothesis. Approaches using size-exclusion chromatography, gel electrophoresis, and atomic force microscopy (AFM) have demonstrated that there are several stable types of oligomers: naturally occurring soluble oligomers (dimers or trimers), AßP-derived diffusible ligands (ADDLs), AβP globulomers, and protofibrils. Walsh et al. found the existence of SDS-stable oligomers in the conditioned medium of cultured cells transfected with the human APP gene. The intracerebral administration of these SDS-stable low-molecular-weight oligomers (dimers, trimers, or tetramers) inhibited long-term potentiation (LTP), which is a form of synaptic information storage that is a well-known paradigm for the mechanisms underlying memory formation (Walsh and Selkoe, 2007). They also demonstrated that LTP was not blocked by AβP monomers or larger aggregates. Natural AβP oligomers derived from the cerebrospinal fluid of AD patients induced the loss of dendritic spines and synapses, and also blocked the oligomers in the conditioned medium. Klein and the colleagues reported that ADDLs obtained by sedimentation with clusterin are highly toxic to cultured neurons. They also reported that ADDLs inhibited LTP and exhibited adverse effects on synaptic plasticity e.g., decreased spine density, abnormal spine morphology, and decreased levels of synaptic proteins (Lacor et al., 2007). Tomiyama et al. found a new AβP variant (AβP E42Δ) that exhibited enhanced oligomerization but no fibrillization (Tomiyama et al., 2008). This unique variant AβP decreased synaptophysin immunostaining and blocked LTP. Since synaptic plasticity is crucial for the process of memory formation and is involved in the early stages of AD, these lines of evidence indicate that the synaptic impairment induced by AβP oligomers is the primary event in the memory impairment observed in AD patients.

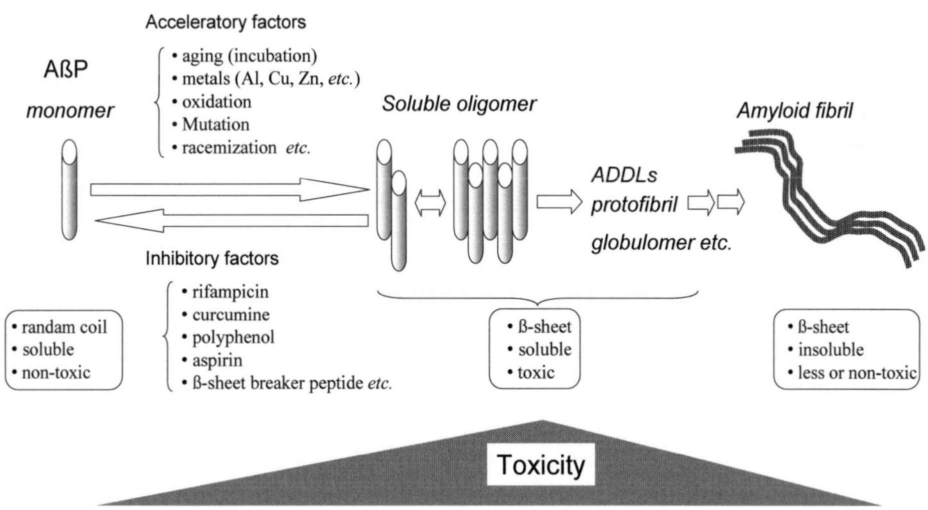

Fig. 1. Oligomerization of AβP

AβP monomers exhibit random-coil structures. However, during aging or in the presence of some acceleratory factors, AβP self-aggregates and forms several types of oligomers (SDS-soluble oligomers, ADDLS, globulomers, protofibrils, *etc.*) and finally forms insoluble aggregates, which are termed amyloid fibrils. Oligomeric soluble AβPs are toxic, although monomers and fibrils are rather nontoxic.

AβP is secreted into the cerebrospinal fluid (CSF) of young individuals as well as in aged or dementia patients (Fukuyama et al., 2000). Therefore, factors that accelerate or inhibit AβP oligomerization may play essential roles in the pathogenesis of AD. Several factors such as peptide concentration, the pH or composition of solvents, and temperature can influence the oligomerization processes. In addition, oxidations, mutations, and racemization of AβP enhance its oligomerization. Substances that can influence the oligomerization processes, e.g., cholesterol or its oxidation products, transthyretin, rifampicin, curcumin, aspirin, docosahexaenoic acid (DHA) and peptides such as the β-sheet breaker peptide, reportedly inhibit AβP oligomerization *in vitro*.

Among these factors, Al is of particular interest considering its epidemiological link with AD (Kawahara and Kato-Negishi, 2011). Al^{3+} has strong positive charges and a relatively small ionic radius in comparison to other metal ions; thus, Al^{3+} firmly binds to metal-binding amino acids (e.g. histidine, tyrosine, arginine *etc.*) or phosphorylated amino acids and acts as a cross-linker. Owing to this property, Al can cause the aggregation of various proteins and induce the conformational changes. Exposure to Al causes the accumulation of AβP in cultured neurons and in the brains of experimental animals and humans (Pratico et al., 2002; Exley and Esiri, 2006).

3. Alzheimer's Disease and calcium homeostasis

Ca^{2+} is required for various normal brain functions and is a component of key enzymes such as kinases, phosphatases, and proteases, it is highly possible that Ca^{2+} dyshomeostasis could be the earliest adverse event among AβP-induced various adverse effects such as ROS production, cytokine induction, endoplasmic reticulum (ER) stresses induction. Once neuronal Ca^{2+} homeostasis is disrupted and $[Ca^{2+}]_i$ is changed, various apoptotic pathways, such as Ca^{2+}-activated neutral protease (calpain) and caspase, are activated, leading to neuronal death. The disruption of Ca^{2+} homeostasis can trigger membrane disruption, the formation of free radicals, and the induction of other adverse effects, which are often observed after exposure to AβP. It is widely recognized that an increase in $[Ca^{2+}]_i$ induces changes in the number and morphology of synapses and spines, and that an imbalances of Ca^{2+} in synapses directly influences neuronal activity and synaptic impairment. Considering that APP localizes in synapses and that AβP is secreted from APP into synaptic clefts by neuronal excitation, the adverse effects caused by AβP-induced Ca^{2+} dyshomeostasis can occur in synaptic compartments and induce synaptotoxicity. Therefore, the influx of Ca^{2+} is tightly controlled and $[Ca^{2+}]_i$ levels are strictly regulated by various mechanisms including voltage-dependent Ca^{2+} channels (VDCC), and neurotransmitter receptors e.g., glutamate (Glu) and acetylcholine (ACh) (Zorumski and Thio, 1992). Moreover, the ER and mitochondoria represent the major intracellular stores of Ca^{2+} (Green and LaFerla, 2008; Leuner et al., 2007).

An increasing amount of data indicates that exposure to AβP causes an abnormal increase in $[Ca^{2+}]_i$ in intoxicated neurons. There is considerable interest regarding the mechanism by which AβPs interact with neurons and disrupts Ca^{2+} homeostasis (Demuro et al., 2010). There are several possible mechanisms that account for AβP-induced Ca^{2+} dyshomeostasis, e.g., interaction with endogenous Ca^{2+}-permeable ion channels, disruption of membrane integrity, and formation of Ca^{2+}-permeable channels (pores) by the direct membrane incorporation of AβP (Fig.6). It is possible that AβP directly binds to membranes and causes their disruption, or that AβP-induced ROS impairs membrane structures.

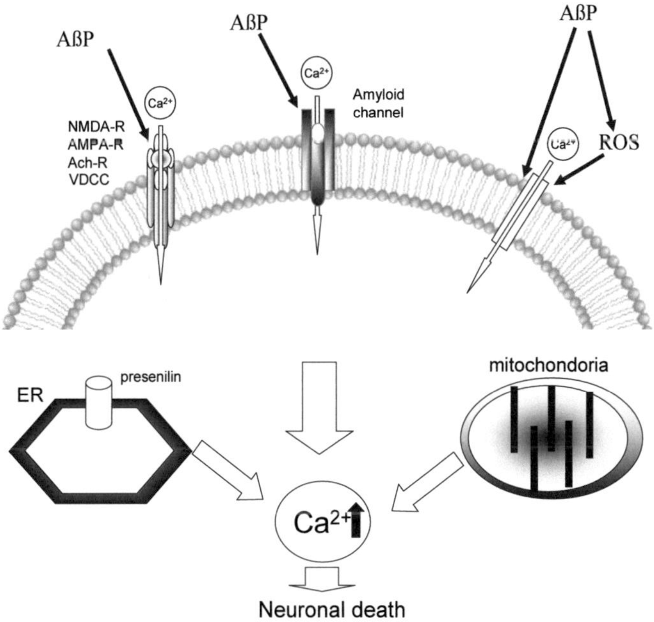

Fig. 2. AβP-induced calcium dyshomeostasis in neurons. It is possible that AßP-induced Ca^{2+} dyshomeostasis by (i) its interactions with endogenous Ca^{2+}-permeable ion channels, (ii) disruption of membrane integrity, and (iii) formation of Ca^{2+} permeable channels (pores) by the direct membrane incorporation of AβP. AβP can directly cause membrane disruption, or AβP-induced ROS can impair membrane structure. Presenilins in the ER or mitochondria can participate in the abnormal increase in $[Ca^{2+}]i$ in neurons

AβP reportedly binds to *N*-methyl D-aspartate (NMDA)-, and α-amino-3-hydroxy-5-methylisoxazole-4-propionic acid (AMPA) -type glutamate receptors (Parameshwaran et al., 2008), and nicotinic ACh receptors (Parri and Dineley, 2010). All of these receptors contain Ca^{2+} channels and regulate $[Ca^{2+}]_i$ during membrane depolarization. AβP also influences voltage-gated Ca^{2+} channels and the inositol triphosphate (IP_3) receptor. The influx of Ca^{2+} from the ER is regulated by ryanodine-type Ca^{2+} channels, the sarcoplasmic reticulum Ca-ATPase (SERCA), and presenilins (Green et al., 2008). Presenilins are found in the ER membrane, and are involved in capacitative Ca^{2+} entry, ER Ca^{2+} signaling, Ca^{2+} leakage from the ER, and mitochondrial Ca^{2+} signaling (Querfurth and LaFerla, 2010).

4. Formation of Ca^{2+} permeable pores by AßP

Our and other numerous studies have demonstrated that AβPs are directly incorporated into the surfaces of cellular membrane and create unregulated cytotoxic pore-like channels. In 1993, Arispe et al. first demonstrated that AβP(1–40) directly incorporates into artificial lipid bilayer membranes and forms cation-selective ion channels (Arispe et al., 1993a, 1993b). These channels termed amyloid channels were revealed to be giant multilevel pores that can facilitate the transport of large amounts of Ca^{2+}. Their activity was blocked by Zn^{2+} ions, which are abundant in the brain (Arispe et al., 1996). Electrophysiological studies have revealed that other neurotoxic peptide fragments of AβP including AβP(25–35) and

AβP(1–42) form Ca^{2+}-permeable pores in artificial lipid bilayers. The C-terminal fragment of APP (CT_{105}) including AβP also formed ion channels in Xenopus oocytes (Fraser et al., 1996).

Durell et al. proposed a 3-D structural model of amyloid channels obtained from a computer simulation of the secondary structure of AβP(1–40) in membranes that showed the aggregation of 5- to 8-mers to form pore-like structures on the membranes (Durell et al., 1994). Jang et al. established a model for amyloid channels on membranes and observed the pentameric AβP forms pores (Jang et al, 2009). Strodel et al. proposed a model of AβP(1–42) pores which consist of tetrameric and hexameric β-sheet subunits from the observations in NMR (Strodel et al., 2010). The dimension, shape, and subunit organization of these models were in good agreement with the morphological observations using high resolution AFM that demonstrated that AβPs form pore-like structures on mica plates or on reconstituted membranes (Lal et al., 2007, Jang et al., 2010). Furthermore, the presence of pore-like structures of AßPs *in vivo* was demonstrated in the neuronal cell membrane of the brains of AD patients and of AD-model mice. Using high resolution transmission electron microscopy, Inoue observed in situ AßP pores in the neuronal cell membrane in AD brains (Inoue, 2008). Kayed *et al.* reported that the annular protofibrils (APFs) of AßP exhibit ring-shaped and pore-like structures (Kayerd, et al., 2009). The age-dependent accumulation of APFs was observed on the membranes of AD model mice (APP transgenic mice; APP23) (Kokubo et al., 2009).

It is important to determine whether AβPs form channels in neuronal cell membranes in addition to artificial lipid bilayers. To address this issue, we employed membrane patches from a neuroblastoma cell line (GT1-7 cells), and found that AβP(1–40) formed amyloid channels on GT1-7 cell membranes (Kawahara et al., 1997). GT1-7 cells (immortalized hypothalamic neurons) are derived from murine hypothalamic neurons by site-directed tumorigenesis and exhibit several neuronal characteristics such as the extension of neurites and the expression of neuron-specific proteins and receptors (Mellon et al., 1990). The features of amyloid channels formed on GT1-7 membranes were considerably similar to those observed in artificial lipid bilayers; cation-selective, multilevel, voltage-independent, and long-lasting; channel activity was inhibited by the addition of Zn^{2+}, and recovered by the addition of zinc chelator *o*-phenanthroline. Moreover, Sepulveda et al. revealed that AβP(1-40) formed perforations on membranes excised from hippocampal neurons and induced currents (Sepulveda et al., 2010). The effect of AβP was similar to that of gramicidin and amphotericin which are commonly used to perforate neuron membranes.

Furthermore, we have revealed that AβP directly caused the disruption of liposomal membrane vesicles by observing the release of fluorescent dye (Kawahara et al., 2011b). These results are consistent with the findings that AßP causes membrane disruption, increases membrane permeability, causes hemolysis, and changes membrane fluidity (Eckert et al., 2005).

These results strongly support the hypothetical idea termed amyloid channel hypothesis namely, that the direct incorporation of AβPs and the subsequent imbalances of Ca^{2+} and other ions through amyloid channels may be the primary event in AßP neurotoxicity.

5. Disruption of calcium homeostasis by amyloid channels

In order to test the validity of the amyloid channel hypothesis more precisely, we examined whether AβP alters the $[Ca^{2+}]_i$ levels of GT1-7 cells under the same conditions, using a high-resolution multi-site video imaging system with Ca^{2+}-sensitive fluorescent dye (fura-2) (Kawahara et al., 2000; Kawahara & Kuroda, 2001). We also observed AβP-induced abnormal increases in $[Ca^{2+}]_i$ in primary cultured rat hippocampal neurons (Kato-Negishi & Kawahara, 2008). Shown in figure 3 are temporal changes of $[Ca^{2+}]_i$ in GT1-7 cells before and after exposure to AβP(1-40) and related peptides. Although a marked increase in $[Ca^{2+}]_i$ was caused by AβP(1–40) (*line (a)*), AβP(1–42) (*line (c)*), and AβP(25–35) (*line (e)*), no remarkable changes were induced by AβP(40–1), control peptide with no toxicity (*line (b)*). There is controversy over whether the AβP-induced $[Ca^{2+}]_i$ changes occur through receptor-mediated pathways or amyloid channels formed by direct incorporation of AβP. To clarify the precise characterization of the AβP-induced $[Ca^{2+}]_i$ changes, we performed detailed and quantitative analysis of the AβP-induced Ca^{2+} influx using a high-resolution multi-site video imaging system. This multisite fluorometry system enables the simultaneous long-term observation of temporal changes in $[Ca^{2+}]_i$ in more than 50 neurons. There are 5 major pieces of evidence supporting the hypothesis that AßP-induced $[Ca^{2+}]_i$ changes occur through amyloid channels. *First,* the AβP-induced $[Ca^{2+}]_i$ rise was highly heterogeneous among genetically identical GT1-7 cells. Even in the same field of view, exposure to the same peptide solution produced differential changes in the $[Ca^{2+}]_i$ levels (Fig. 4A). Considering the heterogeneity, we compared the peak increase in $[Ca^{2+}]_i$ ($\Delta[Ca^{2+}]_i$) induced by AβPs, and its latency (the lag between the $[Ca^{2+}]_i$ increase and the time of AβP addition) in each cell to quantitatively analyze Ca^{2+} influx.

Although AβP (1–40) induced an increase in $[Ca^{2+}]_i$ levels either instantly or after some delay, the magnitude and latency differed. In addition, some adjacent cells still did not exhibit any responses. *Second,* the average $\Delta[Ca^{2+}]_i$ was increased and the average latency was shortened in a dose-dependent manner (Fig. 4B and C). These features are considerably similar to those observed in relation to toxic peptide channels formed on membranes. *Third,* the AβP-induced increase in $[Ca^{2+}]_i$ was not influenced by the addition of a Na^+ channel blocker (tetrodotoxin), a Ca^{2+} channel blocker (nifedipine), a glutamate receptor antagonist (D-APV), or a γ-aminobutyric acid (GABA) antagonist (bicuculline). However, antibodies to AβP remarkably inhibited the $[Ca^{2+}]_i$ increase resulting from AβP (Kawahara, 2004). *Fourth,* D-AβP(1–40), AβP(1–40) composed of D-amino acid residues, also caused the elevation of $[Ca^{2+}]_i$ in a manner similar to AβP(1–40) (see Fig. 3, *line (d)*). *Fifth,* the vulnerability of primary cultured rat hippocampal neurons to AβP was changed during the culture period, despite that the expression and the function of neurotransmitter are not changed (Kato-Negishi and Kawahara, 2008). On the basis of these lines of evidence, we conclude that AβP causes the disruption of Ca^{2+} homeostasis *via* the formation of amyloid channels in membranes, ultimately resulting in neuronal death.

Pore formation-induced cytotoxicity is commonly observed in our biological system, particularly in the presence of certain toxins and venoms including the α-toxin of *Staphylococcus aureus,* magainin 2, a 26-residue antimicrobial peptide obtained from *Xenopus laevis,* melitin, a bee venom composed of 28 amino acids, or antibiotics such as amphotericin and gramicidin (Bechinger, 1997). In this respect, AβPs may share the similar toxicity mechanism as various antimicrobial or antifungal peptides that exhibit pore-forming ability and cell toxicity. Indeed, Soscia et al. demonstrated that AβP exerts antimicrobial activity against 8 common and clinically relevant microorganisms (Soscia et al., 2010).

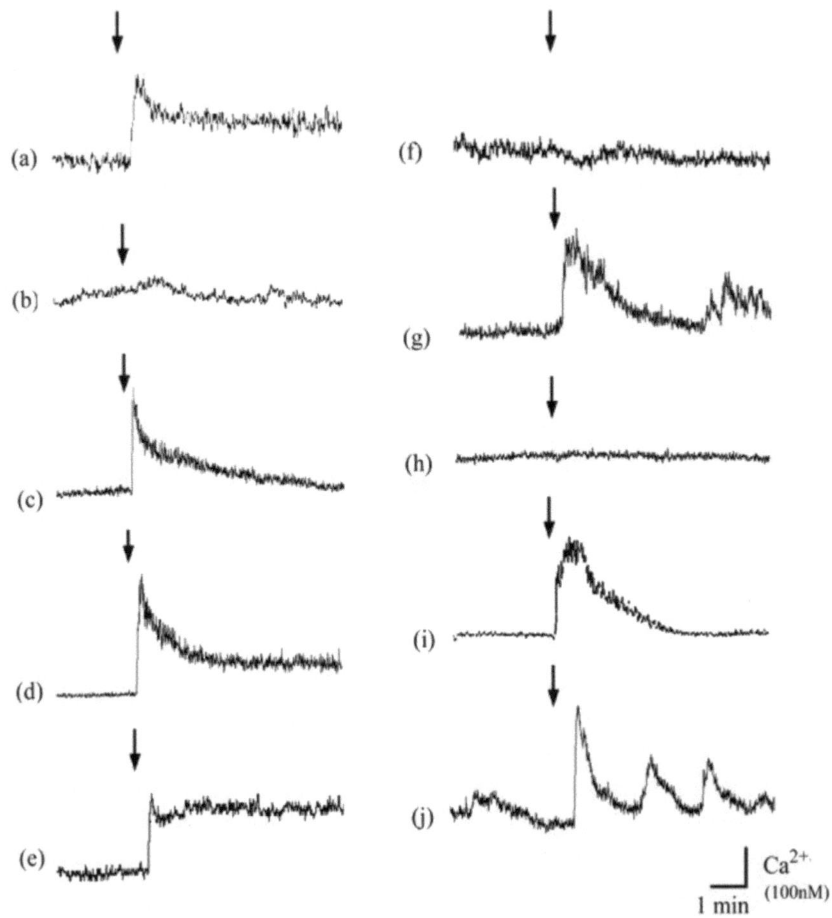

Fig. 3. Characteristics of the elevations in $[Ca^{2+}]_i$ induced by AβP and other amyloidogenic proteins. Typical time course of $[Ca^{2+}]_i$ at 2 min prior to and at 3 min after the application of the peptide is depicted. (a) AßP(1-40); (b) AßP(40-1); (c) AßP(1-42); (d) D-AßP(1-40); (e) PrP106-126; (f) scramble PrP106-126; (g) human amylin; (h) rat amylin; (i) NAC; and (j) magainin 2. All peptides were at 10 μM. The arrow indicates the time of peptide addition

Recently, a new concept of "conformational disease," had been proposed, suggesting that the conformation of disease-related proteins (amyloidogenic proteins) is an important determinant of their toxicity, and consequently, the disease development (Carrell and Lomas, 1997). The conformational diseases includes prion diseases, triplet-repeat diseases, e.g., Huntington's disease, Parkinson's disease and other neurodegenerative diseases that can be categorized under dementia with Lewy bodies (DLB). Increasing evidence indicates that most of these disease-related amyloidogenic proteins or their peptide fragments are directly incorporated into membranes to form ion channels as well as AβP (Lashuel and Lansbury, 2002; Kawahara et al., 2011b). It was also demonstrated that AßP (1–40), α-synuclein, amylin, ABri, or other amyloidogenic peptides morphologically similar common ion channel-like structures and elicit single channel currents using AFM, CD, gel electrophoresis, and electrophysiological recordings (Quist et al., 2005; Lal et al., 2007).

We have also demonstrated that these amyloidogenic peptides including PrP106-126 (a peptide fragment of prion protein), human amylin, NAC, or antimicrobial peptide magainin2 also caused an elevation in the $[Ca^{2+}]_i$ levels similar to that induced by AβPs (Kawahara et al., 2000; Kawahara, 2004). However, rat amylin and a peptide a randomized PrP106-126 sequence (scrambled PrP106-126) did not induce any $[Ca^{2+}]_i$ changes (Fig. 3). We have also demonstrated that PrP106-126 forms β-sheet structures and exhibits neurotoxicity as well as AβP (Kawahara et al., 2011a). In addition, oligomeric α-synuclein causes neuronal death *via* the Ca^{2+} influx (Danzer et al., 2007). Considering these results

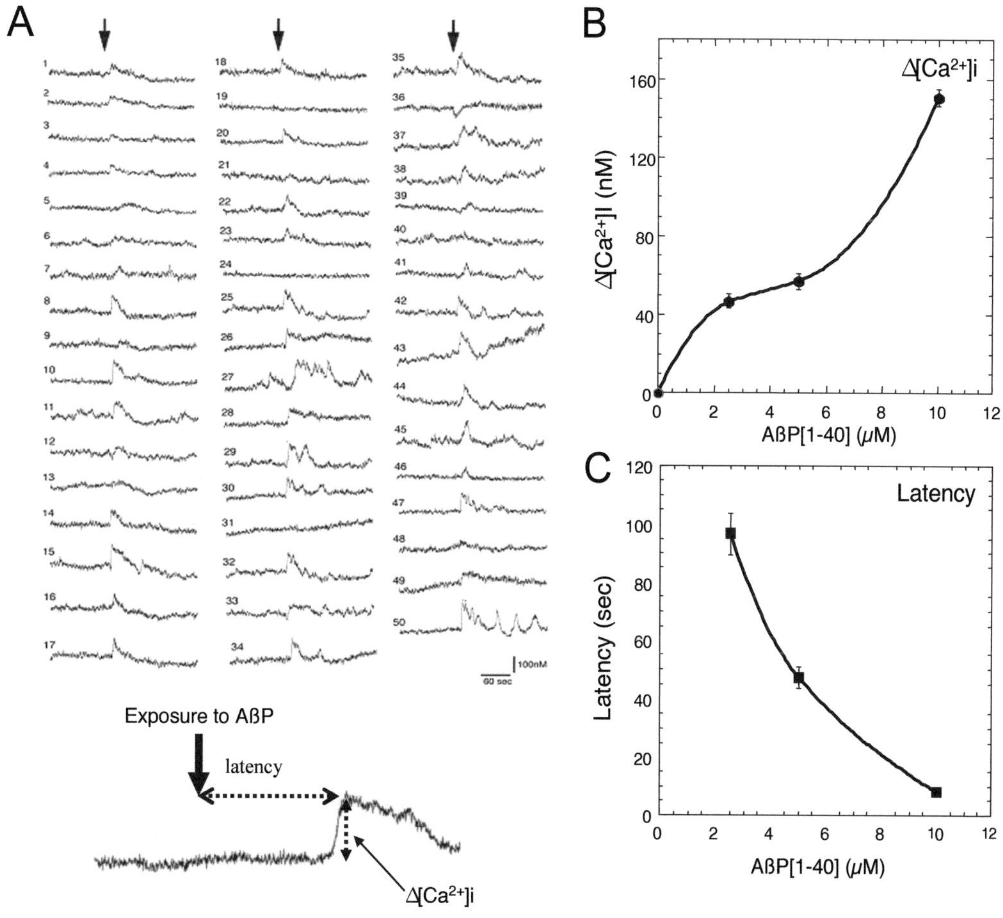

Fig. 4. (A) Heterogeneity of AβP-induced changes in $[Ca^{2+}]_i$ Temporal changes of 50 randomly chosen GT1-7 cells in the same field of view before and after the exposure to AβP(1–40). The arrow indicates the time of peptide addition. B~C: The peak increase in $[Ca^{2+}]_i$ ($\Delta[Ca^{2+}]_i$) in each cell and the latency after exposure to AβP (1–40) were analyzed (B) in more than 50 cultured neurons in a single field of view (360×420 μm³) (mean ± S.E.M., n=300). Typical responses of $[Ca^{2+}]_i$ in cultured neurons following exposure to various concentrations of AβP (1–40) (2.5~10 μM). The peak increase in $[Ca^{2+}]_i$ ($\Delta[Ca^{2+}]_i$) in each cell (C) and the latency (D) after exposure to AßP (1–40)

together, it is plausible that these disease-related amyloidogenic proteins share similarities in channel formation and the disruption of Ca^{2+} homeostasis as well as β-sheet formation and cytotoxicity. Table 1 summarizes the common properties of these proteins.

Disease	Amyloidogenic protein or its fragment peptide and the primary sequence	ß-sheet formation	Cytotoxicity	Channel formation	Morphological pores	$[Ca^{2+}]_i$ rise
Alzheimer's disease	*AßP(1-40)* DAEFRHDSGYEVHHQKLVFFAEDVGSNKGAIIGL MVGGVV	+	+	+	+	+
	AßP(40-1) VVGGVMLGIIAGKNSGVDEAFFVLKQHHVEYGS DHRFEAD	–	–	–	n.d.	–
	AßP(25-35) DVGSNKGAII	+	+	+	+	+
	AßP(1-42) DAEFRHDSGYEVHHQKLVFFAEDVGSNKGAIIGL MVGGVVIA	+	+	+	n.d.	+
Prion disease	*PrP106-126 (prion protein fragment)* KTNMKHMAGAAAAGAVVGGLG	+	+	+	n.d.	+
	Scramble PrP106-126 NGAKALMGGHGATKVMVGAAA	–	–	–		–
Parkinson's disease (DLB; diseases with Lewy bodies)	*α-synuclein* *NAC (α fragment of α-synuclein)* EQVTNVGGAVVTGVTAVAQKTVEGAGSIAAATGFV	+	+	+	+	+
Triplet-repeat disease	*Polyglutamine* QQQQQQQQ------------------	+	+	+	n.d.	n.d.
Familial British dementia	*ABri35* ASNCPAIRHPGNKPAVGTLICSRTVKKNIIGGN	+	+	+	+	n.d.
Diabetes mellitus	*Human amylin* KCNTATCATQRLANFLVHSSNNFGAILSSTNVGS NTY	+	+	+	+	+
	Rat amylin KCNTATCATQRLANFLVRSSNNLGPVLPPTNVGS NTY	–	–	–		–
Medullary carcinoma of the thyroid	Calcitonin CGNLSTCMLGTYTQDFNKFHTFPQTAIGVGAP	+	+	+	+	+

n.d.: not determined

Table 1. Characteristics of amyloidogenic proteins and the related peptides

6. Possible candidates for the treatment of AD

The search for protective agents against AβP-induced neurotoxicity is of great importance. Substances that prevent the oligomerization of AβP such as rifampicin, curcumin, aspirin, DHA can be potential candidates against AβP neurotoxicity (Fig. 2). Reduction of AβP production using BACE or γ-secretase inhibitors is reportedly effective for the treatment of AD. In addition, even though AβP vaccines had been associated with adverse effects, they may be considered as a potential treatment alternative. Conversely, trace metals such as Al, Zn, and Cu enhance AβP oligomerization; thus, chelation therapy with clioquinol, deferoxamine, or silicates has been proposed to be effective in the treatment of AD (Lannfelt et al., 2008; Exley, 2007).

Here, we focused on substances that inhibit the formation of amyloid channels. As discussed, the elevation of $[Ca^{2+}]_i$ by its permeation through amyloid channels is considered to be the primary event of AβP-induced neurotoxicity; therefore, such compounds could serve as the foundation for the new and effective drugs with fewer adverse effects.

Inorganic cations such as Zn^{2+} inhibit the current induced by amyloid channels. Zn is abundant in presynaptic terminal vesicles and is secreted into synaptic clefts following neuronal excitation. Considering that Zn binds to the His residues of AβP, Arispe et al. found that His-related peptide derivatives, such as His-His, effectively inhibit the current through amyloid channels, attenuate AβP-induced $[Ca^{2+}]_i$ changes, and protect neurons from AβP toxicity (Arispe et al., 2008). They also developed new compounds with pyrimidine structures that inhibit the amyloid channels and investigated its efficacy for treatment (Diaz et al., 2009, Arispe et al., 2010).

We focused substances which modify the membrane properties and inhibit amyloid channels. It is widely accepted that the composition of membrane lipids strongly influences the direct incorporation of peptides into membranes and consequent channel formation (Bechinger and Lohner, 2006; Simakova & Arispe, 2007). In particular, electrostatic interactions between peptides and lipids, namely, the net charges of the membrane surface, and membrane fluidity play crucial roles in the affinity for peptides (Seelig et al., 1994). Several AβP residues (e.g., Arg^5, Lys^{16}, and Lys^{28} residues) have a positive charge at a neutral pH; thus, AβP has an affinity for negatively charged phospholipids, such as phosphatidylserine (PS) or phoshatidylglycerol (PG), but not for neutral phospholipids such as phosphatidylcholine (PC). The formation of ß-sheet structures by AβP (1–40) was increased after the addition of PG. Meanwhile, substances that decrease membrane fluidity are known to enhance membrane stiffness and influence pore formation by toxins (Tomita et al., 1992). Gangliosides also contribute to the net charge of the outer membrane surface and to the binding to AβPs. Micro-circumstances on the membranes, such as rafts, containing gangliosides and cholesterol, may provide suitable locations that facilitate this process (Matsuzaki et al., 2010). Indeed, disruption of raft protected neurons from AβPs-induced neurotoxicity (Malchiodi-Albedi et al., 2010).

Thus, we have developed a screening system for compounds that influence membrane properties by observing the AβP-induced influx of Ca^{2+}. Among tested, we demonstrated that several lipophilic substances such as phloretin, cholesterol, 17β-estradiol, 17α-estradiol, and neurosteroids including dehydroepiandrosterone (DHEA), DHEA sulfate (DHEA-S), and pregnenolone, significantly inhibit AβP-induced $[Ca^{2+}]_i$ elevation (Kawahara and Kuroda, 2001, Kato-Negishi and Kawahara, 2008). Figure 5 exhibits the structures of these compounds.

Phloretin, a plant-derived flavonoid, decreases the membrane potential and inhibits the electrostatic interaction between AβP and membrane lipids (Hertel et al., 1997). Cholesterol decreases membrane fluidity and inhibits channel formation by peptides such as α-toxin, gramicidine, amylin, and AβP. The pretreatment with phloretin or cholesterol significantly inhibited the AßP-induced increase in $[Ca^{2+}]_i$ in cultured neurons. Meanwhile, 6-ketocholestanol, which increases the membrane dipole potential, did not influence the AβP-induced increase in $[Ca^{2+}]_i$.

Furthermore, 17β-estradiol, a female hormone, is neuroprotective and affects membrane fluidity (Schwartz et al., 1996). Considering that both of 17β-estradiol and 17α-estradiol inhibit the AβP-induced $[Ca^{2+}]_i$ elevation, this inhibition may depend on their membrane modifying effects (Whiting et al, 2000). All of these compounds inhibit AβP neurotoxicity.

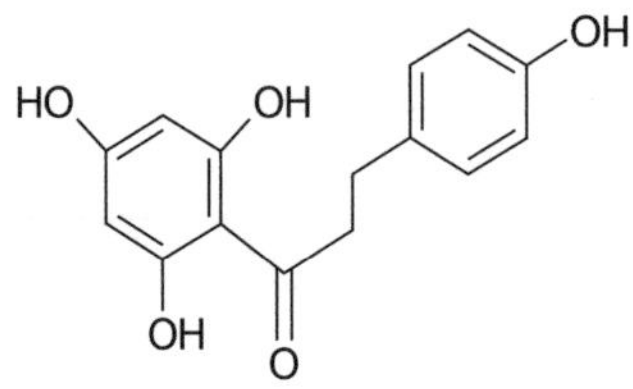

Phloretin (PH)

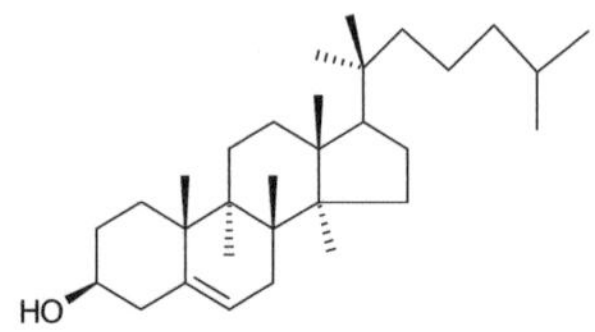

Cholesterol (Chol)

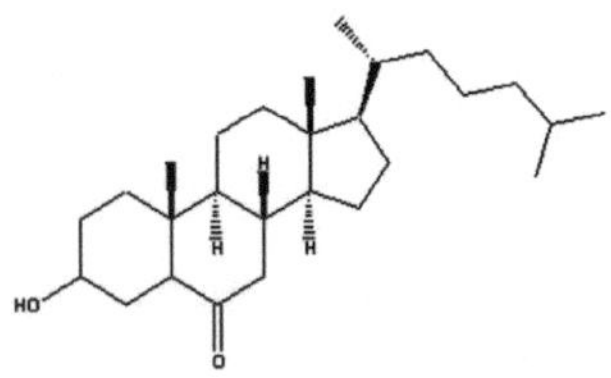

6-ketocholestanol(6KC)

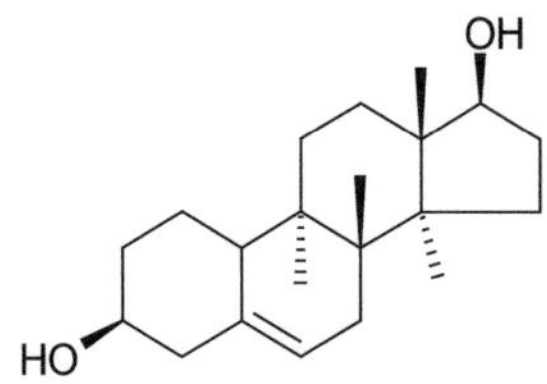

17-ß estradiol

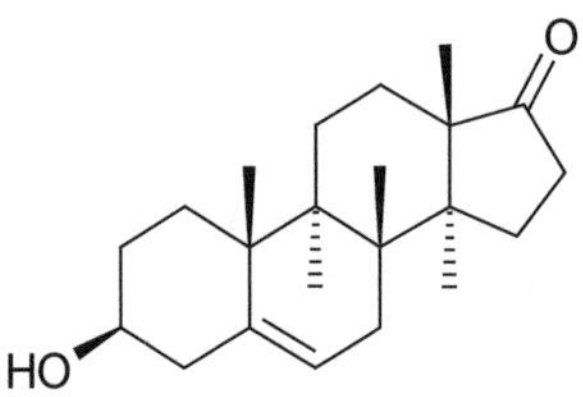

DHEA

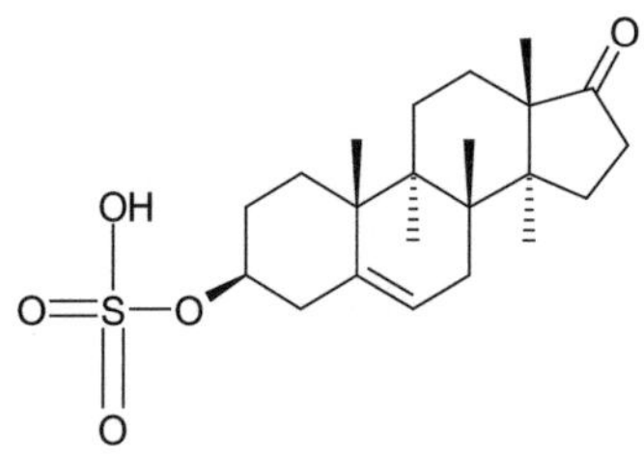

DHEA-S

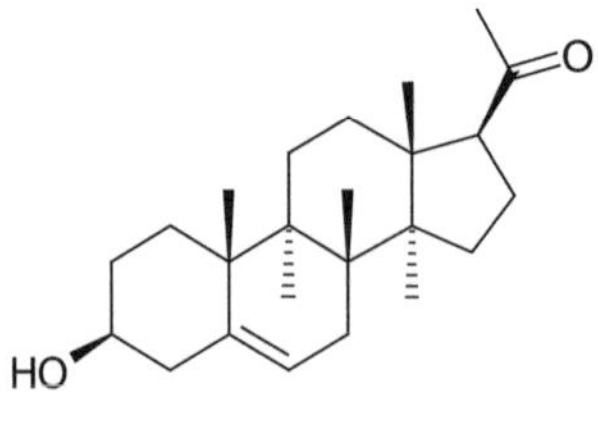

pregnenolone

Fig. 5. Chemical structures of substances which influence AβP-induced $[Ca^{2+}]_i$ elevation

Neurosteroids are steroid hormones synthesized *de novo* in the central nervous system from cholesterol or from peripheral steroid precursors (Tsutuki et al., 2000). Several lines of evidence suggest that neurosteroids modulate various functions of the brain and exhibit neuroprotective activitiy (Mellon, 2007). Thus, neurosteroids have been recognized as anti-aging hormones, and are widely used as supplements to improve the impaired cognitive functions of the elderly (Huppert et al., 2000). Considering that plasma DHEA-S levels are reduced in healthy individuals in an age-dependent manner and in AD patients (Hillen et al., 2000; Aldred and Mecocci, 2010), neurosteroids may have an important role in the pathogenesis of AD.

7. Amyloid channel hypothesis

Considering the results of our study together with those of the others, we propose the following hypothetical scheme of AβP-induced neurodegeneration (Fig. 6).

AβPs are normally secreted following the cleavage of APP in the synaptic compartment into the cerebrospinal fluid. The secreted AβPs are usually degraded proteolytically within a short period. However, the upregulation of AβP secretion from APP, or an increased ratio of AβP(1–42) to AβP(1–40), which are influenced by APP or presenilin gene mutations, may facilitate the retention of AβP in the brain.

As descried previously, the net charge of the outer membrane surface may be a determinant when secreted AβPs bind to cellular membranes. The distribution of phospholipids on cellular membranes is usually asymmetrical; neutral lipids such as PC usually exist on the outer surface of plasma membranes, whereas negatively charged phospholipids such as PS exist on the inner membrane surface. When this asymmetric distribution is disrupted by apoptotic conditions or aging, AβPs can bind to the membrane surfaces (Fig. 6, step (A)). After incorporation into the membrane, the conformation of AβPs change and the accumulated AβPs aggregate on the membranes. The ratio of cholesterol to phospholipids in the membrane may alter membrane fluidity, thereby affecting the process from step (A) to (B). Considering that apoE, its phenotype is a risk factor of AD, is a cholesterol-binding protein, the relationship between cholesterol and AD is important in the pathogenesis of AD.

Finally, aggregated AβP oligomers form ion channels (Fig. 6 (C)), leading to the various neurodegenerative processes. Once AβP channels are formed in neuronal membranes, the homeostasis of Ca^{2+} and other ions is disrupted. Unlike endogenous Ca^{2+} channels, these AβP channels are not regulated by the usual channel blockers; thus, once formed on the membrane, a continuous flow of Ca^{2+} is initiated. However, Zn^{2+} ions, which are secreted into the synaptic cleft in a neuronal activity-dependent manner, inhibit AβP-induced Ca^{2+} entry, and thus have a protective function in AD. Disruption of Ca^{2+} homeostasis triggers several apoptotic pathways and promotes numerous degenerative processes, including free radical formation and tau phosphorylation, thereby accelerating neuronal death. Presenilins can influence Ca^{2+} homeostasis through the disturbances of the capacitive Ca^{2+} entry or other pathways, and may influence these pathways. Free radicals also induce membrane disruption, by which further amplifies unregulated Ca^{2+} influx. The disruption of Ca^{2+} homeostasis influences the production and processing of APP. Thus, a vicious cycle of neurodegeneration is initiated.

The velocity of channel formation will be regulated by the binding of AßP on membranes and its concentration, considering that *in vitro* aging can enhance the neurotoxicity of AβP and natural oligomers (dimmers or trimers) are more toxic as compared to monomers, it is provable that AßP oligomerization *in vitro* accelerates the velocity from (A) to (B), and enhances the formation of tetrameric or hexameric pores on membranes. These oligomers might easily form tetrameric or hexameric pores and exhibit neurotoxicity. Indeed, O'Nuallain

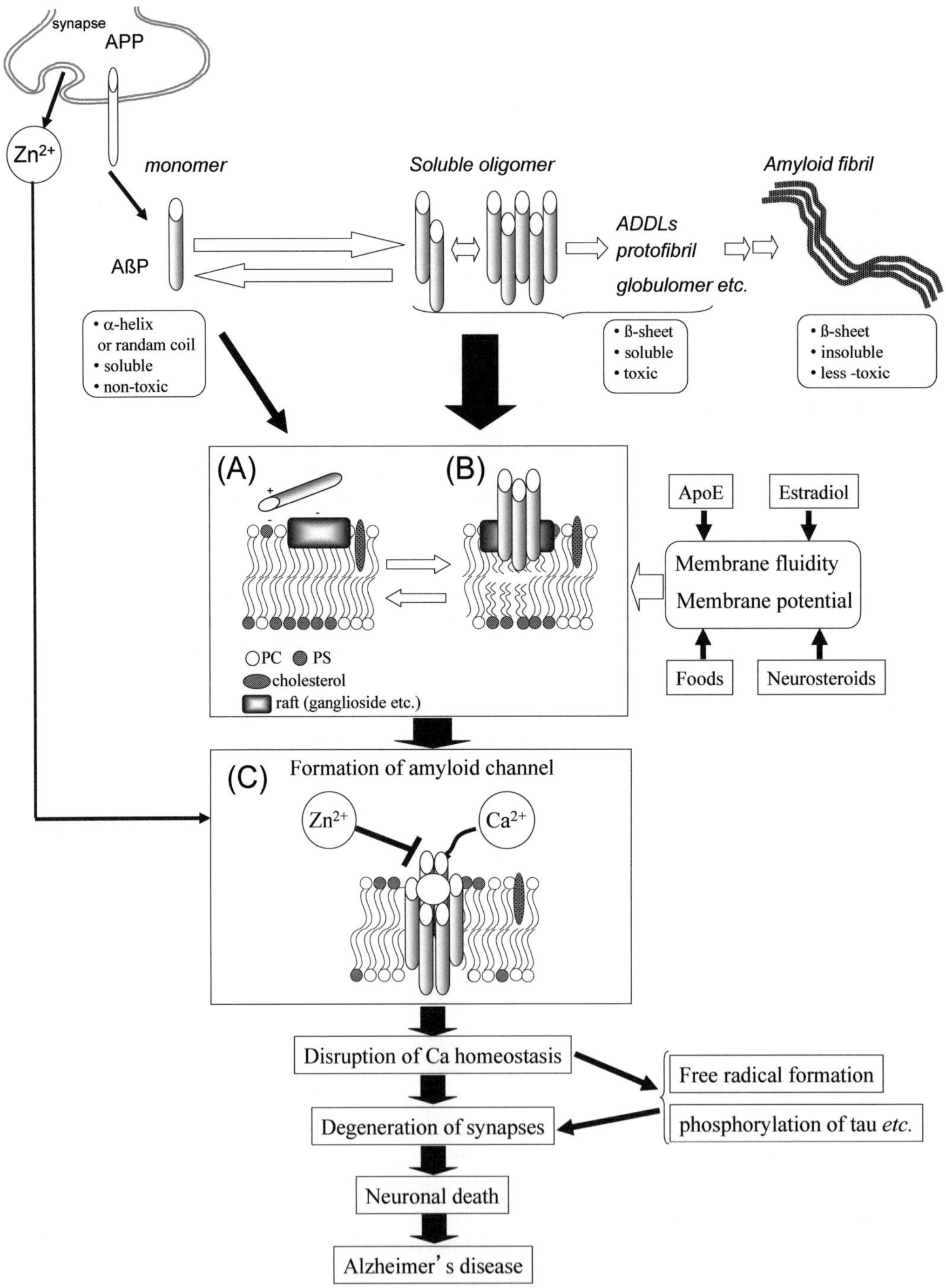

Fig. 6. Hypothesis concerning amyloid channels in the pathogenesis of Alzheimer's disease. AβPs are secreted from into synapses following the cleavage of APP, and then directly incorporated into membranes. The hypothetical scheme for the formation of oligomeric amyloid channels is depicted. Details are shown in the text

et al. demonstrated that AßP dimmers formed toxic protofibrils more rapidly compared to monomer (O'Nuallain et al., 2010). In spite that the exposure to relatively high concentration of AβP *in vitro* causes the acute elevation of $[Ca^{2+}]_i$ and exhibits neurotoxicity, the concentration of the AβP are low and it is difficult to bind to outer membranes. Thus, the processes required for channel formation (from steps (A) to (C)) in our brains may require a long life span and determine the rate of the entire process. This amyloid channel hypothesis explains the long delay in AD development; AD occurs only in aged subjects despite the fact that AβPs are normally secreted in younger or normal subjects. Various environmental factors, such as foods or trace metals, as well as genetic factors will influence these processes and contribute to AD pathogenesis.

8. Conclusion

Despite the immense efforts to develop a therapeutic drug for AD, the results have not been satisfactory. However, we believe that if we can understand the precise pathogenic mechanism more clearly, then potential therapeutic drugs (such as supplements) will be developed in the future. The amyloid channel hypothesis may improve the precise understanding of AD and the development of drugs for AD treatment. Further, it might be worthwhile to consider the application of dietary supplements such as estrogen or neurosteroids for the prevention of AD. Our efforts in developing new drugs will certainly be fruitful for the economy of the nation and the health of the population.

9. Acknowledgement

This work was partially supported by a Grant-in-Aid for Scientific Research from the Ministry of Education, Culture, Sports, Science and Technology of Japan.

10. References

Aldred, S. & Mecocci, P. (2010). Decreased dehydroepiandrosterone (DHEA) and dehydroepiandrosterone sulfate (DHEAS) concentrations in plasma of Alzheimer's disease (AD) patients, *Arch. Gerontol. Geriatr.*, vol. 51, pp. e16-8, 2010.

Arispe, N.; Rojas, E. & Pollard, H.B. (1993a) Alzheimer disease amyloid β protein forms calcium channels in bilayer membranes: Blockade by tromethamine and aluminum. *Proc Natl Acad Sci USA*, vol. 90, pp. 567-571.

Arispe, N.; Rojas, E. & Pollard, H.B. (1993b) Giant multilevel cation channels formed by Alzheimer disease amyloid β protein [AßP-(1-40)] in bilayer membranes. *Proc Natl Acad Sci USA*, vol. 90, pp. 10573-10577.

Arispe, N.; Pollard, H.B. & Rojas, E. (1996) Zn^{2+} interactions with Alzheimer's amyloid β protein calcium channels. *Proc Natl Acad Sci USA*, vol. 93, pp. 1710-1715.

Arispe, N.; Diaz, J.C. & Simakova, O. (2007) Aβ ion channels. Prospects for treating Alzheimer's disease with Aβ channel blockers. *Biochim Biophys Acta*, vol. 1768, pp. 1952-65.

Arispe, N.; Diaz, J.C. & Flora, M. (2008) Efficiency of histidine-associating compounds for blocking the alzheimer's Aβ channel activity and cytotoxicity. *Biophys J*, vol. 95, pp. 4879-4889.

Arispe, N.; Diaz, J.; Durell, S.R. ; Shafrir, Y. & Guy, H.R. (2010) Polyhistidine peptide inhibitor of the Aβ calcium channel potently blocks the Aβ-induced calcium response in cells. Theoretical modeling suggests a cooperative binding process. *Biochemistry*, vol. 49, pp. 7847-53.

Bechinger, B. (1997) Structure and functions of channel-forming peptides: Magainins, cecropins, melittin and alamethicin. *Journal of Membrane Biology*, vol. 156, pp. 197-211.

Bechinger, B. & Lohner, K. (2006). Detergent-like actions of linear amphipathic cationic antimicrobial peptides. *Biochim. Biophys. Acta.*, vol. 1758, pp. 1529-39.

Carrell, R.W. & Lomas, D.A. (1997) Conformational disease. *The Lancet*, vol. 350, pp. 134-138.

Danzer, K.M.; Haasen, D.; Karow, A.R.; Moussaud, S.; Habeck, M.; Giese, A.; Kretzschmar, H.; Hengerer, B.; Kostka, M. (2007). Different species of alpha-synuclein oligomers induce calcium influx and seeding. *J Neurosci.* vol. 27, pp. 9220-32.

Demuro, A.; Parker, I. & Stutzmann, G.E. (2010). Calcium signaling and amyloid toxicity in Alzheimer disease. *J. Biol. Chem.*, vol. 285, pp. 12463-8.

Diaz, J.C.; Simakova, O.; Jacobson, K.A., et al., (2009). Small molecule blockers of the Alzheimer Aβ calcium channel potently protect neurons from Aβ cytotoxicity. *Proc Natl Acad Sci USA*, vol. 106, pp. 3348-53.

Durell, S.R.; Guy, H.R.; Arispe, N.; Rojas, E. & Pollard, H.B. (1994). Theoretical models of the ion channel structure of amyloid β-protein. *Biophys J*, vol. 67, pp. 2137-3145.

Eckert, G.P.; Wood, W.G. & Müller, W.E. (2005). Membrane disordering effects of β-amyloid peptides. *Subcell Biochem.*, vol. 38, pp. 319-37.

Exley, C. & Esiri, M.M. (2006). Severe cerebral congophilic angiopathy coincident with increased brain aluminium in a resident of Camelford, Cornwall, UK. *J Neurol Neurosurg Psychiatry*, vol. 77, pp. 877-9.

Exley, C. (2007). Organosilicon therapy in Alzheimer's disease? *J Alzheimers Dis*, vol. 11, pp. 301-2.

Fraser, S.P.; Suh, Y.H.; Chong, Y.H. & Djamgoz, M.B. (1996). Membrane currents induced in *Xenopus* oocytes by the C-terminal fragment of the β-amyloid precursor protein. *J. Neurochem.*, vol. 66, pp. 2034-40.

Fukuyama, R.; Mizuno, T.; Mori, S.; Nakajima, K.; Fushiki, S. & Yanagisawa, K. (2000). Age-dependent change in the levels of Aβ40 and Aβ42 in cerebrospinal fluid from control subjects, and a decrease in the ratio of Aβ42 to Aβ40 level in cerebrospinal fluid from Alzheimer's disease patients. *Eur. Neurol.* vol. 43, pp. 155-60.

Goate, A. ; Chartier-Harlin, M.C. ; Mullan, M. *et al.*. (1991). Segregation of a missense mutation in the amyloid precursor protein gene with familial Alzheimer's disease. *Nature* vol. 349, pp. 704-706.

Green, K.N.; Demuro, A.; Akbari, Y., et al. (2008). SERCA pump activity is physiologically regulated by presenilin and regulates amyloid beta production. *J. Cell Biol.*, vol. 181, pp. 1107-16.

Green, K.N. & LaFerla, F.M. (2008). Linking calcium to Aβ and Alzheimer's disease. *Neuron*, vol. 59, pp. 190-4.

Hardy J. & Selkoe, D.J. (2002). The amyloid hypothesis of Alzheimer's disease: progress and problems on the road to therapeutics. *Science*, vol.297, pp. 353-356.

Hertel, C.; Terzi, E.; Hauser, N., et al. (1997). Inhibition of the electrostatic interaction between β-amyloid peptide and membranes prevents ß-amyloid-induced toxicity. *Proc Natl Acad Sci USA*, vol. 94, pp. 9412-9416.

Hillen, T.; Lun, A.; Reischies, F.M.; et al. (2000). DHEA-S plasma levels and incidence of Alzheimer's disease. *Biol Psychiatry*, vol. 47, pp. 161-163.

Huppert, F.A.; van Niekerk, J.K.; Herbert, J. (2000). Dehydroepiandrosterone (DHEA) supplementation for cognition and well-being. *Cochrane Database Syst Rev*, vol. 2, CD000304.

Inoue, S. (2008). In situ Aβ pores in AD brain are cylindrical assembly of Aß protofilaments. *Amyloid*, vol. 15, pp. 223-33.

Jang, H.; Arce, F.T.; Capone, R.; Ramachandran, S.; Lal, R.; Nussinov, R. (2009). Misfolded amyloid ion channels present mobile ß-sheet subunits in contrast to conventional ion channels. *Biophys J*, vol. 97, pp. 3029-37.

Jang, H.; Arce, F.T.; Ramachandran, S. et al. (2010). β-Barrel topology of Alzheimer's β-amyloid ion channels. *J. Mol. Biol.* vol. 404, pp. 917-34.

Jarrett J.T. & Lansbury, P.T. Jr (1993). Seeding "one-dimensional crystallization" of amyloid: a pathogenic mechanism in Alzheimer's disease and scrapie? *Cell*, vol. 73, pp. 1055-1058.

Kato-Negishi, M. & Kawahara, M. (2008). Neurosteroids block the increase in intracellular calcium level induced by Alzheimer's β-amyloid protein in long-term cultured rat hippocampal neurons. *Neuropsychiatr Dis Treat*, vol. 4, pp. 209-218.

Kawahara, M.; Arispe, N.; Kuroda, Y.; Rojas, E. (1997). Alzheimer's disease amyloid β-protein forms Zn^{2+}-sensitive, cation-selective channels across excised membrane patches from hypothalamic neurons. *Biophys J*, vol. 73, pp. 67-75.

Kawahara, M., Arispe, N., Kuroda, Y.; Rojas, E. (2000). Alzheimer's β-amyloid, human islet amylin and prion protein fragment evoke intracellular free-calcium elevations by a common mechanism in a hypothalamic GnRH neuronal cell-line. *J Biol Chem*, vol. 275, pp. 14077-14083.

Kawahara, M. & Kuroda, Y. (2001). Intracellular calcium changes in neuronal cells induced by Alzheimer's β-amyloid protein are blocked by estradiol and cholesterol. *Cell Mol Neurobio*, vol. 21, pp. 1-13.

Kawahara, M. (2004). Disruption of calcium homeostasis in Alzheimer's disease and other conformational disease. *Current Alzheimer Research*, vol. 1, pp. 87-95.

Kawahara, M. (2010). Role of calcium dyshomeostasis *via* amyloid channels in the pathogenesis of Alzheimer's disease. *Current Pharmaceutical Design*, vol. 16, pp. 2779-2789.

Kawahara, M.; Koyama, H.; Nagata, T.; Sadakane, Y. (2011a). Zinc, copper, and carnosine attenuate neurotoxicity of prion fragment PrP106-126, *Metallomics*, vol. 3, pp. 726-734.

Kawahara, M.; Ohtsuka, I.; Yokoyama, S.; Kato-Negishi, M. & Sadakane, Y. (2011b). Membrane incorporation, channel formation, and disruption of calcium homeostasis by Alzheimer's β-amyloid protein, *Int. J. Alzheimer Dis.*, 304583.

Kawahara, M. & Kato-Negishi, M. (2011) Link between aluminum and the pathogenesis of Alzheimer's disease: the integration of the aluminum and amyloid cascade hypotheses, *Int. J. Alzheimer Dis.*, 276393.

Kayed, R.; Pensalfini, A.; Margol, L.; Sokolov, Y.; Sarsoza, F.; Head, E.; Hall, J.; Glabe, C. (2009)Annular protofibrils are a structurally and functionally distinct type of amyloid oligomers. *J. Biol. Chem.* vol. 284, pp. 4230-7.

Kokubo, H.; Kayed, R.; Glabe, C.G.; Staufenbiel, M.; Saido, T.C.; Iwata, N. & Yamaguchi, H.(2009). Amyloid ß annular protofibrils in cell processes and synapses accumulate with aging and Alzheimer-associated genetic modification. *Int. J. Alzheimers Dis.* vol. 2009, Pii, 689285.

Lacor, P.N.; Buniel, M.C.; Furlow, P.W.; Clemente, A.S.; Velasco, P.T.; Wood, M.; Viola, K.L.; Klein, W.L. (2007). Aβ oligomer-induced aberrations in synapse composition, shape, and density provide a molecular basis for loss of connectivity in Alzheimer's disease. *J. Neurosci.* Vol. 27, pp. 796-807.

Lal, R.; Lin, H. ; Quist, A.P. (2007). Amyloid β ion channel: 3D structure and relevance to amyloid channel paradigm. *Biochim Biophys Acta*, vol. 1768, pp. 1966-75.

Lannfelt, L.; Blennow, K.; Zetterberg, H.et al. (2008). Safety, efficacy, and biomarker findings of PBT2 in targeting Aβ as a modifying therapy for Alzheimer's disease: a phase IIa, double-blind, randomised, placebo-controlled trial. *Lancet Neurol*, vol. 7, pp. 779-86.

Lashuel, H.A. & Lansbury, P.T. Jr. (2002). Are amyloid diseases caused by protein aggregates that mimic bacterial pore-forming toxins? *Q Rev. Biophys.*, vol. 39, pp. 167-201.

Leuner, K.; Hauptmann, S.; Abdel-Kader, R.; Scherping, I.; Keil, U.; Strosznajder, J.B.; Eckert, A.; Müller, W.E. (2007). Mitochondrial dysfunction: the first domino in brain aging and Alzheimer's disease? *Antioxid. Redox. Signal.* vol. 9, pp. 1659-75.

Lin, H.; Bhatia, R. & Lal, R. (2001). Amyloid β protein forms ion channels: implications for Alzheimer's disease pathophysiology. *FASEB J.* vol. 15, pp. 2433-44.

Malchiodi-Albedi, F.; Contrusciere, V.; Raggi, C.; Fecchi, K.; Rainaldi, G.; Paradisi, S.; Matteucci, A.; Santini, M.T.; Sargiacomo, M.; Frank, C.; Gaudiano, M.C. & Diociaiuti, M. (2010). Lipid raft disruption protects mature neurons against amyloid oligomer toxicity", *Biochim. Biophys. Acta.*, vol. 1802, pp. 406-15.

Matsuzaki, K.; Kato, K. & Yanagisawa, K. (2010). Aβ polymerization through interaction with membrane gangliosides. *Biochim. Biophys. Acta.*, vol. 1801, pp. 868-77.

Mellon, P.L.; Windle, J.J.; Goldsmith, P.C., et al. (1990). Immortalization of hypothalamic GnRH neurons by genetically targeted tumorigenesis. *Neuron*, vol. 5, pp. 1-10.

Mellon, S.H. (2007). Neurosteroid regulation of central nervous system development. *Pharmacol Ther*, vol. 116, pp. 107-24.

O'Nuallain, B.; Freir, D.B.; Nicoll, A.J.; Risse, E.; Ferguson, N.; Herron, C.E.; Collinge, J.; Walsh D.M., "Amyloid beta-protein dimers rapidly form stable synaptotoxic protofibrils", *J. Neurosci.*, vol. 30, 14411-9, 2010.

Parameshwaran, K.; Dhanasekaran, M.; Suppiramaniam, V. (2008). Amyloid beta peptides and glutamatergic synaptic dysregulation. *Exp Neurol.*, vol. 210, pp. 7-13.

Parri, R.H. & Dineley, T.K. (2010). Nicotinic acetylcholine receptor interaction with beta-amyloid: molecular, cellular, and physiological consequences. *Curr. Alzheimer Res.*, vol. 7, pp. 27-39.

Pike, C.J.; Walencewicz, A.J.; Glabe, C.G.; Cotman, C.W. (1991). In vitro aging of beta-amyloid protein causes peptide aggregation and neurotoxicity. *Brain Res.*, vol. 563, pp. 311-4.

Pratico, D.; Uryu, K.; Sung, S.; Tang, S.; Trojanowski, J.Q.; Lee, V.M. (2002). Aluminum modulates brain amyloidosis through oxidative stress in APP transgenic mice. *FASEB J*, vol. 16, pp. 1138-40.

Querfurth, H.W. & LaFerla, F.M. (2010). Alzheimer's disease. *N. Engl. J. Med.*, vol. 362, pp. 329-44.

Quist, A.; Doudevski, I.; Lin, H.; Azimova, R.; Ng, D.; Frangione, B.; Kagan, B.; Ghiso, J.; Lal, R. (2005). Amyloid ion channels: a common structural link for protein-misfolding disease. *Proc Natl Acad Sci USA*, vol. 102, pp. 10427-32.

Schwartz, Z.; Gates, P.A.; Nasatzky, E.; et al. (1996). Effect of 17β-estradiol on chondrocyte membrane fluidity and phospholipid metabolism is membrane-specific, sex-specific, and cell maturation-dependent. *Biochim Biophys Acta* , vol. 1282, pp. 1-10.

Seelig, J.; Lehrmann, R.; Terzi, E. (1994). Domain formation induced by lipid-ion and lipid-peptide interactions. *Mol Membr Biol*, vol. 12, pp. 51-57.

Selkoe, D.J. (1991). The molecular pathology of Alzheimer's disease. *Neuron*, vol. 6, pp. 487-498.

Selkoe, D.J. & Wolfe, M.S. (2007). Presenilin: running with scissors in the membrane. *Cell* vol. 131, pp. 215-221.

Sepulveda, F.J.; Parodi, J.; Peoples, R.W.et al., (2010). Synaptotoxicity of Alzheimer β amyloid can be explained by its membrane perforating property. *PLoS One*, vol. 27, e11820.

Sherrington, R.; Rogaev, E.I.; Liang, Y. et al. (1995). Cloning of a gene bearing missense mutations in early-onset familial Alzheimer's disease. *Nature*, vol. 375, pp. 754-760.

Simakova O. and Arispe, N. (2007). The cell-selective neurotoxicity of the Alzheimer's Aβ peptide is determined by surface phosphatidylserine and cytosolic ATP levels. Membrane binding is required for Aß toxicity. *J. Neurosci.* vol. 27, pp. 13719-29.

Simmons, L.K.; May, P.C.; Tomaselli, K.J. *et al.*(1994). Secondary structure of amyloid β peptide correlates with neurotoxic activity in vitro. *Mol. Pharmacol*, vol. 45, pp. 373-379.

Small, D.H.; Mok, S.S. & Bornstein, J.C. (2001). Alzheimer's disease and Aβ toxicity: from top to bottom. *Nat. Rev. Neurosci.* vol. 2, pp. 595-8.

Soscia, S.J.; Kirby, J.E.; Washicosky, K.J. et al. (2010). The Alzheimer's disease-associated amyloid beta-protein is an antimicrobial peptide. *PLoS One*. Vol. 5, e9505.

Strodel, B.; Lee, J.W.; Whittleston, C.S.; Wales, D.J. (2010). Transmembrane structures for Alzheimer's Aβ(1-42) oligomers. *J. Am. Chem. Soc.* vol.132, pp. 13300-12.

Terry, R.D.; Masliah, E. Salmon, D.P.et al., (1991). Physical basis of cognitive alterations in Alzheimer's disease: synapse loss is the major correlate of cognitive impairment. *Ann. Neurol.* vol. 30, pp. 572-580.

Tomita, T.; Watanabe, M.; Yasuda, T. (1992). Influence of membrane fluidity on the assembly of Staphylococcus aureus alpha-toxin, a channel-forming protein, in liposome membrane. *J Biol Chem* vol. 267, pp. 13391-13397.

Tomiyama, T.; Nagata, T.; Shimada, H. et al. (2008). A new amyloid β variant favoring oligomerization in Alzheimer's-type dementia. *Ann. Neurol. vol.* 63, pp. 377-387.

Tsutsui, K.; Ukena, K.; Usui, M.; et al. (2000). Novel brain function: biosynthesis and actions of neurosteroids in neurons. *Neurosci Res* vol. 36, pp. 261-273.

Walsh, D.M. & Selkoe, D.J. (2007). Aβ oligomers - a decade of discovery. *J. Neurochem.* vol. 101, pp. 1172-1184.

Whiting, K.P.; Restall, C.J.; Brain, P.F. (2000). Steroid hormone-induced effects on membrane fluidity and their potential roles in non-genomic mechanisms. *Life Sci.*, vol. 67, pp. 743-57.

Yankner, B.A.; Duffy, L.K. & Kirschner, D.A. (1990). Neurotropic and neurotoxic effects of amyloid β protein: reversal by tachykinin neuropeptides. *Nature,* vol. 250, pp. 279-282.

6

Recent Developments in Molecular Changes Leading to Alzheimer's Disease and Novel Therapeutic Approaches

Vijaya B. Kumar
VA Medical Center and St. Louis university Health Sciences Center, St. Louis, MO USA

1. Introduction

Alzheimer's disease (AD) is a debilitating progressive neurological disease affecting significant number of individuals above the age of 65 years and even those who are as young as 30 years, around the globe. According to the Alzheimer's Association 2011 facts and figures report, Alzheimer's is the sixth leading cause of death and approximately 5.4 million people age 65 and older suffer from Alzheimer's disease in USA alone. Of all Americans over the age of 65, one out of every eight has AD. As the age advances, the risk of developing AD increases to as much as 47-50% by the age of 85. Risk is even greater if both parents suffer the disease (Bachman *et al*, 1992). Two types of AD have been described. The sporadic form of AD is a general deterioration of intra-neuronal contact without any association to any genetic element. Familial AD (FAD) on the other hand is associated with mutations in amyloid precursor protein (APP) on chromosome 21 (Goates A.M *et al*, 1991), apolipoprotein E gene on chromosome 19 (Cedazo-Minguez & Cowburn, 2001), presenilin 1 (PS1) on chromosome 14 (Sudoh *et al*, 1998), and presenilin 2 (PS2) on chromosome 1 (Jayadev *et al*, 2010). In addition, high phosphorylation that results in tangle formation is also attributed to mutations in the gene of microtubule associated protein Tau, located on chromosome 17 (Hanger *et al*, 1992). Among these, deposition of amyloid is widely accepted as the leading cause of AD. Although, amyloid plaque formation was observed in AD brains as early as 1907 (Alzheimer *et al*, 1995), it was only recently the toxicity (Yankner & Lu, 2009; Yankner *et al*, 1990) and the contents (Tokutake, 1988; Vital, 1988; Pardridge *et al*, 1987) have been established. It has been a common observation in several investigations that a single or multiple mutations in any of these proteins alone can affect the performance of other proteins resulting in neurodegeneration. Each mutation in any single protein may differentially affect its function. Therefore, some of the mutations have more drastic consequences than others such as a quintessential mutation in PS2 described by Yu (Yu *et al*, 2010). In addition some of the mutations appear to cause greater harm than the others by shutting down a whole complex of protein activity such as specific presenilin 1 mutation (Heilig *et al*, 2010), suggesting that lethality and onset of AD is not a simple process. That said, the converse also appears to be true. That is, if the damage of any one of the affected proteins is reversed, it may be sufficient to alleviate the distress caused by the disease process (Kumar *et al*, 2000a). In light of the fact that reversal of the changes observed due to or as a consequence of AD in any one or two proteins may have beneficial effects has opened a possibility to target these proteins to develop therapeutic agents *inter alia* (Tokutake, 1988; Vital, 1988; Pardridge *et al*, 1987; Lee, 2002; Morley *et al*, 2002; Okura & Matsumoto, 2007; Ohno, 2006; Schenk *et al*, 1999; Roggo, 2002; Evin *et al*, 2006; Hussain *et al*, 2007; Thompson *et al*, 2005; Kumar *et al*, 2000a; Santacruz *et al*, 2005; Kumar *et al*, 2000b). Despite so many targets for the development of agents that may alleviate the symptoms or even cure the disease, the available products to treat the disease are marginal.

Among various approaches that are made to reduce or enhance any of the affected proteins during AD, this chapter deals with regulating some of these proteins by antisense oligonucleotide technology developed in my laboratory.

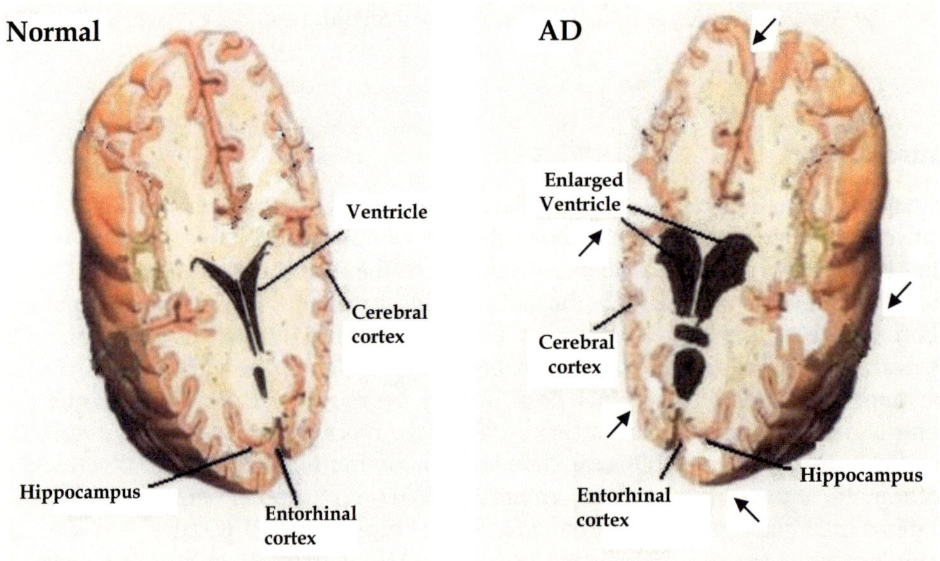

Fig. 1. Cartoon of normal and AD brains. In AD, there is overall shrinkage of the brain and ventricular enlargement. Arrows indicate some changes. The morphology of AD brain itself suggests that the disease is more complex involving multiple factors

2. Areas of the brain affected in AD

There are two major changes that can be observed in the brain upon the onset of AD. The morphological appearance of affected brain is significantly different compared to a normal brain due to the shrinkage of several areas of the brain and enlargement of the ventricles (Fig. 1). This shrinkage of some areas and enlargement of others in AD brain are dramatically different from the changes in cerebral cortex of a normal brain that occur due to normal aging. The cerebral cortex is the outer surface of the brain. It is responsible for all intellectual functioning. Although we find the effect on the overall brain being affected both in size and biology in AD, mostly memory associated regions such as hippocampus (Puolivali *et al*, 2002), amygdala and septum show considerable degeneration in AD which also have shown an increased amounts of amyloid precursor protein (APP) (Kumar *et al* unpublished). Atrophy of the parietal and temporal lobes is observed in AD. Secondly, AD is characterized by the presence of numerous senile plaques and neurofibrillaray tangles

(Chen & Fernandez, 1999; Goedert & Crowther, 1989). AD is associated with disorientation, loss of language and memory due to these changes. The memory associated region, mostly hippocampus suffers a progressive neuronal dysfunction and denigration of the neurons (Gibson, 1987). For this reason, my laboratory concentrated on the hippocampal areas in an animal model of AD (Kumar *et al.*, 1999). It has been shown that increase in hippocampal APP correlates with memory loss in mice that exhibit early loss of memory (Morley *et al.*, 2000). While the cortex, and the memory centers show physical and biochemical changes, the overall brain itself shows a shrinkage and enlargement of the ventricles. This may be due to the drastic changes in the membrane fluidity which follows the changes in the fatty acid composition as observed by Kumar et al (Kumar *et al*, 1999) in a senescence accelerated mouse brain. The histological features of AD in the brain are well characterized and three major hypotheses are currently in vogue for pharmaceutical agent development to combat this disease. The earliest hypothesis proposes a deficiency in cholinergic signaling. This is attributed to be the primary cause of initiation of the disease. The second hypothesis suggests that Tau protein alone or in combination with amyloid beta fragment begin the neuronal tangles and loss neuronal communication that initiate the disease. Thirdly APP is aberrantly processed resulting the plaque formation. Currently there is no clear accepted hypothesis for the initiation of AD. While current therapeutic agents are based on the first hypothesis, vigorous research to develop novel agents to combat the disease in many institutions, including my laboratory, is dependent on the amyloid beta hypothesis. This hypothesis provides several molecular targets to develop agents which may alleviate the disease symptoms, even though one cannot claim that they serve as preventive drug therapies. Therefore, it is essential to study in depth the molecular factors that are either the cause or manifestation of the disease to develop preventive or totally disease curing drugs.

3. Molecular factors attributed to the manifestation of AD

Deposition of amyloid plaques in AD patients was described as early as 1907 by Alzheimer -English translation (Alzheimer *et al*, 1995). Molecular analysis of the plaque (Pardridge *et al*, 1987) and understanding its toxicity is of recent origin (Yankner *et al*, 1990). The degeneration of neurons is attributed largely to a gradual accumulation of small molecular weight fragment derived from the proteolytic cleavage of APP (Blom & Linnemann, 1992). This peptide fragment which varies in size from 38-43 amino acids is called amyloid beta protein (Aß). When this fragment is less than 42 amino acids, it is considered to be soluble and less harmful to the neuronal communications. At 42 amino acid level it can essentially precipitate and form plaques with increased propensity in the brain bringing down other Aß fragments and disrupt the cell-cell communication consequently causing the death of the neurons (Suzuki *et al*, 1994). As Aß is obtained by the cleavage of APP by the proteases called the secretases, these secretases are the targets for AD therapy (Hendriksen *et al*, 2002; Citron, 2000; Dewachter & Van, 2002). These amyloid peptides are not independently translated although the ß-peptide region starts with an ATG codon. No independent mRNA for this peptide thus far is isolated that opens an investigation to study a possibility of an independent translation for the Aß fragment(s). Therefore, it appears that the amount of this peptide is dependent on the amount of APP and the rate of elimination of Aβ from the brain.
PS1 and PS2 mutations and levels seem to affect the processing of APP thus increasing Aβ concentrations. We measured PS1 levels and attributed this to the increased APP processing to cause early loss of memory in senescence accelerated mouse (SAMP8) (Kumar *et al.*, 2009).

We have also shown that one of the types of Tau increased with age in the SAMP8 mice (unpublished). Suppression of Tau in transgenic mice is shown to increase memory (Santacruz *et al.*, 2005).
Increased risk of AD is associated with one or both apolipoprotein, APOE e4 (Green et al., 2002) alleles. However, the presence of APOE e4 alleles in itself is neither necessary nor sufficient to establish it as a diagnosis method of AD.

4. Currently available therapies for Alzheimer's disease

The clinical manifestation of Alzheimer's disease (AD) is dementia that typically begins with subtle and poorly recognized failure of memory and slowly becomes more severe and, eventually, incapacitating the individual. Other common findings include confusion, poor judgment, language disturbance, agitation, withdrawal, and hallucinations (Bacanu *et al*, 2005). Several strategies to counter these symptoms with various pharmaceutical agents are currently being used which essentially employ either acetylcholine esterase inhibition or glutamate pathway modification.
Various approaches are currently being taken to combat AD. The "cholinergic hypothesis" proposes that AD is initiated by a deficiency in the production of acetylcholine (an ester of acetic acid and choline, $CH_3COOCH_2CH_2N(CH_3)$. As this is an important neurotransmitter, early therapeutic agents were developed to increase or protect acetylcholine levels. Mode of action of Donepezil (commonly known as Aircept) is that it serves as an acetylcholine esterase inhibitor, thus acts by increasing the levels of acetylcholine. It is shown to be effective in mild cognitive impairments and Schizoprenia, and attention deficit disorder. Galantamine (commonly called Reminyl, Razadyne) is obtained from Narcissus pseudonarcissus, a tertiary alkaloid acts to inhibit acetyl choline esterase to increase the neurotransmitter, acetylcholine levels. This is a recently approved drug for AD treatment. Memantine is useful for many neurological disorders which includes AD. The mechanism of action of this drug is to act as an antagonist of the channels of N-methyl-d-aspartate (NMDA) receptors. The glutamate receptor subfamily is ubiquitously involved in several brain functions; therefore, this has a broader function for neurological disorders. The next available drug is rivastigmine tartrate (commonly known as Exelon) is a new generation acetylcholine esterase inhibitor. Lastly, tarcine (1,2,3,4-tetrahydro-5aminiacridine) is presumed to have several modes of actions to reverse the cognitive impairments. This is the earliest FDA approved drug for the treatment of AD. Its structure allows it to easily penetrate the cell membrane. The exact mechanism of its action is unknown. It enhances cholinergic function and several clinical studies with this drug have been done (Summers, 2006; Summers *et al*, 1989).
These medications, though beneficial, have not led to a cure. In all cases, they have served to only treat symptoms of the disease and have neither completely prevented nor reversed the disease. These results and other research have led to the conclusion that acetylcholine deficiencies may not be the direct cause but a result of neurodegeneration. Recently cholinergic effects have been proposed as a potential cause for the generation of the amyloidal plaques and tangles leading to neuroinflammation (Wenk, 2006).
Recent techniques of developing pharmacological agents for AD depend on the amyloid theory. Thus, the aim of the agents generated is to reduce the amount of Aß peptide formed. This is achieved, at least in the animal models, either by using some plant extracts or by the molecular targets that reduce the amount of secretases, or APP or Tau expression. In the

herbal treatments, Chinese medicine leads the filed by offering several plant products for reducing the amyloid plaque formation. *Danggui Shaoyao San* (Hu et al, 2010) or *Ginko biloba* (Gold et al, 2003) are leading plant products in this area. Several large pharmaceutical companies are developing organic chemical agents that modulate the expression of proteins involved in the increase of plaque formation.

I will describe our approach that uses antisense oligonucleotide technology to achieve the same goal of prevention of plaque formation by reducing the amount of amyloid produced. This chapter essentially is dedicated to the approaches for the regulation of amyloid precursor protein (APP) and the proteases that generate plaque forming small molecular beta protein (Aß) using antisense oligonucleotides to specific regions of relevant mRNA(s) designed in my laboratory. Further, I will also describe a novel hybrid antisense technique which might open a new approach to regulate more than one message with a single antisense oligonucleotide. These hybrid antisense oligonucleotides have also been tested by my collaborators who confirmed their efficacy in animal models.

5. Molecular techniques to counter the factors that induce AD symptoms

At molecular level, several targets have been identified to develop new drugs. The approach of the large pharmaceutical agencies is to inhibit γ secretase (Eli Lilly, Merk), blocking Receptor for advanced glycation end products (RAGE-by Pfizer), beta secretase-1 block (CoMentis pharma), 5-HT1A receptor antagonish development (Wyeth etc labs) in addition to immunization against Aß protein (Melnikova, 2007).

In my laboratory we have altered the levels of APP, Tau PS1, γ and β secretases which have direct or indirect role in the generation of insoluble plaque forming $A\beta_{42}$ by using antisense oligonucleotide and siRNA technologies. We have shown their potency and beneficial effects in the cell culture and as well as animal models. We have successfully reversed the symptoms of memory loss and behavioral alterations (Banks *et al*, 2000; Kumar *et al*, 2000a). Even by reducing the levels of just APP, improvement to memory have been observed.

Recently we also developed what is named as hybrid antisense technology (unpublished) which has successfully affected more than one protein at molecular level. This novel technology will open new methods to possible successful therapies not only for AD but also other diseases, neurological or otherwise, which involves more than one gene.

6. Antisense nucleotide technology

Gene regulation can be achieved by several methods. Among these, ribozyme (Macpherson *et al*, 1999), small molecular weight interfering RNAs (siRNA/RNAi) (Koutsilieri *et al*, 2007) and antisense oligonucleotide technologies (Helene & Toulme, 1990; Toulme *et al*, 1990) have been extensively studied. These techniques use a relatively simple concept that a complementary sequence can make a Watson-Crick base pairing with corresponding message thus preventing the translation. In the case of ribozyme which has a clover leaf structure, called as hammer head or hair pin, seeks out the targeted mRNA using complementary sequences, binds to mRNA and cleaves it, acting as a nuclease. RNA interference by SiRNAs and miRNAs are more complex. A dicer generates a double stranded structure of 21-23 nucleotides in length which gets separated and the complementary strand is amplified by RdRP (RNA dependent RNA polymerase). The single strand complexes with RISC (RNA induced silencing complex) and binds to target sequences and cleaves the mRNA which gets inactivated. Although the ribozyme and RNAi technologies are powerful techniques, their utility is largely confined to cell culture and *in vitro* studies due to the difficulties in their transport to specific sites without nuclease induced degradation. Antisense oligonucleotide technology on the other hand has more flexibility for regulation of messages both in *vitro* and *in vivo*. This technique utilizes a set of complementary oligonucleotides to a specific mRNA, to block its translation. The use of complementary deoxyribonucleotide sequences to halt mRNA translation has been described as early as 1977 (Paterson *et al*, 1977). In fact we have shown around the same time that RNA molecules and oligonucleotides could prevent RNA transcription *in vitro* (Kumar *et al*, 1977). Simplest method by which complementary sequences bind to a segment of a given mRNA block the translation of the mRNA is given in fig. 2. The mechanism of action of an antisense oligonucleotide is generally by RNase H cleavage of the double stranded region created by the complementary oligonucleotide that forms a hybrid with specific sequences on the mRNA. RNase H is rather ubiquitous enzyme. Alternatively, the hybrid formed by the complementary oligonucleotide may serve as a block to ribosome from proceeding to complete peptide synthesis. If the complementary sequences are made to 5′ un-translated region near or on the ribosome binding site, the ribosome would not even bind to initiate the translation or can be halted from movement. However, an internal antisense oligonucleotide generally works by RNase H mechanism, as assessed by the detection of incomplete mRNA molecules. Antisense oligonucleotide technology is not limited to preventing translation, but can be used to target the gene itself and prevent mRNA transcription thus preventing RNA splicing itself.

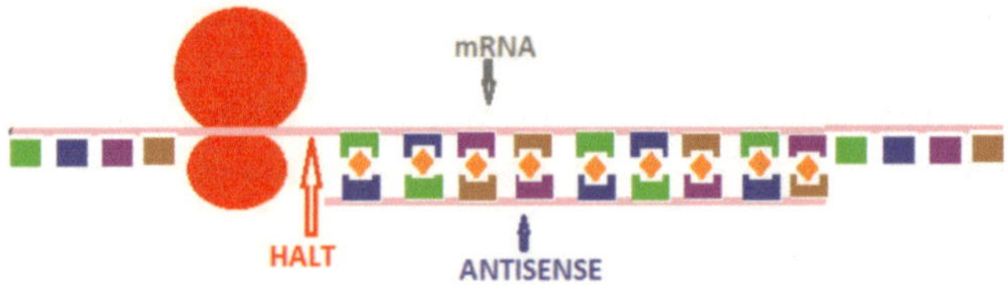

Fig. 2. A cartoon of complementary sequence (antisense) blockade of mRNA translation. This cartoon shows the steric hindrance of to the ribosome to prevent further completion of protein translation

There are several advantages in using antisense technology as opposed to RNAi technology. First of all, the antisense oligonucleotides are deoxy oligonucleotides, therefore, are more stable than RNA based antisense as in RNAi technology which uses ribonucleotide backbone in the complementary sequences. Therefore, it is more vulnerable to RNases. Secondly, the phosphate back bone and deoxyribose sugar can be modified in the antisense technology as these are made synthetically. This is done by substituting various other groups (Fig. 3) making the oligonucleotide more resistant to deoxyribonucleases. Thirdly, the quantity of antisense oligonucleotide can be manipulated so that the extent of mRNA regulation can be controlled. Further, sequences selected on the target mRNA, also give a handle to modulate the mRNA translation. In the case of RNA interference, such controls cannot be exerted. In the RNAi technology, the complementary sequences along with coding sequences need to be cloned into a vector, which generates the double stranded molecules continuously. Further, the double stranded molecule needs to be converted to single strand by cellular machinery to generate the antisense molecules which in turn inactivate the targeted message (Moazed, 2009). For all practical purposes, using deoxyoligonucleotides with altered sugar or phosphate bone appear to be more practical to modulate messages than SiRNA/RNAi techniques which have the same goal. However, the latter ones which have been shown to be more effective in cell cultures may become potent therapeutic agents once techniques to regulate their expression are developed. Currently, in a whole animal, including man, oligonucleotide technology may be more manageable to modulate gene activity. I generally used phophorothiated antisense oligonucleotides for *in vivo* studies (in the animal and cells) successfully (Kumar *et al*, 2000c; Kumar *et al*, 2001). We have shown that phosphorothiated antisense molecules did reverse the memory loss caused by aging or amyloid accumulation. Further, many laboratories used this technology against cancer (Dolnick, 1991), amyotrophic lateral sclerosis (ALS) (Smith *et al*, 2006), Ebola (Swenson *et al*, 2009; Enterlein *et al*, 2006), HIV Aids (Stein *et al*, 1989; Matsukura *et al*, 1989; Rossi *et al*, 2007), diabetes (Machen *et al*, 2004), Duchenne muscular dystrophy (Bremmer-Bout *et al*, 2004; Aartsma-Rus *et al*, 2004), Asthma (Nyce & Metzger, 1997) etc. This technique has been applied for a variety of diseases including neurological diseases.

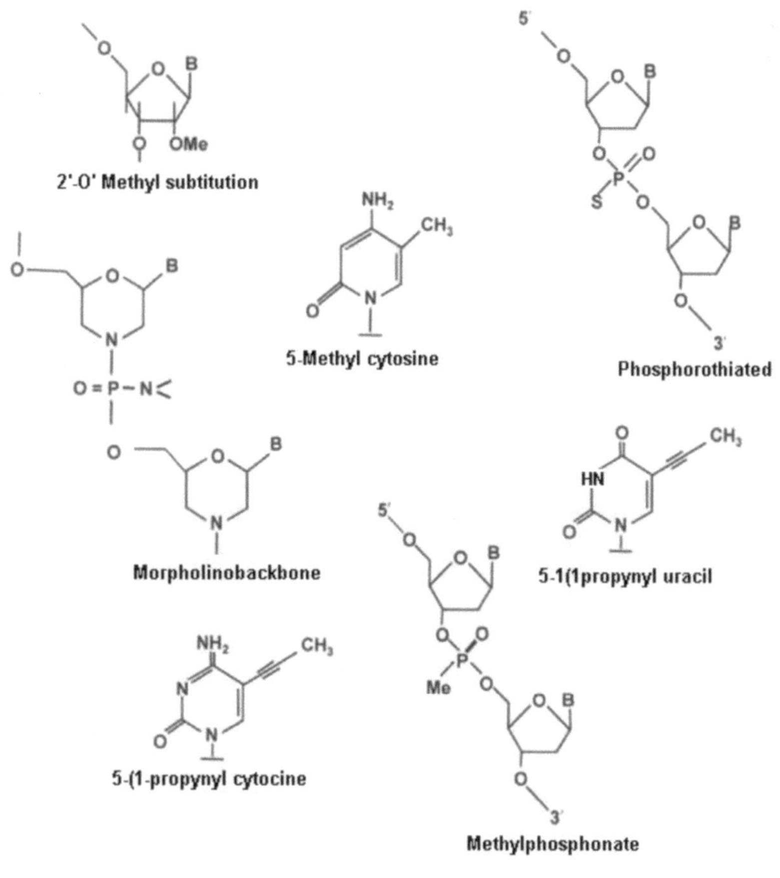

Fig. 3. Substitutions that make the oligonucleotides resistant to nuclease degradation. Figure shows currently available base substitutions that confer resistance to nuclease resistance to the oligonucleotide backbone

7. Uptake of antisense oligonucleotides

Antisense oligonucleotides are easily taken up into the eukaryotic cells across cell membrane by active transport which is temperature dependent (Loke *et al*, 1989). However, the transport into neuronal cells is not a passive transport and needs help with external agents. Fig. 4 shows various agents that we used for transport across PC 12 cell line to test the efficacy of antisense oligonucleotides. In this experiments a 42 mer antisense against human APP. Amphotericin B was first used by us to transport DNA (Kumar *et al*, 1974) and later shown to be a valuable agent for the transport of oligonucleotides into 3T3 cells (Garcia-Chaumont *et al*, 2000). Using $CaCl_2$ or Amphotericin B would cause some cell death if we cross concentrations above 1mM and 10 μM respectively. In the figure we have used lower than these concentrations. DMSO concentration was 1%. Lipid encapsulation transporter, lipofectamine did not cause any cell damage even at concentrations higher than suggested by the manufacturer.

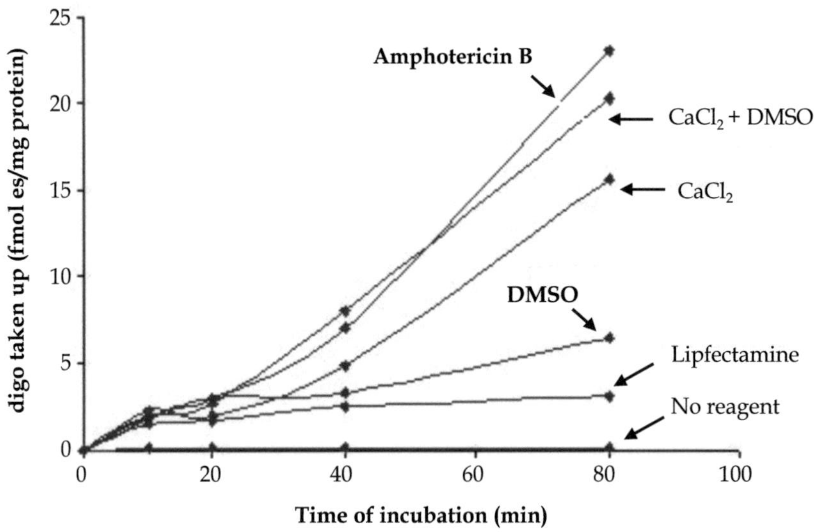

Fig. 4. Efficiency of transport of a 42 mer oligonucleotide into HTB 11 cells in the presence of various agents. The oligonucleotide was labeled with ^{32}P and purified by ethanol precipitation and tested for homogeneity on a 15% polyacrylamide gel. The cells were incubated with known amount of labeled oligonucleotide for specified times, washed, homogenized and counted. Notice that minimal concentrations of $CaCl_2$ in combination with DMSO or Amphotericin B are of great advantage in the transport of oligonucleotides

When a mouse is administered an antisense oligonucleotide by any route, it can reduce the translation of corresponding mRNA. In the animal system, the neuronal cells have the ability to transport the oligonucleotide without the additional aid by cationic reagents. However, in both neuronal cells in culture and in the animal, the transport of oligonucleotide occurs by binding to specific receptor(s). When the cells were incubated with ^{32}P labeled oligonucleotide in the presence of DMSO+$CaCl_2$ as in fig. 5 and cell extracts were subjected gel retardation assay (Scott *et al*, 1994) by 12% polyacrylamide gel, we observed higher size bands suggesting its association with a protein(s) which may serve as receptors to transport the oligonucleotide (Fig. 5). Such an association is observed in the brain tissues of the animals which were administered the oligonucleotide. We have noticed that there are receptors in the brain that may be facilitating the transport of oligonucleotides.

Fig. 5. Association of oligonucleotide with cellular receptor protein. HTB 11 human neuronal cells were incubated for 60 minutes and the cell extracts were run on 12% polyacrylamide gels in Trisborate buffer and subjected to autoradiography. Notice the association of majority of oligonucleotide with protein(s)

In the case of animals, the delivery of antisense oligonucleotides by three routes was tested. When the delivery was made by icv (intra crebrovascular), minimum amounts (as low as 60 ng/antisense oligonucleotides of 20-40 nucleotides) was very effective in reversing the loss of memory or acquisition. This is because most of the antisense oligonucleotide could be targeted to hippocampal area which is involved in memory. When an antisense oligonucleotide made against some sequences at Aβ region of APP (5′ GGCGCCTTTGTTCGAACCCACATCTTCAGCAAAGAACACCAG - Kumar-US patent 6310048-2001) was administered by icv, its levels were considerably reduced (Kumar *et al*, 2000b). The transport of oligonucleotide though to a lesser extent occurs also by iv (intra venous) and reverses memory loss in mice (Banks *et al*, 2000). The transport into brain could also be achieved by oral or peritoneal routes (Kumar unpublished). For therapy, oral administration is most preferred. The distribution of orally and intraperitoneally administered oligonucleotide of 42 nucleotides is given in Figs. 6 and 7 respectively. Notice that by both routes of administration the percentage of the administered oligonucleotide recovered in the brain is same. But the distribution of the oligonucleotide in various organs is different. The behavioral studies are yet to be performed to quantify the efficacy of the oral or intraperitoneal administrations. But, the stability of the oligonucleotide was tested by extracting the oligonucleotide from these tissues by polyacrylamide gels. The oligonucleotide does undergo some degradation in all the tissues in spite of the fact that the oligonucleotide was phosphorothiated. However, what was extracted from brain did not seem to be degraded and is associated with a protein as it runs at a higher molecular weight than the monomer on polyacrylamide gels.

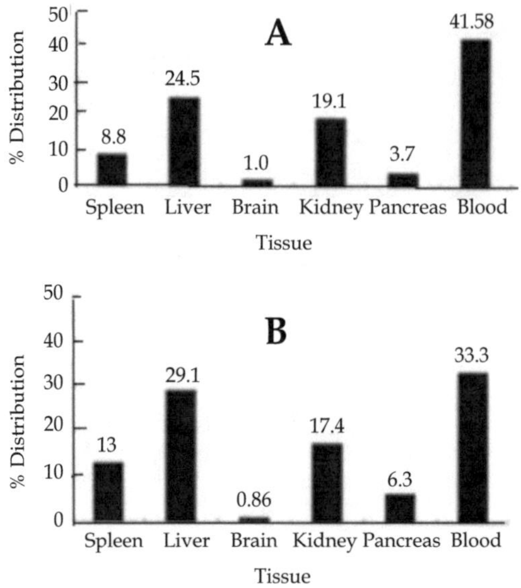

Fig. 6. Distribution short (20 mer-panel A) and long (42 mer-panel B) ^{32}P-labled oligonucleotide 4hrs after *oral* administration in C57 black mice. 6 month old C57 black mice were administrated ^{32}P-labled oligonucleotides and their distribution is similar irrespective of the size of the oligonucleotide

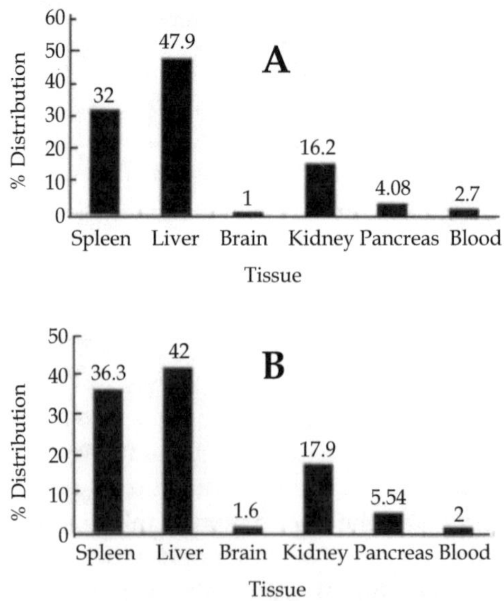

Fig. 7. Distribution short (20 mer-panel A) and long (42 mer-panel B) ^{32}P-labled oligonucleotide 4hrs after *intraperitoeneal* administration in C57 black mice. 6 month old C57 black mice were administrated ^{32}P-labled oligonucleotides and their distribution was determinated as percent of a total/mg of protein. The distribution is similar irrespective of the size of the oligonucleotide

If antisense oligonucleotides have become effective therapeutic agents, the efficacies of administration by different routes have to be established. Although, there is no evidence for any adverse effect in animal models used, in humans more experiments have to be performed to confirm that there will be no adverse effect. As oligonucleotides are natural products, adverse effects if any are likely to be minimal, if oral, nasal or intraperitoneal are the routes of administration.

8. New antisense oligonucleotide technology to regulate multiple genes products with a single oligonucleotide

Variety of neurological diseases including AD, involve altered transcriptional and translational processes of more than one gene. If we consider Alzheimer's disease, a direct linkage exists for disease manifestation and altered expression of secretases, APP, apolipoprotein E, presenilins 1 and 2 and Tau phosphorylation. The changes in the expression of so many genes may be due to a single or multiple mutations in the corresponding genes or due to onset of disease. Therefore, these gene products are the rational molecular targets for the development of therapeutic agents. The results obtained by antisense molecules developed in my laboratory that modulated the expression of some of these proteins showed that this technology may be used to down regulate the specific mRNAs both *in vivo* and *in vitro* with surprisingly positive out come. In the case of methionine enkephalin, we have successfully used more than one antisense molecule to regulate the levels of this protein, as this protein has repetitive sequences (Banks *et al*, 2004). However, when two or more antisense oligonucleotides are used to regulate the messages, there is a high probability of developing anti nucleic acid antibodies (Isenberg *et al*, 2007;Hahn, 1998). In order to avoid such possibility, a technique where one single antisense oligonucleotide molecule can down regulate more than one mRNA is developed in my laboratory. It has been shown that even hexa and decamers have the ability to down regulate a targeted mRNA (Wagner, 1994;Wagner, 1995). Thus two phosphorothiated antisense oligonucleotides of ten nucleotide lengths against PS1 (5'TCTCTGTCAT) and APP (5'TGGGCAGCAT) mRNAs were constructed. A random oligonucleotide (5'GATCACGTAC) was used as control. Their ability to down regulate APP and PS1 proteins in COS 7 cells transfected with respective cDNAs in a co-transfected cell system was tested (Fig. 8, 9). Immunoblotting technique was used to quantify the expression (Kumar *et al*, 2009). In each of these cases there is 40-50% reduction in protein expression.
Based on the above observation A 20 mer hybrid antisense molecule was constructed with a combined sequence of anti APP (blue) and anti PS1 (Purple) (5' TGGGCAGCATTCTCTGTCAT). The hybrid consists of the first ten nucleotides are anti to APP message and the next ten are to anti to PS1 message. The fist 10 nucleotides, when binding to APP mRNA, there will be a 5' over hang of 10 nucleotides and when it is binding to PS1 mRNA, it will have a 3' over hang of the 10 nucleotides. Theoretically, such an over hang need not weaken the antisense blockade or RNase H degradation of the mRNA preventing it from translation. Random oligonucleotide (5'GATCACGTACACATCGACAC) along with the hybrid antisense described above was tested in a COS 7 cell transfected with the APP and PS1 cDNAs. The hybrid antisense molecule could effectively reduce the expression of both APP and PS1 almost as efficiently as individual 10 mers (Fig. 10) in 24 hours. The hybrid antisense oligonucleotides were successfully used in the animals to reverse the loss of memory in animal models of AD (*Kumar et al* unpublished).

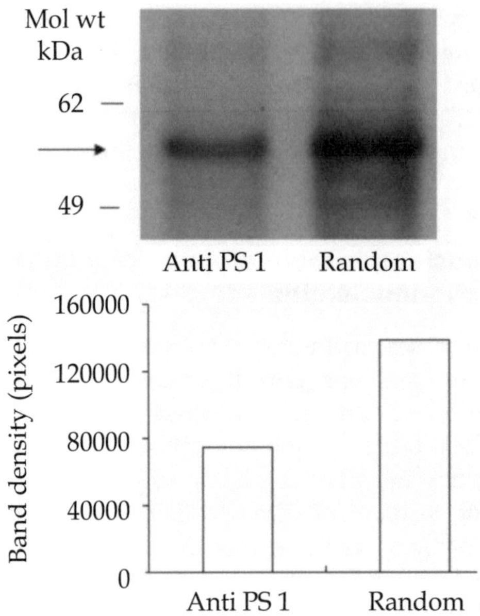

Fig. 8. Down regulation of PS1 with a 10 nucleotide antisense oligonucleotide in COS 7 cells. COS 7 cells were transfected with PS1 cDNA in pCDNA expression vector and a 10 mer antisense or a random oligonucleotide was co-transfected. Cells were grown for 24 hrs and the 10 μg of protein was subjected to immunoblotting. Lower panel gives band densities

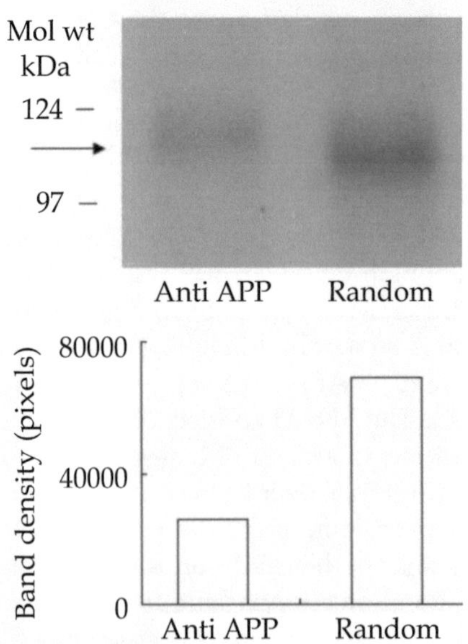

Fig. 9. Down regulation of APP with a 10 nucleotide antisense oligonucleotide in COS 7 cells. COS 7 cells were transfected with APP cDNA in pCDNA expression vector and a 10 mer antisense or random oligonucleotide was co-transfected. Cells were grown for 24 hrs and the 10 μg of protein was subjected to immunoblotting. Lower panel gives band densities

Using a single antisense oligonucleotide molecule containing antisense sequences to two mRNAs to down regulate both mRNAs at the same time may have an advantage in avoiding possible auto antibody induction that may be caused if two different antisense molecules are administered at the same time. We have further extended this technique by using an oligonucleotide which has antisense oligonucleotide sequences against three mRNAs (PS1, APP and Tau).

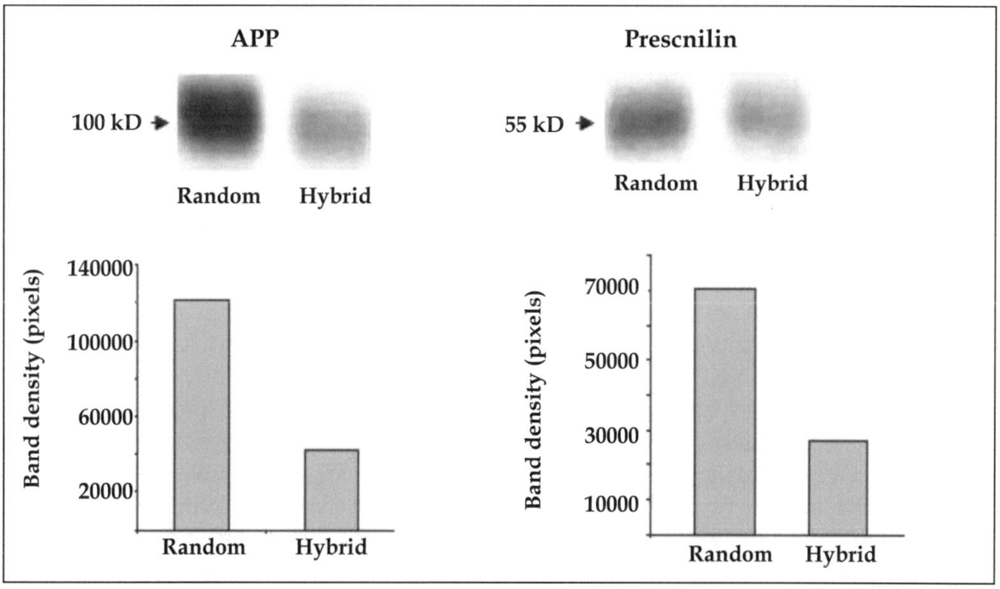

Fig. 10. Down regulation of APP and PS1 mRNAs by a hybrid antisense oligonucleotide. COS7 cells transfected with cDNAs of APP and PS1 were co-transfected with hybrid antisense oligonucleotide and a random control of 20 nucleotides. 24hrs after transfection, 10 µg of cell extracts were subjected to immunoblotting. Notice the reduction of protein expression in antisense transfected cells

Despite the fact that the antisense sequence for one of the messages is embedded in the middle of the oligonucleotide the tribrid antisense molecule thus generated down regulated the translational products of all the three targeted messages (data not given). This approach of one oligonucleotide to regulate multiple messages may serve as an invaluable tool in antisense technology. This would also offset the fear of developing autoimmunity.

9. Conclusion

The use of complementary oligonucleotides to prevent translation of a given message was described as early as 1977 (Paterson *et al*, 1977). Using small RNA or oligonucleotides to block transcription by RNA polymerases was described by Kumar et al in 1977 (Kumar *et al*, 1977). Popular use of complementary synthetic deoxyribonucleitides took another 20 plus years. For a variety of reasons such as the low cost synthesis of oligonucleotides, relative stability, ease of transport, reproducible down regulation of a specific message, relatively simple method for base modification to generate nuclease resistant backbone etc. made antisense technology against a disease state became more common. Extensive use of antisense oligonucleotides in a variety of diseases is not therapeutically ubiquitous after the advent of more powerful RNA interference technology. Various methods are being developed to achieve a viable transport of SiRNA, miRNA (micro RNA) or ShRNA (short hairpin RNA) for clinical use (Leng *et al*, 2009). In this technology also, to increase the stability of interfering RNAs, base modifications such as 2′-O-methyl or morpholino are being developed (Behlke, 2008;Robbins *et al*, 2009). Despite increasing the stability, and billions of dollars spent to develop the agents to down regulate mRNAs by RNA interference, still a targeted and controlled delivery of SiRNA is a far cry. In addition, a viral/bacterial vector usage, while attractive, regulation of the amount produced is difficult. Therefore, currently complementary oligonucleotide therapy is an attractive practical method.

In this article, a novel method is proposed where by more than one gene product may be regulated by a single complementary sequence is described. This procedure is a valuable tool in combating diseases where more than one gene product is shown to be affected due to disease manifestation or as the cause for the disease. This technique will be of great use due to the fact that possible autoimmunity against DNA will be less compared to administering more than one antisense oligonucleotide. It is possible to envisage that this hybrid technology be combined with the currently available SiRNA technology for effective down regulation of several messages at the same time. My laboratory is currently developing such possible products. Novel oligonucleotides that enhance one gene and reduce another are also being developed in my laboratory. Such structures will naturally have a tremendous potential as therapeutic agents, as any disease state is not only accompanied by over expression, but also involves decreased expression of one or more mRNAs. As for the delivery of such molecules in humans, I would suggest nasal delivery instead of oral, intravenous or intra peritoneal. Results of such delivery using an animal model is not presented here, but that route appeared be very effective in preliminary experiments. As oligonucleotides may be considered natural to the biological systems, the possible side effects by antisense delivery may be expected to be rather insignificant. In conclusion, although RNA interference by small molecular weight or micro RNA and ShRNA is of great importance, direct antisense oligonucleotide technology should not be completely ignored, particularly because of its simplicity and ease with which such interfering molecules can be synthesized and administered for relatively low cost. Further, the demand from the cellular machinery by synthetic oligonucleotide for their processing is minimal compared to RNA interference technology which requires dicer mechanism. A combinational therapy of RNA interference and the hybrid technology may also be speculated for an efficient therapeutic intervention of over/under produced transcription and translational products. Such molecules are contemplated and designed by me in my laboratory. A note in proof: Craft et al (Archives of neurology on line Sep. 2011) reported an effective intranasal insulin therapy for AD and mild cognitive impairments, which further suggests that nasal administration suggested in this article may be the ideal route of administration for neurological impairments.

10. Acknowledgements

The author wishes to acknowledge the critical reading by Dr. Vijaya Lakshmi. The laboratory work done by Mr. Mark Franko, only a small sample of which is presented in this article is invaluable. The cells used in culture were donated by Dr. Girdhar Sharma of

Washington University of St. Louis, for which the author is grateful. Thanks are due to Elaine Kosick and Connie Young of the illustration department of VA medical Center, St. Louis, for some of the illustrations used in this manuscript. The help rendered by Tamly J. Farrar is gratefully acknowledged.

11. References

Aartsma-Rus,A., Janson,A.A., Kaman,W.E., Bremmer-Bout,M., van Ommen,G.J., den Dunnen,J.T., & van Deutekom,J.C. (2004) Antisense-induced multiexon skipping for Duchenne muscular dystrophy makes more sense. *American Journal of Human Genetics*, 74, 83-92.

Alzheimer,A., Stelzmann,R.A., Schnitzlein,H.N., & Murtagh,F.R. (1995) An English translation of Alzheimer's 1907 paper, "Uber eine eigenartige Erkankung der Hirnrinde". *Clinical Anatomy*, 8, 429-431.

Bacanu,S.A., Devlin,B., Chowdari,K.V., DeKosky,S.T., Nimgaonkar,V.L., & Sweet,R.A. (2005) Heritability of psychosis in Alzheimer disease. *American Journal of Geriatric Psychiatry*, 13, 624-627.

Bachman,D.L., Wolf,P.A., Linn,R., Knoefel,J.E., Cobb,J., Belanger,A., D'Agostino,R.B., & White,L.R. (1992) Prevalence of dementia and probable senile dementia of the Alzheimer type in the Framingham Study. *Neurology*, 42, 115-119.

Banks,W.A., Farr,S.A., Butt,W., Kumar,B.V., Franko,M., & Morley,J.E. (2000) Delivery of antisense directed against amyloid beta across the blood-brain barrier: reversal of learning and memory deficits in mice overexpressing APP. *Journal of Pharmacolgy and experimental therapeutics*, 297, 1113-1121.

Banks,W.A., Kumar,V.B., & Morley,J.E. (2004) Influence of ethanol dependence and methionine enkephalin antisense on serum endomorphin-1 and methionine enkephalin levels. *Alcoholism: Clinical & Experimental Research.*, 28, 792-796.

Behlke,M.A. (2008) Chemical modification of siRNAs for in vivo use. *Oligonucleotides*, 18, 305-319.

Bremmer-Bout,M., Aartsma-Rus,A., de Meijer,E.J., Kaman,W.E., Janson,A.A., Vossen,R.H., van Ommen,G.J., den Dunnen,J.T., & van Deutekom,J.C. (2004) Targeted exon skipping in transgenic hDMD mice: A model for direct preclinical screening of human-specific antisense oligonucleotides. *Molecular Therapeutics*, 10, 232-240.

Cedazo-Minguez,A. & Cowburn,R.F. (2001) Apolipoprotein E: a major piece in the Alzheimer's disease puzzle. *Journal of Cellular & Molecular Medicine*, 5, 254-266.

Chen,M. & Fernandez,H.L. (1999) The Alzheimer's plaques, tangles and memory deficits may have a common origin. Part V: why is Ca2+ signal lower in the disease? *Frontiers in Bioscience*, 4, 9-15.

Citron,M. (2000) Secretases as targets for the treatment of Alzheimer's disease. *Molecular Medicine Today*, 6, 392-397.

Dewachter,I. & Van,L.F. (2002) Secretases as targets for the treatment of Alzheimer's disease: the prospects. *Lancet Neurology*, 1, 409-416.

Dolnick,B.J. (1991) Antisense agents in cancer research and therapeutics. *Cancer Investigation*, 9, 185-194.

Enterlein,S., Warfield,K.L., Swenson,D.L., Stein,D.A., Smith,J.L., Gamble,C.S., Kroeker,A.D., Iversen,P.L., Bavari,S., & Muhlberger,E. (2006) VP35 knockdown inhibits Ebola virus amplification and protects against lethal infection in mice. *Antimicrobial Agents and Chemotherapy*, 50, 984-993.

Evin,G., Sernee,M.F., & Masters,C.L. (2006) Inhibition of gamma-secretase as a therapeutic intervention for Alzheimer's disease: prospects, limitations and strategies. *CNS Drugs*, 20, 351-372.

Garcia-Chaumont,C., Seksek,O., Jolles,B., & Bolard,J. (2000) A cationic derivative of amphotericin B as a novel delivery system for antisense oligonucleotides. *Antisense & Nucleic Acid Drug Development*, 10, 177-184.

Gibson,P.H. (1987) Ultrastructural abnormalities in the cerebral neocortex and hippocampus associated with Alzheimer's disease and aging. *Acta Neuropathologica*, 73, 86-91.

Goates A.M, Hayens,A.R., & Owens,M.J.e.a. Segregation of missense mutation in the amyloid precursor protein with familial Alzheimer's disease. Nature, 349, 704-706. 1991.

Goedert,M. & Crowther,R.A. (1989) Amyloid plaques, neurofibrillary tangles and their relevance for the study of Alzheimer's disease. *Neurobiology of Aging*, 10, 405-6.

Gold,P.E., Cahill,L., & Wenk,G.L. (2003) The lowdown on Ginkgo biloba. *Scientific American*, 288, 86-91.

Hahn,B.H. (1998) Antibodies to DNA. *New England Journal of Medicine*, 338, 1359-1368.

Hanger,D.P., Mann,D.M., Neary,D., & Anderton,B.H. (1992) Tau pathology in a case of familial Alzheimer's disease with a valine to glycine mutation at position 717 in the amyloid precursor protein. *Neuroscience Letters*, 145, 178-180.

Heilig,E.A., Xia,W., Shen,J., & Kelleher,R.J., III (2010) A presenilin-1 mutation identified in familial Alzheimer disease with cotton wool plaques causes a nearly complete loss of gamma-secretase activity. *Journal of Biological Chemistry*, 285, 22350-22359.

Helene,C. & Toulme,J.J. (1990) Specific regulation of gene expression by antisense, sense and antigene nucleic acids. *Biochimica et Biophysica Acta*, 1049, 99-125.

Hendriksen,J.V., Nottet,H.S., & Smits,H.A. (2002) Secretases as targets for drug design in Alzheimer's disease. *European Journal of Clinical Investigation*, 32, 60-68.

Hu,Z.Y., Liu,G., Yuan,H., Yang,S., Zhou,W.X., Zhang,Y.X., & Qiao,S.Y. (2010) Danggui-Shaoyao-San and its active fraction JD-30 improve Abeta-induced spatial recognition deficits in mice. *Journal of Ethnopharmacology*, 128, 365-372.

Hussain,I., Hawkins,J., Harrison,D., Hille,C., Wayne,G., Cutler,L., Buck,T., Walter,D., Demont,E., Howes,C., Naylor,A., Jeffrey,P., Gonzalez,M.I., Dingwall,C., Michel,A., Redshaw,S., & Davis,J.B. (2007) Oral administration of a potent and selective non-peptidic BACE-1 inhibitor decreases beta-cleavage of amyloid precursor protein and amyloid-beta production in vivo. *Journal of Neurochemistry*, 100, 802-809.

Isenberg,D.A., Manson,J.J., Ehrenstein,M.R., & Rahman,A. (2007) Fifty years of anti-ds DNA antibodies: are we approaching journey's end? *Rheumatology.(Oxford)*, 46, 1052-1056.

Jayadev,S., Leverenz,J.B., Steinbart,E., Stahl,J., Klunk,W., Yu,C.E., & Bird,T.D. (2010) Alzheimer's disease phenotypes and genotypes associated with mutations in presenilin 2. *Brain*, 133, 1143-1154.

Koutsilieri,E., Rethwilm,A., & Scheller,C. (2007) The therapeutic potential of siRNA in gene therapy of neurodegenerative disorders. *Journal of Neural Transmission. Supplementum*, 72., 43-90.

Kumar,B.V., McMillian,R., Medoff,G., Schlessinger,D., & Kobayashi,G.S. (1977) Mechanism of the inhibition by RNA of the RNA polymerases of Histoplasma capsulatum. *Biochimica et Biophysica Acta*, 478, 192-200.

Kumar,B.V., Medoff,G., Kobayashi,G., & Schlessinger,D. (1974) Uptake of Escherichia coli DNA into HeLa cells enhanced by amphotericin B. *Nature*, 1974 250, 323-325.

Kumar,V.B., Farr,S.A., Flood,J.F., Kamlesh,V., Franko,M., Banks,W.A., & Morley,J.E. (2000a) Site-directed antisense oligonucleotide decreases the expression of amyloid precursor protein and reverses deficits in learning and memory in aged SAMP8 mice. *Peptides*, 21, 1769-1775.

Kumar,V.B., Farr,S.A., Flood,J.F., Kamlesh,V., Franko,M., Banks,W.A., & Morley,J.E. (2000b) Site-directed antisense oligonucleotide decreases the expression of amyloid precursor protein and reverses deficits in learning and memory in aged SAMP8 mice. *Peptides*, 21, 1769-1775.

Kumar,V.B., Farr,S.A., Flood,J.F., Kamlesh,V., Franko,M., Banks,W.A., & Morley,J.E. (2000c) Site-directed antisense oligonucleotide decreases the expression of amyloid precursor protein and reverses deficits in learning and memory in aged SAMP8 mice. *Peptides*, 21, 1769-1775.

Kumar,V.B., Franko,M., Banks,W.A., Kasinadhuni,P., Farr,S.A., Vyas,K., Choudhuri,V., & Morley,J.E. (2009) Increase in presenilin 1 (PS1) levels in senescence-accelerated mice (SAMP8) may indirectly impair memory by affecting amyloid precursor protein (APP) processing. *Journal of Experimental Biology*, 212, 494-498.

Kumar,V.B., Vyas,K., Buddhiraju,M., Alshaher,M., Flood,J.F., & Morley,J.E. (1999) Changes in membrane fatty acids and delta-9 desaturase in senescence accelerated (SAMP8) mouse hippocampus with aging. *Life Sciences*, 65, 1657-1662.

Kumar,V.B., Vyas,K., Franko,M., Choudhary,V., Buddhiraju,C., Alvarez,J., & Morley,J.E. (2001) Molecular cloning, expression, and regulation of hippocampal amyloid precursor protein of senescence accelerated mouse (SAMP8). *Biochemistry and Cell biology*, 79, 57-67.

Lee,V.M. (2002) Amyloid binding ligands as Alzheimer's disease therapies. *Neurobiology of Aging*, 23, 1039-1042.

Leng,Q., Woodle,M.C., Lu,P.Y., & Mixson,A.J. (2009) Advances in Systemic siRNA Delivery. *Drugs Future*, 34, 721.

Loke,S.L., Stein,C.A., Zhang,H., Mori,A., Nakanishi,M., Subasinghe,C., Cohen,J.S., & Neckers,L.M. (1989) Characterization of oligonucleotide transport into living cells. *Proceedings of the National Academy of Sciences of the United States of America*, 86, 3474-3478.

Machen,J., Harnaha,J., Lakomy,R., Styche,A., Trucco,M., & Giannoukakis,N. (2004) Antisense oligonucleotides down-regulating costimulation confer diabetes-preventive properties to nonobese diabetic mouse dendritic cells. *Journal of Immunology*, 173, 4331-4341.

Macpherson,J.L., Ely,J.A., Sun,L.Q., & Symonds,G.P. (1999) Ribozymes in gene therapy of HIV-1. *Frontiers in Bioscience*, 4, D497-D505.

Matsukura,M., Zon,G., Shinozuka,K., Robert-Guroff,M., Shimada,T., Stein,C.A., Mitsuya,H., Wong-Staal,F., Cohen,J.S., & Broder,S. (1989) Regulation of viral expression of human immunodeficiency virus in vitro by an antisense phosphorothioate oligodeoxynucleotide against rev (art/trs) in chronically infected cells. *Proc.Natl.Acad.Sci.U.S.A*, 86, 4244-4248.

Melnikova,I. (2007) Therapies for Alzheimer's disease. *Nature Reviews Drug Discovery*, 6, 341-342.

Moazed,D. (2009) Small RNAs in transcriptional gene silencing and genome defence. *Nature*, 457, 413-420.

Morley,J.E., Farr,S.A., & Flood,J.F. (2002) Antibody to amyloid beta protein alleviates impaired acquisition, retention, and memory processing in SAMP8 mice. *Neurobiology of Learning & Memory*, 78, 125-138.

Nyce,J.W. & Metzger,W.J. (1997) DNA antisense therapy for asthma in an animal model. *Nature*, 385, 721-725.

Ohno,M. (2006) Genetic and pharmacological basis for therapeutic inhibition of beta- and gamma-secretases in mouse models of Alzheimer's memory deficits. *Reviews in the Neurosciences*, 17, 429-454.

Okura,Y. & Matsumoto,Y. (2007) Development of anti-Abeta vaccination as a promising therapy for Alzheimer's disease. *Drug News & Perspectives.*, 20, 379-386.

Pardridge,W.M., Vinters,H.V., Yang,J., Eisenberg,J., Choi,T.B., Tourtellotte,W.W., Huebner,V., & Shively,J.E. (1987) Amyloid angiopathy of Alzheimer's disease: amino acid composition and partial sequence of a 4,200-dalton peptide isolated from cortical microvessels. *Journal of Neurochemistry*, 49, 1394-1401.

Paterson,B.M., Roberts,B.E., & Kuff,E.L. (1977) Structural gene identification and mapping by DNA-mRNA hybrid-arrested cell-free translation. *Proceedings of the National Academy of Sciences of the United States of America*, 74, 4370-4374.

Puolivali,J., Wang,J., Heikkinen,T., Heikkila,M., Tapiola,T., van Groen,T., & Tanila,H. (2002) Hippocampal A beta 42 levels correlate with spatial memory deficit in APP and PS1 double transgenic mice. *Neurobiology of Disease.*, 9, 339-347.

Robbins,M., Judge,A., & MacLachlan,I. (2009) siRNA and innate immunity. *Oligonucleotides*, 19, 89-102.

Roggo,S. (2002) Inhibition of BACE, a promising approach to Alzheimer's disease therapy. *Current Topics in Medicinal Chemistry*, 2, 359-370.

Rossi,J.J., June,C.H., & Kohn,D.B. (2007) Genetic therapies against HIV. *Nature Biotechnology*, 25, 1444-1454.

Santacruz,K., Lewis,J., Spires,T., Paulson,J., Kotilinek,L., Ingelsson,M., Guimaraes,A., DeTure,M., Ramsden,M., McGowan,E., Forster,C., Yue,M., Orne,J., Janus,C., Mariash,A., Kuskowski,M., Hyman,B., Hutton,M., & Ashe,K.H. (2005) Tau suppression in a neurodegenerative mouse model improves memory function. *Science*, 309, 476-481.

Schenk,D., Barbour,R., Dunn,W., Gordon,G., Grajeda,H., Guido,T., Hu,K., Huang,J., Johnson-Wood,K., Khan,K., Kholodenko,D., Lee,M., Liao,Z., Lieberburg,I., Motter,R., Mutter,L., Soriano,F., Shopp,G., Vasquez,N., Vandevert,C., Walker,S., Wogulis,M., Yednock,T., Games,D., & Seubert,P. (1999) Immunization with amyloid-beta attenuates Alzheimer-disease-like pathology in the PDAPP mouse [see comments]. *Nature*, 400, 173-177.

Scott,V., Clark,A.R., & Docherty K. Protocols for Gene Analysis. *Methods in Molecular Biology*, 31, 339-347. 1994.

Smith,R.A., Miller,T.M., Yamanaka,K., Monia,B.P., Condon,T.P., Hung,G., Lobsiger,C.S., Ward,C.M., McAlonis-Downes,M., Wei,H., Wancewicz,E.V., Bennett,C.F., & Cleveland,D.W. (2006) Antisense oligonucleotide therapy for neurodegenerative disease. *Journal of Clinical Investigation*, 116, 2290-2296.

Stein,C.A., Matsukura,M., Subasinghe,C., Broder,S., & Cohen,J.S. (1989) Phosphorothioate oligodeoxynucleotides are potent sequence nonspecific inhibitors of de novo infection by HIV. *AIDS Research and Human Retroviruses*, 5, 639-646.

Sudoh,S., Kawamura,Y., Sato,S., Wang,R., Saido,T.C., Oyama,F., Sakaki,Y., Komano,H., & Yanagisawa,K. (1998) Presenilin 1 mutations linked to familial Alzheimer's disease increase the intracellular levels of amyloid beta-protein 1-42 and its N-terminally truncated variant(s) which are generated at distinct sites. *Journal of Neurochemistry*, 71, 1535-1543.

Summers,W.K. (2006) Tacrine, and Alzheimer's treatments. *Journal of Alzheimer's Disease*, 9, 439-445.

Summers,W.K., Tachiki,K.H., & Kling,A. (1989) Tacrine in the treatment of Alzheimer's disease. A clinical update and recent pharmacologic studies. *European Neurology*, 29 Suppl 3, 28-32.

Suzuki,N., Cheung,T.T., Cai,X.D., Odaka,A., Otvos,L.J., Eckman,C., Golde,T.E., & Younkin,S.G. (1994) An increased percentage of long amyloid beta protein secreted by familial amyloid beta protein precursor (beta APP717) mutants. *Science*, 264, 1336-1340.

Swenson,D.L., Warfield,K.L., Warren,T.K., Lovejoy,C., Hassinger,J.N., Ruthel,G., Blouch,R.E., Moulton,H.M., Weller,D.D., Iversen,P.L., & Bavari,S. (2009) Chemical modifications of antisense morpholino oligomers enhance their efficacy against Ebola virus infection. *Antimicrobial Agents and Chemotherapy*, 53, 2089-2099.

Thompson,L.A., Bronson,J.J., & Zusi,F.C. (2005) Progress in the discovery of BACE inhibitors. *Current Pharmaceutical Design.*, 11, 3383-3404.

Tokutake,S. (1988) [Biochemical and immunological properties of senile plaque amyloid]. [Japanese]. *Nippon Ronen Igakkai Zasshi - Japanese Journal of Geriatrics*, 25, 352-357.

Toulme,J.J., Verspieren,P., Boiziau,C., Loreau,N., Cazenave,C., & Thuong,N.T. (1990) [Antisense oligonucleotides: tools of molecular genetics and therapeutic agents]. *Ann.Parasitol.Hum.Comp*, 65 Suppl 1, 11-14.

Vital,C. (1988) [Cerebral amyloid angiopathy]. [French]. *Revue de Medecine Interne*, 9, 12-17.

Wagner,R.W. (1994) Gene inhibition using antisense oligodeoxynucleotides. *Nature*, 372, 333-335.

Wagner,R.W. (1995) The state of the art in antisense research. *Nature Medicine*, 1, 1116-1118.

Wenk,G.L. (2006) Neuropathologic changes in Alzheimer's disease: potential targets for treatment. *Journal of Clinical Psychiatry*, 67 Suppl 3, 3-7.

Yankner,B.A., Duffy,L.K., & Kirschner,D.A. (1990) Neurotrophic and neurotoxic effects of amyloid beta protein: reversal by tachykinin neuropeptides. *Science*, 250, 279-282.

Yankner,B.A. & Lu,T. (2009) Amyloid beta-protein toxicity and the pathogenesis of Alzheimer disease. *Journal of Biological Chemistry*, 284, 4755-4759.

Yu,C.E., Marchani,E., Nikisch,G., Muller,U., Nolte,D., Hertel,A., Wijsman,E.M., & Bird,T.D. (2010) The N141I mutation in PSEN2: implications for the quintessential case of Alzheimer disease. *Archives of Neurology*, 67, 631-633.

7

Clinical Profile of Alzheimer's Disease Non-Responder Patient

Alessandro Martorana[1,2], Roberta Semprini[3] and Giacomo Koch[1,2]
[1]*Dipartimento di Neuroscienze, Università di Roma Tor Vergata, Rome*
[2]*Fondazione Santa Lucia IRCCS, Rome*
[3]*IRCCS San Raffaele, Pisana-Rome*
Italy

1. Introduction

Alzheimer's disease (AD) is a disabling neurodegenerative disorder typical of old age. Recent advances led to the development of drugs which effectively alleviate cognitive symptoms. About one-third of patients however do not respond to current pharmacological treatment (Ryu et al., 2005). Reasons of such lack of efficacy of available drugs may represent a step ahead in the understanding of this disabling disorder. To define a non responder profile is the aim of this work.

Accordingly, authors will deal with pathogenesis of AD, neuro-behavioural symptoms, brain imaging and CSF characteristics in order to extract from each section the most relevant features helpful for identification of non responder profile. Such work is difficult and may meet disagreement among specialists, however authors strongly believe that this work may represent a sort of starting point contributing to better understand AD pathophysiology.

1.1 Apathy and Alzheimer's disease

Apathy is a behavioural syndrome common in normal physiological aging, is also part of the psychiatric spectrum of mental illness, and often is part of clinical symptoms of neurodegenerative disorders like AD, fronto-temporal dementia, Parkinson's disease. The opportunity to discuss about its presence during AD lead to start from its definition and anatomical substrates, to better understand possible pathologic reasons of its occurrence.

Apathy is an observable behavioural syndrome consisting in a quantitative reduction of voluntary (or goal-directed) behaviours (Levy and Dubois, 2006). Therefore, apathy occurs when the systems that generate and control voluntary actions are altered. In this view apathy can be defined as the quantitative reduction of self-generated voluntary and purposeful behaviour. Accordingly, apathy is not to be considered a clinical aspect of depression, although they may co-exist (Marin et al., 1993;1994).

Anatomical circuits of apathy are generally represented by cortical areas like the prefrontal cortex (neo-, paleo- and archeo-cortex), amygdala and hippocampus and the ventral basal ganglia (limbic striatum or better the nucleus accumbens, midbrain ventral tegmental area, medial tip of subthalamic nucleus, centro-median and para-fascicular nuclei of the thalamus) (Haber et al., 1995; Deniau et al., 1997; Haber et al., 2010) (Fig. 1). In general, prefrontal cortex (PFC) has an essential role in cognitive and executive processes that involve

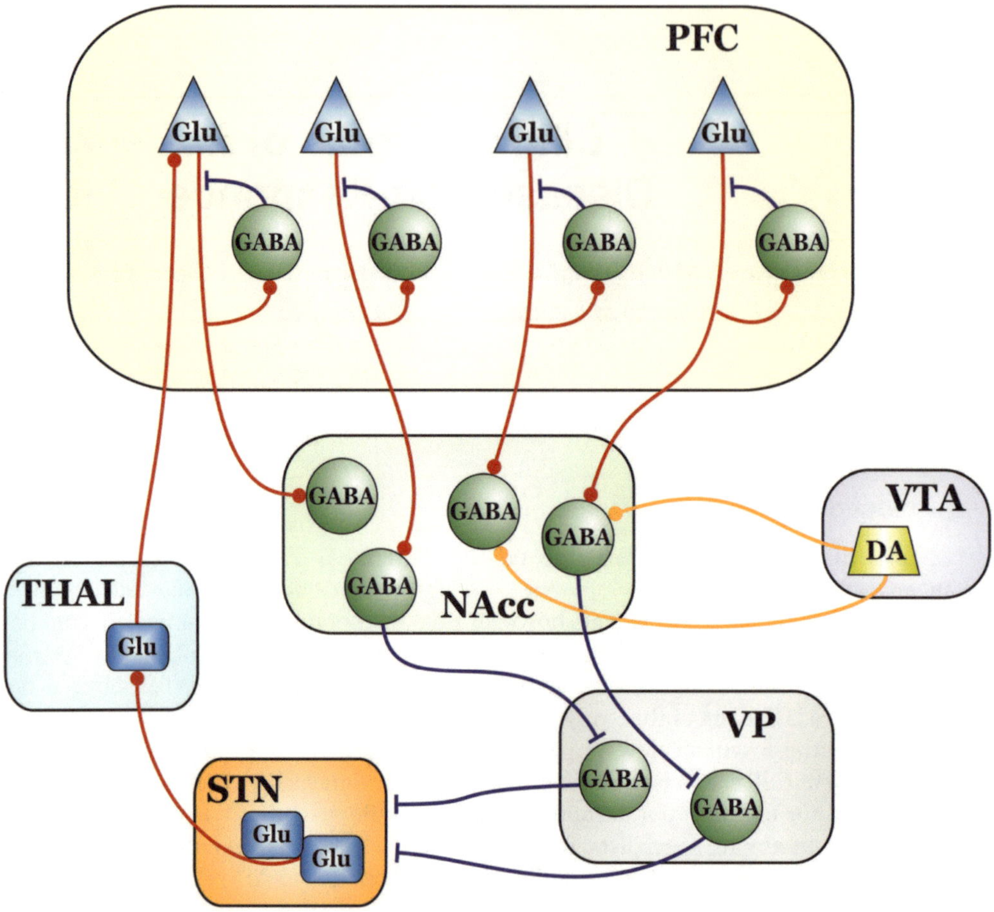

PFC: prefrontal cortex; NAcc: nucleus accumbens; VP: ventral pallidum; VTA: ventral tegmental area; STN: subthalamic nucleus; THAL: thalamus; Glu: glutamatergic excitatory neurons; GABA: GABA-ergic inhibitory neurons; DA: dopaminergic neurons.

Fig. 1. Schematic representation of ventral aspects of the cortical-basal ganglia circuit. Prefrontal cortex envy inputs to the main afferent nuclei of the system, the NAcc, which in turn envy inputs to the VP. Then information flow pass through the STN to the Parafascicular and Centro-Median nuclei of the thalamus and then again to the cortex

motivation, emotion learning and memory. PFC integrates sensory and limbic information and promotes goal-directed behavior through efferent projections to the nucleus accumbens (NAcc). In addition, PFC sends outputs to other limbic areas such as the hippocampus and amygdala, which in turn modulate the activity of the NAcc through excitatory-glutamatergic projections. NAcc has been proposed to play a role in emotion, and more generally in limbic-motor integration (Nicola et al., 2007). This hypothesis has been based on the anatomical organization of the NAcc which suggests that this nucleus is an interface through which limbic (glutamatergic) structures influence motor activity, and that these limbic influences on behavior could in part be controlled by meso-limbic (dopaminergic structures) and cholinergic systems (Haber et al., 1997; Amalric et al., 1993) (Fig. 2).

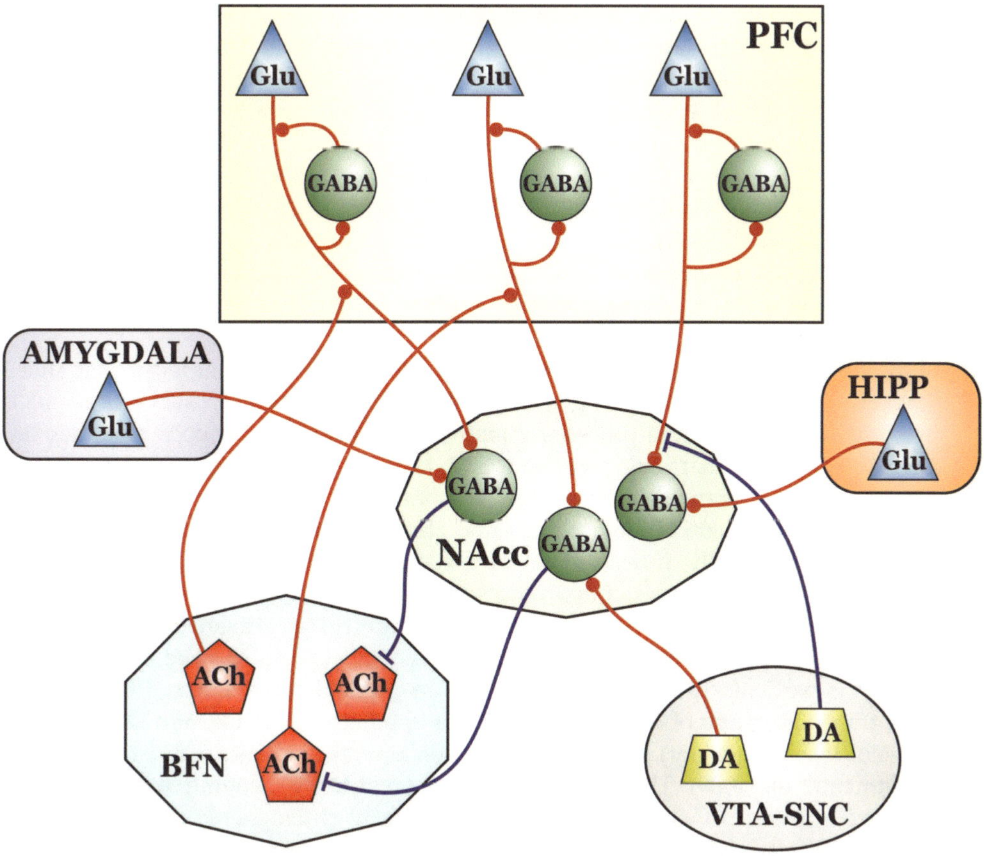

PFC: prefrontal cortex; HIPP: hippocampus; NAcc: nucleus accumbens; SN-VTA: substantia nigra and ventral tegmental area; BFN: basal forebrain nucleus.

Fig. 2. Schematic representation of the complex relationship among NAC(nucleus accumbens) and cortical areas (amygdale, hippocampus and prefrontal cortex), dopamine-nuclei (substantia nigra and ventral tegmental area) and basal forebrain cholinergic neurons (Meinert's nucleus). NAC is in a position to modulate excitatory drive from cortical areas, cholinergic inputs to the cortex through basal forebrain neurons, modulated by dopamine inputs from the ventral midbrain

Inputs from the cortex convey through the multiple organization of the basal ganglia into the pallidum and then back to the cortex. Such arrangement is organized to extract (selection) relevant signals from background noise and to amplify it throughout the final pathway. The final selection is then transferred back to the PFC, which in turn generates inputs in output targets such as cognitive, limbic and even motor territories (Haber et al., 2010).

Over all, PFC and nucleus NAcc are considered the main structures responsible for apathy. In this view, apathy may be distinct at least in three different phenomena related to cortico-basal ganglia topography (Levy and Dubois, 2006): the first, that involves the affective-emotional processing, is topographically related to the ventral-medial PFC and its connection with NAcc and amygdala. This circuit integrates the affective or emotional value of a given stimulus into ongoing behaviour. The second, involving cognitive processing, is topographically related to lateral PFC and to the dorsal caudate nucleus. This circuit is responsible for executive elaboration of a plan of action and involved in a goal-directed behaviour. The third, is observed in severe cases of apathy, is characterised by difficulties in self-initiating actions or thoughts, contrasting with relatively spared externally driven response. This pattern which was called the "auto-activation" deficit is the result of bilateral lesion of the pallidum (Starkstein et al., 1989; Lugaresi et al., 1990) or after extensive damage of the PFC (Kumral et al., 2002).

Within these perspectives, apathy observed in AD patients is more likely to be the result of a dysfunction of affective-emotional processing, thus involving the medial PFC and its connection with amigdala and NAcc.

During normal aging as well as during AD, it is conceivable to suppose that due to morphological and metabolic changes of cortical neurons and of subcortical nuclei, disorder of emotional-affective processing may appear. PFC and hippocampus has been demonstrated to show particular vulnerability during normal aging. Subtle regional changes of dendritic branching or altered mechanisms of neural plasticity has been experimentally demonstrated in lab animals and also in humans (Hof et al., 2004; Petanjek et al., 2008; Bloss et al., 2010; Juraska et al., 2011; Kalpouzos et al., 2011). These changes are also associated to reduced levels of neurotransmitters like acetylcholine, glutamate, GABA and dopamine with age (Chen et al., 2011). Such alterations may reasonably be responsible for appearance of apathetic behavior. Moreover, several reports showed that dopamine transmission is particularly vulnerable with age. In particular reduction of the accumbal dopamine transporter, and of cortical dopamine receptors (both D1-like and D2-like, where D2-like seem to be prevalent) in aged subjects (Volkow et al., 1994,1996; Ishibashi et al., 2009; Backman et al., 2009). These changes were related to PFC cognitive deficits and in particular were related to executive function impairment (Mizoguchi et al., 2009). Given the particular deficits of dopamine transmission and the role played by this transmitter in the control of PFC-basal ganglia circuit, it is conceivable to suppose that such changes could be responsible for apathetic behavior in old subject. Moreover, apathy increases with age in healthy old population (Brodaty et al., 2010), and its presence is considered an early sign of cognitive decline (Onyike et al., 2007). Contrarily to what expected bio-physical and also metabolic differences between AD brain and aged brain are very subtle (Hof et al., 2004). Myth of neuronal loss during aging is not confirmed, and pathologic metabolism of APP and hyper-phosphorylation of tau protein do represent the real difference with age related changes (Giannakopoulos et al., 2008 and 2009; Dickstein et al., 2010). Although many neurotransmitters dysfunction were found in AD brain, interest on dopaminergic transmission has been recently developed with relevant results (McNeil et al., 1984; Martorana et al., 2009; Martorana et al., 2010; Koch et al., 2011-b). However, apathy is usually recognized as part of AD symptoms, being considered the most common behavioral symptom in AD. Apathy increases with severity of AD (yet from conversion from MCI to AD) and has been associated with poorer initiative and executive functions (Drijgers et al., 2011). More importantly, apathy could be an early manifestation of a more aggressive AD phenotype, in which a faster cognitive decline occur (Starkstein et al.,2010). Studies of correlation between dopamine deficits and apathy in AD are needed to better interpret this behavioral syndrome. Of note is the concept that presence of apathy may render difficult the pharmacological approach to AD patients (See Boyle et al., 2004; Robert et al., 2010).

In conclusion, to define apathy simply a neuropsychiatric symptom common in AD, as well as in other dementias or degenerative disorders of the brain, or whether it may represent a clinical predictor of the turn-over (thus worsening) of a defined clinico-pathologic entity (like AD) actually represent a challenge for neurologists studying cognitive decline.

1.2 Neuroimaging morphometric predictors

The effectiveness of current pharmacological treatment of AD, by using AchEIs on cognitive decline symptoms can be highly variable. Genetic factors like the presence of 1 or 2 apolipoprotein E4 (APOE4) alleles are considered predictive of poorer response to therapy, while demographic factor like sex, or culture of the subject revealed some importance if related or associated to APOE status.

Recently, the development of neuro-morphometric measures of regional blood flow and also brain metabolism provided a new possible biomarker of the AD pathologic process. In particular, volumetric analysis of different brain regions showed that hippocampal volume loss is present in patients with mild AD, and the progression of volume loss parallels the worsening of clinical symptoms, and may also be used to predict to the pharmacological response of patients (Csernansky et al., 2005).

Moreover, during AD neuro-psychiatric symptoms are usually persistent, although with variable intensity, and can also be resistant to treatment (Ryu et al., 2005). The physio-pathological and psychological mechanisms involved in the development of neuro-psychiatric symptoms are still poorly understood. Thus, several neuro-anatomical correlative studies have been made, and association between discrete regional pathologies and psychiatric symptoms emerged (Mega et al., 2000; Sweet et al., 2003; Rosen et al., 2005; Sultzer et al., 2003; Shanks and Venneri, 2004; Migneco et al., 2001). Most of recent literature tried to correlate neuro-psychiatric symptoms to morphological features, particularly in early stages of AD. Delusions and agitation, more frequent at late stages of AD, are associated primarily with atrophy of the right fronto-parietal regions (matching with results obtained with metabolic and cerebral blood flow studies) (se Staff et al., 1999 ; Sultzer et al., 2003). Agitation was observed in about one third of AD patients and associated to atrophy of left insula and bilaterally of anterior cingulate cortex (Bruen et al., 2008).

Apathy which is the most frequent symptom of early AD, may be also an early indicator of the disease and is detectable in a high proportion of patients with mild cognitive impairment (Palmer et al., 2007; Lyketos et al., 2007). Presence of apathy was correlated with atrophy of sub-cortical nuclei like putamen bilaterally and of left caudate nucleus. Significant correlations were also found with atrophy of anterior cingulated cortex bilaterally, inferior frontal and orbito-frontal regions of both hemispheres (Gado et al., 1983; Jack et al., 2005; Shiino et al., 2006; Bruen et al., 2008). Apathy has also been linked to dysfunction or atrophy of ventral frontal areas (Rosen et al, 2005; Marshall et al., 2007). Apathy is often seen in early presentation of AD and is sometimes described even before memory deficits become noticeable.

In conclusion morphometric analysis of AD brains indicate that variable degrees of atrophy in selected brain regions could represent a potential and reliable predictor of clinical-type of presentation and may also be used as predictor of pharmacological response to treatment.

1.3 Cerebrospinal fluid analysis

Biochemical changes in the brain extracellular fluid are reflected in the cerebrospinal fluid (CSF). Levels of biological markers like Aβ42, total-tau (t-Tau) and hyper-phosphorylated tau (p-Tau) are currently measured in clinical settings of many western countries, and used as diagnostic tool for diagnosis and for stratification of patients useful for pharmacological trials (Mattsson et al., 2009; Blennow and Zettemberg 2009). In AD patients typically levels of CSF Aβ42 is lower (370 ng/L in AD vs 670 ng/L in controls), while t-Tau (559 ng/L in AD vs 280 ng/L in controls) and p-Tau (82 ng/L in AD vs 51 ng/L in controls) are higher than in healthy controls (Blennow et al., 2007; Mattsson et al., 2009). Low levels of Aβ42 reflect a disturbance of the metabolism of this protein.

Aβ is produced mainly in neurons and is secreted in the CSF 12 hs later, then excreted through the blood-brain barrier 24 hs later into blood (clearance of Aβ), and finally degraded in the reticulo-endothelial system (Shoij et al., 2001). These different phases are in equilibrium among them. In AD patients, Aβ42 forms insoluble aggregates and accumulates in form of fibrils in extracellular space of the brain (Bateman et al., 2009). The reason why Aβ42 levels are decreased in CSF of these patients is believed to be caused by the impairment of the physiologic clearance mechanism above described.

Major biological function of tau is to promote microtubule assembly and maintain the stability of the microtubules, play also crucial roles in signal transduction of neurons (Wang et al.,; 2008; Fanara et al., 2010), and in neural plasticity mechanisms (Avila et al., 2004; Boekhoorn et al., 2006). In AD patients, where plasticity mechanisms are altered, t-Tau levels increase three-fold than the age-matched controls. It's increase in CSF is considered as the result of degenerating process of neurones. Thus, increase of tau protein may leak from the degenerating neurons into the CSF as disease progresses (Blom et al., 2009; Mattson et al., 2009). P-Tau is considered a marker of NFT tangles production, and is strictly associated to the patho-physiological process of AD. Thus, p-Tau is increased in the CSF of AD in relation to neuronal degeneration degree (Blennow and Hampel, 2003).

Whether CSF biomarkers could be used as predictors for progression rate or treatment response was investigated only recently (Wallin et al., 2010; Blom et al., 2009; de Souza et al., 2011). In general, results of recent studies indicate that CSF biomarkers are not considered useful as predictors of treatment response (Wallin et al., 2009), nor were ever considered as markers for pharmacological response. From these studies has emerged that increased levels of t-Tau and p-Tau are associated to rapid progression rate of disease (Kester et al., 2009; Van Der Vlies et al., 2009), in particular for patients converting from MCI to AD (Blom et al., 2009), and also for patients with malignant form of AD (Wallin et al., 2010). In the latter condition was characterised by very high levels of t-Tau(> 800 ng/L) in the CSF, and by higher risk of mortality.

More recently high levels of tau (both total and hyper-phosphorylated) were also associated to hippocampal atrophy (de Souza et al., 2011), or with forms of pathologic neural plasticity (Koch et al., 2011a), indicating again for these proteins possible role as markers of rapid cognitive deficits observed in course of AD. Therefore, heterogeneity of AD patients reflects heterogeneity also in CSF biomarkers, thus the need to deepen the relationship between CSF biomarkers and different subgroups of AD emerges. Within these perspective, association between biomarkers and clinical and/or biochemical data could in turn provide new insight of our understanding of patho-physiology of AD and also of an appropriate pharmacological treatment.

2. Non responder profile

The current approach to cognitive deficits of AD patients derives from the so-called "cholinergic hypothesis", where major cholinergic deficit was suggested to characterise AD, similarly to dopamine for Parkinson's disease. The cholinergic deficiency is currently a target of therapy since cholinesterase inhibitors treatment enhance the cholinergic transmission in AD and shows beneficial effects on cognition in both placebo controlled and open studies (Birks et al., 2006; Wallin et al., 2007). Despite several studies provided the efficacy of pharmacological treatment on cognition, however long-term treatment showed unsatisfactory results. Reasons of such interpretation of data were individuated in the progressive degeneration of cortical and sub-cortical neurons, as the consequence of the abnormal accumulation of Aβ42 and NFT formation.

Interestingly, during the treatment trials of the first cholinesterase inhibitor tacrine, heterogeneity in treatment response was observed. About one-third of the patients evaluated resulted to respond to treatment, one-third remained unchanged and one-third resulted to not respond to pharmacological treatment (Minthon et al., 1993; Eagger and Harvey, 1995; Wallin et al., 2004). The discussion of these results showed clearly the need to define a treatment response, that was extended also to the AchEIs of second generation, however a consensus for how to define a response treatment do not exist.

Such difficulty may justify a sort of "lack of interest" for non responders and moreover may render obscure and hard to define the non responder profile. Many variables (genetic, metabolic, vascular, biochemical, etc) may be considered responsible for pharmacological treatment un-efficacy, and in recent years several studies investigated the importance of these factors. Among others, as possible predictors to treatment response were included cognitive impairment severity (Pakrasi et al., 2003; Van Der Putt et al., 2006; Wallin et al., 2005 and 2009), frontal lobe blood flow (Hanyu et al., 2003), age (Schneider et al., 1991; Evans et al., 2000), gender (Macgowan et al., 1998; Winblad et al., 2001), APOE genotype (Almkvist et al., 2001; Winblad et al., 2001). Unfortunately conflicting results were obtained, and reliable predictors are still unavailable.

However, taking in account the anatomical, clinical and biochemical consideration made above, a profile of "non responder" AD patients may be outlined.

In general patients that do not respond to treatment present with rapidly progressive cognitive decline, not dependent on age, gender, years of education, baseline instrumental activities of daily living, or APOE genotype. The neuropsychological assessment of these patients show involvement of executive functions associated to memory deficits, and the presence of severe apathy. No other behavioural symptoms do occur in these cases. CSF analysis show low levels of Aβ42, and very high levels of t-Tau (> 800 ng/L). Gross morphology remains unaltered in neuro-imaging assessment, although changes of grey matter volumes in frontal-temporal areas were recently described (Serra et al., 2010). It is interesting to note that such transition from responder to non responder state coincide with described changes occurring in MCI converters (Hansson et al., 2009; Mattsson et al., 2009; Blom et al., 2009; Palmer et al., 2010), and also in a subset of AD patients with moderate AD showing rapidly progressive rate of cognitive decline (van Der Vlies et al., 2009; Kester et al., 2009; Wallin et al., 2010; Musicco et al., 2011; Stepaniuk et al., 2011). Thus, from these results appear that the efficacy of current pharmacological treatment with AchEIs could depend on the rate of progression of cognitive decline (fast or slow), which in turn appear as to be associated to signs of frontal lobe dysfunction (indicative of faster decline), hence with the appearance of severe apathy and of executive functions alterations.

Impairment of executive functions and also neurobehavioral symptoms are often observed in course of AD. Their occurrence is typical of more advanced stages and is associated to greater impairment of daily activities in these patients (Boyle et al., 2003; Marshall et al.,

2011; Carter et al., 2011). In this view non responders might represent a clinico-pathological variant of AD (as identified by Back-Madruga et al., 2002), not rare, in which frontal lobe degeneration prevails. Moreover, the reason why the cognitive decline become faster may reside in the interaction between Aβ42 and Tau. Yet at intracellular level Aβ42 has been demonstrated to induce tau fragments formation, which are particularly toxic for mitochondria, leading rapidly to cell dysfunction (Amadoro et al., 2010; 2011). Such interaction would happen also at post-synaptic site leading to cell death via excitotoxic mechanisms (Ittner et al., 2010; Roberson et al., 2011). Such condition could be sufficient to explain the reason of AchEIs treatment un-effectiveness. As alternative hypothesis, it may be supposed that the frontal lobe dysfunction could be due to the direct interaction of Aβ peptides with neurotransmitters system, leading to impairment of cross-talk between transmitters (Palop et al., 2010).

From the patho-physiological point of view, frontal lobe function depends on the anatomical integrity of neurotransmitters network and cross-talk (acetylcholine, dopamine, glutamate, GABA) which function regulating memory, behaviour and emotions (see Martorana et al., 2010). Recent experimental evidences show that such modulatory role is played by interaction between acetylcholine, and other major transmitters like glutamate or dopamine (Moore et al., 2009; Gulledge et al., 2009; Dasari et al., 2011; Livingstone et al., 2010). Thus, frontal lobe dysfunction, particularly in cases of AD would be the result of an impairment among transmitters, particularly of acetylcholine, glutamate, and dopamine, thus likely responsible for faster cognitive decline. Interestingly, recent papers showed marked changes of glutamatergic as well as of dopaminergic systems in frontal lobe of AD brains (Kashani et al., 2008; Kirvell et al., 2007; Kumar and Patel, 2007), suggesting also that involvement of frontal lobe in AD might occur earlier than supposed. Moreover recent transcranial magnetic stimulation studies showed that in AD central cholinergic transmission was restored by L-dopa administration (Martorana et al., 2009), and further showed that L-dopa was unable to modulate neural plasticity mechanisms in AD patients (Koch et al., 2011-b). Within these perspectives it is conceivable to suppose that impaired neurotransmitter systems could account for lack of response to AchEIs.

Remain to be established whether frontal lobe dysfunction represent a reversible condition, and whether alternative treatments, like memantine or dopamine agonists could interfere with this event.

3. Acknowledgements

We want to express our gratitude to Graziano Bonelli for his contribution to the work.

4. References

Almkvist O, Jelic V, Amberla K, Hellström-Lindahl E, Meurling L, Nordberg A. Responder characteristics to a single oral dose of cholinesterase inhibitor: a double-blind placebo-controlled study with tacrine in Alzheimer patients. Dement Geriatr Cogn Disord. 2001 Jan-Feb;12(1):22-32.

Amadoro G, Corsetti V, Stringaro A, Colone M, D'Aguanno S, Meli G, Ciotti M, Sancesario G, Cattaneo A, Bussani R, Mercanti D, Calissano P. A NH2 tau fragment targets neuronal mitochondria at AD synapses: possibile implications for neurodegeneration. J Alzheimers Dis. 2010;21(2):445-70.

Amadoro G, Corsetti V, Ciotti MT, Florenzano F, Capsoni S, Amato G, Calissano P. Endogenous Aβ causes cell death via early tau hyperphosphorylation. Neurobiol Aging. 2011 Jun;32(6):969-90.

Amalric M, Koob GF. Functionally selective neurochemical afferents and efferents of the mesocorticolimbic and nigrostriatal dopamine system. Prog Brain Res. 1993;99:209-26.

Avila J, Pérez M, Lucas JJ, et al. Assembly in vitro of tau protein and its implications in Alzheimer's disease. Curr Alzheimer Res. 2004;1:97-101.

Back-Madruga C, Boone KB, Briere J, Cummings J, McPherson S, Fairbanks L, Thompson E. Functional ability in executive variant Alzheimer's disease and typical Alzheimer's disease. Clin Neuropsychol. 2002 Aug;16(3):331-40.

Bateman RJ, Klunk WE. Measuring target effect of proposed disease-modifying therapies in Alzheimer's disease. Neurotherapeutics. 2008 Jul;5(3):381-90.

Blennow and Hampel. CSF markers for incipient Alzheimer's disease. Lancet Neurol. 2 (2003), pp. 605–613.

Blennow K, Zetterberg H, Minthon L, Lannfelt L, Strid S, Annas P, Basun H, Andreasen N. Longitudinal stability of CSF biomarkers in Alzheimer's disease. Neurosci Lett. 2007 May 23;419(1):18-22.

Blennow K, Zetterberg H. Cerebrospinal fluid biomarkers for Alzheimer's disease. J Alzheimers Dis. 2009;18(2):413-7.

Blom ES, Giedraitis V, Zetterberg H, et al. Rapid progression from mild cognitive impairment to Alzheimer's disease in subjects with elevated levels of tau in cerebrospinal fluid and the APOE epsilon4/epsilon4 genotype. Dement Geriatr Cogn Disord. 2009;27(5):458-64.

Bloss EB, Janssen WG, McEwen BS, Morrison JH. Interactive effects of stress and aging on structural plasticity in the prefrontal cortex. J Neurosci. 2010 May 12;30(19):6726-31.

Boekhoorn K, Terwel D, Biemans B, Borghgraef P, Wiegert O, Ramakers GJ, de Vos K, Krugers H, Tomiyama T, Mori H, Joels M, van Leuven F, Lucassen PJ. Improved long-term potentiation and memory in young tau-P301L transgenic mice before onset of hyperphosphorylation and tauopathy. J Neurosci. 2006;26(13):3514-23.

Boyle PA, Malloy PF, Salloway S, Cahn-Weiner DA, Cohen R, Cummings JL. Executive dysfunction and apathy predict functional impairment in Alzheimer disease. Am J Geriatr Psychiatry. 2003 Mar-Apr;11(2):214-21.

Bruen PD, McGeown WJ, Shanks MF, Venneri A. Neuroanatomical correlates of neuropsychiatric symptoms in Alzheimer's disease. Brain. 2008 Sep;131(Pt9):2455-63.

Carter SF, Caine D, Burns A, Herholz K, Lambon Ralph MA. Staging of the cognitive decline in Alzheimer's disease: insights from a detailed neuropsychological investigation of mild cognitive impairment and mild Alzheimer's disease. Int J Geriatr Psychiatry. 2011 May 25.

Chen KH, Reese EA, Kim HW, Rapoport SI, Rao JS. Disturbed Neurotransmitter Transporter Expression in Alzheimer's Disease Brain. J Alzheimers Dis. 2011 Jul 8.

Colom LV, Castañeda MT, Bañuelos C, Puras G, García-Hernández A, Hernandez S, Mounsey S, Benavidez J, Lehker C. Medial septal beta-amyloid 1-40 injections alter septo-hippocampal anatomy and function. Neurobiol Aging. 2010 Jan;31(1):46-57.

Csernansky JG, Wang L, Miller JP, Galvin JE, Morris JC. Neuroanatomical predictors of response to donepezil therapy in patients with dementia. Arch Neurol. 2005 Nov;62(11):1718-22.

Dasari S, Gulledge AT. M1 and M4 receptors modulate hippocampal pyramidal neurons. J Neurophysiol. 2011 Feb;105(2):779-92.

de Souza LC, Chupin M, Lamari F, Jardel C, Leclercq D, Colliot O, Lehéricy S, Dubois B, Sarazin M. CSF tau markers are correlated with hippocampal volume in Alzheimer's disease. Neurobiol Aging. 2011 Apr 11.

Dickstein DL, Brautigam H, Stockton SD Jr, Schmeidler J, Hof PR. Changes in dendritic complexity and spine morphology in transgenic mice expressing human wild-type tau. Brain Struct Funct. 2010 Mar;214(2-3):161-79.

Drijgers RL, Verhey FR, Leentjens AF, Köhler S, Aalten P. Neuropsychological correlates of apathy in mild cognitive impairment and Alzheimer's disease: the role of executive functioning. Int Psychogeriatr. 2011 Jun 28:1-7.

Eagger SA, Harvey RJ. Clinical heterogeneity: responders to cholinergic therapy. Alzheimer Dis Assoc Disord. 1995;9 Suppl 2:37-42.

Fanara P, Husted KH, Selle K, Wong PY, Banerjee J, Brandt R, Hellerstein MK. Changes in microtubule turnover accompany synaptic plasticity and memory formation in response to contextual fear conditioning in mice. Neuroscience. 2010 Jun 16;168(1):167-78.

Gado M, Hughes CP, Danziger W, Chi D. Aging, dementia, and brain atrophy: a longitudinal computed tomographic study. AJNR Am J Neuroradiol. 1983 May-Jun;4(3):699-702.

Giannakopoulos P, Kövari E, Gold G, von Gunten A, Hof PR, Bouras C. Pathological substrates of cognitive decline in Alzheimer's disease. Front Neurol Neurosci. 2009;24:20-9.

Giannakopoulos P, Bouras C, Hof PR. Clinicopathologic correlates in the oldest-old: Commentary on "No disease in the brain of a 115-year-old woman". Neurobiol Aging. 2008 Aug;29(8):1137-9.

Gulledge AT, Bucci DJ, Zhang SS, Matsui M, Yeh HH. M1 receptors mediate cholinergic modulation of excitability in neocortical pyramidal neurons. J Neurosci. 2009 Aug 5;29(31):9888-902.

Haber SN, Fudge JL. The primate substantia nigra and VTA: integrative circuitry and function. Crit Rev Neurobiol. 1997;11(4):323-42.

Haber SN, Kunishio K, Mizobuchi M, Lynd-Balta E. The orbital and medial prefrontal circuit through the primate basal ganglia. J Neurosci. 1995 Jul;15(7Pt 1):4851-67.

Haber SN, Knutson B. The reward circuit: linking primate anatomy and human imaging. Neuropsychopharmacology. 2010 Jan;35(1):4-26.

Hanyu H, Shimuzu T, Tanaka Y, Takasaki M, Koizumi K, Abe K. Effect of age on regional cerebral blood flow patterns in Alzheimer's disease patients. J Neurol Sci. 2003 May 15;209(1-2):25-30.

Hartmann J, Kiewert C, Klein J. Neurotransmitters and energy metabolites in amyloid-bearing APP(SWE)xPSEN1dE9 Mouse Brain.J Pharmacol Exp Ther. 2010 Feb;332(2):364-70.

Henny P, Jones BE. Projections from basal forebrain to prefrontal cortex comprise cholinergic, GABAergic and glutamatergic inputs to pyramidal cells or interneurons. Eur J Neurosci. 2008 Feb;27(3):654-70.

Hof PR, Morrison JH. The aging brain: morphomolecular senescence of cortical circuits. Trends Neurosci. 2004 Oct;27(10):607-13.

Hollerman JR, Tremblay L, Schultz W. Involvement of basal ganglia and orbitofrontal cortex in goal-directed behavior. Prog Brain Res. 2000;126:193-215.

Huang YZ, Edwards MJ, Rounis E, Bhatia KP, Rothwell JC. Theta burst stimulation of the human motor cortex. Neuron. 2005;45:201-6.

Ishibashi K, Ishii K, Oda K, Kawasaki K, Mizusawa H, Ishiwata K. Regional analysis of age-related decline in dopamine transporters and dopamine D2-like receptors in human striatum. Synapse. 2009;63(4):282-90.

Juraska JM, Lowry NC. Neuroanatomical Changes Associated with Cognitive Aging. Curr Top Behav Neurosci. 2011 Jun 14.

Kalpouzos G, Persson J, Nyberg L. Local brain atrophy accounts for functional activity differences in normal aging. Neurobiol Aging. 2011 Apr 23.

Kashani A, Lepicard E, Poirel O, Videau C, David JP, Fallet-Bianco C, et al.Loss of VGLUT1 and VGLUT2 in the prefrontal cortex is correlated with cognitive decline in Alzheimer disease. Neurobiol Aging. 2008; 29(11):1619-30.

Kester MI, van der Vlies AE, Blankenstein MA, et al. CSF biomarkers predict rate of cognitive decline in Alzheimer disease. Neurology. 2009;73(17):1353-8.

Kirvell SL, Esiri M, Francis PT. Down-regulation of vesicular glutamate transporters precedes cell loss and pathology in Alzheimer's disease. J Neurochem. 2006 Aug;98(3):939-50.

Klingner M, Apelt J, Kumar A, Sorger D, Sabri O, Steinbach J, Scheunemann M, Schliebs R. Alterations in cholinergic and non-cholinergic neurotransmitter receptor densities in transgenic Tg2576 mouse brain with beta-amyloid plaque pathology. Int J Dev Neurosci. 2003 Nov;21(7):357-69.

Koch G, Esposito Z, Kusayanagi H, Monteleone F, Codecá C, Di Lorenzo F, Caltagirone C, Bernardi G, Martorana A. CSF Tau Levels Influence Cortical Plasticity in Alzheimer's Disease Patients. J Alzheimers Dis. 2011 May 23.

Koch G, Esposito Z, Codecà C, Mori F, Kusayanagi H, Monteleone F, Di Lorenzo F, Bernardi G, Martorana A. Altered dopamine modulation of LTD-like plasticity in Alzheimer's disease patients. Clin Neurophysiol. 2011 Apr;122(4):703-7.

Kumar U, Patel SC. Immunohistochemical localization of dopamine receptor subtypes (D1R-D5R) in Alzheimer's disease brain. Brain Res. 2007; 1131:187-96.

Levy R, Dubois B. Apathy and the functional anatomy of the prefrontal cortex-basal ganglia circuits. Cereb Cortex. 2006 Jul;16(7):916-28.

Livingstone PD, Dickinson JA, Srinivasan J, Kew JN, Wonnacott S. Glutamate-dopamine crosstalk in the rat prefrontal cortex is modulated by Alpha7 nicotinic receptors and potentiated by PNU-120596. J Mol Neurosci. 2010 Jan;40(1-2):172-6.

Livingstone PD, Srinivasan J, Kew JN, Dawson LA, Gotti C, Moretti M, Shoaib M, Wonnacott S. alpha7 and non-alpha7 nicotinic acetylcholine receptors modulate dopamine release in vitro and in vivo in the rat prefrontal cortex. Eur J Neurosci. 2009 Feb;29(3):539-50.

Lyketsos C. Apathy and agitation: challenges and future directions. Am J Geriatr Psychiatry. 2007 May;15(5):361-4.

MacGowan SH, Wilcock GK, Scott M. Effect of gender and apolipoprotein E genotype on response to anticholinesterase therapy in Alzheimer's disease. Int J Geriatr Psychiatry. 1998 Sep;13(9):625-30.

McNeill TH, Koek LL, Haycock JW. The nigrostriatal system and aging. Peptides 1984.;5 Suppl 1:263-8.

Marin RS, Firinciogullari S, Biedrzycki RC. The sources of convergence between measures of apathy and depression. J Affect Disord. 1993 Jun;28(2):117-24.

Marin RS, Firinciogullari S, Biedrzycki RC. Group differences in the relationship between apathy and depression. J Nerv Ment Dis. 1994 Apr;182(4):235-9.

Marshall GA, Rentz DM, Frey MT, Locascio JJ, Johnson KA, Sperling RA; Alzheimer's Disease Neuroimaging Initiative. Executive function and instrumental activities of daily living in mild cognitive impairment and Alzheimer's disease. Alzheimers Dement. 2011 May;7(3):300-8.

Martorana A, Mori F, Esposito Z, Kusayanagi H, Monteleone F, Codecà C, et al. Dopamine modulates cholinergic cortical excitability in Alzheimer's disease patients. Neuropsychopharmacology 2009; 34(10):2323-8.

Martorana A, Esposito Z, Koch G. Beyond the cholinergic hypothesis: do current drugs work in Alzheimer's disease? CNS Neurosci Ther. 2010; 16(4): 235-245.

Mattsson N, Zetterberg H, Hansson O, et al.CSF biomarkers and incipient Alzheimer disease inpatients with mild cognitive impairment. JAMA. 2009; 302(4):385-93.

Maurice N, Deniau JM, Menetrey A, Glowinski J, Thierry AM. Position of the ventral pallidum in the rat prefrontal cortex-basal ganglia circuit. Neuroscience. 1997 Sep;80(2):523-34.

Mega MS, Lee L, Dinov ID, Mishkin F, Toga AW, Cummings JL. Cerebral correlates of psychotic symptoms in Alzheimer's disease. J Neurol Neurosurg Psychiatry. 2000 Aug;69(2):167-71.

Migneco O, Benoit M, Koulibaly PM, Dygai I, Bertogliati C, Desvignes P, Robert PH, Malandain G, Bussiere F, Darcourt J. Perfusion brain SPECT and statistical parametric mapping analysis indicate that apathy is a cingulate syndrome: a study in Alzheimer's disease and nondemented patients. Neuroimage. 2001 May;13(5):896-902.

Minthon L, Gustafson L, Dalfelt G, Hagberg B, Nilsson K, Risberg J, Rosén I,Seiving B, Wendt PE. Oral tetrahydroaminoacridine treatment of Alzheimer's disease evaluated clinically and by regional cerebral blood flow and EEG. Dementia. 1993 Jan-Feb;4(1):32-42.

Moore SJ, Cooper DC, Spruston N. Plasticity of burst firing induced by synergistic activation of metabotropic glutamate and acetylcholine receptors. Neuron. 2009 Jan 29;61(2):287-300.

Musicco M, Salamone G, Caltagirone C, Cravello L, Fadda L, Lupo F, Mosti S, Perri R, Palmer K. Neuropsychological predictors of rapidly progressing patients with Alzheimer's disease. Dement Geriatr Cogn Disord. 2010;30(3):219-28.

Nicola SM. The nucleus accumbens as part of a basal ganglia action selection circuit. Psychopharmacology (Berl). 2007 Apr;191(3):521-50.

Pakrasi S, Mukaetova-Ladinska EB, McKeith IG, O'Brien JT. Clinical predictors of response to Acetyl Cholinesterase Inhibitors: experience from routine clinical use in Newcastle. Int J Geriatr Psychiatry. 2003 Oct;18(10):879-86.

Palmer K, Berger AK, Monastero R, Winblad B, Bäckman L, Fratiglioni L. Predictors of progression from mild cognitive impairment to Alzheimer disease. Neurology. 2007 May 8;68(19):1596-602.

Palop JJ, Mucke L. Amyloid-beta-induced neuronal dysfunction in Alzheimer's disease: from synapses toward neural networks. Nat Neurosci 2010;13:812-8.

Petanjek Z, Judas M, Kostović I, Uylings HB. Lifespan alterations of basal dendritic trees of pyramidal neurons in the human prefrontal cortex: a layer-specific pattern. Cereb Cortex. 2008 Apr;18(4):915 29

Petkova-Kirova P, Rakovska A, Della Corte L, Zaekova G, Radomirov R, Mayer A. Neurotensin modulation of acetylcholine, GABA, and aspartate release from rat prefrontal cortex studied in vivo with microdialysis. Brain Res Bull. 2008 Sep 30;77(2-3):129-35.

Robert PH, Mulin E, Malléa P, David R. Apathy diagnosis, assessment, and treatment in Alzheimer's disease. CNS Neurosci Ther. 2010 Oct;16(5):263-71.

Rosen HJ, Narvaez JM, Hallam B, Kramer JH, Wyss-Coray C, Gearhart R, Johnson JK, Miller BL. Neuropsychological and functional measures of severity in Alzheimer disease, frontotemporal dementia, and semantic dementia. Alzheimer Dis Assoc Disord. 2004 Oct-Dec;18(4):202-7.

Schneider LS, Pollock VE, Zemansky MF, Gleason RP, Palmer R, Sloane RB. A pilot study of low-dose L-deprenyl in Alzheimer's disease. J Geriatr Psychiatry Neurol. 1991 Jul-Sep;4(3):143-8.

Shoji M, Kanai M, Matsubara E, Tomidokoro Y, Shizuka M, Ikeda Y, Ikeda M, Harigaya Y, Okamoto K, Hirai S. The levels of cerebrospinal fluid Abeta40 and Abeta42(43) are regulated age-dependently. Neurobiol Aging. 2001 Mar-Apr;22(2):209-15.

Shanks MF, Venneri A. Delusional thoughts in Alzheimer's disease. Am J Psychiatry. 2004 Apr;161(4):764.

Staff RT, Shanks MF, Macintosh L, Pestell SJ, Gemmell HG, Venneri A. Delusions in Alzheimer's disease: spet evidence of right hemispheric dysfunction. Cortex 1999 Sep;35(4):549-60.

Shiino A, Watanabe T, Maeda K, Kotani E, Akiguchi I, Matsuda M. Four subgroups of Alzheimer's disease based on patterns of atrophy using VBM and a unique pattern for early onset disease. Neuroimage. 2006 Oct 15;33(1):17-26.

Shoji M, Kanai M, Matsubara E, Tomidokoro Y, Shizuka M, Ikeda Y, Ikeda M, Harigaya Y, Okamoto K, Hirai S. The levels of cerebrospinal fluid Abeta40 and Abeta42(43) are regulated age-dependently. Neurobiol Aging. 2001 Mar-Apr;22(2):209-15.

Staff RT, Shanks MF, Macintosh L, Pestell SJ, Gemmell HG, Venneri A. Delusions in Alzheimer's disease: spet evidence of right hemispheric dysfunction. Cortex 1999 Sep;35(4):549-60.

Starkstein SE, Berthier ML, Leiguarda R. Psychic akinesia following bilateral pallidal lesions. Int J Psychiatry Med. 1989;19(2):155-64.

Starkstein SE, Brockman S, Bruce D, Petracca G. Anosognosia is a significant predictor of apathy in Alzheimer's disease. J Neuropsychiatry Clin Neurosci. 2010 Fall;22(4):378-83.

Stepaniuk J, Ritchie LJ, Tuokko H. Neuropsychiatric impairments as predictors of mild cognitive impairment, dementia, and Alzheimer's disease. Am J Alzheimers Dis Other Demen. 2008 Aug-Sep;23(4):326-33.

Sultzer DL, Brown CV, Mandelkern MA, Mahler ME, Mendez MF, Chen ST, Cummings JL. Delusional thoughts and regional frontal/temporal cortex metabolism in Alzheimer's disease. Am J Psychiatry. 2003 Feb;160(2):341-9.

Sweet RA, Nimgaonkar VL, Devlin B, Jeste DV. Psychotic symptoms in Alzheimer disease: evidence for a distinct phenotype. Mol Psychiatry. 2003 Apr;8(4):383-92.

Ryu SH, Katona C, Rive B, Livingston G. Persistence of and changes in neuropsychiatric symptoms in Alzheimer disease over 6 months: the LASER-AD study. Am J Geriatr Psychiatry. 2005 Nov;13(11):976-83.

Van Der Putt R, Dineen C, Janes D, Series H, McShane R. Effectiveness of acetylcholinesterase inhibitors: diagnosis and severity as predictors of response in routine practice. Int J Geriatr Psychiatry. 2006 Aug;21(8):755-60.

van der Vlies AE, Verwey NA, Bouwman FH, Blankenstein MA, Klein M, Scheltens P, van der Flier WM. CSF biomarkers in relationship to cognitive profiles in Alzheimer disease. Neurology. 2009 Mar 24;72(12):1056-61.

Volkow ND, Ding YS, Fowler JS, Wang GJ, Logan J, Gatley SJ, Hitzemann R, Smith G, Fields SD, Gur R. Dopamine transporters decrease with age. J Nucl Med. 1996 Apr;37(4):554-9.

Volkow ND, Fowler JS, Wang GJ, Logan J, Schlyer D, MacGregor R, Hitzemann R,Wolf AP. Decreased dopamine transporters with age in health human subjects. Ann Neurol. 1994 Aug;36(2):237-9.

von Gunten A, Bouras C, Kövari E, Giannakopoulos P, Hof PR. Neural substrates of cognitive and behavioral deficits in atypical Alzheimer's disease. Brain Res Rev. 2006 Aug;51(2):176-211.

Wallin AK, Gustafson L, Sjögren M, Wattmo C, Minthon L. Five-year outcome of cholinergic treatment of Alzheimer's disease: early response predicts prolonged time until nursing home placement, but does not alter life expectancy. Dement Geriatr Cogn Disord. 2004;18(2):197-206.

Wallin AK, Blennow K, Andreasen N, Minthon L. CSF biomarkers for Alzheimer's Disease: levels of beta-amyloid, tau, phosphorylated tau relate to clinical symptoms and survival. Dement Geriatr Cogn Disord. 2006;21(3):131-8.

Wallin AK, Hansson O, Blennow K, Londos E, Minthon L. Can CSF biomarkers or pre-treatment progression rate predict response to cholinesterase inhibitor treatment in Alzheimer's disease? Int J Geriatr Psychiatry. 2009 Jun;24(6):638-47.

Wallin AK, Blennow K, Zetterberg H, et al. CSF biomarkers predict a more malignant outcome in Alzheimer disease. Neurology. 2010; 74:1531-7.

Wang XF, Dong CF, Zhang J, Wan YZ, Li F, Huang YX, Han L, Shan B, Gao C, Han J, Dong XP. Human tau protein forms complex with PrP and some GSS- and fCJD-related PrP mutants possess stronger binding activities with tau in vitro. Mol Cell Biochem. 2008 Mar;310(1-2):49-55.

Winblad B. Maintaining functional and behavioral abilities in Alzheimer disease. Alzheimer Dis Assoc Disord. 2001 Aug;15 Suppl 1:S34-40.

8

Construction of Drug Screening Cell Model and Application to New Compounds Interfering Production and Accumulation of Beta-Amyloid by Inhibiting Gamma-Secretase

Xiao-Ning Wang[1], Jie Yang[1], Ping-Yue Xu[1], Jie Chen[1,2], Dan Zhang[1], Yan Sun[1] and Zhi-Ming Huang[1]
[1]*State Key Laboratory of Pharmaceutical Biotechnology, Department of Biochemistry, College of Life Sciences, Nanjing University, Nanjing 210093,*
[2]*Department of Pathology, The University of Hong Kong, Queen Mary Hospital, Pokfulam Road,*
[1]*P.R.China*
[2]*Hong Kong*

1. Introduction

Alzheimer's disease (AD) is a tenacious neurodegenerative dementia, characterized clinically by progressive loss of memory, cognitive dysfunction, and behavioral abnormalities, accompanied by the accumulation of intracellular neurofibrillary tangles (NFTs), neuropil threads, as well as extracellular amyloid-beta containing senile plaques, cerebrovascular amyloid-beta deposits, and selective nerve cell and synapse loss (Kelliher et al, 1999; Tanzi, 1999; Solertea et al, 2000). The last two decades have witnessed an expanding body of research that elucidated the central role of amyloid precursor protein (APP) processing and amyloid beta (Abeta) production in the risk, onset, and progression of AD (Findeis, 2007). The accumulation of insoluble aggregates of Abeta peptide 1–42 (Abeta42) derived from APP is believed to play an important role in AD (Hardy, 1997; Kelliher et al, 1999). The generation of Abeta peptides requires two sequential proteolytical cleavages of APP by beta-secretase (BACE1) (Roßner et al, 2006) and gamma-secretase, composed of four integral membrane proteins, presenilins (PS1/2), APH-1 (anterior pharynx-defective 1), PEN-2 (presenilin enhancer 2) and nicastrin (NCT) (Kaether et al, 2006; Zhang & Koo, 2006). Previous evidence points to the involvement of the endoplasmic reticulum (ER) in AD pathogenesis owing to the fact that it is an important site for generating Abeta42 in neurons (Hartmann et al, 1998) and that presenilins are predominantly localized in this cellular compartment (Kovacs et al, 1996; Cook et al, 1996). Cleavage of the APP ectodomain by beta-secretase at the amino-terminus of Abetą is followed by cleavage of the beta-secretase-generated carboxyl-terminal fragment (beta-CTF, C99) at the carboxyl terminus of Abetą by gamma-secretase. A third activity, referred to as alpha-secretase, cleaves otherwise the APP ectodomain within the Abetą sequence, and subsequent cleavage of the alpha-secretase-derived APP CTF (alpha-CTF, C83) by gamma-secretase results in production of P3

(Abeta17-40/42) (McLendon, et al., 2000; Roßner et al, 2006; Walsh, et al., 2007). Studies in molecular pathology have indicated that the accumulation of Abeta leads to Abeta fibril deposition or beta-sheet amyloid deposition, whereas the dye molecular Congo red can interfere with beta-amyloid fibril formation as well as bind to preformed fibrils and prevent in vitro cytotoxicity, which is supported by the results of Carter DB and Chou KC (1998).
On the other hand, nicotine produces its actions on mammalian tissue via interactions with a family of ligand-gated ion channels that modulate the effects of the alkaloid on nervous, cardiovascular, immune, and neuromuscular system function (Wei, et al, 2005). The neuronal nicotinic acetylcholine receptors (nAChRs) are named on the basis of their subunit components and are thought to have a pentameric functional motif formed from a variety of subunits that comprise an ion channel similar to that of the neuromuscular junction nAChR. Two of the most abundant brain nAChRs are the heteromeric alpha4beta2 and homomeric alpha7 subtypes and the latter is an important target for Abeta-mediated neurotoxicity (Wang, et al, 2000). Abeta42 activation of alpha7 receptors expressed in the *Xenopus laevis* oocyte was prevented by two alpha7 ligands, the antagonist methyllycaconitine and a metabolite of GTS-21 (Wei, et al, 2005). The alpha7 receptor agonists enhance cognition and auditory-gating processes and thus are attractive drug candidates for the treatment of senile dementias and schizophrenia. Chou KC group has screened and found new drug candidates for treating Alzheimer's disease using GTS-21 as a template to search the Traditional Chinese Medicines Database by DOCK module based on the structure of alpha7 nicotinic acetylcholine receptor (Wei, et al, 2005). In addition, a key hallmark for AD is the decreased level of acetylcholine, a neurotransmitter playing a decisive role in memory and learning (Whitehouse, et al, 1982). Acetylcholinesterase (AChE), which degrades acetylcholine to its inactive metabolite choline, has emerged as a promising target for the management of AD. We have characterized some novel poly-phenols from the stem bark of *Hopea hainanensis*, especially hopeahainol A as AchE inhibitors with an IC_{50} value of 4.33 μM (Ge, et al, 2008). We have even made progress with the interaction between AD-related proteins and other proteins focused attention upon as potential drug targets (Jiang, et al, 2006). Moreover, the identification of the cell type-specific expression and activation of NF-kB, Sp1 and YY1 transcription factors may provide a basis to specifically interfere with BACE1 expression and, thereby, to lower the concentrations of Abeta peptides, which may prevent neuronal cell loss and cognitive decline in AD patients (Roßner et al, 2006).
It is clear that the accumulation of Abeta initiates a series of downstream neurotoxic events. As a result, considerable attention is being focused on attempts to develop therapies for Alzheimer's disease that are directed towards metabolic pathways that involve Abeta. One way is to reduce production of Abeta through the upstream processing enzymes (beta-secretase and gamma-secretase). gamma-secretase is a multi-subunit protease complex, minimally consists of four individual proteins: presenilin, nicastrin, APH-1, and PEN-2. Consequently, several gamma-secretase inhibitors have recently been described, including transition state analogs that mimic the gamma-secretase cleavage site on the immediate Abeta precursor (C99) and presumably compete with it for binding to the gamma-secretase enzymatic site (Netzer, et al., 2003). Here express gamma-secretase's substrate (such as EGFP-tagged C99 of APP) in the cultured cells (CHO) under control of tetracycline inducible system (Tet-off system) and then evaluate the efficiency of the inhibitors by ELISA (Enzyme-Linked Immunosorbnent Assay) and Western blot. This paper focuses on construction of a drug screen model for AD's gamma-secretase inhibitors and further finds some active compounds possessing gamma-secretase inhibition activity.

2. Materials and methods

2.1 Materials

The expression plasmids pcDNA3.1 (-), pEGFP, T vector (pBluescript II SK (+)), and tetracycline inducible expression system (pUHD30F and p15-1neo) were kindly provided by Prof Xue-Liang Zhu (Institute of Biochemistry and cell Biology, Chinese Academy of Sciences). The restriction endonucleases, SacII, XbaI, EcoRI, BamHI, HindIII and Cfr9I, and T4 DNA ligase were purchased from MBI Ferments (MD, USA). NdeI, SacI, XbaI, BspE I (AccIII) and ExTaq polymerase were obtained from TAKARA Bio Inc. Taq DNA polymerase and Pfu-Taq DNA polymerase were purchased from Shanghai Bioasia Biotechnology Co., Ltd (China). UNIC-10 trizol total RNA extraction kit, RT-PCR kit, DNA gel extraction kit, Uniq-10 DNA retraction kit, and plasmid mini preparation kit were from Shanghai Sangon Biotechnology Company (China). Methylenebisacrylamide, acrylamide, BSA, EDTA, and standard molecular weight protein marker were purchased from Nanjing Shengxing Biotechnology Co., Ltd (China). DNA marker was from MBI Company. The primers for PCR were synthesized by Shanghai Bioasia Biotechnology Co., Ltd (China).
The Chinese hamster cell lines CHO (ATCC 9096) was kindly provided by Prof Xue-Liang Zhu (Institute of Biochemistry and cell Biology, Chinese Academy of Sciences). Transfast™ reagent (eukaryotic cell transfection kit) was obtained from Promega Company (Madison, WI., USA). DMEM (Dulbecco's Modified Eagels' Medium) was obtained from GIBCO. New Zealand fetal bovine serum (FBS), *L*-glutamine, Trypsin, sodium pyruvate, ampicillin (Amp), and aminoglycosides (i.e. neomycin and kanamycin) were purchased from Hyclone (Logan, UT, USA). G418 (geneticin) was obtained from Ameresco Inc. PC152 (anti-beta-amyloid (15-30) rabbit pAb), recognizing three beta-amyloid peptides (Abeta40, Abeta42, and Abeta43), was obtained from Merck Co. Inc. Bovine insulin, bovine GSA (G-protein's alpha), and 3-(4,5-dimethylthiazol-2-yl)-2,5-diphenyltetrazolium bromide (MTT), and were obtained from Sigma Co. (St. Louis, MO, USA). BCA (bicinchoninic acid), ELISA TMB (3,3′,5,5′- tetramethylbenzidine), PBS buffer (PH7.4), Hepes, $CaCl_2$, Na_2HPO_4, and NaH_2PO_4 were purchased from Shanghai Sagon Company (China). 2-substituted-1,2,3,4-tetrahydro-isoquinoline derivatives (compound **I1-I6** and **II1-II6**) were designed and synthesized by our laboratory.

2.2 Design and construction of expression plasmids

2.2.1 Construction of expression plasmid pcDNA-C99 of human APP segment

Human total RNA was extracted from brain using UNIC-10 trizol total RNA extraction kit. Then obtain cDNA by reverse transcription using RT-PCR kit. C99 includes gamma-secretase active sites as gamma- secretase substrate. Taking cDNA as a template, the region of the gene encoding C99 of human APP (Homo sapiens amyloid beta (A4) precursor protein, NM_000484) was amplified by PCR using the following oligonucleotides: 5′-GCT GGATCC gcagaattccgacatgactc-3′ as the 5′ forward primer and 5′-AGC AAGCTT ctagttctgcatctgctcaaag-3′ as the 3′ reverse primer (restriction sites for BamHI and HindIII are underlined, respectively) according to Goo and Park (2004). The PCR product was purified using agarose gel DNA extraction kit and confirmed by sequencing analysis. The sequencing analysis is consistent with the gene sequence (1986-2282) of human APP (NM_201414.1), which codes residue 661-759 segment of human APP (NM_201414.1), namely residue 672-770 of APP770 (Fig. 1a). The PCR product was restricted with BamHI and HindIII, identified by 10g/L agarose gel electrophoresis and cloned into expression vector pcDNA3.1(-), named pcDNA-C99. The expression vector was transformed into Escherichia coli DHalpha5 fertilized on LB (30μg /ml Amp included) plate at 37°C overnight for amplification screening. Single clone was selected to be cultured in LB liquid overnight and then purified using plasmid mini preparation kit. The expression vector was verified by PCR, digestion and sequencing (Fig. 1b).

```
  1 MLPGLALLLL AAWTARALEV PTDGNAGLLA EPQIAMFCGR LNMHMNVQNG KWDSDPSGTK
 61 TCIDTKEGIL QYCQEVYPEL QITNVVEANQ PVTIQNWCKR GRKQCKTHPH FVIPYRCLVG
121 EFVSDALLVP DKCKFLHQER MDVCETHLHW HTVAKETCSE KSTNLHDYGM LLPCGIDKFR
181 GVEFVCCPLA EESDNVDSAD AEEDDSDVWW GGADTDYADG SEDKVVEVAE EEEVAEVEEE
241 EADDDEDDED GDEVEEEAEE PYEEATERTT SIATTTTTTT ESVEEVVREV CSEQAETGPC
301 RAMISRWYFD VTEGKCAPFF YGGCGGNRNN FDTEEYCMAV CGSAMSQSLL KTTQEPLARD
361 PVKLPTTAAS TPDAVDKYLE TPGDENEHAH FQKAKERLEA KHRERMSQVM REWEEAERQA
421 KNLPKADKKA VIQHFQEKVE SLEQEAANER QQLVETHMAR VEAMLNDRRR LALENYITAL
481 QAVPPRPRHV FNMLKKYVRA EQKDRQHTLK HFEHVRMVDP KKAAQIRSQV MTHLRVIYER
541 MNQSLSLLYN VPAVAEEIQD EVDELLQKEQ NYSDDVLANM ISEPRISYGN DALMPSLTET
601 KTTVELLPVN GEFSLDDLQP WHSFGADSVP ANTENEVEPV DARPAADRGL TTRPGSGLTN
661 IKTEEISEVK MDAEFRHDSG YEVHHQKLVF FAEDVGSNKG AIIGLMVGGV VIATVIVITL
721 VMLKKKQYTS IHHGVVEVDA AVTPEERHLS KMQQNGYENP TYKFFEQMQN
```

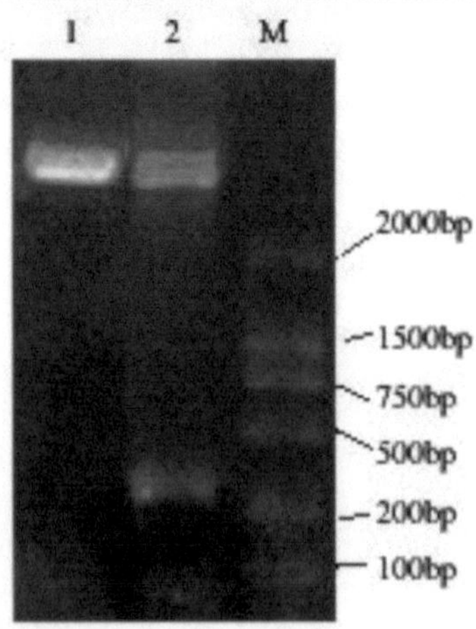

Fig. 1. Amino acid sequence of APP770, in which the single-underlined amino acid sequence means APP695. a) The amino acid sequence double-underlined displays Abeta42, while that shaded (D_{672}-N_{770}) figures C-terminal fragment of APP of 99 amino acids (C99, includeing gamma- secretase active sites). b) Southern blot of recombinant APP fragment by Agarose gel electrophoresis. Note: 1. Empty pcDNA3.1(-); 2. Not digested pcDNA3.1(-)-C99; M. DNA Marker. C99 gene fragment is about 300bp. DNA marker are 100, 200, 500, 750, 1000 and 2000bp

2.2.2 Construction of LGC (leading peptide -EGFP-C99) fusion gene

Construction of LGC fusion gene was based on APP leading peptide, pEGFP-C1, and pcDNA-C99, which is able to express a EGFP-tagged C99 segment under control of the tetracycline-responsive system (Zhu, 1999). Schematic diagrams of all constructs are shown in Fig. 2A. To construct pLGC, the region coding for APP leading peptid, containing nucleotides 195 to 245 (NM_201414_1), was synthetized as the 5′ forward primer of LGC fusion; the region coding for EGFP was from pEGFP-C1 (Clontech); and the region coding for C99 was from pcDNA-C99. To link EGFP to C99, BspE I (AccIII or BspM II) restriction sit was introduced into 3′ reverse primer of EGFP and 5′ forward primer of C99, respectively. To render membrance localization of LGC fusion produced by pLGC, a sequence coding for APP's signal peptide (nucleotides 195 to 245) was introduced in frame into the *Nhe*I site located before the EGFP-coding sequence and C99 cDNA to form pLGC-EGFP. The region of the gene encoding APP's leading peptide-EGFP fusion segment (LG) was amplified by PCR with primers: 5′-GTGCTAGC atgctgcccggtttggcactgctcctgctggccgcctggacggctcgggcg ctggaggtacccact gatatggtgagcaagggcgaggag-3′ as the 5′ forward primer and 5′-GATCCGGA cttgtacagctcgtccatgc-3′ as the 3′ reverse primer (restriction sites for NheI and BspEI are capital letters underlined, respectively, while the signal peptide of APP is small letters underlined). The PCR fragment was cleaved with NheI and BspE I and then was ligated to replace the *Nhe*I-BspEI restriction fragment of pEGFP-C1 (nucleotides 592 to 1330). Similarly, the encoding region of C99 was amplified by PCR using the following oligonucleotides: 5′-GCTCCGGA gcagaattccgacatgactc-3′ as the 5′ forward primer and 5′-AGCAAGCTT ctagttctgcatctgctcaaag-3′ as the 3′ reverse primer (restriction sites for BspEI and HindIII are underlined, respectively). The PCR fragment was digested with BspE I and HindIII and then was ligated to replace the BspEI-HindIII restriction fragment of pEGFP-C1 (nucleotides 1331 to 1352). The resulting plasmid was named pLGC-EGFP. The PCR fragment in pLGC-EGFP was sequenced. The sequence coding for the 17-residue leading peptide of APP was inserted as previously described. pLGC-EGFP was constructed from pEGFP-C1 to express LGC fusion with a signal peptide at N termini as in APP.

Then, the region of the gene encoding LGC fusion segment was amplified by PCR using the following oligonucleotides: 5′-CCTCCGCGGatgctgcccggtttggcactg-3′ as the 5′ forward primer and 5′-TCCTCTAGActagttctgcatctgctcaaag-3′ as the 3′ reverse primer (restriction sites for SacII and XbaI are underlined, respectively). The PCR product was restricted with SacII and XbaI; the resultant ~ 1.1kb fragment was ligated to replace the SacII-XbaI fragment of pUHD30F, a vector derived from pUHD20 (Zhu et al, 1997), to create pLGC-30F. The PCR fragment in pLGC-EGFP was sequenced and identified by 10g/L agarose gel electrophoresis.

The expression vectors (pLGC-EGFP and pLGC-30F) was transformed into Escherichia coli DHalpha5 fertilized on LB (30μg /ml Amp included) plate at 37°C overnight for amplification screening. Picked monoclonal to amplify, extracted plasmids, and tested positive clones by PCR, enzymatic detection, and sequencing of positive clones (Fig. 2).

a. Construction of LGC fusion gene;
b. Construction of expression plasmid pLGC-EGFP;
c. Construction of tetracycline-inducible expression system (pLGC-30F);
d. Southernblot of recombinant plasmid pLGC-EGFP (left) and pLGC-30F (right) by agarose gel electrophoresis. 1. DNA marker; DNA marker are 100, 250, 500, 750, 1000

and 2000bp. Left: 2-3. PCR analysis; 4-5. Digested pLGC-E by NheI and HindIII. Right: 2-3. Digested pLGC-30F by SacII and XbaI; 4-5. PCR analysis.

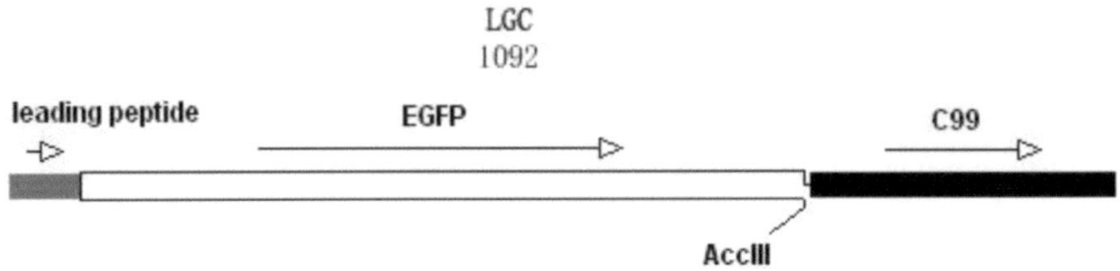

(a)

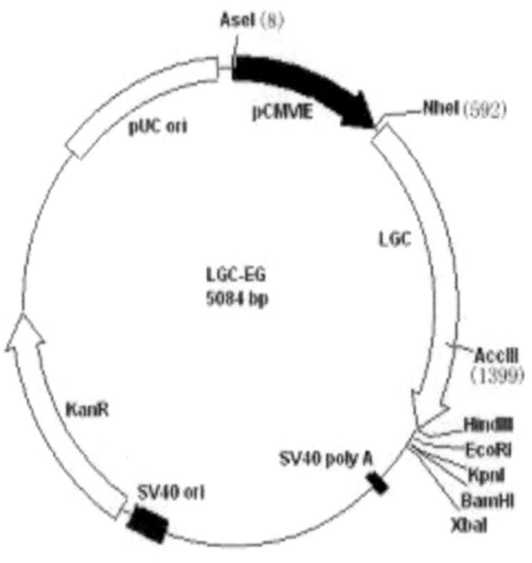

(b)

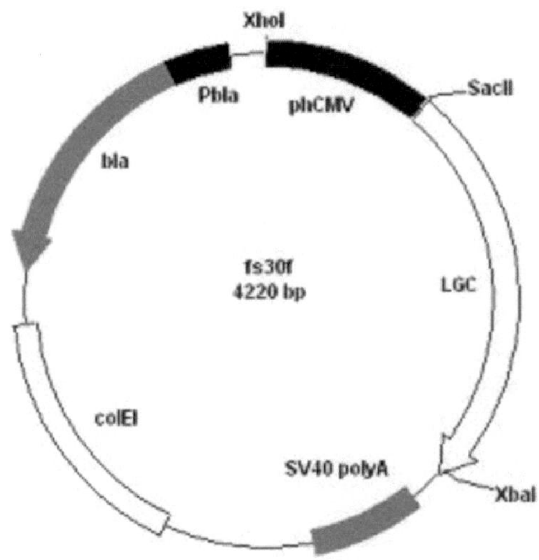

(c)

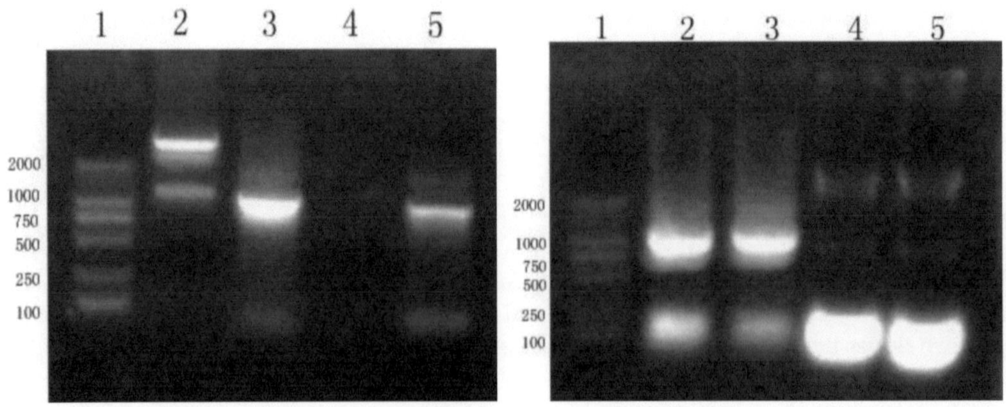

(d)

Fig. 2. Construction of LGC fusion gene and recombinant plasmids pLGC-EGFP and pLGC-30F

2.3 Stable expression of LGC fusion in CHO cells

2.3.1 Cell culture

Chinese hamster ovary (CHO) cells were cultured in a humidified atmosphere of 5% CO2, 95% air at 37 °C with DMEM (Dulbecco's modified Eagle medium) growth media supplemented with 10% FBS, 3% glutamine and 20 µg/ml kanamycin (Basani et al., 2001; Basani et al., 2000; Pabón et al., 2006). After 7-10 days of culture, colonies with CHO morphology were passed to fresh feeder layers for subculture. Resulting colonies were dissociated for 10 min with 0.25% trypsin and passed to fresh feeder layers at 5-10-day intervals, depending on the proliferation rate. The CHO cell lines at a stage of rapid proliferation were chosen for the following transgenic experiment.

2.3.2 Transfection and selection of stably transfected cells under control of Tet-off system

Stable transfection of tTA into CHO cells was done via the calcium phosphate coprecipitation (CPP) method (Resnitzky et al, 1994; Zhu et al, 1997; Baron et al, 1997; Ryoo et al, 1997). For stable expression, CHO cells were transfected and selected with G418 as described previously (Yang et al, 2009). Briefly, CHO cells were incubated in 24-well plates at a density of 5.5×105 cells per well for 24 h before transfection. CHO cells were transfected with 20 µg of pLGC-30F in combination with 2 µg of p15-1neo (modified by P.L. Chen and W.-H. Lee by inserting a G418-resistant gene into p15-1, one of the two plasmids required for the tetracycline system) using the calcium phosphate method (Zhu et al, 1997). For transient expression, cells were assayed 48 h after transfection. Clones were selected in the presence of G418 (1 mg/ml), cells were extracted, and proteins were analyzed by sodium dodecyl sulfate (SDS)-polyacrylamide gel electrophoresis and then by immunoblotting with anti-amyloid monoclonal antibody (Resnitzky et al, 1994). Positive clone was found to induce expression from both plasmids in the absence of Tet and was chosen to be used in the subsequent experiments.

Cells were subsequently cultured in presence of G418 (1 mg/ml) for 3 weeks. We replenished the selective media every 3-4 days, and observed the percentage of surviving cells. Viable colonies were subcultured to test inducible expression of the EGFP-tagged C99 by ELISA, fluorescence assay and western blot analysis. Cells stably transfected with the empty pUHD-30F vector were selected with G418 and used as a control (Appendix 1). Tetracycline (1 µg/ml) was always included in the culture medium until expression of exogenous LGC fusion was required (Gossen and Bujard, 1992; Resnitzky et al, 1994). G418-resistant colonies were then cultured as a whole in DMEM containing 0.2 mg of G418/ml. To prevent unscheduled expression, all the transfected cells were maintained in DMEM containing tetracycline (1 mg/ml) (Zhu et al, 1997; Zhu, 1999). G418-resistant CHO colonies expressing LGC under control of tetracycline (tetracycline-inducible expression system, Tet-off system), named Tet-CHO.

2.3.3 ELISA using anti-beta-amyloid

2.0×10^5 cells were plated in 96-well plates and incubated with primary rabbit anti-beta-amyloid (15-30) antibody (PC152) (1:2000 dilution) in PBS buffer with 1%BSA followed by 10 mins incubation of HRP-conjugated goat anti-rabbit IgG (1:20000 dilution) in PBS buffer with 1%BSA. Optical density (OD) determined by ultraviolet spectrophotometry was measured with an ELISA plate reader at test wavelength of 450nm (table 1). Absorbance value (A_{450}) was used for calculating cell survival rate as follows: survival rate=(A_{450} for experimental group/A_{450} for control group) ×100%.

Clones	ELISA [a]										WB [b]	F-EGFP [c]
	1	2	3	4	5	6	7	8	9	Mean±S.D.	Anti-Abeta	Fluorescence
A (control)	0.0528	0.0550	0.0537	0.0514	0.0515	0.0509	0.0532	0.0532	0.0519	0.0526±0.0013*		
B (control)	0.0560	0.0511	0.0519	0.0504	0.0508	0.0507	0.0536	0.0528	0.0551	0.0525±0.0020*		
C	0.1410	0.1543	0.1342	0.1428	0.1429	0.1397	0.1397	0.1399	0.1306	0.1406±0.0065*	+	+
D	0.1821	0.1881	0.1712	0.1654	0.1566	0.1694	0.1564	0.1568	0.1695	0.1684±0.0113*	+	+
E	0.5514	0.5017	0.4982	0.5439	0.4578	0.5834	0.4290	0.4423	0.5021	0.5011±0.0521*	++	+
F	0.3410	0.3325	0.3869	0.3478	0.4421	0.4019	0.3908	0.4063	0.3566	0.3784±0.0363*	+	+

Note: CHO cells were cultured in DMEM medium supplemented with 10% fetal bovine serum. cDNAs encoding human LGC fusion were cloned into pUHD-30F and were introduced into the CHO cells using Transfast™ according to the manufacturer's instructions. Two days after transfection, the cells were transferred to selection medium containing 0.722 M (500 mg/ml) G418. After 3 weeks of selection, LGC expression was detected and assessed by ELISA, Western blot, and Fluorescence (and RT-PCR) using anti-beta-amyloid antibody, respectively. The cells were then sorted by fluorescence-activated cell sorting to obtain cell lines expressing high levels of LGC fusion.

[a] The ELISA result of expressed proteins in CHO with rabbit anti-beta-amyloid as the first antibody by accounting fluorescence (A_{450}) of the transfected CHO cells; * $P < 0.001$.

[b] Using western blot detecting the fluorescence (A_{450}) of the transfected CHO cells with rabbit anti-beta-amyloid antibody.

[c] Using microplate reader detecting the fluorescence (OD_{488}) of the transfected CHO cells with EGFP.

Table 1. The detected result of expressed proteins in CHO cells

2.3.4 Western blot using anti-beta-amyloid

The positive cells were detected by Western blotting using rabbit anti-beta-amyloid as the first antibody and HRP-labeling goat anti-rabbit IgG as the secondary antibody. Confluent cultures of CHO cells grown in 60-mm diameter dishes were rinsed with PBS. Following a brief rinse with PBS, cells were harvested by gentle scraping into 5 ml PBS and centrifuged at 200*g*. LGC fusion was extracted with 100μl cell lysis buffer for Western containing protease inhibitors cocktail (e.g. PMSF), but without reducing agents, followed by a 5 sec sonication to eliminate DNA viscosity. Protein concentration in extracts was determined using BCA reagent. Equal amounts of LGC were loaded and resolved on 18% SDS polyacrylamide gels. Proteins separated by SDS-PAGE were electrotransferred on PVFD (polyvinylidene fluoride) membranes and probed with anti-beta3 antibodies (1:2000 dilution). Immunoreactivity was detected with a corresponding secondary anti-IgG antibody conjugated with HRP (1:10000 dilution) and with an enhanced chemiluminescent (ECL) substrate (Fig. 3).

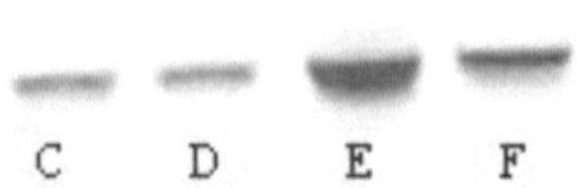

Fig. 3. Western blot results of LGC expressed in CHO cells using anti-amyloid antibody after ELISA results of the transfected CHO cells show positive with anti-amyloid as the first antibody

2.3.5 Fluorescence test

The following detection of LGC fusion stably expressed in CHO cells was determined by fluorescent microscopy. The CHO cells expressing LGC were inoculated in 96-well plate. The fluorescence was read with Tecan Safir microplate reader (excitation at 488 nm wavelength; emission at 507 nm wavelength) at excitation and emission wavelengths of 488 and 507 nm, respectively (table 2). Absorbance value (A_{488}) was used for calculating cell survival rate as follows: survival rate=(A_{488} for experimental group/A_{488} for control group) ×100%.

	1	2	3	4	5	6	7	8	Mean±S.D.
C	29286	30382	28562	30082	25511	32003	20826	30505	28395±3599*
D	23461	31222	26847	32466	29306	29002	26725	29544	28572±2838*
E	30597	32319	29415	33785	30984	30679	30350	27999	30766±1743*
F	22019	32479	31875	33087	32355	29952	25670	29211	29581±3899*
control	19996	23069	22992	18006	23385	23408	20639	22474	21746±1984*

* $P<0.001$ vs group control with the same concentration.

Table 2. The fluorescence values (OD_{488}) of expressed proteins in CHO cells

2.3.6 RT-PCR test

Total RNA was isolated from CHO cells expressing LGC using UNIC-10 trizol total RNA extraction kit. PowerScript reverse transcriptase (Invitrogen) was used to synthesize the first-strand cDNA from an equal amount of the RNA sample. The newly synthesized cDNA templates were further amplified by Platinum *Taq* DNA polymerase (Invitrogen). cDNA sequence of LGC was obtained by the following PCR procedure with plasmid pLGC-30F as template: (1) 95°C for 5 min; (2) 30 cycles at 95°C for 30 sec, 57°C for 60 sec, 72°C for 75 sec; (3) 72°C for 10 min (Yang, et al, 2005; Yang, et al, 2006; Li, et al, 2006). The LGC gene-specific primers 5′-CCTCCGCGGatgctgcccggtttggcactg-3′ and 5′-TCCTCTAGActagttctgcatctgctcaaag-3′ were used to amplify LGC gene fragment. The samples were restricted with SacII and XbaI and further analyzed on 10g/L agarose gel electrophoresis (Fig. 4).

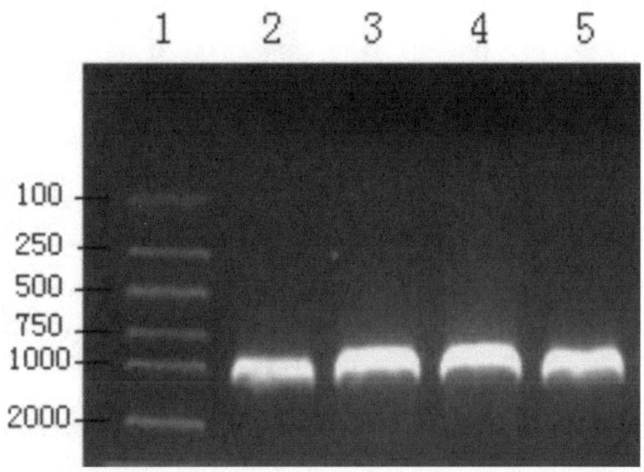

Fig. 4. RT-PCR products on 10g/L agarose gel electrophoresis. Right: 1. DNA marker; DNA marker are 100, 250, 500, 750, 1000 and 2000bp. Left: 2-5. RT-PCR products

2.4 Lithium chloride assay

After CHO cells were transfected with pLGC-30F by CPP method, positive cell colonies were isolated by the selective medium containing geneticin (G418). G418-resistant colonies were limiting dilution in 96 well flat bottomed culture plates at a density of 1.25×10^4 cells per well in the absence of tetracycline to induce expression. Stocks of lithium chloride (LiCl) were prepared in sterile water, whereas compounds were prepared in dimethylsulphoxide. LiCl were added to cells in fresh medium at the final concentrations 0.25 and 0.5 mM, respectively, and media and cells were collected 48 h later. Abeta determinations from media were made by fluorescence assay and ELISA. The fluorescence intensity of CHO cells expressing LGC fusion with EGFP was detected using the microplate reader at an excitation and emission wavelength of 488 nm and 507 nm, respectively. Optical density (OD) determined by ultraviolet spectrophotometry was detected with an ELISA microplate reader at test wavelength of 450nm (table 3).

mM	The fluorescence values (OD_{488}) by EGFP											Mean±S.D.
0.00	41169	43903	42605	41551	44615	46157	45805	48343	42045	42422	43622	43840±2220*
0.25	39132	38565	40417	39567	42697	39193	40993	40909	43352	39795	42658	40662±1626*
0.50	27879	28683	30744	29829	31154	29915	30797	29832	29722	29626	29208	29763±951*
	OD_{450} by ELISA											
0.00	0.2681	0.2384	0.2354	0.2337	0.2272	0.2348	0.231	0.244	0.2571	0.2375	0.2333	0.2400±0.00015*
0.25	0.1731	0.1613	0.1427	0.151	0.1263	0.1122	0.1196	0.1092	0.1341	0.1315	0.1171	0.1344±0.00043*
0.50	0.1309	0.1384	0.1092	0.112	0.0966	0.0761	0.0946	0.1213	0.1254	0.1315	0.1310	0.1152±0.00038*

* P<0.001 vs group control with the same concentration.

Table 3. Test of the CHO cell model expressing LGC fusion by LiCl

	C (M)	OD570					Inhibiting rate
		1	2	3	4	Mean±S.D.	(%)
Pepstatin A	8.00×10^{-4}	0.48	0.4959	0.4504	0.4876	0.4785±0.0198*	>100
	5.36×10^{-4}	0.3777	0.3765	0.3312	0.3425	0.3570±0.0237*	>100
	2.64×10^{-4}	0.2293	0.2315	0.2498	0.2477	0.2396±0.0107*	>100
	8.00×10^{-5}	0.2011	0.2086	0.202	0.2086	0.2051±0.0041*	90.63
	5.36×10^{-5}	0.175	0.1711	0.1765	0.1651	0.1719±0.0051*	59.82
	2.64×10^{-5}	0.1457	0.1413	0.1469	0.1564	0.1476±0.0064*	37.18
	8.00×10^{-6}	0.1386	0.1357	0.1398	0.1317	0.1365±0.0036*	26.84
Control	0	0.1119	0.1079	0.1007	0.1098	0.1076±0.0049*	

* P<0.001 vs group control with the same concentration.

Table 4. Activity of Pepstatin A by MTT assay

2.5 MTT assay

2.5.1 Activity of pepstatin A

Pepstatin A was aspartic proteinase inhibitor (PDB filecode 2RMP) (Yang & Quail, 1999) as well as beta-secretase inhibitor with IC_{50} value of 50 mM (Michelle, et al, 2001), which was reported to block solubilized gamma-secretase activity with IC_{50} value of 4.0 and 5.9 μM, respectively (Li et al, 2000; Zhang et al, 2001).

Tet-CHO cells were incubated in 96 well plates at a density of 2.0×10^4 cells per well overnight. Pepstatin A was prepared in dimethylsulphoxide (DMSO). Pepstatin A was added to cells in fresh medium in the presence of 1 μg/ml Tet (Gossen and Bujard, 1992; Liang et al, 2004) at the final concentrations 8.0×10^{-4}, 5.36×10^{-4}, 2.64×10^{-4}, 8.0×10^{-5}, 5.36×10^{-5}, 2.64×10^{-5}, and 8.0×10^{-6} M, respectively (table 4). 5mg/ml MTT at 20 μl per well were added to the pepstatin-treated or -untreated cells 48 h later. After 4 h, DMSO was added to dissolve the formed formazan crystals. Absorbance of the final product was examined by measuring the optical density at 570 nm using the microplate reader. Absorbance value was used for calculating cell survival rate as follows: survival rate=(A_{570} for experimental group/A_{570} for control group) ×100%.

2.5.2 Screening of some compounds

Some compounds (I1-I6 and II1-II6) under test were prepared in DMSO. Similarly, Tet-CHO cells were incubated into 96-well plates and cultured in DMEM supplemented with 10% FBS. These compounds were added to Tet-CHO cells in fresh medium in the presence of 1 μg/ml Tet at different final concentrations (table 5). After incubation at 37 °C in a 5% CO2 atmosphere for 48 h, Abeta determinations from media were made by fluorescence assay. The fluorescence intensity of Tet-CHO cells expressing LGC fusion with EGFP was detected using the microplate reader at an excitation and emission wavelength of 488 nm and 507 nm, respectively.

On the other hand, incubated at 37 °C for 48 h later, MTT was added (final concentration 0.5 μg/ml) to the compound-treated or -untreated cells for 4 h, then DMSO was added to dissolve the formed formazan crystals. Optical density (OD) was measured with the microplate reader at test wavelength of 570nm. Absorbance value was used for calculating cell survival rate as follows: survival rate=(A_{570} for experimental group/A_{570} for control group) ×100%.

2.5.3 Cytotoxicity

The cytotoxic effect of these compounds on normal CHO cells were tested by MTT assay and the IC_{50} values were calculated from the dose-response curves (Basani et al., 2001; Yang et al., 2009). CHO were incubated into 96-well plates and cultured in DMEM supplemented with 10% FBS. The compounds (Table 5) were added to CHO cells. After incubation at 37 °C for 48 h, MTT was added (final concentration 0.5 μg/ml) to the compound-treated or -untreated cells for 4 h, then DMSO was added to dissolve the formed formazan crystals. Absorbance of the final product was examined by measuring the optical density at 570 nm.

2.6 Statistics

Data are expressed as mean±standard deviation (S.D.) throughout this paper. All experiments were performed independently at least thrice. Statistical analyses were performed with Student's *t*-test where significant ($P<0.01$) differences were found between mean values.

3. Results

3.1 Plasmid pLGC

The consecutive cleavage of APP by beta- and gamma-secretase constitutes the amyloidogenic pathway as it generates Abeta, which plays a critical role in the pathogenesis

No		Structure	Anti-beta-amyloid aggregation		Cell toxicity (CHO)
		R	MTT (IC_{50}, mM) [a]	Fluorescence[b]	IC_{50} (mM) [c]
Type I 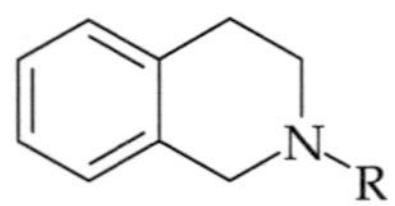	I-1	$C_6H_5SO_2$-	0.9563	+	7.71± 0. 87
	I-2	p-CH_3-$C_6H_4SO_2$-	8.047	+	8.65 ±1.04
	I-3	o-NO_2-C_6H_4CO-	2.625	+	5.39 ± 0. 55
	I-4	m-NO_2-C_6H_4CO-	4.448	+	6.22 ±0. 38
	I-5	p-NO_2-C_6H_4CO-	10.610	+	7.54 ±0. 79
	I-6 [24]	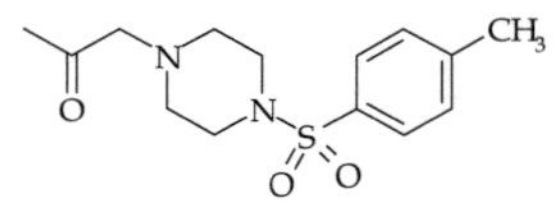	9.684	+	8.81±1. 63
Type II 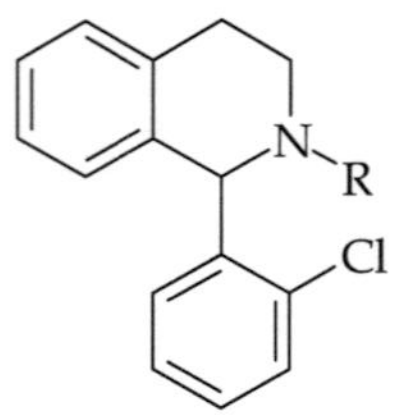	II-1	$C_6H_5CH_2$-	2.428	+	8.86±1. 33
	II-2	m-Cl-C_6H_4CO-	5.399	+	9.11±1. 18
	II-3 [42]	m-Br-C_6H_4CO-	87.520	+	8.42±0. 77
	II-4	o-Cl-C_6H_4CO-	0.8191	+	6.69±0. 86
	II-5	p-Cl-C_6H_4CO-	5.317	+	5.79±0. 57
	II-6	$C_6H_5SO_2$-	1.225	+	8.67±1. 05

[a] The inhibitory concentrations (IC_{50}) of these compounds for anti-beta-amyloid aggregation were evaluated by MTT assay based on Tet-CHO cells expressing EGFP-tagged C99 (LGC fusion). P<0.01; n=3.
[b] Using microplate reader detecting the fluorescence (OD_{488}) of the transfected CHO cells with EGFP.
[c] The inhibitory concentrations (IC_{50}) of these compounds for cell toxicity were evaluated by MTT method using flow cytometry accounting absorbance (A_{570}) of CHO cells and Hela cells. P<0.01; n=5.

Table 5. The biological activities of some compounds

of Alzheimer's disease. C99 is derived from cleavage of APP by the protease beta-secretase at the N-terminus of the Abeta-domain, which is further cleaved within its transmembrane domain by gamma-secretase, leading to the secretion of the Abeta peptide. beta-secretase might generate Abeta peptides by cleavage of APP between position Met671 and Asp672 of APP770 as well as gamma-secretase by cleavage of Val711-Ile712 or Ala713-Thr714 of APP770 (Fig. 1). To construct cell model of gamma-secretase inhibitors, we introduced C99 sequence into the structure of gamma-secrease's substrate (LGC fusion), composed of APP's signal peptide, EGFP and C99. The resultant 1.1kb LGC fragment was ligated to replace the *Nhe*I-HindIII restriction fragment of pEGFP-C1 to form pLGC-EGFP. In addition, to utilize the tetracycline-responsive system to express EGFP-tagged C99, the resultant 1.1kb fragment was ligated to replace the SacII-XbaI fragment of pUHD30F to create pLGC-30F. The expression vectors were transformed into E. coli DHalpha5 and confirmed by sequencing analysis (Fig. 2).

3.2 Stable expression of LGC in CHO cells

Tetracycline-inducible expression system includes pUHD30F (vacancy vector for expressing target gene) and p15-1neo (expressing tTA). CHO cells were cultured in DMEM medium supplemented with 10% FBS. pLGC-30F mentioned above in combination with 2 μg of p15-1neo was introduced into the CHO cells via CPP method (Zhu et al, 1997; Zhu, 1999). Cells were subsequently cultured in presence of G418 (1 mg/ml) for 3 weeks and then were detected and assessed by ELISA, fluorescence assay and western blot using anti-beta-amyloid antibody (Table 1). Tetracycline (1 μg/ml) was always included in the culture medium until expression of exogenous LGC fusion was required. G418-resistant colonies, Tet-CHO, were then cultured as a whole in DMEM containing 0.2 mg/ml of G418 and 1 mg/ml of tetracycline.

The ELISA was used to validate LGC expression in transfected cell colonies. The A_{450} of the negative control proteins from 9 CHO cells was 0.0526 ± 0.0013 (mean ± S.D.). The total range of the A_{450} was 0.1406 to 0.5011 (Table 1). The t test reveals that four samples (C-F clones) are positive, whose A_{450} values were significantly higher than the negative serum sample ($P < 0.001$).

The positive cells were chosen for the identification of LGC by Western blotting using mouse anti-beta-amyloid as the first antibody and HRP-congulated goat anti-rabbit IgG as the second antibody (Fig. 3). Comparison of the assay results between ELISA and western blot displayed that three samples (C, D, E and F clones) are positive; the protein expression amount of E is higher than that of C, D and F, which is supported by fluorescence assay (Table 2) and RT-PCR analyses (Fig. 4).

LiCl were added to Tet-CHO cells in fresh medium at different concentrations. After 48 h, Abeta determinations from media were made by fluorescence assay (A_{488}) and ELISA (A_{450}) (Table 3). The A_{488} and A_{450} of the negative control were 43840 ± 2220 and 0.2400 ± 0.00015, respectively. The t test shows that LiCl at a concentration of 0.25 and 0.5 nM are positive, whose A_{450} values were significantly higher than the control sample ($P < 0.001$).

The extent of inhibiting Abeta generation and assembly of pepstatin A was measured by MTT assay. Inhibiting rate of different concentrations of pepstatin A are >100%, 90.63%, 58.82%, 37.18% and 26.84%, respectively, whose IC_{50} (half-maximal inhibitory concentration) values is approximately 35.83 μM (Table 4), which is consist with the research results (pepstatin A with IC_{50} value of 35 μM) of Campbell's group (Campbell et al, 2002). This also verified that Tet-CHO cell model can be used for detection of gamma-secretase inhibitor activity.

3.3 Activity of some new compounds

To determine their molecular basis, the ability of these compounds to inhibit EGFP-tagged C99 binding to gamma-secrease were measured based on the Tet-CHO cells. Fluorescence assay reveals that these compounds inhibited production of Abeta by interfering gamma-secrease. Similarly, the IC_{50} values for inhibiting Abeta generation and assembly of compounds **I1-I6** and **II1-II6** were 0.819 to 81.920 mM (Table 5), while IC_{50} of pepstatin A is 35.83 μM, which is consistent with Campbell's results (pepstatin A with IC_{50} value of 35 μM) (Campbell et al, 2002).

Cytotoxicity profiles of compounds **I-1-I-6** and **II-1-II-6** treated on Tet-CHO cells were compared with the standard CHO cell-based MTT assay. Their cytotoxicity assay on Tet-CHO cells was more sensitive than that on the standard CHO cells, and nine compounds **I-1, I-2, I-3, I-4, II-1, II-2, II-4, II-5** and **II-6** with IC_{50} values of 5.39 to 9.91 mM (Table 5). Especially, compounds **I-1, I-3, II-1, II-4,** and **II-6** show higher anti- Abeta activities with a sort order of **I-1 > II-4 > II-6 > II-1 > I-3**. Further evaluation is under investigation.

Comparison of their anti-Abeta activities with their cytotoxicities displayed that nine compounds **I-1, I-2, I-3, I-4, II-1, II-2, II-4, II-5** and **II-6** are positive, especially compounds **I1, I3, II1, II4,** and **II6** show higher anti-Abeta activities but lower than pepstatin A.

4. Discussion

A system for tetracycline-regulated inducible gene expression has been described which relies on constitutive expression of a tetracycline-controlled transactivator (tTA) fusion protein combining the tetracycline (Tet) repressor (tetR) and the transcriptional activation domain of virion protein 16 (VP16). In the Tet-Off expression system, *tTA* regulates expression of a target gene that is under transcriptional control of a tetracycline-responsive promoter element (TRE), which is made up of Tet operator (tetO) sequence concatemers fused to the human cytomegalovirus (hCMV) immediate-early promoter (Gossen, & Bujard, 1992). The specificity of the Tet repressor-operator-effector interaction and the pharmacological characteristics of Tet's make this autoregulatory system well suited for the control of gene activities both in cultured cells and in transgenic animals (Gossen, et al, 1995; Shockett, et al, 1995). For example, Zhu's group has researched regulation of cell motilities by expression of nuclear distributions (Nud) (Yan et al, 2003; Liang et al, 2004; Liang et al, 2007; Ma et al, 2009), mitosin (Zhu, 1999; Zhou et al, 2005; Yang et al, 2003), etc. (Shen et al, 2008; Shan et al, 2009; Ding et al, 2009; Zhang et al, 2009), under the control of tetracycline-inducible Tet-off system.

Additionally, the green fluorescent protein (GFP) from the jellyfish *Aequorea victoria* has become a useful tool in molecular and cell biology, as its intrinsic fluorescence can be visualized in living cells (Elsliger, et al., 1999), especially the enhanced green fluorescent protein (EGFP) widely used as a molecular tag in cell biology (Pan, et al., 2009). GFP emits a bright green light when expressed in either eukaryotic or prokaryotic cells and illuminated by blue or UV light. GFP has generated intense interest as a marker for gene expression and localization of gene products (Ormoe, et al., 1996). The crystal structure of recombinant wild-type GFP reveals also that the protein is in the shape of a cylinder, comprising 11 strands of beta-sheet with an alpha-helix inside and short helical segments on the ends of the cylinder. The fluorophore (chromophore), resulting from the spontaneous cyclization and oxidation of the sequence -Ser65 (or Thr65)-Tyr66-Gly67-, are protected inside the cylinders and requires the native protein fold for both formation and fluorescence emission (Ormoe, et al., 1996; Yang, et al., 1996). Up to now, the numerous applications include: using GFP as a reporter for gene expression, as a marker to study cell lineage during development and as a tag to localize proteins in living cells (Gerdes & Kaether, 1996). Here we focus on the use of EGFP as a protein tag and upon those applications of this new tool in which EGFP promises to be truely superior to conventional methods.

This experiment is to design a drug screening cell model for gamma-secretase inhibitors. So far, the specific components of gamma-secretase, composed of PS, APH-1, PEN-2 and nicastrin, and its mechanism have not yet established. In view of the wide distribution of gamma-secretase in a variety of cell lines and tissues, as well as testing of new beta-secretory inhibitors or gamma-secretase inhibitors using APP transgenic cell or APP transgenic animal, we utilized the tetracycline-responsive system to express EGFP-tagged C99 fusion as a gamma-secretase substrate in the cultured CHO cells and validated by ELISA and Western blot for the following evaluation of the efficiency of some compounds.

To further contruct cell model for screening gamma-secrease inhibitors, we designed a novel fusion as gamma-secrease's substrate based on the structural basis of the proteolytical cleavages of APP. C99 was further defined as the domain of APP for gamma-secrease's substrate due to APP processing pathways and Abeta production, resulting from sequential cleavage of APP by proteases named beta- and gamma-secretases (Walsh, et al., 2007; Mouradian, 2007; Roßner et al, 2006). BACE1 (beta-secretase) might generate Abeta peptides by cleavage of APP between position Met671 and Asp672 of APP770 as well as gamma-secretase by cleavage of Val711-Ile712 or Ala713-Thr714 of APP770 (Fig. 1). Elevated Abeta42 levels, as well as particularly the elevation of the ratio of Abeta42 to Abeta40, has been identified as important in early events in the pathogenesis of AD (Mouradian, 2007). Here, C99 sequence was introduced into the structure of gamma-secrease's substrate (LGC fusion). The region coding for EGFP was from pEGFP-C1, added to the structure of gamma-secrease's substrate. To link EGFP to C99, BspE I restriction sit was introduced into 3' reverse primer of EGFP and 5' forward primer of C99, respectively. To render membrance localization of LGC fusion, a sequence coding for APP's signal peptide was introduced by the 5' forward synthesized primers in frame into the *Nhe*I site located before the EGFP-coding sequence and C99 cDNA. The resultant 1.1kb fragment was ligated to replace the *Nhe*I-HindIII restriction fragment of pEGFP-C1 (nucleotides 592 to 1352) to form pLGC-EGFP (Fig. 2). pLGC-EGFP was constructed from pEGFP-C1 to express LGC fusion with a signal peptide at N termini as in APP. To utilize the tetracycline-responsive system (Zhu, 1999) to express EGFP-tagged C99, the resultant 1.1kb fragment was ligated to replace the SacII-XbaI fragment of pUHD30F to create pLGC-30F. The expression vectors (pLGC-EGFP and pLGC-30F) were transformed into Escherichia coli DHalpha5 in order to verify the correct sequence through sequence analysis (Fig. 2). It is necessary to connect EGFP gene to the N-terminal of the gamma-secretase substrate C99 in order to facilitate screening. Only the pair of plasmids were stably transfected into CHO cells, target gene was able to expressed and the cells show fluorescent. EGFP fluoresces under certain wavelengths of ultraviolet excitation can be easily detected, but also its molecular weight is relatively small so that the basic structures of the proteins fused with EGFP do not been affected and the proteins can play their normal function.

In a previous study, our group has constructed the drug screening cell model applied to some compounds inhibiting FITC-fibrinogen binding to human alphaIIbbeta3 expressed in CHO cells (Yang et al, 2009). We utilized the tetracycline-responsive system (Zhu, 1999) to express EGFP-tagged C99 fusion as a gamma-secretase substrate. Expression levels were indeed reduced under control of either the cytomegalovirus promoter or the tetracycline-responsive promoter. p15-1 neo included is essential for activation of the tetracycline-responsive promoter in the pUHD30F vector. Moreover, the tetracycline inducible system (pUHD30F and p15-1 neo) contains switching mechanism, and close the expression of substrate (pUHD30F-C99) by adding Tet (or Dox) in Tet-off system to avoid generation of Abeta and its cell toxicity. The dual-plasmid system of the Tet-off system transfected CHO cells to build a cell model for anti-Abeta drug screen. G418-resistant cell lines were screened for conditional expression of LGC and the stable expression cell lines (Tet-CHO) was obtained. Cell lines transfected with just the expression vector were isolated as controls. Clones displaying highly regulated expression were obtained for LGC. It should be noted, however, that all clones exhibited a low basal level of LGC expression in the presence of tetracycline, which was detectable in most of the experiments performed. Then, added positive drugs (LiCl and pepstatin A) to validate whether this cell model has the effect of function for detection of gamma-secretase inhibitors. Finally, the cell model was capable of screening other compounds for discovery of new gamma-secretase inhibitors.

Glycogen synthase kinase 3 (GSK3) is a constitutively active, proline-directed serine/threonine kinase that plays a part in a number of physiological processes ranging from glycogen metabolism to gene transcription. GSK3 also plays a pivotal and central role in the pathogenesis of both sporadic and familial forms of AD. The over-activity of GSK3 accounts for memory impairment, tau hyper-phosphorylation, increased beta-amyloid production and local plaque-associated microglial-mediated inflammatory responses; all of which are hallmark characteristics of AD. The inhibitors of GSK3 would provide a novel avenue for therapeutic intervention in this devastating disorder (Hooper, et al., 2008). Inhibition of GSK3 by LiCl has been reported to reduce Abeta (Phiel, et al., 2003; Sun, et al., 2002), perhaps through presenilin-dependent gamma-secretase inhibition (Netzer, et al., 2003). Abeta peptides are derived from APP by sequential proteolysis, catalysed by beta-secretase, followed by presenilin-dependent gamma-secretase cleavage (Phiel, et al., 2003). Besides interaction with nicastrin, APH-1 and PEN-2 required for gamma-secretase function, presenilins also interact with alpha-catenin, beta-catenin and GSK-3 (Francis et al, 2002). The therapeutic concentrations of LiCl, a GSK3 inhibitor, block the production of Abeta peptides by interfering with APP cleavage at the gamma-secretase step, but do not inhibit Notch processing. Importantly, lithium also blocks the accumulation of Abeta peptides in the brains of mice that overproduce APP. The target of lithium in this setting is GSK-3, which is required for maximal processing of APP. Since GSK-3 also phosphorylates tau protein, the principal component of NFTs, inhibition of GSK-3 offers a new approach to reduce the formation of both amyloid plaques and NFTs, two pathological hallmarks of AD (Phiel, et al., 2003). Here, we added LiCl to Tet-CHO cells expressing EGFP-tagged C99 fusion. The results of ELISA and fluorescence assay revealed that LiCl inhibited the production of Abeta at a concentration of 0.25 and 0.5 mM with the inhibiting rates of 7.25% and 32.11% by fluorescence assay, respectively (or 44% and 52% by ELISA, respectively) (Table 3), which is supported by the research results of Phiel's group (LiCl with an IC_{50} of 1-2mM) (Phiel, et al., 2003), and consistent with a report using transient overexpression of the APP carboxy terminus C100 in COS7 cells (Sun, et al., 2002).

Pepstatin A was aspartic proteinase inhibitor (PDB filecode 2RMP) (Yang & Quail, 1999) as well as beta-secretase inhibitor with IC_{50} value of 50 mM (Michelle, et al, 2001), which was reported to block solubilized gamma-secretase activity (Li et al, 2000). When C100Flag was used as a gamma-secretase substrate in an in vitro assay, the IC_{50} for pepstatin A to inhibit Abeta40 and Abeta42 generation was 4.0 and 5.9 μM, respectively (Li et al, 2000). A cell-free assay on membrane vesicles derived from C99-transfected cells showed that the IC_{50} of pepstatin A for inhibition of both Abeta40 and Abeta42 was estimated at ~ 4μM (Zhang et al, 2001). Because both C100Flag and C99 are immediate substrates for gamma-secretase, it is not surprising to see an IC_{50} for pepstatin A at 35 μM when Campbell and co-worker used microsomes derived from full length (FL) APP expressing cells (Campbell et al, 2002). Here, we built Tet-CHO cells expressing EGFP-tagged C99 fusion (LGC) with 17-residue signal peptide of APP and obtained an IC_{50} for pepstatin A at 35.83 μM employing MTT assay, similar to Campbell's method. And Campbell et al have found that pepstatin A was shown to bind to PS1 with higher affinity to FL PS1 than to PS1 fragments. The high efficacy of pepstatin A binding to FL PS1 may lead to efficient inhibition of endoproteolysis compared to the low efficacy of binding to functional NTF/CTF complexes and inhibition of gamma-secretase cleavage in the Golgi/TGN (Campbell et al, 2002).

Fluorescence and MTT assay revealed that twelve new 2-substituted-1,2,3,4-tetrahydroisoquinoline derivatives (**I-1-I-6** and **II-1-II-6**) inhibited production and assemblage of Abeta to some extent by interfering gamma-secrease (Table 5). Especially, compounds **I-1, I-3, II-1, II-4,** and **II-6** showed higher anti-Abeta activities while their cytotoxicity assay on Tet-CHO cells was more sensitive than that on the standard CHO cells. However, their IC_{50} values (from 0.819 to 81.920 mM) for inhibiting Abeta assembly (Table 5) were smaller than that of pepstatin A. Our results displayed that their anti-Abeta activities depended on the substitutes at position 2 of the tetrahydroisoquinoline nucleus. Phenylsulfonyl, benzyl or ortho-substituted benzoyl derivatives have higher anti-Abeta activities, such as compounds **I-1, I-3, II-1, II-4,** and **II-6**, which is supported by our previous research results that the phenylsulfonye group is necessary (Yang et al., 2009). Electron-withdrawing groups (EWG) at the position ortho of benzene are propitious to anti-Abeta activities, such as chlorine (**II-4**) and nitryl groups (**I-3**). Similarly, electron-donating groups (WDG) at the position para of phenylsulfonyl group are not beneficial to their anti-Abeta activities, such as compound **I-2**. The anti-Abeta activities of unsubstituted phenylsulfonyl derivatives (**I-1** and **II-6**) are evidently higher than that of **I-2**. We have reported that the nitrogen atom at 2 position of 1,2,3,4-tetrahydroisoquinoline interacted with the carboxyl group at the side chain of Asp179 of integrin alpha2b in the fashion of electrostatic interaction (Yang et al, 2009). Here the sulphonyl and carbonyl group at 2 position of 1,2,3,4-tetrahydroisoquinoline may interact with gamma-secrease in the same fashion to exhibit anti-Abeta activities. On the other hand, our previous research has also exhibited that compound **I-6** possessed higher anti-platelet aggregation by inhibiting fibrinogen binding to its receptor GPIIbIIIa (integrin alpha2bbeta3) with IC_{50} value of approximately 37.13 μM (Yang et al, 2009). Molecular modeling indicated that this compound might interact with fibrinogen receptor by Thr125 residue of beta3, Tyr166 and Asp179 residues of alpha2b, especially the hydroxyl groups of Thr125 and Tyr166 and the carboxyl group at side chain of Asp179. Interestingly, the anti-platelet aggregation activities of type II compounds have ever reported as well as ticlopidine (Yang et al, 2004). Their antiplatelet aggregatory activity is related to the sizes of substitutes, as well as charge or electronegativity, which is consistent with the CoMFA study results: the steric and electrostatic interactive energy is the major contribution to antiplatelet aggregatory activity, and an area accomodating a small weak-polar group exists near the 7 position of the tetrahydroisoquinoline nucleus.

Interestingly, these compounds possessed anti-Abeta activities as well as anti-platelet aggregation activites, and they may play important roles in AD therapy by fibrin-guided signal pathway (Adams, et al, 2004). Merkle and co-worker have indicated that vascular deposition of Abeta is associated with recurrent intracerebral hemorrhages in certain disease states and revealed a network of fibrin (Fn) and amyloid fibers formed in the presence of Abeta with significantly decreased lateral Fn-Fn interactions using electron microscopic analysis, namely Abeta significantly altering the nature of the Fn obtained in its presence (Merkle et al, 1996). Since platelets are the principal source of both APP and Abeta in human blood, AD platelet activation may reflect or even contribute to the pathogenesis of the disease (Sevush et al, 1998). These results suggest that fibrin is a mediator of inflammation and may impede the reparative process for neurovascular damage in AD. Fibrin and the mechanisms involved in its accumulation and clearance may present novel therapeutic targets in slowing the progression of AD (Paul et al, 2007). Fibrin receptors are defined as membrane-bound proteins that can transduce intracellular signals upon fibrin binding, whereas fibrin binding proteins are either soluble or anchored molecules that bind fibrin but have no documented ability to directly transduce intracellular signals upon fibrin binding. The functional consequences of these protein–fibrin interactions range from blood coagulation and initiation of angiogenesis, to inflammation and propagation of infection (Adams, et al, 2004). Fibrin binds several families of integrins, including $beta_1$, $beta_2$, and $beta_3$ subtypes. Fibrin–integrin interactions mediate a variety of cellular responses, including clotting and inflammation via the mitogen-activated protein kinase (MAPK), the phosphoinositide-3 kinase (PI3K), or the NF-κB signal pathways. Moreover, reducing fibrinogen, a circulating protein critical in hemostasis, provides a significant decrease in the neurovascular damage, blood-brain barrier permeability and neuroinflammation present in AD. These studies implicate fibrinogen as a possible contributor to AD (Cortes-Canteli & Strickland, 2009). In addition, platelet-derived growth factor (PDGFs) has been indicated that it can induce the beta-gamma-secretase-mediated cleavage of APP through a Src-Rac-dependent pathway (Gianni et al, 2003). Studies of PDGFs and their receptors have revealed roles for PDGF signaling in gastrulation and in the development of the cranial and cardiac neural crest, gonads, lung, intestine, skin, CNS, and skeleton as well as blood vessel formation and early hematopoiesis (Andrae et al, 2008). PDGF signaling is implicated in a range of diseases, such as certain gliomas, sarcomas, leukemias, epithelial cancers, vascular disorders, and fibrotic diseases, involving tumor growth, angiogenesis, invasion, and metastasis. How these compounds to inhibit both platelet aggregation and Abeta accumulation and its mechanism are under investigation.

5. Conclusion

This experiment is to design a drug screening cell model (Tet-CHO) for gamma-secretase inhibitors. In view of the specific components of gamma-secretase, we utilized the tetracycline-inducible Tet-off system to express EGFP-tagged C99 fusion as a gamma-secretase substrate in the cultured CHO cells and validated by ELISA and Western blot for the following evaluation of the efficiency of some compounds. Additionally, twelve

2-substituted 1,2,3,4-tetrahydroisoquinoline derivatives were designed and synthesized by the aid of computer drug design, based on the principles of isosterism and the reported SAR of synthesized tetrahydroisoquinoline derivatives. These compounds have anti-Abeta accumulation activity by inhibiting gamma-secretase interaction with its substrate, EGFP-tagged C99. The phenylsulfonyl derivatives (compound **I-1** and **II-6**), the benzyl derivative **II-1**, and the benzoyl derivatives (**I-3** and **II-4**) showed higher anti-Abeta activities, which is supported by our previous research results that the phenylsulfonye group is necessary (Yang et al., 2009). Especially compound **I-6** has not only anti-Abeta accumulation activity but also anti-platelet aggregation activity, suggesting a potential role of fibrin-guided signal pathway in AD therapy.

6. Acknowledgments

This work is supported by Nature Science Fund of China (No. 30171094 and No. 30271497).

Appendix 1. The growth properties of G418-resistant cells during three weeks

time		Annotation	time		Annotation
2 days	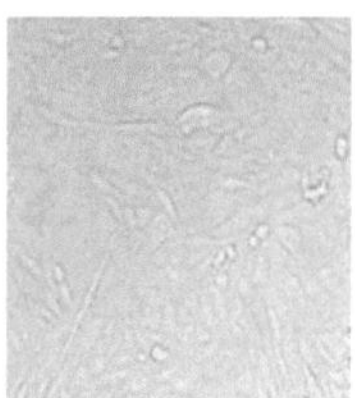	Some cells begin to age and cell rounding.	8 days	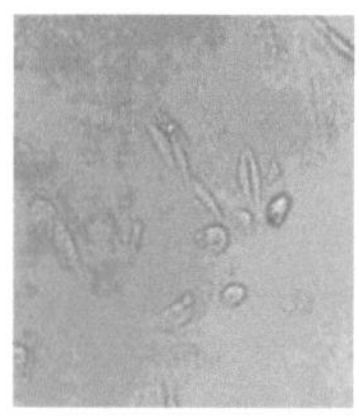	The drug-resistant cell lines survive.
5 days	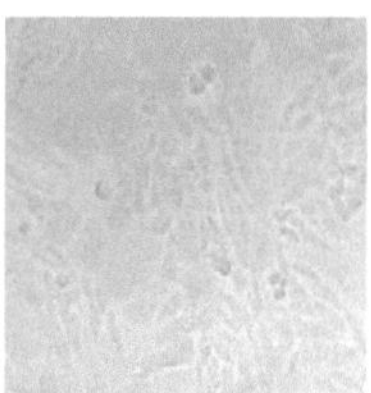	Cells begin to die.	12 days	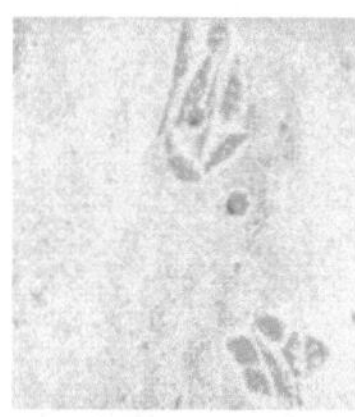	Single cells began to amplification
15 days	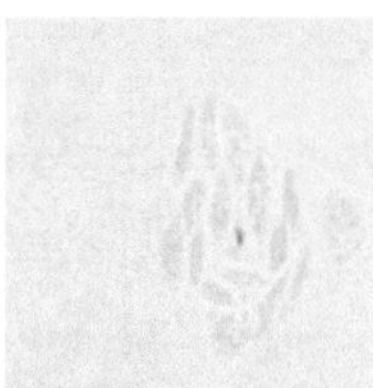	cells amplifi-cation and colony-forming unit	21 days	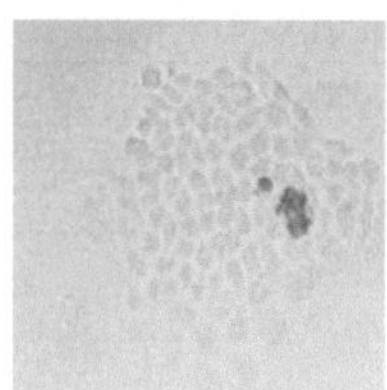	Form a stable clone.
18 days	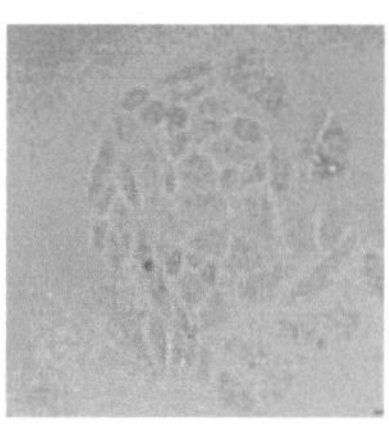	Colony-forming unit			

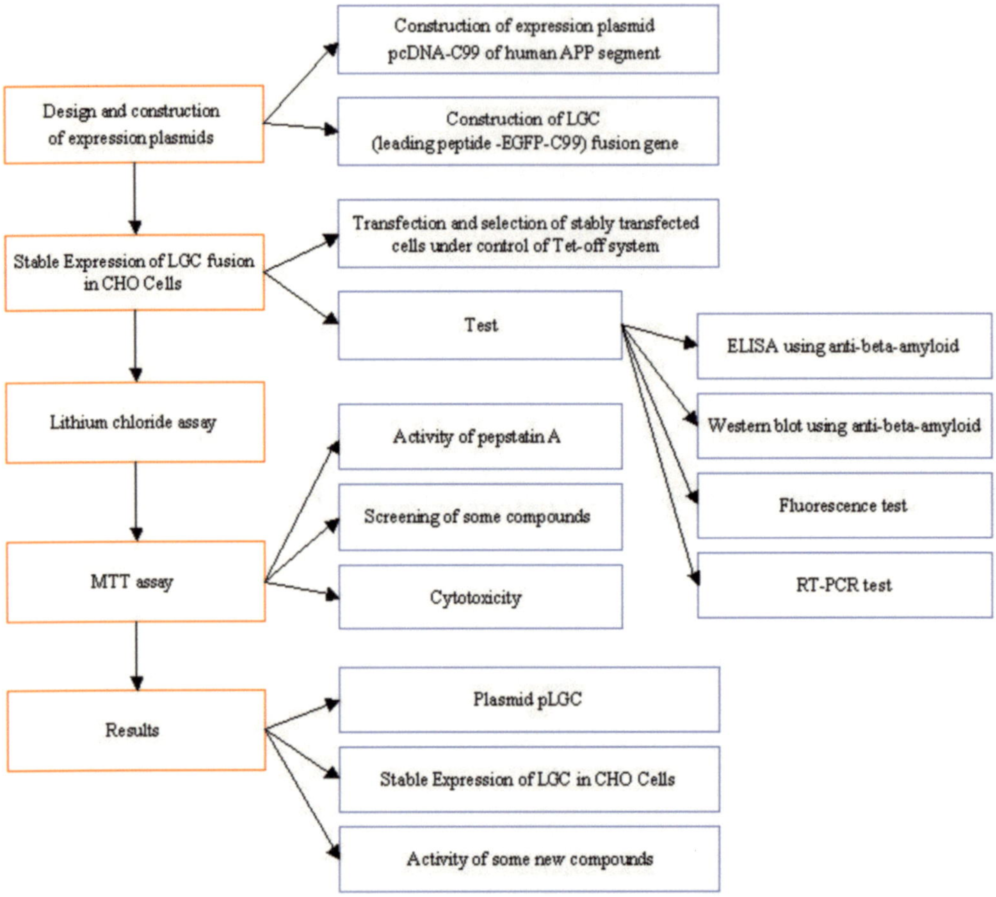

Flowchart for construction of drug screening cell model and its application

7. References

Adams, R. A.; Passino, M.; Sachs, B.D.; Nuriel, T. & Akassoglou, K. (2004). Fibrin Mechanisms and Functions in Nervous System Pathology. *Mol. Interv.*, Vol. 4, No. 3, (Jun 2004), pp163-176, ISSN 1534-0384.

Andrae, J.; Gallini, R. & Betsholtz C. (2008). Role of platelet-derived growth factors in physiology and medicine. *Genes Dev.*, Vol. 22, No. 10, (May 2008), pp1276-1312, ISSN 0890-9369.

Baron, U.; Gossen, M. & Hermann Bujard, H. (1997). Tetracycline-controlled transcription in eukaryotes: novel transactivators with graded transactivation Potential. *Nucleic Acids Research*, Vol. 25, No. 14, (Jul 1997), pp 2723–2729, ISSN 0305-1048.

Campbell, W.A.; Iskandar, M.-K.; Reed, M.L.O. & Xia, W. (2002). Endoproteolysis of Presenilin in Vitro: Inhibition by gamma-Secretase Inhibitors. *Biochemistry*, Vol. 41, No. 10, (May 2002), pp3372-3379, ISSN 0006-2960.

Carter, D.B.; Chou, K.C. (1998). A model for structure dependent binding of Congo Red to Alzeheimer beta-amyloid fibrils. *Neurobiol. Aging*, Vol. 19, No. 1, (Jan.-Feb 1998), pp37-40, ISSN 0197-4580.

Cook, D.G.; Sung, J.C.; Golde, T.E.; Felsenstein, K.M.; Wojczyk, B.S.; Tanzi, R.E.; Trojanowski, J.Q.; Lee, V.M.-Y. & Doms, R.W. (1996). Expression and analysis of presenilin 1 in a human neuronal system: localisation in cell bodies and dendrites. *Proc. Natu. Acad. Sci. U.S.A.*, Vol. 93, No. 17, (Aug 1996), pp9223-9228, ISSN 0027-8424.

Ding, C.; Liang, X.; Ma, L.; Yuan, X. & Zhu, X. (2009). Opposed effect of Ndel1 and alpha1/2 on cytoplasmic dynein functions through competitive binding to Lis1. *J Cell Sci.*, Vol. 122, No. 16, (Aug 2009), pp 2820-2827, ISSN 0021-9533.

Elsliger, M.A.; Wachter, R.M.; Hanson, G.T.; Kallio, K. & Remington, S.J. (1999). Structural and spectral response of green fluorescent protein variants to changes in pH. *Biochemistry*, Vol. 38, No. 17, (Apr 1999), pp 5296-5301, ISSN 0006-2960.

Findeis, M.A. (2007). The role of amyloid beta peptide 42 in Alzheimer's disease. *Pharmacology & Therapeutics*, Vol. 116, No. 2, (Jul 2007), pp 266-286, ISSN 0163-7258.

Francis, R.; McGrath, G.; Zhang, J.; Ruddy, D.; Sym, M.; Apfeld, J.; Nicoll, M.; Maxwell, M.; Hai, B.; Ellis, M.; Parks, A.L.; Xu, W.; Li, J.; Gurney, M.; Myers, R.L.; Himes, C.S.; Hiebsch, R.; Ruble, C.; Nye, J.S. & Curtis, D. (2002). aph-1 and pen-2 are required for Notch pathway signalling, g-secretase cleavage of bAPP, and presenilin protein accumulation. *Dev. Cell*, Vol. 3, No. 1, (Jul 2002), pp 85-97, ISSN 1534-5807.

Ge, H.M.; Zhu, C.H.; Shi, D.H.; Zhang, L.D.; Xie, D.Q.; Yang, J.; Ng, S.W. & Tan, R.X. (2008). Hopeahainol A, An Acetylcholinesterase Inhibitor from Hopea hainanensis. *Chem. Eur. J.*, Vol. 14, No. 1, (Jan 2008), pp376-381, ISSN 1521-3765.

Gerdes, H.-H. & Kaether,C. (1996). Green fluorescent protein: applications in cell biology. *FEBS Lett.*, Vol. 389, No. 1, (Jun 1996), pp 44-47, ISSN 0014-5793.

Gianni, D.; Zambrano, N.; Bimonte, M.; Minopoli, G.; Mercken, L.; Talamo, F.; Scaloni, A. & Russo, T. (2003). Platelet-derived Growth Factor Induces the beta-gamma-Secretase-mediated Cleavage of Alzheimer's Amyloid Precursor Protein through a Src-Rac-dependent Pathway. *J. Biol. Chem.*,Vol. 278, No. 11, (Mar 2003), pp 9290-9297, ISSN 0021-9258.

Goo, J.H. & Park, W.J. (2004). Elucidation of the Interactions between C99, Presenilin, and Nicastrin by the Split-Ubiquitin Assay. *DNA Cell Biol.*, Vol. 23, No. 1, (Jan 2004), pp 59-65, ISSN 1044-5498.

Gossen M, Bujard H. Tight control of gene expression in mammalian cells by tetracycline-responsive promoters. *Proc Natl Acad Sci U S A., Vol. 89, No. 12, (Jun* 1992), pp 5547-5551, ISSN 0027-8424.

Gossen, M.; Freundlieb, S.; Bender, G.; Muller, G.; Hillen, W. & Bujard, H. (1995). Transcriptional activation by tetracyclines in mammalian cells. *Science*, Vol. 268, No. 5218, (Jun 1995), pp 1766-1769, ISSN 0036-8075.

Hardy, J. (1997). Amyloid, the presenilins and Alzheimer's disease. *Trends Neurosci.*, Vol. 20, No. 4, (Apr 1997), pp 154-159, ISSN 0166-2236.

Hartmann, T.; Bieger, S.C.; Bruhl, B.; Tienari, P.J.; Ida, N.; Allsop, D.; Roberts, G.W.; Masters, C.L.; Dotti, C.G.; Unsicker, K. & Beyreuther, K. (1998). Distinct sites of intracellular production for Alzheimer's Ab40/42 amyloid peptides. *Nature Med.*, Vol. 3, No. 9, (Sep 1998), pp 1016–1020, ISSN 1078-8956.

Hooper, C.; Killick, R. & Lovestone, S. (2008). The GSK3 hypothesis of Alzheimer's disease. *J Neurochem.*, Vol. 104, No. 6, (Mar 2008), pp 1433-1439, ISSN 0022-3042.

Jiang, X.F.; Yang, J. & Wang, W. (2006). The Complex Network of Protein-Protein Interaction of Alzheimer's Disease Associated Proteins and an Interaction Predicting. *Journal of Nanjing University (Natural Science)*, Vol. 42, No. 5, (May 2006), pp 479-489, ISSN 0469-5097.

Kaether, C.; Haass, C. & Steiner, H. (2006). Assembly, trafficking and function of gamma-secretase. *Neurodegener Dis.*, Vol. 3, No. 4-5, (Oct 2006), pp 275-283, ISSN 1660-2854.

Kelliher, M.; Fastbom, J.; Cowburn, R.F.; Bonkale, W.; Ohm, T.G.; Ravid, R.; Sorrentino, V. & O'Neill, C. (1999). Alterations in the ryanodine receptor calcium release channel correlate with Alzheimer's disease neurofibrillary and beta-amyloid pathologies. *Neuroscience*, Vol. 92, No. 2, (May 1999), pp 499-513, ISSN 0306-4552.

Kovacs, D.M.; Fausett, H.J.; Page, K.J.; Kim, T.-W.; Moir, R.D.; Merriam, D.E.; Hollister, R.D.; Hallmark, O.G.; Mancini, R.; Felsenstein, K.M.; Hyman, B.T.; Tanzi, R.E. & Wasco, W. (1996). Alzheimer-associated presenilins 1 and 2: neuronal expression in brain and localization to intracellular membranes in mammalian cells. *Nature Med.*, Vol. 2, No. 2, (Feb 1996), 224–229, ISSN 1078-8956.

Li, Y.M.; Lai, M.T.; Xu, M.; Huang, Q.; DiMuzio-Mower, J.; Sardana, M.K.; Shi, X.P.; Yin, K.C.; Shafer, J.A. & Gardell, S.J. (2000). Presenilin 1 is linked with gamma-secretase activity in the detergent solubilized state. *Proc. Natl. Acad. Sci. U.S.A.*, Vol. 97, No. 11, (May 2000), pp 6138-6143, ISSN 0027-8424.

Liang, Y.; Yu, W.; Li, Y.; Yang, Z.; Yan, X.; Huang, Q. & Zhu, X. (2004). Nudel functions in membrane traffic mainly through association with Lis1 and cytoplasmic dynein. *J. Cell Biol., Vol.* 164, No. 4, (Feb 2004), pp 557-566, ISSN 0021-9525.

Liang, Y.; Yu, W.; Li, Y.; Yu, L.; Zhang, Q.; Wang, F.; Yang, Z.; Du, J.; Huang, Q.; Yao, X. & Zhu, X. (2007). Nudel modulates kinetochore association and function of cytoplasmic dynein in M phase. *Mol. Biol. Cell.*, Vol. 18, No. 7, (Jul 2007), pp 2656-2666, ISSN 0270-7306.

Cortes-Canteli, M. & Strickland, S. (2009). Fibrinogen, a possible key player in Alzheimer's disease. *J. Thromb. Haemost.*, Vol. 7, Suppl. 1, (Jul 2009), pp 146-150, ISSN 1538-7933.

Ma, L.; Tsai, M.-Y.; Wang, S.; Lu, B.; Chen, R.; Yates, III JR.; Zhu, X. & Zheng, Y. (2009). Requirement for Nudel and dynein for assembly of the lamin B spindle matrix. *Nat. Cell Biol.*, Vol. 11, No. 3, (Mar 2009), pp 247-256, ISSN 1465-7392.

McLendon, C.; Xin, T.; Ziani-Cherif, C.; Murphy, M.P.; Findlay, K.A.; Lewis, P.A.; Pinnix, I.; Sambamurti, K.; Wang, R.; Fauq, A. & Golde, T.E. (2000). Cell-free assays forgamma-secretase activity. FASEB J., Vol. 14, No. 15, (Dec 2000), pp 2383-2386, ISSN 0892-6638.

Merkle, D.L.; Cheng, C.H.; Castellino, F.J. & Chibber, B.A. (1996). Modulation of fibrin assembly and polymerization by the beta-amyloid of Alzheimer's disease. *Blood Coagul Fibrinolysis*, Vol. 7, No. 6, (Sep 1996), pp 650-658, ISSN 09575235.

Michelle, L.S.; Turner, R.S. & James, R.G. (2001). The protease inhibitor, MG132, blocks maturation of the amyloid precursor protein Swedish mutant preventing cleavage bybeta-secretase. *J. Biol. Chem.*, Vol. 276, No. 6, (Feb 2001), pp 4476-4484, ISSN 0021-9258.

Mouradian, M.M. (2007). The role of amyloid beta peptide 42 in Alzheimer's disease. *Pharmacology & Therapeutics*, Vol. 116, No. 2, (Nov 2007), pp 266-286, ISSN 0163-7258.

Netzer, W.J.; Dou, F.; Cai, D.; Veach, D.; Jean, S.; Li, Y.; Bornmann, W.G.; Clarkson, B.; Xu, H. & Greengard, P. (2003). Gleevec inhibits beta-amyloid production but not Notch cleavage. Proc. Natl. Acad. Sci. U. S. A., Vol. 100, No. 21, (Oct 2003), pp 12444-12449, ISSN 0027-8424.

Ormoe, M.; Cubitt, A.B.; Kallio, K.; Gross, L.A.; Tsien, R.Y. & Remington S.J. (1996). Crystal structure of the Aequorea victoria green fluorescent protein. *Science*, Vol. 273, No. 5, (Nov 1996), pp 1392-1395, ISSN 0036-8075.

Paul, J.; Strickland, S. & Melchor, J.P. (2007). Fibrin deposition accelerates neurovascular damage and neuroinflammation in mouse models of Alzheimer's disease. *J Exp Med.*, Vol. 204, No. 8, (Aug 2007), pp 1999-2008, ISSN 0022-1007.

Phiel, C.J.; Wilson, C.A.; Lee, V. M. & Klein, P.S. (2003). GSK-3alpha regulates production of Alzheimer's disease amyloid-beta peptides. *Nature*, Vol. 423, No. 6938, (May 2003), pp 435–439, ISSN 0028-0836.

Resnitzky, D.; Gossen, M.; Bujard, H. & Reed, S.I. (1994). Acceleration of the G(1)/S phase-transition by expression of Cyclin-D1 and Cyclin-E with an inducible system. *Molecular and Cellular Biology*, Vol. 14, No. 3, (Mar 1994), pp 1669-1679, ISSN 0270-7306.

Roßner, S.; Sastre, M.; Bourne, K. & Lichtenthaler, S.F. (2006). Transcriptional and translational regulation of BACE1 expression—Implications for Alzheimer's disease. *Progress in Neurobiology*, Vol. 79, No. 2, (Jun 2006), pp 95-111, ISSN 0301-0082.

Ryoo, H.M.; Hoffmann, H.M.; Beumer, T.; Frenkel, B.; Towler, D.A,; Stein, G.S.; Stein, J.L.; van Wijnen, A.J. & Lian, J.B. (1997). Stage-Specific Expression of Dlx-5 during Osteoblast Differentiation: Involvement in Regulation of Osteocalcin Gene Expression. *Molecular Endocrinology*, Vol. 11, No. 11, (Oct 1997), pp 1681-1694, ISSN 0888-8809.

Sevush, S.; Jy, W.; Horstman, L.L.; Mao, W.W.; Kolodny, L. & Ahn, Y.S. (1998). Platelet activation in Alzheimer disease. *Arch Neurol.*, Vol. 55, No. 4, (Apr. 1998), pp 530-6, ISSN 0096-6886.

Shan, Y.; Yu, L.; Li, Y.; Pan, Y.; Zhang, Q.; Wang, F.; Chen, J. & Zhu, X. (2009). Nudel and FAK as antagonizing strength modulators of nascent adhesions through Paxillin. *PLoS Biol.*, Vol. 7, No. 5, (May 2009), pp e1000116, ISSN 1544-9173.

Shen, Y.; Li, N.; Wu, S.; Zhou, Y.; Shan, Y.; Zhang, Q.; Ding, C.; Yuan, Q.; Zhao, F.; Zeng, R. & Zhu, X. (2008). Nudel binds Cdc42GAP to modulate Cdc42 activity at the leading edge of migrating cells. *Dev. Cell*, Vol. 14, No. 3, (Mar 2008), pp 342-353, ISSN 1534-5807.

Shockett, P.; Difilippantonio, M.; Hellman, N. & Schatz, D.G. (1995). A modified tetracycline-regulated system provides autoregulatory, inducible gene expression in cultured cells and transgenic mice. *Proc Natl Acad Sci U S A.*, Vol. 92, No. 14, (Jul 1995), pp 6522-6, ISSN 0027-8424.

Solertea, S.B.; Ceresinib, G.; Ferraria, E. & Fioravantia, M. (2000). Hemorheological changes and overproduction of cytokines from immune cells in mild to moderate dementia of the Alzheimer's type: adverse effects on cerebromicrovascular system. *Neurobiology of Aging*, Vol. 21, No. 2, (Mar-Apr 2000), pp 271–281, ISSN 0197-4580.

Sun, X.; Sato, S.; Murayama, O.; Murayama, M.; Park, J.M.; Yamaguchi, H. & Takashima, A. (2002). Lithium inhibits amyloid secretion in COS7 cells transfected with amyloid precursor protein C100. *Neurosci. Lett.*, Vol. 321, No. 1-2, (Mar 2002), pp 61–64, ISSN 0304-3940.

Tanzi, R,E. (1999). A genetic dichotocny model for the inheritance of Alzheimer's disease and common age- related disorders. *J. Clin. Invest.*, Vol. 104, No. 9, (Nov 1999), pp 1175-1179, ISSN 0021-9738.

Walsh, D.M.; Minogue, A.M.; Frigerio, C.S.; Fadeeva, J.V.; Wasco, W. & Selkoe, D.J. (2007). The APP family of proteins: similarities and differences. *Biochemical Society Transactions*, Vol. 35, Pt 2, (Apr 2007), pp 416-420, ISSN 0300-5127.

Wang, H.-Y.; Lee, D.H.S.; Davis, C.B. & Shank, R.P. (2000). Amyloid peptide Abeta 1-42 binds selectively and with picomolar affinity to alpha7 nicotinic receptors. *J. Neurochem.*, Vol. 75, No. 3, (Sep 2000), pp 1155-1161, ISSN 0022-3042.

Wei, D.Q.; Sirois, S.; Du, Q.S.; Arias, H.R. & Chou, K.C. (2005). Theoretical studies of Alzheimer's disease drug candidate [(2,4-dimethoxy) benzylidene]-anabaseine dihydrochloride (GTS-21) and its derivatives. *Biochem. Biophy. Res. Commun.*, Vol. 338, No. 2, (Dec 2005), pp 1059-1064, ISSN 0006-291X.

Whitehouse, P.J.; Price, D.L.; Struble, R.G.; Clark, A.W.; Coyle, J.T. & DeLong, M.R. (1982). Alzheimer's disease and senile dementia: loss of neurons in the basal forebrain. *Science*, Vol. 215, No. 4537, (Mar 1982), pp 1237-1239, ISSN 0036-8075.

Yan, X.; Li, F.; Liang, Y.; Shen, Y.; Zhao, X.; Huang, Q.; & Zhu, X. (2003) Human Nudel and NudE as Regulators of Cytoplasmic Dynein in Poleward Protein Transport along the Mitotic Spindle. *Mol. Cell. Biol.*, Vol. 23, No. 4, (Feb 2003), pp 1239-50, ISSN 0270-7306.

Yang, F.; Moss, L.G. & Phillips, G.N. Jr. (1996). The molecular structure of green fluorescent protein. *Nat. Biotechnol.*, Vol. 14, No. 10, (Oct 1996), pp 1246-1251, ISSN 1087-0156.

Yang, J.; Yao, J.; Chen, J.; Wang, X.N.; Zhu, T.Y.; Chen, L.L. & Chu, P. (2009). Construction of drug screening cell model and application to new compounds inhibiting FITC-fibrinogen binding to CHO cells expressing human alphaIIbbeta3. *European Journal of Pharmacology*, Vol. 618, No. 1-3, (Sep 2009), pp 1-8, ISSN 0014- 2999.

Yang, J.B.; Yao, J.; Chen, L.L. & Yang, J. (2006). The Amino-Terminal Domain of Integrin beta3 Functions as a Transcriptional Activator in Yeast. *Molecular and Cellular Biochemistry*, Vol. 288, No. 1-2, (Jan 2006), pp 1-5, ISSN 0300-8177.

Yang, J.B.; Yao, J.; Yang, K.; Hua, Z.C. & Yang, J. (2005). Expression, Purification and Activity Assay of new recombinant antagonists of fibrinogen receptor. *Am. J. Biochem. Biotech.*, Vol. 1, No. 2, (Feb 2005), pp 69-73, ISSN 1553-3468.

Yang, Z.; Guo, J.; Li, N.; Qian, M.; Wang, S. & Zhu, X. (2003). Mitosin/CENP-F is a conserved kinetochore protein subjected to cytoplasmic dynein-mediated poleward transport. *Cell Res.*, Vol. 13, No. 4, (Aug 2003), pp 275-283, ISSN 1001-0602.

Yang, J. & Quail, J.W. (1999). Structure of the Rhizomucor miehei aspartic proteinase complexed with the inhibitor pepstatin A at 2.7 A resolution. *Acta Crystallogr., Sect. D*, Vol. 55, No. Pt 3, (Mar 1999), pp 625-630, ISSN 0907-4449.

Zhang, Q.; Wang, F.; Cao, J.; Shen, Y.; Huang, Q.; Bao, L. & Zhu, X. (2009). Nudel promotes axonal lysosome clearance and endo-lysosome formation via dynein-mediated transport. *Traffic.*, Vol. 10, No. 9, (May 2009), pp 1337-1349, ISSN 1600-0854.

Zhang, H. & Koo, E.H. (2006). The amyloid precursor protein: beyond amyloid. *Molecular Neurodegeneration*, Vol. 1, No. 1, (Jan 2006), pp 5-12, ISSN 1750-1326.

Zhang, L.; Song, L.; Terracina, G.; Liu, Y.; Pramanik, B. & Parker, E. (2001). Biochemical characterization of the gamma-secretase activity that produces beta-amyloid peptides. *Biochemistry*, Vol. 40, N0. 16, (Apr 2001), pp 5049-5055, ISSN 0006-2960.

Zhou, X.; Wang, R.; Fan, L.; Li, Y.; Ma, L.; Yang, Z.; Yu, W.; Jing, N. & Zhu, X. (2005). Mitosin/CENP-F as a negative regulator of activating transcription factor-4. *J. Biol. Chem.*, Vol. 280, No. 14, (Apr 2005), pp 13973-13977, ISSN 0021-9258.

Zhu, X. (1999). Structural requirements and dynamics of mitosin-kinetochore interaction in M phase. *Mol. Cell. Biol.*, Vol. 19, No. 2, (Feb 1999), pp 1016-1024, ISSN 0270-7306.

Zhu, X.; Ding, L. & Pei, G. (1997). Carboxyl terminus of mitosin is sufficient to confer spindle pole localization. *J. Cell. Biochem.*, Vol. 66, No. 4, (Sep 1997), pp 441-449, ISSN 0730-2312.

9

Therapeutics of Alzheimer's Disease

Marisol Herrera-Rivero[1] and Gonzalo Emiliano Aranda-Abreu[2]
[1]*Doctorado en Ciencias Biomédicas, Centro de Investigaciones Biomédicas,*
[2]*Programa de Neurobiología, Universidad Veracruzana,*
Xalapa, Veracruz,
Mexico

1. Introduction

Alzheimer's disease (AD) is the most common age-related neurodegenerative disorder, its prevalence is increasing along with population longevity and there is no cure for this disease so far, despite of the amount of information research has provided. This leads us to seek for better treatments able to improve the patient's and caregivers' quality of life. In this chapter we will review some of the main aspects of those proteins playing a key role in the pathological processes of Alzheimer's disease, as well as the therapeutic strategies currently in use and those that have been developing in the last few years for the treatment of this disease.

We will take a look on the processes of formation of the characteristic lesions of the Alzheimer's brain and sum up some of the properties of the main proteins involved in such processes leading to neuronal damage and death and the resulting cognitive decline. We will also have an overview of the current drugs of choice for Alzheimer's treatment and discuss about the latest therapies research has been developing to treat AD in its different stages, such as a therapy of our own proposal for the repair of neuronal membranes prior to initiate a conventional drug treatment and the advantages these strategies would provide combined on patients with a mild to moderate neuronal damage. At last we will focus on the importance of an integral care of Alzheimer's patients.

2. A quick view into the Alzheimer's brain

Two characteristic lesions develop within the brain of an AD patient, namely neuritic plaques and neurofibrillary tangles, both responsible for the symptomatology due to neuronal damage and death. We will take now a short look into these lesions.

2.1 Neuritic plaques

The so called neuritic or amyloid plaques are mainly extracellular aggregates of insoluble filaments of β-amyloid peptides with adjacent microglia, frequently surrounded by astrocytes. The dystrophic neurites are located into and around these amyloid deposits. Plaques are largely found in the limbic and association cortices, where they slowly start to develop over the years preceding the onset of the disease.

2.1.1 β-amyloid formation

β-amyloid peptides (Aβ) are the result of the sequential actions of the secretases over the amyloid precursor protein (APP). When APP is cleaved by the β- and γ-secretases the insoluble amyloid species are released (Figure 1). Some authors suggest a physiological role for Aβ in memory processes and as a regulator of the potassium channels expression and neuronal excitability (Ohno et al., 2004; Plant et al., 2006).

2.1.2 The amyloid precursor protein

APP is a type I membrane protein member of a small family with a large extracellular domain and a short cytoplasmic one, APP presents three main isoforms (695, 751 and 770 residues) and is the only protein containing the Aβ sequence. The 695 residues is the most abundant isoform in neurons, but other brain cells also express variable amounts of APP and non-neural cells express mainly the 751 and 770 residues APP isoforms. The APP gene is located in chromosome 21 and over 25 mutations to this gene have been described as responsible for familial forms of AD (Thinakaran & Koo, 2008; Hung & Selkoe, 1994; Haas et al., 1991). APP undergoes a variety of post-translational modifications and proteolitic cleavages along and after its pass through the secretory pathway, releasing its derivatives into the lumen of secretory vesicles and the extracellular space (Selkoe, 2001). This protein has a poorly understood physiological role, but there have been autocrine and paracrine growth functions as well as trophic functions described, it is involved in neurite growth and synaptogenesis (Hung et al., 1992; Muresan et al., 2009; Chan et al., 2002).

2.1.3 The secretases

The α-, β- and γ-secretases cleave APP in several sites generating soluble peptides and membrane fragments as well as the insoluble Aβ peptides ($A\beta_{40}$ and $A\beta_{42}$) of amyloid plaques, these last as a result of the sequential actions of β-secretase (beta-site APP cleaving enzyme-1, BACE1) and the γ-secretase complex (composed by the presenilines-PS1 or PS2-, APH-1, PEN-2 and nicastrin).

The β-secretase gene is localized in chromosome 11 and it responds to stress conditions. Almost every tissue expresses BACE1, nevertheless its highest levels of expression are found in the brain. This enzyme has a 501 amino acids sequence containing two aspartil protease active sites and is located within cholesterol rich lipid rafts; it is believed BACE1 plays a role in synaptic function and the myelination process (Riddell et al., 2001; Ma et al., 2007; Cole & Vassar, 2007). On the other hand, γ-secretase is an enzymatic complex formed by four essential protein subunits necessary for an active mature complex. Mutations in either of the two preseniline genes (PS1, chromosome 14 and PS2, chromosome 1) have been described in cases of familial AD (Yu et al., 2000; Thinakaran & Koo, 2008). This secretase cleaves APP in several sites within its transmembrane domain perhaps to regulate programmed cell death, there is some evidence supporting a relationship between APP and PS expression levels and apoptotic activity (Vito et al., 1996).

2.2 Neurofibrillary tangles

These lesions are mainly the result of the intracellular aggregation of hyperphosphorylated protein tau in the form of paired helical filaments (PHFs) in the brain regions affected by AD, such as the enthorrinal cortex, hippocampus, parahippocampal gyrus, amygdala and frontal, temporal, parietal and occipital association cortices and subcortical nuclei projecting to these regions (Brion et al., 1985; Grundke-Iqbal et al., 1986; Kosik et al., 1986; Nukina & Ihara, 1986; Wood et al., 1986).

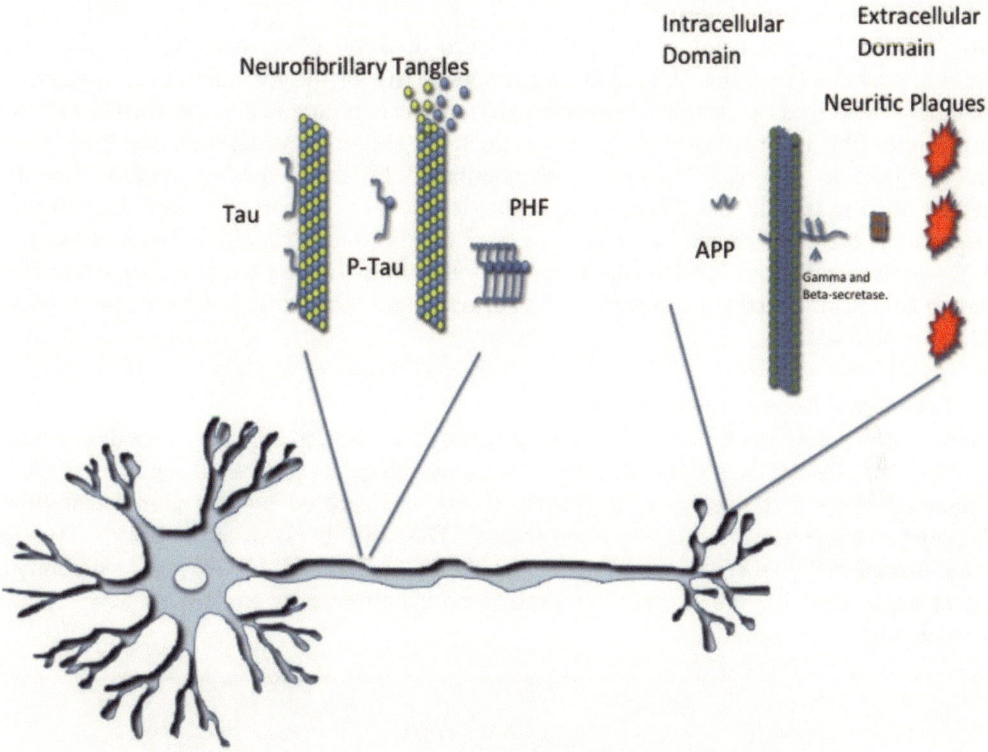

Fig. 1. Processes of formation of neuritic plaques and neurofibrillary tangles

Microtubule-associated protein tau (MAPT) promotes the microtubule assembly and stabilization required for morphogenesis and axonal transport in neurons, but it is also found in other cell lines (Johnson & Hartigan, 1999; Ingelson et al., 1996; Thurston et al., 1996). Tau gene is localized in chromosome 17. This protein controls microtubule stability in two ways: isoforms and phosphorylation. Tau phosphorylation in several sites regulates in a negative manner the protein's ability to bind to microtubules (Pope et al., 1994; Preuss et al., 1995; Preuss & Mandelkow, 1998; Illenberger et al., 1998), being this one the reason why the hyperphosphorylation of tau is a crucial event in the pathophysiology of AD. When tau gets hyperphosphorylated, it dissociates from microtubules and forms the PHFs which aggregate in the perinucleic cytoplasm, leaving a destabilized membrane to deform and lose synaptic activity (Figure 1). While neuritic plaques are thought to develop in a minor amount within the normal aging brain, the hyperphosphorylation of tau is almost an exclusive event of AD and the so called tauophaties.

3. The Alzheimer's therapeutic strategies

As we shall remember there is no cure for AD, however drug treatments are available to help with the symptomatology in several aspects of the disease and researchers keep making efforts around the world to find better treatments as well as preventive strategies and ultimately a cure for AD.

3.1 Available drug treatments

Now we will review some of the characteristics of those drugs most widely used and approved by the Food and Drug Administration (FDA) for the treatment of AD, these are mainly divided into two groups: the acetylcholinesterase inhibitors and the NMDA receptor antagonists (this last represented by Memantine). We should consider here that these drugs are designed to diminish the symptoms originated by the neurodegeneration but that neither of them targets the plaques and/or tangles to destroy them or to stop the processes responsible for their formation and progress; they provide cognitive improvement by different means. It is also convenient here to say that these are not the only drugs that have shown beneficial effects on AD patients, nevertheless no other drug has been approved for AD treatment so far.

3.1.1 Acetylcholinesterase inhibitors

Diminished cholinergic function is a normal feature in aging, in AD and other dementias it becomes of special severity however. The physiological processes underlying AD's pathology cause a decline in acetylcholine levels, exacerbated by the neurotransmitter's degrading enzyme, the acetylcholinesterase. The members of this group support communication between nerve cells by increasing the acetylcholine levels and availability at the synaptic cleft (Figure 2), they suppress acetylcholinesterase to prevent acetylcholine degradation.

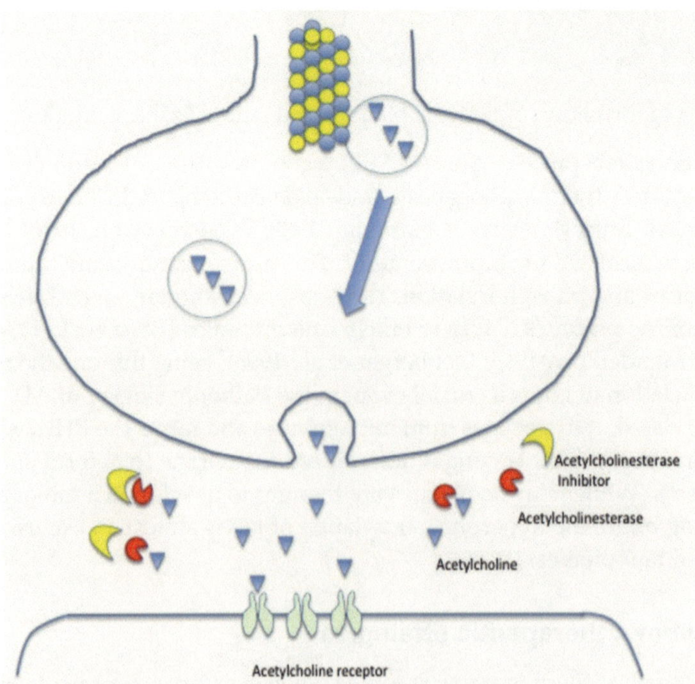

Fig. 2. Action mechanism of acetylcolinesterase inhibitors

There are three types of acetylcholinesterase inhibitors: short-acting, medium-duration and irreversible inhibitors; the difference between each other is the way they interact with the active site of the enzyme (Rang et al., 2001). The general side effects of these drugs may include diarrhea, nausea, dizziness, fatigue, loss of appetite and insomnia; the treatment with any of them should be monitored and start with low initial doses progressively increased until the maximum recommended daily dosage is reached. Precautions must be taken with concomitant (cardiovascular, gastrointestinal, pulmonary, urinary, neurological) diseases (De la Vega-Cotarelo & Zambrano-Toribio, 2011).

A. Tacrine (Cognex)

Derived from acridine, tacrine was one of the first drugs developed to help with the main symptoms of AD such as memory problems, cognitive decline and behavioral changes. Tacrine has been approved for the treatment of mild-to-moderate AD. Besides its acetylcholinesterase inhibiting activity, tacrine may also act as a potassium channel blocker which would increase the release of acetylcholine by functional cholinergic neurons. It should be noticed that tacrine has been associated with increased levels of transaminases (40-50% of patients) although its damage mechanism and efficacy remain controversial. This drug is contraindicated in conditions including cardiovascular disease, asthma, hyperthyroidism, urinary obstruction, prostatic hypertrophy, peptic ulcer and hepatic disease. The treatment with tacrine initiates with 10 mg/6h for at least 6 weeks and progressively increases every 6 weeks until a 30 mg/6h dosage; this treatment must be monitored for drug interactions, liver toxicity, severe side effects and efficacy to identify the need for interruption due to highly adverse conditions induced by tacrine administration.

B. Galantamine (Razadyne)

It is a natural compound derived from *Galanthus nivalis*. Galantamine directly stimulates nicotinic receptors to acetylcholine (which are especially important for learning and short-term memory processes) allosterically, avoiding receptor desensitization and down-regulation, although these receptors are damaged in AD. The main characteristics of galantamine are the protective role it has shown in cortical neurons, preventing these cells from the cytotoxicity of the amyloid peptides and from suffering oxidative stress, and the inhibition of Aβ aggregation; besides, galantamine increases acetylcholine release and modulates the levels of other neurotransmitters such as GABA, serotonin and glutamate. Galantamine is approved for mild-to-moderate stages of the disease. Its administration depends on the pharmaceutical presentation but usually dose does not exceed 24 mg/day with a regular evaluation of side effects and clinical benefit.

C. Donepezil (Aricept)

This drug is a piperidine derivative, being a reversible acetylcholinesterase inhibitor with good specificity it shows few side effects, there is no risk for hepatotoxicity with this drug. Donepezil has been approved for moderate-to-severe AD with a maximum administration of 10 mg/day every night before going to bed.

D. Rivastigmine (Exelon)

It is a carbamate compound which, compared to donepezil, shows better tolerance by patients and fewer side effects; however, its effectiveness is more limited than that of donepezil and the main concern about its use is the possibility of severe gastric damage and hepatotoxicity after its prolonged consumption. Rivastigmine has been approved for mild-to-moderate AD in a low dosage (depending on the route of administration, until 12 mg/day). This drug is also used to treat dementia linked to Parkinson's disease.

3.1.2 Memantine

This non-competitive, voltage-dependent and of moderate affinity N-methyl-D-aspartate (NMDA) receptor antagonist regulates glutamate activity and prevents neuronal cells of an excessive income of calcium ions (Figure 3). Memantine (Namenda) is the only drug of its kind that has been approved by the FDA for the treatment of moderate-to-severe AD; its side effects may include hallucinations, confusion, dizziness, headaches and debilitation. Some authors have reported a decreasing activity for memantine of the amyloid peptide aggregation and prevention of synaptic dysfunction as well. Besides, it has been suggested by studies in transgenic mice inhibiting and reversing activities of the abnormal hyperphosphorylation of tau by a mechanism involving protein phosphatase-2A (Aronov et al., 2001).

The treatment of AD with memantine, as with acetylcholinesterase inhibitors, requires low initial dosages (5 mg/day) which will be progressively increased depending on the patient's tolerance until the maximum recommended is reached (20 mg/day), with constant monitoring of drug interaction, toxicity, efficacy and adverse side effects (Table 1). Memantine is contraindicated in cases of renal insufficiency, epilepsy, concomitant administration of amantadine, ketamine and dextromethorphan and conditions leading to an increase in urinary pH.

3.1.3 Auxiliary drugs

Symptoms of AD are often divided into cognitive, behavioral and psychiatric and thus exists a wide variety of symptoms accompanying the disease. Cognitive symptomatology affects memory, judgment, language, attention, planning and thinking processes while behavioral and psychiatric symptomatology affects the way a patient acts and feels and amongst these last are included anxiety, restlessness, hallucinations and delirium; besides there are other physical problems AD patients are prone to present and the side effects of primary drug treatments and drug interactions. For this reason it becomes of importance to attend the whole range of symptoms accompanying the disease.

For psychiatric symptoms should always be tried first a non-pharmacologic therapy followed, if necessary, by a pharmacologic treatment. Treatable conditions include, as we mentioned before, side effects of the primary drugs and interactions between drugs, symptoms of some common diseases and vision and hearing problems. Medication must target specific symptoms to contribute to the control of behavioral changes due to anxiety and restlessness originated by the accompanying symptomatology of AD (Table 2).

3.2 Developing therapies

A wide variety of research groups around the globe focus their investigations on the discovery of new biomarkers that serve as tools for an early diagnosis of AD in order to make treatments more effective when applied at the very first stages of the disease, where neuronal loss is not that significant for patients to present marked cognitive decline and it could be still possible to delay the neurodegenerative process. Along with that, many research groups are making efforts to develop new therapies for the treatment of AD using pharmacologic and non-pharmacologic strategies. Our group is currently investigating both

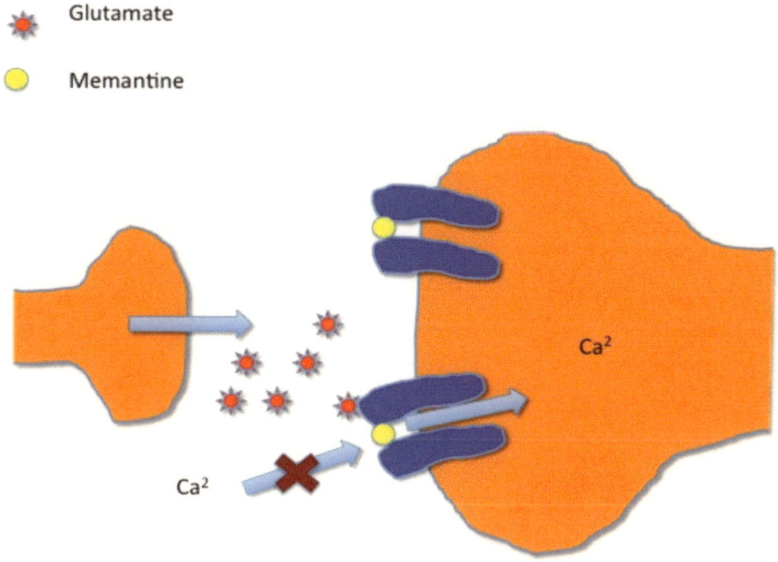

Fig. 3. Action mechanism of memantine

Group	Drug	AD stage	Beneficial effect	Risk	Dosage
Acetilcholinesterase inhibitor	Tacrine	Mild-to-moderate	Improves cognition and behavior	Hepatotoxicity	Initial: 10 mg/6h Maintenance: 30 mg/6h
	Galantamine	Mild-to-moderate	Improves learning and memory, cor-tical protection, in-hibition of Aβ aggregation	Nausea, vomi-ting, weight loss	Solution- Initial: 4 mg/12h Maintenance: 8 mg/12h Capsules-Initial: 8mg/day Maintenance: 16 mg/day Maximum: 24 mg/day
	Donepezil	Moderate-to-severe	Improves cognition Good tolerance	Muscle weakness	Initial: 5 mg/day Maintenance: 10 mg/day
	Rivastigmine	Mild-to-moderate	Improves cognition Good tolerance	Gastric damage Hepatotoxicity	Oral-Initial: 1,5 mg/12h Maintenance: 3-6 mg/12h Transdermic-Initial: 4,6 mg/day Maintenance: 9,5 mg/day
NMDA receptor antagonist	Memantine	Moderate-to-severe	Decreases Aβ aggregation, pre-vents synaptic dys-function, inhibits tau hyperphospho-rylation	Hallucinations Confusion Debilitation	Initial: 5 mg/day Maintenance: 20 mg/day

Table 1. Drugs approved for the AD treatment

the identification of gene expression-based peripheral biomarkers and the effectiveness of a neuronal rehabilitating therapy based mostly on natural products.

Conditions to control	Drugs	Examples
Humor, Irritability	Antidepressants	Citalopram, Fluoxetine, Paroxetine, Sertraline, Trazodone
Anxiety, Verbal problems, Resistance, Restlessness	Anxiolytics	Loracepam, Oxacepam
Hallucinations, Delirium, Aggression, Agitation, Hostility, Lack of cooperation	Antipsychotics	Aripiprazole, Clozapine, Haloperidol, Olanzapine, Ketiapine, Risperidone, Ziprasidone

Table 2. Auxiliary drugs in the treatment of AD's symptomatology

There has been studied the possibility of using anti-inflammatory drugs in the treatment of AD due to the evidence on the importance of inflammatory processes in the pathophysiology of AD. We shall notice two aspects in this subject: the presence of immune response in the AD brain and the immune response originated peripherally in these patients. Neuro-inflammation is a silent process occurring with morphological changes in activated microglia, the generation of reactive oxygen species (ROS) and other toxic materials, complement activation and cytokine release (Rogers et al., 1996; P.L. McGeer & E.G. McGeer, 1999, 2002); it is suggested that this inflammatory process might be due to the amyloid aggregation and damage to the blood brain barrier (BBB) (Hickey, 2001). The stress-induced production of pro-inflammatory cytokines and stress hormones by lymphocytes associates with several age-related diseases. In the AD, these peripheral processes may enhance the amyloid-induced inflammation in the brain. Because all of these, non-steroidal anti-inflammatory drugs (NSAIDs) (Anthony et al., 2000) and berberine (Zhu et al., 2006) have been investigated with therapeutic purposes for AD.

Immunotherapeutic approaches seek for the induction of an immune response against amyloid deposits. Three modalities are distinguished: passive immunization, active immunization and genetic vaccination; the last meaning the transfection of genes which produce the antigen. Immunization has proven efficient in animal models of AD, with several epitopes presenting different immunological properties being tested, as well as the mechanisms by which they exert an effect on Aβ clearance (Menéndez-González et al., 2005). Although clinical trials have failed so far, they rendered some relevant observations for the improvement of these strategies.

Other therapeutic strategies in development involve several methods to restore lipid homeostasis, promote synaptogenesis and regeneration and reduce Aβ production in the AD brain based on ApoE manipulation (Cedazo-Mínguez et al., 2007). Also, an increase in insulin stimuli in the brain could help improve memory in AD patients (Benedict et al., 2007). Nerve growth factor (NGF) and insulin-like growth factor-1 have shown a reduction of cognitive impairment and improvement of neurological functions in models of AD (Alzheimer's Research Center, 2008). Antioxidants, ginkgo biloba, estrogens and omega-3 fatty acids, among some other natural products, have also been investigated for therapeutic effects on AD. Despite the promising results of several of these studies, there still is a long way to go until some of these strategies could be available for the general population; nevertheless, each and every day we could be a step closer to develop a really effective treatment for such a complex disease as AD.

3.2.1 Neuro-rehabilitation in Mild-to-Moderate AD stages

AD treatment with both acetylcholinesterase inhibitors and Memantine has a quite reduced period of about six months of true effectiveness and noticeable results in patients, probably because of two reasons. Neither of these drugs is designed to stop the pathophysiological processes occurring within the AD brain, thus in one hand neurons keep degenerating and lesions growing in a slowly but progressive manner and synaptic connections are interrupted; on the other hand, the plasma membrane of neural cells is suffering a loss in stability and shape what we believe leads to the misplacement of receptors at the cell surface, leaving them unreachable for the neurotransmitter binding or even that both the neurotransmitter cannot be released and its receptor might not be properly carried to the cell surface because of the resulting damaged anterograde and retrograde transports. Thus despite of the neurotransmitter's maintained availability at the synaptic cleft, it is not able to reach the postsynaptic neuron and bind to its receptor or even the amount of neurotransmitter released from the presynaptic neuron is not enough to generate an adequate action in the postsynaptic neuron (Figure 4).

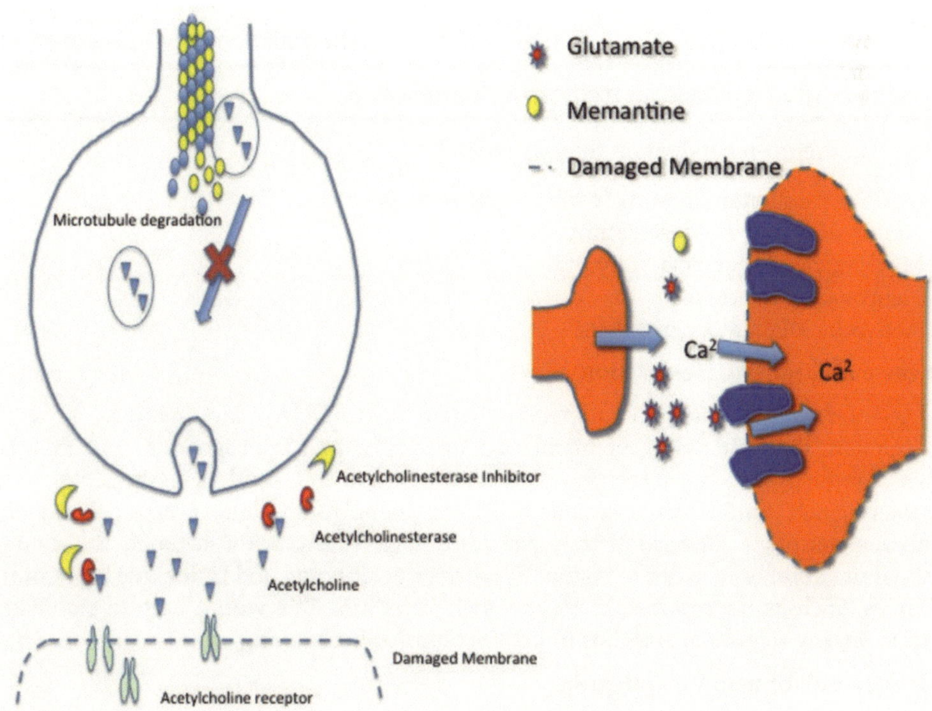

Fig. 4. Drugs do not function because of the damaged membrane

Because of all the above, our group proposed an alternative therapy for AD focused on neuronal membrane repair what would restore its functionality, including the transport of molecules such as neurotransmitters and their receptors, the availability of receptors binding domains and the correct placing of membrane molecules (receptors, enzymes and carriers). This therapy is based on a daily consumption of natural products including omega-3 and folic acids, ginkgo biloba and resveratrol which cause no side effects and have shown to provide good advantages for neuronal functionality, in addition of their easy accessibility. We also include Nimesulide for the inflammatory component of AD, and Fluoxetine or Escitalopram to promote neuronal reconnection. We suggest that a rehabilitation of neuronal membranes followed by or combined with the conventional drug treatments (Table 3) would enhance and prolong the beneficial effects of the treatment in AD patients. This therapy has shown good results so far (Aranda-Abreu et al., 2011) and there are currently more subjects initiating the protocol to test this therapy including normally aged individuals, AD patients and patients suffering from neurological disorders and dementias different from AD.

Day	Omega-3	600 – 1000 mg	(Membrane repair)
	Resveratrol	60 mg	(Antioxidant)
	Ginkgo biloba	60 mg	(Memory processes)
	Escitalopram	10 mg	(Neuronal reconnection)
Night	Folic acid	1 mg	(Neuronal integrity maintenance)
	Nimesulide	100 mg	(Anti-inflammatory – If necessary)
Alzheimer's drug treatment as medical doctor indicated			

Table 3. The Neuro-rehabilitation therapy recipe*

The neuro-rehabilitation therapy involves four aspects:

A. Neuronal membrane restoration.
B. Maintenance of neuronal integrity.
C. Neuronal reconnection.
D. Activation of memory processes.

A. Neuronal membrane restoration

Omega-3 fatty acids, such as docosahexaenoic acid (DHA), are involved in neurite development, the remodeling of membrane lipid rafts and neurogenesis, and they have shown a reduction in the hyperphosphorilation of tau and amyloid aggregation in AD. Cholesterol rich lipid rafts associate with the stabilization and proper clustering of membrane receptors. Because of this, we use omega-3 fatty acids to repair the damaged neuronal membranes in order to restore the correct positioning and trafficking of membrane molecules, such as neurotransmitters and their receptors; this would help to stabilize the synaptic activity (Figure 5) and thus improve cognitive functioning.

B. Maintenance of neuronal integrity

The integrity of neuronal membranes should be maintained in both the remaining healthy neurons and those already restored. This is important because we shall remember here that we are not making the damaging processes to stop and thus membranes would tend to degenerate if we do not help to delay these processes. With this purpose we included folic acid in the neuro-rehabilitation therapy as it plays an important role in neuroplasticity and the maintenance of neuronal integrity by a mechanism involving one-carbon metabolism, which associates with neurological and psychiatric pathologies when deranged.

* From Aranda-Abreu et al., 2011, Dovepress.

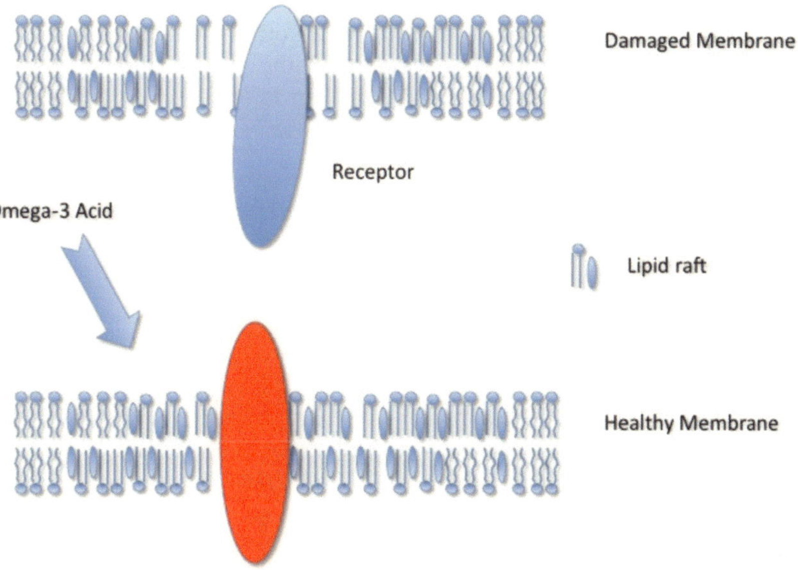

Fig. 5. Membrane restoration by the remodeling of lipid rafts

Resveratrol is also included in this therapy with the purpose of maintaining neuronal integrity. Resveratrol belongs to a group of molecules known as phytophenols, which act as free radical scavengers. Resveratrol is found in grape extracts and its use as antioxidant has become very popular nowadays because it protects against ROS toxicity and provides beneficial effects on inflammatory and neoplastic processes. In addition, resveratrol has shown a protective effect against Aβ toxicity in neuronal cell lines. The protection resveratrol provides to neuronal cells makes it a good agent to guard the integrity of these cells.

C. Neuronal reconnection

Neurons should be capable of making new connections between each other to re-establish cognitive processes. Some drugs such as Fluoxetine (Wang et al., 2008) and Escitalopram (Alboni et al., (2010) could help in this task by the induction of serotonin reuptake. Serotonin regulates neuronal morphology and its recapture is involved in the formation of new synapses, which would reconnect newly restored neurons (Figure 6). With their membranes repaired neurons regain the ability to receive and transmit impulses, thus once they make new inter-neuronal connections, the damaged AD brain would improve its functionality and cognitive impairment might be diminished.

D. Activation of memory processes

Ginkgo biloba is known for its beneficial effects on memory processes as well as its antioxidant activity. Among the pharmacological effects of ginkgo biloba are its antagonism to the platelet activation factor and the increase in GABA levels, glutamic decarboxylase and muscarinic receptors. Although consumption of ginkgo biloba with a therapeutic purpose for AD patients has brought inconclusive results, numerous authors report an improvement of the cognitive impairment in AD patients by the treatment with ginkgo biloba and we have observed good results in these patients after a follow up of one year from initiation of our neuro-rehabilitation therapy, which includes ginkgo.

Despite of the effects of ginkgo biloba on memory, we shall bear in mind that brain stimulation helps to keep it healthy. In AD, as in other neurodegenerative disorders, cognitive stimulation becomes of great importance for the rehabilitation process, improving memory and cognitive impairment. We will point out later the importance of stimulating the brain, along with other aspects, in order to assure the best possible outcome with this or any other AD treatment chosen.

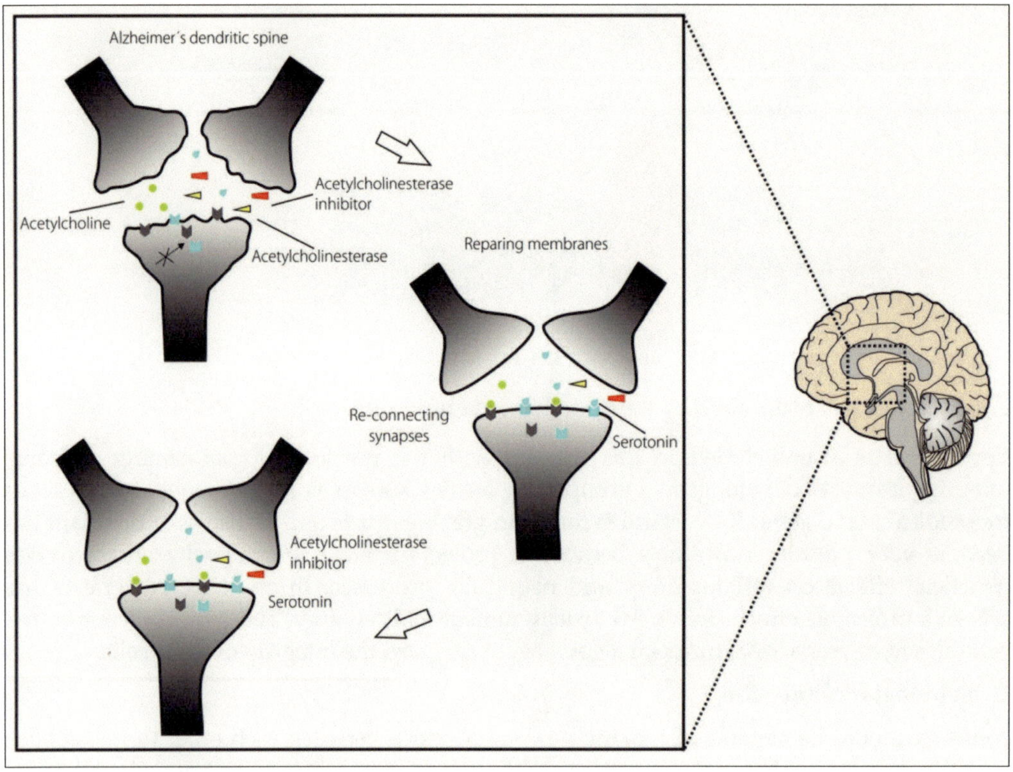

Fig. 6. Neuronal reconnections by serotonin recapture

3.2.2 Stem cells and advanced AD

Nowadays we have all heard about new therapies for all kinds of pathologies based on stem cells and AD is not the exception. In fact, the therapeutic strategy most widely investigated and, probably, promising for the severe cases of AD involves the growingly popular stem cells.

As we know, in AD there is a progressive loss of neuronal cells and thus in advanced stages of the disease the loss in brain mass is very significant, reason why no other pharmacological treatment or non-pharmacological therapy could promise much of an improvement. At this point, the alternative would be to replace the already lost neurons with new ones of the same type, the last being the main problem encountered by researchers in this area. As some groups have been able to successfully proliferate and differentiate stem cells from different sources into neurons of several types in culture, they found this to be difficult to reproduce into the brain. The conditions required *in vivo* for stem cells to differentiate into specific lineages are yet to be unraveled and only then effective and reproducible protocols could be developed to produce healthy and functional stem/progenitor cell-derived neurons (Wicklund et al., 2010). But even if we are to accomplish this task effectively another concern shall rise: would these cells be also affected by the disease in time? And, if so, how long would they provide an actual improvement on cognition before facing the pathophysiological processes of AD?

In AD, a stem cell-based approach should be able to replace several types of neuronal cells in different brain regions (Figure 7) and show a significant rescue of cognitive functions, some studies in animal models have suggested an improvement of cognition by means of a variety of mechanisms different to the direct alteration of either tau or Aβ pathologies (Blurton-Jones et al., 2009).

Another path to be taken would consist of protocols developed for endogenous stem cells stimulation. The main issue on this matter is the prevalent controversy about discrepant results on the effects of Aβ over stem cells and neurogenesis, as some studies suggest a neurogenic effect while others show neurotoxicity on stem/progenitor cells. Hence, modulation of the microenvironment within the AD brain would be crucial for the feasibility of this and other related approaches (Wicklund et al., 2010).

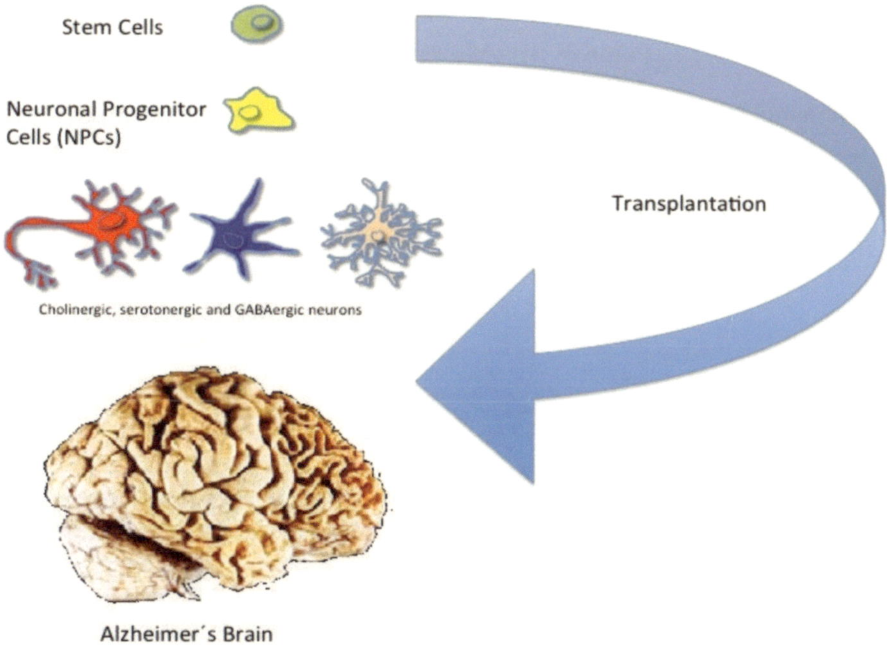

Fig. 7. Stem cell transplantation into the AD brain

4. Integral care of AD patients

There are many aspects we should keep an eye on once an individual is diagnosed with AD, for such a complex disease must be attacked in all possible directions; as there is no magic treatment for AD one could use all the help one can possibly get (Table 4). In our present study we are instructing the caregivers of our patients on the best way to assure an integral care able to render the best outcome for the therapy as it is not enough to repair the damaged neuronal membranes, to seek for neurogenesis, cognitive stimulation and the maintenance of neuronal functionality actually is the best way to enhance and prolong the positive effects of any AD therapy.

	Characteristics	Recommendations
Nutrition	Required for brain metabolism and synaptic function.	HAD, EPA, vitamins (E, K, C, B6, B12), minerals (iron, iodine, manganese, copper, zinc), unsaturated fatty acids, fish, 5 small meals.
Sleep	Helps neurogenesis, neuronal plasticity, learning and memory	No daytime naps, full 8 hr nighttime sleep, watch for sleep apnea, same bedtime every day.
Physical exercise	Good for metabolism, inflammation, memory, learning, information processing, neurogenesis, neuronal plasticity, neurotransmission	Exercise for 30 minutes, 3 times a week, at least.
Cognitive stimulation	Improvement of learning, memory and praxis, and socialization and mood	Reading, puzzles, crosswords, figure-recognition and problem-solving games, chess, Pictionary, drawing, bingo, etc.
Enriched environment	Regulates stress, mood, behavior, sleep-wake cycle and sensory stimulation	Comfortable, clean and ordered space, social and cultural activities, music, lightning, no loud noises, company, affection
Neuro-rehabilitation	Repairs neuronal membranes, synaptogenesis, improves memory and learning	Daily consumption, monitoring of patients.
Treatment	Helps neurotransmission.	Continue drug treatment as indicated by medical doctor. Monitor for potentially risky side effects.
General health	Improves restlessness, humor, vision and hearing, sleep, etc.	Often checkups, treatment of concomitant diseases, correction of vision and hearing problems.

Table 4. Integral care of the AD patient

4.1 Nutrition

The structure and function of the brain is affected by the nutrients in our diet as up to 50% of carbohydrates are consumed by the brain, lipids constitute neuronal membranes and amino acids, vitamins and some minerals are required for neurotransmitter synthesis and the maintenance of cognitive functions (Lanyau-Domínguez, 2009). Therefore, a healthy diet becomes important not only for preventing neuronal deterioration in non-demented

individuals, but for the maintenance of the remaining healthy neurons in demented patients. For example, glucose intake in the brain requires vitamin B_1, and vitamin B_{12} is necessary for myelination, this last together with vitamin B_6 are involved in neurotransmitter synthesis, vitamin E protects neuronal membranes; iron and iodine are required for cellular metabolism and manganese, copper and zinc are cofactors in the protection against free radicals and ROS; a high consumption of mono- and polyunsaturated fatty acids, DHA and EPA, together with a low consumption of saturated and trans-saturated ones, has been associated with a better cognitive functionality.
AD patients have demonstrated to be prone to develop nutrient deficiency due to loss of independence, disorientation and altered eating behavior which could lead not only to an exacerbation of cognitive decline but to recurrent infectious diseases, anemia and an increase in morbidity and mortality (Finley, 1997; Morley, 1996; Franzoni et al., 1996; Riviére et al., 1999).
We recommend caregivers to implement with the therapy the following diet:

A. Fish or tuna fish at least twice a week.
B. Legumes one to three times per week.
C. Highly energetic meals including bread, pasta, rice and potatoes.
D. Two portions of dairy products.
E. Two portions of meat, chicken and eggs, one portion when fish is included.
F. Five portions of fruits and vegetables.
G. Vegetable oils.
H. Distribute in 5 small meals per day.

4.2 Sleep

In AD, as in other neurological disorders, age-related sleep disorders are exacerbated by several factors including homeostatic alterations in the circadian rhythms, medication side effects, environmental factors and medical illness. The different sleep stages have a role in learning and memory processes as well as in neurogenesis and neuronal plasticity. Furthermore, it is suggested that sleep disturbances could exacerbate Aβ aggregation and that the optimization of sleep time may slow the progression of AD (Kang et al., 2009). Fluoxetine or Escitalopram in our therapy could help to modulate sleep disorders, although we also suggest caregivers to pay attention to the patient's sleep-wake cycle to try to avoid naps during the daytime and wakefulness during the night to promote a better nighttime sleep.

4.3 Physical exercise

Exercise helps keeping our bodies healthy and that includes our brains, it increases cerebral blood flow by the improvement of vascular function, improves metabolism, reduces inflammation and regulates several brain chemicals, but it does not stop here. It has been suggested that exercise may also improve memory and learning, delay age-related memory loss, speed information processing, aid neurogenesis and synaptic plasticity, enhance the glutamatergic system, increase brain derived neurotrophic factor and dendritic spines and reduce cell death (van Praag, 2009; Cotman et al., 2007, as cited in Wollen, 2010). Therefore we ask the participants in our therapy program to include at least 30 minutes of exercise 3 times a week, this would help improve the mood of patients and facilitate cognitive functions.

4.4 Cognitive stimulation

It is crucial to stimulate the brain while following the neuro-rehabilitation therapy as we shall remember our ultimate purpose is to reconnect neuronal networks in order to improve cognition. A higher degree of education and regular reading have proven to decrease the risk to develop AD, thus stimulating the brain helps to keep it healthy ("use it or lose it"). As our therapy is designed to be accessible to our patients' family members or professional caregivers, this aspect is covered with activities that are both stimulating and recreational. Board games and other challenging activities could help activate memory, learning, sensory, motor and language processes and, when performed as a group, they may also contribute to socialization and mood. Therefore we ask our participants to ensure that at least one hour per every day will be destined to activities such as reading, solving crosswords, making puzzles, playing picture-recognition games, pictionary, bingo, chess, etc., and that they will be performed in group at least 3-4 times per week.

4.5 Environment

Studies have shown a significant improvement of cognition by environmental enrichment in models of AD (Jankowsky et al., 2005). Environmental enrichment here seeks for stress reduction, mood improvement, behavioral management, sleep-wake cycle regulation and sensory stimulation. In this aspect it is important to enrich the environment where our patients live within not only by social and recreating activities as we mentioned before, but by making them feel comfortable physically and emotionally. We ask our participants to create a harmonious, quiet and familial environment with an adequate lighting, music, order and affection. Social and cultural activities are also suggested.

4.6 Rehabilitation

The neuro-rehabilitation therapy should be followed as indicated. For it could take some time to show an improvement, maintenance and patience are needed. As we previously reported (Aranda-Abreu et al., 2011), we observed good outcomes with patients followed up to one year after the incorporation of our therapy to their AD treatment and thus we ask for our patients' family members to be patient and follow the instructions to ensure the best possible response to the therapy. We also promote preventive precautions between patients' family members, caregivers and between people above 50 years old because we believe prevention is currently the best weapon we could use to fight the increasing prevalence of AD and other age-related diseases.

4.7 Treatment

For all our participants that have already been diagnosed with AD by the time of initiation of the therapy, we recommend their relatives not to discard the drug treatment previously prescribed by the physician; the neuro-rehabilitation therapy should help these drugs to work more properly when combined. It is important to understand that these drugs do work and provide some benefits for AD patients, but their effect decreases as neurodegeneration continues; when neuronal membranes are repaired and synapses re-established these drugs should exacerbate the positive effects of the neuro-rehabilitation therapy.

4.8 General health care

Our recommendation to provide the best health care is to visit the physician with certain frequency to make sure concomitant diseases, drug side effects and possible limiting organic conditions are attended adequately. Comorbidity could speed up the rate of cognitive decline and discomfort due to physical or psychological illness might exacerbate behavioral and mood changes. Health care must be multidisciplinary in order to attend the whole range of the patients' needs.

5. Conclusion

Alzheimer's is a complex disease due to the presence of diverse pathological processes, it does not only involve plaque and tangle formation but inflammation, immune response, mitochondrial dysfunction, altered membrane traffic and positioning of molecules and a whole series of mechanisms leading to neuronal degeneration and death. Because of this diversity of events drug treatments remain scarcely effective which highlights the need for therapeutic strategies seeking for an integral care of every aspect of the patient's life. In attendance to this need, our group has proposed a neuro-rehabilitation therapy based mostly on natural products for the repair of neuronal membranes and the formation of new synapses in order to re-establish communication and cognitive processes. This therapy involves a change in the patient's lifestyle that would enhance the positive effects and provide a better quality of life for both patients and their families.

Our overall purpose is to identify a fingerprint of the disease detectable in an accessible sample and test its ability to proportion a suitable tool for an early diagnosis of AD, as we offer a choice for the prevention and treatment of the disease. Our work is not quite done yet and our efforts to improve the quality of life for people suffering from AD will continue. There is still a long way to go until the day research finds a cure for AD; meanwhile, alternative diagnostic and therapeutic approaches are being developed by a number of groups around the globe to offer actual and long lasting improvements in patients' cognition. Results have been promising so far and we hope in a future not so far the general population could find access to these approaches, though preventive strategies should be promoted especially for those individuals with a presumed higher risk to develop AD.

6. Acknowledgments

The authors would like to thank to Consejo Nacional de Ciencia y Tecnología (CONACyT, Mexico) for the doctoral fellowship number 223277 in biomedical sciences granted to M.H.R., as well as to the nursing home "Emperatríz de las Américas" for the support to our work.

7. References

Alboni S, Benatti C, Capone G, Corsini D, Caggia F, Tascedda F, Mendlewicz J, Brunello N. (2010). Time-dependent effects of escitalopram on brain derived neurotrophic factor (BDNF) and neuroplasticity related targets in the central nervous system of rats. *Eur J Pharmacol*, Vol. 643, No. 2-3, (Sep 2010), pp. (180-187).

Alzheimer's Research Center. (n.d.). Intranasal nerve growth factor research, In: *Alzheimer's Reasearch Center current research*, 2008, Available from: <http://www.alzheimersinfo.org>.

Anthony JC, Breitner JC, Zandi PP, Meyer MR, Jurasova I, Norton MC, et al. (2000). Reduced prevalence of AD in users of NSAIDs and H2 receptor antagonists: the Cache County study. *Neurology*, Vol. 54, No. 11, (Jun 2000), pp. (2066-2071).

Aranda-Abreu GE, Hernández-Aguilar ME, Manzo-Denes J, García-Hernández LI, Herrera-Rivero M. (2011). Rehabilitating a brain with Alzheimer's: a proposal. *Clinial Interventions in Aging*, Vol. 6, (February 2011), pp. (53-59).

Aronov S, Aranda G, Behar L, Ginzburg I. (2001). Axonal tau mRNA localization coincides with tau protein in living neuronal cells and depends on axonal targeting signal. *J Neurosci*, Vol. 21, No. 17, (Sept 2001), pp. (6577–6587).

Benedict C, Hallschmid M, Schultes B, Born J, Kern W. (2007). Intranasal insulin to improve memory function in humans. *Neuroendocrinology*, Vol. 86, No. 2, (Jul 2007), pp. (136-142).

Blurton-Jones M, Kitazawa M, Martinez-Coria H, Castello NA, Müller FJ, Loring JF, Yamasaki TR, Poon WW, Green KN & LaFerla FM. (2009). Neural stem cells improve cognition via BDNF in a transgenic model of Alzheimer disease. *PNAS*, Vol. 106, No. 32, (Aug 2009), pp. (13594-13599).

Brion J, Passareiro E, Nunez J, Flament-Durand J. (1985). Mise en evidence immunologique de la protein tau au niveau des lesions de degenerescence neurofibrillaire de la maladie D'Alzheimer. *Arch Biol*, Vol. 95, No. 2, (1985), pp. (229–235). ISSN: 0003-9624.

Cedazo-Mínguez A. (2007). Apolipoprotein E and Alzheimer's disease: molecular mechanisms and therapeutic opportunities. *J Cell Mol Med*, Vol. 11, No. 6, (Nov-Dec 2007), pp. (1227-1238).

Chan SL, Furukawa K, Mattson MP. (2002). Presenilins and APP in neuritic and synaptic plasticity: Implications for the pathogenesis of Alzheimer's disease. *Neuromolecular Med*, Vol. 2, No. 2, (2002), pp. (167-196).

Cole SL & Vassar R. (2007). The Alzheimer's disease β-secretase enzyme, BACE1. *Mol Neurodegener*, Vol. 2, No. 22, (Nov 2007).

De la Vega-Cotarelo R & Zambrano-Toribio A. (2011). Glosario-Vademécum, In: *La Circunvalación del Hipocampo*. May 2011, Available from: <http://www.hipocampo.org/glosarioa.asp>

Finley B. (1997). Nutritional needs of the person with Alzheimer's disease: practical approaches to quality care. *J Am Diet Assoc*, Vol. 97, No. 10 suppl 2, (Oct 1997), pp. (S177–80).

Franzoni S, Frisoni GB, Boffelli S, Rozzini R, Trabucchi M. (1996). Good nutritional oral intake is associated with equal survival in demented and nondemented very old patients. *J Am Geriatr Soc*, Vol. 44, No. 11, (Nov 1996), pp. (1366–1370).

Grundke-Iqbal I, Iqbal K, Tung YC, Quinlan M, Wisniewski HM, Binder LI. (1986). Abnormal phosphorylation of the microtubule-associated protein t (tau) in Alzheimer cytoskeletal pathology. *Proc Natl Acad Sci USA*, Vol. 83, No. 13, (Jul 1986), pp. (4913–4917).

Haass C, Hung AY, Selkoe DJ. (1991). Processing of b-amyloid precursor protein in microglia and astrocytes favors a localization in internal vesicles over constitutive secretion. *J Neurosci*, Vol. 11, No. 12, (Dec 1991), pp. (3783–3793).

Hickey W. F. (2001). Basic principles of immunological surveillance of the normal central nervous system. *Glia*, Vol. 36, No. 2, (Nov 2001), pp. (118–124).

Hung AY, Koo EH, Haass C, Selkoe DJ. (1992). Increased expression of beta-amyloid precursor protein during neuronal differentiation is not accompanied by secretory cleavage. *Proc Natl Acad Sci U S A*, Vol. 89, No. 20, (Oct 1992), pp. 9439-9443).

Hung AY, Selkoe DJ. (1994). Selective ectodomain phosphorylation and regulated cleavage of b-amyloid precursor protein. *EMBO J*, Vol. 13, No. 3, (Feb 1994), pp. (534–542).

Illenberger S, Zheng-Fischofer Q, Preuss U, Stamer K, Baumann K, Trinczek B et al. (1998). The endogenous and cell cycle-dependent phosphorylation of tau protein in living cells: implications for Alzheimer's disease. *Mol Biol Cell*, Vol. 9, No. 6, (Jun 1998), pp. (1495-1512).

Ingelson M, Vanmechelen E, Lannfelt L. (1996). Microtubule-associated protein tau in human fibroblasts with the Swedish Alzheimer mutation. *Neurosci Lett*, Vol. 220, No. 1, (Dec 1996), pp. (9-12).

Jankowsky JL, Melnikova T, Fadale DJ, Xu GM, Slunt HH, Gonzales V et al. (2005). Environmentl enrichment mitigates cognitive deficits in a mouse model of Alzheimer´s disease. *J Neurosci*, Vol. 25, No. 21, (May 2005), pp. (5217-5224).

Johnson GVW, Hartigan JA. (1999). Tau protein in normal and Alzheimer's disease brain: an update. *J Alzheimers Dis*, Vol. 1, No. 4-5, (Nov 1999), pp. (329-51).

Kang JE, Lim MM, Bateman RJ, Lee JJ, Smyth LP, Cirrito JR, Fijiki N, Nishino S & Holtzman DM. (2009). Amyloid-β dynamics are regulated by orexin and the sleep-wake cycle. *Science*, Vol. 326, No. 5955, (Nov 2009), pp. (1005-1007).

Kosik KS, Joachim CL, Selkoe DJ. (1986). Microtubule-associated protein, tau, is a major antigenic component of paired helical filaments in Alzheimer's disease. *Proc Natl Acad Sci USA*, Vol. 83, No. 11, (Jun 1986), pp. (4044–4048).

Lanyau-Domínguez Y. (2009). La dieta en la enfermedad de Alzheimer. *Revista Cubana de Salud Pública*, Vol. 35, No. 4, (Oct-Dec 2009), pp. (55-64). ISSN: 0864-3466.

Ma H, Lesne S, Kotilinek L, Steidl-Nichols JV, Sherman M, Younkin L et al. (2007). Involvement of beta-site APP cleaving enzyme 1 (BACE1) in amyloid precursor protein-mediated enhancement of memory and activity dependent synaptic plasticity. *Proc Natl Acad Sci U S A*, Vol. 104, No. 19, (May 2007), pp. (8167-8172).

McGeer PL, McGeer EG. (1999). Inflammation of the brain in Alzheimer's disease: implications for therapy. *J Leukoc Biol*, Vol. 65, No. 4, (Apr 1999), pp. (409–415).

McGeer PL, McGeer EG. (2002). Innate immunity, local inflammation, and degenerative disease. *Sci Aging Knowledge Environ*, Vol. 29, (Jul 2002), re3.

Menéndez-González M, Pérez-Piñera P, Calatayud MT, Blázquez-Menes B. (2005). Inmunoterapia para la enfermedad de Alzheimer. *Arch Med*, Vol. 1, No. 4, (n.d.) ISSN: 1698-9465.

Morley JE. (1996). Dementia is not necessarily a cause of undernutrition. *J Am Geriatr Soc*, Vol. 44, No. 11, (Nov 1996), pp. (1403–1404).

Muresan V, Varvel MH, Lamb BT, Muresan Z. (2009). The cleavage products of amyloid-β precursor protein are sorted to distinct carrier vesicles that are independently transported within neurites. *J Neurosci*, Vol. 29, No. 11, (Mar 2009), pp. (3565-78).

Nukina N, Ihara Y. (1986). One of the antigenic determinants of paired helical filaments is related to tau protein. *J Biochem*, Vol. 99, No. 5, (May 1986), pp. (1541–1544).

Ohno M, Sametsky EA, Younkin LH, Oakley H, Younkin SG, Citron M, Vassar R, Disterhoft JF. (2004). BACE1 Deficiency Rescues Memory Deficits and Cholinergic Dysfunction in a Mouse Model of Alzheimer's Disease. *Neuron*, Vol. 41, No. 1, (Jan 2004), pp. (27-33).

Plant LD, Webster NJ, Boyle JP, Ramsden M, Freir DB, Peers C, Pearson HA. (2006). Amyloid beta peptide as a physiological modulator of neuronal 'A'-type K+ current. *Neurobiol Aging*, Vol. 27, No. 11, (Nov 2006), pp. (1673-1683).

Pope WB, Lambert MP, Leypold B, Seupaul R, Sletten L, Krafft G, Klein WL. (1994). Microtubuleassociated protein tau is hyperphosphorylated during mitosis in the human neuroblastoma cell line SH-SY5Y. *Exp Neurol*, Vol. 126, No. 2, (Apr 1994), pp. (185-194).

Preuss U, Döring F, Illenberger S, Mandelkow EM. (1995). Cell cycle-dependent phosphorylation and microtubule binding of tau protein stably transfected into chinese hamster ovary cells. *Mol Biol Cell*, Vol. 6, No. 10, (Oct 1995), pp. (1397-410).

Preuss U, Mandelkow EM. (1998). Mitotic phosphorylation of tau protein in neuronal cell lines resembles phosphorylation in Alzheimer's disease. *Eur J Cell Biol*, Vol. 76, No. 3, (Jul 1998), pp. (176-84).

Rang HP, Dale MM and Ritter JM. (2001). Cholinergic transmission, In: *Pharmacology, 4th edition*. pp. (110–138), Harcourt Publishers Ltd, Edinburgh, UK.

Riddell DR, Christie G, Hussain I, Dingwall C. (2001). Compartmentalization of beta-secretase (Asp2) into low-buoyant density, noncaveolar lipid rafts. *Curr Biol*, Vol. 11, No. 16, (Aug 2001), pp. (1288-1293).

Riviére S, Gillette–Guyonnet, Nourhashemi F, Vellas B. (1999). Nutrition and Alzheimer's disease. Nutr Rev, Vol. 57, No. 12, (Dec 1999), pp. (363-367).

Rogers J, Webster S, Lue LF, et al. (1996). Inflammation and Alzheimer's disease pathogenesis. *Neurobiol Aging*, Vol. 17, No.5, (Sep-Oct 1997), pp. (681–686).

Selkoe DJ. (2001). Alzheimer's disease: genes, proteins, and therapy. *Physiol Rev*, Vol. 81, No. 2, (Apr 2001), pp. (741-766).

Thinakaran G, Koo EH. (2008). Amyloid precursor protein trafficking, processing and function. *JBC Papers*, Vol. 283, No. 44, (Oct 2008), pp. (29615-9).

Thurston VC, Zinkowski RP, Binder LI. (1996). Tau as a nucleolar protein in human nonneural cells in vitro and in vivo. *Chromosoma*, Vol. 105, No. 1, (Jul 1996), pp. (20-30).

Vito P, Lacaná E, D'Adamio L. (1996). Interfering with Apoptosis: Ca2+-Binding Protein ALG-2 and Alzheimer's Disease Gene ALG-3. *Science*, Vol. 271, No. 5248, (Jan 1996), pp. (521-525).

Wang JW, David DJ, Monckton JE, Battaglia F, Hen R. (2008). Chronic fluoxetine stimulates maturation and synaptic plasticity of adult-born hippocampal granule cells. *J Neurosci*, Vol. 28, No. 6, (Feb 2008), pp. (1374–1384).

Wollen KA. (2010). Alzheimer's disease: the pros and cons of pharmaceutical, nutricional, botanical, and stimulatory therapies, with a discussion of treatment strategies from the perspective of patients and practitioners. *Altern Med Rev*, Vol. 15, No. 3, (Sep 2010), pp. (223-244).

Wood JG, Mirra SS, Pollock NL, Binder LI. (1986). Neurofibrillary tangles of Alzheimer's disease share antigenic determinants with the axonal microtubule-associated protein tau. *Proc Natl Acad Sci USA*, Vol. 83, No. 11, (Jun 1986), pp. (4040–4043).

Yu G, Nishimura M, Arawaka S, Levitan D, Zhang L, Tandon A et al. (2000). Nicastrin modulates presenilinmediated notch/glp-1 signal transduction and bAPP processing. *Nature*, Vol. 407, No. 6800, (Sep 2000), pp. (48-54).

Zhu F, Qian C. (2006). Berberine chloride can ameliorate the spatial memory impairment and increase the expression of interleukin-1beta and inducible nitric oxide synthase in the rat model of Alzheimer's disease. *BMC Neurosci*, Vol. 7, No. 78 (Dec 2006).

10

Frontotemporal Lobar Degeneration

Johannes Schlachetzki
Molecular Neurology, University Hospital of Erlangen
Germany

1. Introduction

Frontotemporal lobar degeneration (FTLD) comprises diseases with a very diverging spectrum in regards to clinical presentation, genetics, and neuropathology. In 1892 Arnold Pick published the case of 71-year old male with progressive symptoms of aphasia, apathy, and dementia (Pick 1892). The pathological examination revealed cortical atrophy with emphasis on the left temporal lobe (Pick 1892). Pick described another case of a 60-year old male with progressive signs of negligence, apathy, apraxia, and dementia (Pick 1906). This patient had bilateral frontal cortical atrophy on pathological examination (Pick 1906). Both cases demonstrate the main clinical and pathological spectrums while at the same time pointing at the clinical and pathological heterogeneity. Leading clinical symptoms were language deficits and behavioral changes. Both cases showed selective cortical atrophy of the left temporal lobe and both frontal lobes while relatively sparing the parietal and occipital lobes.

The frontal lobes harbor the prefrontal cortex with its three distinct parts that differ in phylogeny, assembly, connectivity and function:

1. dorsolateral convexity
2. medial part: anterior gyrus cinguli
3. limbic orbito-frontal cortex

The dorsolateral convexity is important for the *executive functions*, i.e., anticipatory, analytical and imaginative thinking, as well as cognitive flexibility. The medial part is involved in attention, motivation, empathy, and emotion. The orbito-frontal cortex plays an important role in controlling impulses, emotions, and social behavior. The prefrontal cortex is closely connected with the sensory association cortices, the limbic system, and the basal ganglia.

In the first part of this chapter, focus will be on clinical symptoms, diagnostics including neuropsychological and neuroimaiging findings, and therapy, while the second and third part will highlight recent findings in neurogenetics and neuropathology, respectively.

2. Clinical presentation

FTLD is the second most common cause for dementia before 65 years of age. Mean age of onset is around 45 to 60 years. However, FTLD may also contribute to a high degree in older patients (Seelaar, Kamphorst et al. 2008; Hodges, Mitchell et al. 2010). Up to 50% have a positive family history of FTLD (Stevens, van Duijn et al. 1998; Neary, Snowden et al. 2005).

In the early stage of the disease, changes in behavior and/or deficits in language may indicate FTLD. The onset of the disease is usually subtle and slowly progressive. Typically, no signs of impairment in memory or visiospatial function may be evident. The pronounced changes in behavior and/or language may lead to the diagnosis of FTLD in the early stage of the disease, differences to other variants of FTLD itself but also to Alzheimer's disease may even out at later time points. The various forms of FTLD merge into a later stage characterized by apathy, severely impaired intellectual function, echolalia, and mutism. The duration of the illness and the decline is variable and ranges between 2 and 20 years (Hodges, Davies et al. 2003).

2.1 Clinical variants

FTLD is clinically defined according to the consensus criteria by Neary and colleagues (Neary, Snowden et al. 1998). The site of focal cerebral atrophy, i.e., frontal and/or temporal, left and/or right determines the clinical presentation. *Behavioral variant FTLD* (bvFTLD) is associated with usually a symmetrical frontal dysfunction. The language variants *progressive non-fluent aphasia* (PNFA) and *semantic dementia* (SD) are subsumed under the clinical syndrome of primary progressive aphasia (Mesulam 2001) and show involvement of the left anterior temporal lobe.

2.1.1 Behavioral variant FTLD

BvFTLD is the most common subtype of FTLD. Patients with bvFTLD show progressive personality and behavioral changes. Deficits in executive function, social interpersonal conduct, loss of insight (anosognosia), emotional blunting, stereotyped verbal output, hyperorality, dietary changes with weight gain, mood changes including irritability, depression, fatuous euphoria, tactlessness, loss of concern for feeling for others, lack of empathy, reduced emotional engagement, utilisation behavior, obsessive behavior, and neglect of personal hygiene all encompass the wide spectrum of clinical symptoms in bvFTLD.

BvFTLD can be subdivided into an (1) dorsolateral/medial type with an apathetic profile, and (2) basal type with pronounced behavioral changes (Snowden, Bathgate et al. 2001).

Parkinsonian features like rigidity and bradykinesia can be associated with bvFTLD. In many FTLD patients with Parkinsonism, a genetic linkage to chromosome 17 (*tau, PGRN*) was found, and these cases were termed FTDP-17.

Incontinence, orthostatic dysregulation, and the presence of frontal signs (saccadic eye movements, disturbed upward gaze, paratonia, inexhaustible blink reflex, abnormal Luria sequence) on neurological examination may be present.

CT or MRI may be normal early in the course, but symmetrical atrophy frontal atrophy and involvement and atrophy of the prefrontal cortex, the paralimbic areas anterior cingulum and frontal insula, and thalamus (Grimmer, Diehl et al. 2004). At later stages, atrophy may be observed of the temporal and parietal cortex (Diehl-Schmid, Grimmer et al. 2007). [F18]-FDG-PET and HMPAO-SPECT are useful to establish the clinical diagnosis and show the typical involvement of the frontal and temporal lobes (Mendez, Shapira et al. 2007; Mosconi, Tsui et al. 2008).

2.1.2 Progressive non-fluent aphasia

PNFA patients show apraxia of speech and agrammatism. Sentence repetition may be impaired. Later in the disease, PNFA may present with mutism, alexia, and agraphia. Word comprehension and object knowledge are initially spared. Behavioral changes and anosognosia are uncommon in the disease, but may develop later in the course. On CT or MRI scan, left-sided atrophy of the inferior frontal lobe and anterior insula is often appreciated.

2.1.3 Semantic dementia

Typical signs of patients with SD are *anomia* and *loss of word meaning*. Albeit still having fluent speech, the content of speech is empty and semantic paraphasias can be detected. Semantic memory progressively becomes impaired. Patients with SD may not recognize faces or objects. Writing may be spared and figures may be copied. In contrast to PNFA, SD are more prone to develop behavioural changes and anosognosia early in the disease.
Neuroimaging studies with CT or MRI of SD show bilateral atrophy of the anterior and inferior temporal lobes. The left temporal lobe is usually more affected than the right. Progression of lobar atrophy can be automatically observed over a short period of time (Frings, Mader et al. 2011).

2.2 Associated diseases with FTLD

2.2.1 FTLD-ALS

FTLD may be associated with amyotrophic lateral sclerosis (ALS), termed FTLD-ALS. Signs of motor neuron disease can be found in a small subset of patients with FTLD (Hodges, Davies et al. 2003; Mitsuyama and Inoue 2009). Affection of upper motoneurons is characterized by fasciculations, hyperreflexia, and positive Babinski signs whereas affection of lower motoneurons by muscle atrophy and weakness. Dementia, typically behavioral changes and/or PNFA, is usually rapid and patients have a very short disease duration with only about three years (Hodges, Davies et al. 2003). It has been reported that 5-15% of patients diagnosed with ALS also show signs of deficits in executive function, suggesting that these patients may belong to the FTLD-ALS subtype (Ringholz, Appel et al. 2005). FTLD-ALS is pathologically characterized by TDP-43 positive neuronal cytoplasmic inclusions (Mackenzie, Baborie et al. 2006; Sampathu, Neumann et al. 2006). A genetic linkage to chromosome 9p has been established for some cases of FTLD-ALS.

2.2.2 CBD and PSP

Corticobasal degeneration (CBD) and *progressive supranuclear palsy* (PSP) belong into the same clinical, genetic, and pathological spectrum of FTLD (Kertesz and Munoz 2004; Josephs, Petersen et al. 2006).
Patients with CBD present as atypical Parkinson's disease with strong asymmetry of rigidity and unilateral apraxia (sometimes "alien limb" phenomenon). Sometimes dystonia, myoklonus, sensory deficits, and early speech disturbance like dysphasia can be observed. Behavioral and personality changes are subtler than in FTLD patients early in the course of the disease. Later, apathy, disinhibition, irritability, and subcortical dementia can be present. On neuropathological examination, focal, asymmetrical cortical atrophy and degeneration with loss of pigment of the substantia nigra can be noticed. Because CBD is characterized by the accumulation of tau protein in neurons and glia, it is classified as a tauopathy.
PSP also belongs to the group of tauopathies. Clinically, impaired upward and especially downward gaze and frequent falls indicate a diagnosis of PSP. Decreased verbal fluency

with loss of speech later in the course, apathy, behavioural changes and pseudobulbar palsy may contribute. Macroscopic examination reveals focal atrophy of the midbrain and pontine tegmentum. Microscopically, neuronal and glial accumulation of tau protein can be appreciated.

2.2.3 Rare forms associated with FTLD

Neuronal intermediate filament inclusions disease (NIFID), *basophilic inclusion body disease* (BIBD), and *inclusion body myopathy with Paget's disease and frontal dementia* (IBMPFD) are very rare diseases. They share clinical and pathological similarities with FTLD (Kertesz and Munoz 2004; Josephs, Petersen et al. 2006).

NIFID is characterized as early-onset sporadic bvFTLD with affection of the pyramidal and extrapyramidal motor systems. Neuronal inclusions observed on microscopic examination show immunoreactivity for class IV intermediate filaments and accumulation of the FUS protein (Josephs, Holton et al. 2003; Cairns, Grossman et al. 2004; Neumann, Roeber et al. 2009). BIBD is characterized pathologically by basophilic inclusions on haematoxylin and eosin staining. These inclusions are immunoreactive for FUS (Munoz, Neumann et al. 2009). Clinically, symptoms vary and can present as bvFTLD, ALS or combination of both.

IBMPFD is caused by mutations in the *VCP* gene. Accumulation of TDP-43 can be appreciated on microscopic examination (van der Zee, Pirici et al. 2009). Adult-onset proximal/distal muscle weakness, spine or hip pain and deformity and enlargement of long bones, as well as signs of FTLD characterize IBMPFD.

2.3 Neuropsychological assessment

Standard neuropsychological tests do not provide high sensitivity and specificity for the diagnosis of FTLD, in particular to differentiate form Alzheimer's disease (Walker, Meares et al. 2005; Hutchinson and Mathias 2007). But maybe the most important aspect of neuropsychological assessment is not the test battery itself but the accurate observation of the patient during testing. *General appearance, motor activity, speech,* and *linguistic content* may already be suggestive for FTLD. Patients with bvFTLD often grasp at objects during testing, although they were not asked to do so. This phenomenon can be frequently observed and is called *utilisation*. Patient also *imitate* persons verbally and/or gestural. E.g., they repeat words or sentences (echolalia). *High distractibility, low flexibility, indifference, rule breaking behavior, stereotype behavior, impaired drive and motivation,* and *missing cooperation* during testing are indicative of frontal lobe dysfunction. Disturbed social behavior and anosognosia may be seen as well.

Patients often perform normal on the *Mini mental status examination* (MMSE). Recall of learned verbal and figural information are often without pronounced deficits. Sometimes many false positive answers are given on the recognition part of verbal memory. Copying of figures can be impaired, and bvFTLD patients often draw bizarre pictures.

Tests assessing impairment of executive function including planning, organisation, judgement, problem solving, mental flexibility in FTLD patients may support the diagnosis of FTLD. Usually, memory, visual perception, and spatial skills are relatively well preserved (Hodges, Patterson et al. 1999; Mendez, Shapira et al. 2007; Wittenberg, Possin et al. 2008).

Because of impaired executive function and motivation, FTLD patients can score strikingly low in the verbal fluency test. Patients are asked to name as many words (e.g., animals, words that begin with the letter "S") as he can within 60 seconds. The five-point test may

also help to identify patients with executive dysfunction and tests figural fluency. 5 points are given (4 in the rectangle and 1 in the middle), and participants are required to draw as many patterns by connecting at least 2 points within three minutes. Visual attention and task switching may be also checked by performing Trail Making A and B.
More time consuming is the Wisconsin card sorting test (WCST) tests the cognitive flexibility of the patient. Here, the participant has to match cards either to color, design, or quantity. During the course of the test, the matching rules are changed. Another test for cognitive flexibility and selective attention is the stroop color word test. Here, the participant has to suppress a habitual in favour of a novel response. In this experiment the participant is required to say the color of the word, not what the word says.
A test that requires advanced planning and strategical thinking are the tower of London and tower of Hanoi tests. The participant has to arrange different discs and stacks onto other racks in order to come from one starting position to a certain defined end.
Deficits in speech and language are characteristic for primary progressive aphasia. Spontaneous speech, fluency, comprehension, sentence repetition, naming, and reading need to be evaluated.

2.4 Differential diagnosis

Patients with FTLD can be distinguished from Alzheimer's disease (AD) early in the course of the disease because of remarkable changes in their behavior, personality changes, poor motivation, and/or severe language impairment. AD manifests with early deficits in short-term memory, visuo-spatial deficits. In AD, mediobasal temporal atrophy with enlargement of the temporal horns of the ventricle can be observed on CT and MRI scan. SPECT and PET studies can reveal hypoperfusion and hypometabolism temporo-parietal in AD patients. In FTLD patients, memory is usually not impaired, and normal test values can be found in the MMSE or CERAD. CSF markers (abeta, p-tau) are very sensitive for AD.
Patients with *progressive supranuclear palsy* also demonstrate executive dysfunction, which may precede the typical motor symptoms of PSP, characterized by vertical eye movement paralysis and frequent falls. Another movement disorder may mimic cardinal features of FTLD, *corticobasal degeneration* with unilateral rigidity, bradykinesia, apraxia, dystonia (Lang, Bergeron et al. 1994; Jendroska, Rossor et al. 1995).
Other differential diagnoses are listed in the table 1.

2.5 Pharmacotherapy

Therapeutic options for FTLD are limited and primarily aim at the treatment of somatic and psychiatric symptoms. A disease modifying therapy is not available yet.
A *cholinergic* deficit has not been observed in FTLD (Procter, Qurne et al. 1999). Treatment of FTLD patients with *acetylcholinesterase-inhibitors* such as galantamine and donepezil did not improve cognition (Mendez, Shapira et al. 2007; Kertesz, Morlog et al. 2008). However, rivastigmine was able to attenuate behavioral symptoms in an open label study (Moretti, Torre et al. 2004).
NMDA-receptor antagonist memantine may be promising in the treatment of behavioral disturbances (Swanberg 2007; Diehl-Schmid, Forstl et al. 2008; Vossel and Miller 2008; Kavirajan 2009; Chow, Graff-Guerrero et al. 2011).
The *serotonergic* and *dopaminergic* neurotransmitter systems seems to be affected in FTLD (Procter, Qurne et al. 1999; Yang and Schmitt 2001; Franceschi, Anchisi et al. 2005). Selective

Differential diagnosis	Diagnostic work up
Dementia • Alzheimer's disease • Primary progressive aphasia-logopenic • Vascular dementia • Normal pressure hydropcephalus	 Lumbar puncture (Abeta, tau), SPECT/PET (parietal and temporal lobes bilaterally) Language and memory deficits early in the disease CT/MRI CT/MRI, spinal tab
Affective disorders • Depression • Mania	 Past history, response to antidepressive medication Past history, response to mood stabilizers
Schizophrenia	Past history, response to antipsychotics
Morbus Wilson	CT/MRI, coeruloplasmin
Huntington's disease	Genetic testing
Lues	Syphilis serology
Brain tumors	CT/MRI
Alcohol and drug abuse	Past History, blood work (MCV, liver enzymes)

Table 1.

serotonin-reuptake inhibitors (SSRI) such as paroxetin, fluvoxamine, and trazodone have been shown to be efficious in the treatment of obsessive behaviour, agitation, irritability, and depression (Swartz, Miller et al. 1997; Litvan 2001; Perry and Miller 2001; Moretti, Torre et al. 2003; Lebert, Stekke et al. 2004; Huey, Putnam et al. 2006). E.g., paroxetin improved anxiety, and perseveration (Chow and Mendez 2002), however, conflicting results have been reported (Deakin, Rahman et al. 2004). The *monoamine-oxidase B* inhibitor selegiline improved cognition (Moretti, Torre et al. 2002).

The usage of antipsychoctics should be contained especially when parkinsonian symptoms such as bradykinesia are present (Pijnenburg, Sampson et al. 2003).

2.6 Summary

FTLD should be suspected in younger patients, who present with progressive behavioral/personality changes or language/naming impairment. A positive family history may support the diagnosis. Relatives or caregivers should accompany the patient to the hospital in order to give a detailed history. Physical examination may reveal signs of frontal/executive deficits and parkinsonism. A neuropsychological assessment should be done. Here, MMSE, verbal fluency, verbal and figural memory should be tested and special attention is needed to observe behavior during testing. Imaging studies such as CT or MRI can reveal focal frontal and/or temporal atrophy. However, atrophy may be absent early in the course of the disease. If FTLD is suspected, SPECT/PET should be performed. No specific lab or CSF marker are available yet, but should be performed to exclude differential diagnosis.

A disease-modifying therapy has not been discovered. Main focus lies on the treatment of psychiatric symptoms.

3. Genetics

The overall frequency of positive family history for dementia in a German FTLD patient cohort was 24 % (Schlachetzki, Schmidtke et al. 2009). This proportion is below reported frequencies in several earlier series with a positive family history of up to 40-50% of FTLD cases (Neary, Snowden et al. 2005) (Stevens, van Duijn et al. 1998). The possibility remains that the true proportion of dominantly inherited cases is obscured by instances of early death of mutation carriers in the parental generation, siblings that carry mutations but are yet undiagnosed, or illegitimate descent.

30-50 % of patients with bvFTLD have a positive family history. Patients presenting clinically with SD or PNFA show a lower frequency (Seelaar, Kamphorst et al. 2008; Chow, Miller et al. 1999; (Stevens, van Duijn et al. 1998; Rohrer, Guerreiro et al. 2009).

Mutations in *microtubule associated protein tau (MAP)* and *progranulin (PGRN)* can be found in the majority of cases, whereas mutations in *valosin containing protein (VCP), charged multivesicular body protein 2B (CHMP2B), TDP-43* are rare. In about 30 % of FTLD patients with a positive family history, no mutations have been found so far.

The number of mutations and families of each gene can be found at http://www.molgen.ua.ac.be/admutations/default.cfm?MT=1&ML=0&Page=ADMDB.

3.1 *MAPT*

MAPT gene is located on chromosome 17q21.1 and encodes for the protein tau. It contains 11 exons. Exons 2,3, and 10 are alternatively spliced, allowing for 6 isoforms. In 1998 mutations in the *MAPT* gene were identified in patients presenting clinically with FTLD with Parkinsonism linked to chromosome 17 (FTDP-17) (Hutton, Lendon et al. 1998; Poorkaj, Bird et al. 1998; Spillantini, Crowther et al. 1998). This hereditary tauopathy is a rare clinical syndrome, described in around 120 families worldwide and shows a great intra- and interfamilial clinical heterogeneity. More than 40 different *MAPT* mutations have been described and could be classified into two groups: (i) mutations that change the biochemical properties of tau, and (ii) that alter the alternative splicing of tau mRNA. FTDP-17 cases usually present clinically with behavioral changes associated with motor deficits later in the course of the disease, mainly PSP or CBD like symptoms. FTDP-17 is autosomal dominantly inherited. On pathological examination FTDP-17 cases with *MAPT* mutations have (i) a predominant symmetric atrophy of the frontal and temporal lobes, accounting for the observed behavioral changes, and (ii) of the basalganglia and brainstem nuclei, that explain the parkinsonism observed in these cases (Ghetti, Spina et al. 2008). The microscopic examination reveals cytoplasmic neuronal and/or glial inclusions with immunoreactivity against hyperphosphorylated tau. Depending on the type of *MAPT* mutation, distribution and amount of neurofibrillary tangles, neuropil threads, and glial inclusions composed of insoluble tau vary.

Pathological changes in *MAPT* include missense mutations in exons 9 to 13 (e.g., G272V, P301L and R406W) and mutations in the 5′ splice site of exon 10. Missense mutations in exon 9 to 13 impair the function of tau to promote microtubule assembly, organization, and stabilization. The splice site mutation of exon 10 increases the proportion of 4R tau (four microtubule-binding repeats) in neurons and glia by the increased transcription into tau mRNA that includes exon 10 (Hutton, Lendon et al. 1998).

The rate of whole brain atrophy seems to be bigger in patients with *MAPT* mutations (Whitwell, Weigand et al. 2011).

3.2 *PGRN*

PGRN gene is located on chromosome 17 in close vicinity to *MAPT* locus. At present, *PGRN* mutations exceed the number of *MAPT* mutations in patients with FTLD. Pathogenic mutations include missense and nonsense mutations, or small insertions or deletions in the exons or introns of the gene (Gass, Cannon et al. 2006). Most of the mutations lead to frameshift and premature stop codons. E.g., point mutations were identified in two cases of a German cohort of 79 patients (Schlachetzki, Schmidtke et al. 2009). Pathogenic mutations in *PGRN* invariably lead to mutant mRNA transcripts, which undergo nonsense-mediated decay, thereby resulting in haploinsufficiency (Baker, Mackenzie et al. 2006; Cruts, Gijselinck et al. 2006).

Overall, the frequency of PGRN mutations is similar to that of mutations in *MAPT* (Rosso, Donker Kaat et al. 2003). Prevalence of mutations in PGRN is suggested to account for 1-15 % of all cases with FTLD (Bruni, Momeni et al. 2007; Gass, Cannon et al. 2006; Le Ber, van der Zee et al. 2007; Schlachetzki, Schmidtke et al. 2009), but up to 26 % of familial cases (Pickering-Brown, Baker et al. 2006; Cruts, Kumar-Singh et al. 2006; Bronner, Rizzu et al. 2007). In a large series from the USA, mutations were found in 10 % of all patients with FTLD and 23 % in cases of familial FTLD (Gass, Cannon et al. 2006). Several other studies from France, Italy, the Netherlands, the UK, Belgium, Finland, and the USA have reported lower frequencies of on average 5 % in unselected FTLD groups and 4-10 % in groups of cases of familial FTLD (Le Ber, Camuzat et al. 2008; Le Ber, van der Zee et al. 2007; Bruni, Momeni et al. 2007; Borroni, Archetti et al. 2008; Bronner, Rizzu et al. 2007; Pickering-Brown, Rollinson et al. 2008; Cruts, Gijselinck et al. 2006; Gijselinck, van der Zee et al. 2008; Gass, Cannon et al. 2006; Huey, Grafman et al. 2006). The differences in the reported frequencies may be due to differences in the mode of ascertainment of patients, in ethnic variations as well as to founder effects.

Mean age at onset of FTLD patients with *PGRN* mutations is around 60 years. The majority of patients with PGRN mutations show the behavioural-variant phenotype with apathy and social withdrawal as prominent characteristics (van Swieten, Stevens et al. 1999). *PGRN* mutations have also been found in patients who present with language impairment early in the course of the disease, diagnosed as primary non-fluent progressive aphasia (PPA) (Gass, Cannon et al. 2006; Huey, Grafman et al. 2006; Josephs, Ahmed et al. 2007; Snowden, Neary et al. 2007; Mesulam, Johnson et al. 2007). Patients from different families with the same mutation do not necessarily show the same clinical phenotype or age at onset (Huey, Grafman et al. 2006).

On microscopic examination, all cases with PGRN mutations share a common subtype, characterized by NCIs and irregular dystrophic neurites in the neocortex and subcortical nuclei (Josephs, Ahmed et al. 2007; Gass, Cannon et al. 2006; Behrens, Mukherjee et al. 2007; Lopez de Munain, Alzualde et al. 2008; Mackenzie, Baker et al. 2006; Snowden, Pickering-Brown et al. 2006; Spina, Murrell et al. 2007). This subtype is referred to as type A (Mackenzie, Neumann et al.). Former classifications used different numbers: type I by Mackenzie et al. and type 3 by Sampathu and co-workers (Mackenzie, Baker et al. 2006; Sampathu, Neumann et al. 2006).

Mutations in PGRN may also present clinically also with symptoms of parkinsonism (FTDP-17) (Benussi, Binetti et al. 2008; Boeve and Hutton 2008; Ghetti, Spina et al. 2008; Gabryelewicz, Masellis et al. 2010; Di Fabio, Tessa et al. 2010). First findings may lead to new therapeutic approaches. Inhibitors of vacuolar ATPase like bafiomycin A1 and alkalizing molecules like amiodarone have been shown to significantly increase the concentration of progranulin intra- and extracellularly in an animal model (Capell, Liebscher et al. 2011). This may prevent progranulin-mediated neurodegeneration and may be a feasible therapeutic option. These agents could increase PGRN levels in the serum, plasma or CSF. Concentrations of progranulin in plasma, serum, and CSF are predictive in mutation carriers with and without symptoms (Sleegers, Brouwers et al. 2009; Ghidoni, Benussi et al. 2008; Finch, Baker et al. 2009). Thus, genetic screening could then be performed in patients with altered PGRN levels in plasma or serum.

3.3 *VCP*

VCP is located on chromosome 3 and contains 5 exons. *VCP* encodes for the VCP (VCP/p97) protein, which is a member of the ATPase associated with a variety of activities protein family. VCP is a ubiquitously expressed and is involved in numerous cellular processes including proteasomal ubiquitin-dependent protein degradation. VCP regulates autophagosome maturation under basal conditions and in cells challenged by proteasome inhibition, but not in cells challenged by starvation, suggesting that VCP might be selectively required for autophagic degradation of ubiquitinated substrates.

VCP mutations are a rare cause for FTLD with a variable penetrance and are mainly autosomal-dominant inherited. The first mutation in the *VCP* gene was described in 2004 (Watts, Wymer et al. 2004), since then more mutations have been identified in familial cases (Haubenberger, Bittner et al. 2005; Gidaro, Modoni et al. 2008; Djamshidian, Schaefer et al. 2009; Bersano, Del Bo et al. 2009). A mutation has also been described in a sporadic case (Bersano, Del Bo et al. 2009). There is no evidence, that common variants in *VCP* confer a strong risk to the development of sporadic FTLD (Schumacher, Friedrich et al. 2009). Only missense mutations have been described so far. The mutations are located mainly within the ubiquitin-binding domain, suggesting that the pathological accumulation of TDP-43 may be due to problems within the protein degradation system.

VCP mutations can be found in patients with IBMPFD. About 1/3 of these patients actually present with bvFTLD (Kimonis, Fulchiero et al. 2008). A high degree of clinical heterogeneity has been described within families but also among unrelated families bearing the same VCP mutation.

On neuropathological examination, mutant *VCP* cases are characterized by neuronal nuclear inclusions containing ubiquitin (Schroder, Watts et al. 2005) and TDP-43 (Neumann, Mackenzie et al. 2007). Phosphorylated TDP-43 was detected only in insoluble brain extracts from affected brain regions. Identification of TDP-43, but not VCP protein, within ubiquitin-positive inclusions supports the hypothesis that *VCP* gene mutations lead to a dominant negative loss or alteration of VCP function culminating in impaired degradation of TDP-43 (Neumann, Mackenzie et al. 2007). TDP-43 positive Intranuclear inclusions and dystrophic neurites are characteristic (van der Zee, Pirici et al. 2009; Watts, Thomasova et al. 2007) and are referred to as FTLD-TDP pathology type D (Mackenzie, Neumann et al. 2011). Inclusions are also present in muscle and heart and are immunoreactive for TDP-43 and beta-amyloid (Watts, Thomasova et al. 2007; Kimonis, Fulchiero et al. 2008). Presently, the link between TDP-43 and VCP is unsolved. Transgenic mice with *VCP* mutations have been described which mimic the three cardinal symptoms of the disease. E.g., it has been shown that mutant VCP may result in enhanced activation of the NF-kappaB signaling cascade (Custer, Neumann et al. 2010). In addition, impaired autophagy has been shown (Ju, Fuentealba et al. 2009; Badadani, Nalbandian et al. 2010). It was shown in cell culture models, that mutations in the *VCP* gene relocate TDP-43 from the nucleus into the cytosol, decreases proteasome activity, induces endoplasmic reticulum stress and thereby impairs cell viability (Gitcho, Strider et al. 2009). In a drosophila model, mutant *VCP* leads to a redistribution of TDP-43 to the cytoplasm and thereby induces cytotoxicity, thus implying a toxic gain of function of TDP-43 (Ritson, Custer et al. 2010).

3.4 CHMP2B

CHMP2B is located on chromosome 3, and contains 6 exons. It encodes for the protein charged multivesicular protein 2B. CHMP2B protein is a member of ESCRT-III (endosomal sorting complex required for transport III) and is involved in vesicular fusion events within the endosome - lysosome compartments plays an important role in the process of degradation via autophagy. Mutations in this gene are very rare (Cannon, Baker et al. 2006; van der Zee, Urwin et al. 2008) and have been first described in a Danish family (Skibinski, Parkinson et al. 2005). Pathogenic mutations described so far lead to a partial truncation of the C-terminal region. Patients present clinically with bvFTLD and show pyramidal and extrapyramidal signs later in the course of the disease (Gydesen, Brown et al. 2002) and have an autosomal - dominant family history. Missense mutations in the CHMP2B gene causative for FTLD have not been identified so far and seem to be unlikely (Ferrari, Kapogiannis et al. 2011).

On neuropathological examination, inclusions are ubiquitin-positive but negative for tau, TDP-43, and FUS. Thus, the protein within the inclusion bodies still needs to be determined. *CHMP2B* cases are classified as FTLD-UPS (ubiquitin - proteasomal system). It is noteworthy, that FTLD-UPS also includes cases without *CHMP2B* mutation, suggesting that the full complement of FTLD pathologies is yet to be elucidated.

CHMP2B is involved in the protein degradation system, and mutations *CHMP2B* could cause inclusion bodies and disruption of endosome-lysosome fusion by a defective protein degradation system (Urwin, Authier et al. 2010).

In addition, *CHMP2B* mutant animal showed disrupted integrity of dendritic spines and synapses (Belly, Bodon et al. 2010).

3.5 Linkage to chromosome 9p13.2-21.3

A linkage to chromosome 9p13.2-21.3 has been suggested in many autosomal-dominant families with bvFTLD or FTLD-ALS (Morita, Al-Chalabi et al. 2006; Vance, Al-Chalabi et al. 2006; Valdmanis, Dupre et al. 2007; Luty, Kwok et al. 2008; Le Ber, Camuzat et al. 2009; Gijselinck, Engelborghs et al. 2010; Shatunov, Mok et al. 2010). Genome - wide linkage studies verified an association familial bvFTLD, FTLD-ALS, and ALS cases with the chromosomal locus 9p13.2-21.3 (van Es, Veldink et al. 2009; Laaksovirta, Peuralinna et al. 2010; Shatunov, Mok et al. 2010). However, the responsible gene could not be identified so far. These data confirm that FTLD and amyotrophic lateral sclerosis (ALS) share a common genetic risk factor on chromosome 9p (Rollinson, Mead et al. 2011).

On pathological examination, cases with linkage to chromosome 9p13.2-21.3 show a TDP-43 proteinopathy, classified to type B with moderate neuronal cytoplasmic inclusions and few dystrophic neurites in all layers (Mackenzie, Neumann et al. 2011; Cairns, Neumann et al. 2007). Recently, a hexanucleotide GGGGCC repeat in intron 1 of *C9ORF72* has been identified to be the cause of chromosome 9p13.2-21.3-linked FTLD-ALS (Dejesus-Hernandez, Mackenzie et al. 2011; Renton, Majounie et al. 2011). The function of the *C9ORF72* encoding protein has not been characterized yet. It has been suggested that the repeat expansion may imply loss-of-function and gain-of-function mechanisms by affecting transcription and causing the formation of nuclear RNA foci (Dejesus-Hernandez, Mackenzie et al. 2011).

3.6 TARDBP

TARDBP encodes the protein TDP-43. It includes 7 exons. In 2008 mutations in the *TARDBP* gene on chromosome 1 encoding TDP-43 were first described in ALS patients with a positive family history but also in cases of sporadic ALS (Gitcho and Baloh 2008; Kabashi 2008; Sreedharan 2008). A mutation in *TARDBP* is found in about 4% and 1.5% of patients with sporadic and familial ALS, respectively. After these findings, an extensive search begun to identify mutations in *TARDBP* gene of patients with FTLD. In contrast to ALS, TARDBP mutations may be only a rare cause of FTLD. Mainly missense mutations have been described in patients with bvFTLD (Borroni, Bonvicini et al. 2009), FTLD-MND (Benajiba, Le Ber et al. 2009; Borghero, Floris et al. 2011), and FTLD with supranuclear palsy and choreatic movements (Kovacs, Murrell et al. 2009). Most missense changes involve exon 6, which encodes a Gly-rich region and the C-terminus. This may lead to a toxic gain-of function as well as loss of function of TDP-43 by interfering with protein-protein-interactions due to increased propensity to aggregate and by alteration of the phosphorylation site (Kabashi, Lin et al. 2010). In one family with FTLD-ALS a variant in the 3'-untranslated region (3'-UTR) of the *TARDBP* gene has been described and showed FTLD-TDP pathology on neuropathological examination (Gitcho, Bigio et al. 2009).

3.7 *FUS*

Mutations in the *FUS* gene on chromosome 16 were first identified to be responsible in a few cases with familial ALS (Kwiatkowski, Bosco et al. 2009; Vance, Rogelj et al. 2009). Altogether, FUS mutations account only for a minority of familial ALS patients (4%) and roughly 1% in sporadic cases. One missense mutation in a patient with bvFTLD and negative family history was described (Van Langenhove, van der Zee et al. 2010). No autopsy data is available for this proposed case of FTLD-FUS, so it remains uncertain whether FUS mutations truly cause FTLD.

3.8 Summary

30 to 50% of patients with bvFTLD have a positive family history. The frequency for familial PNFA and SD as well as FTLD-ALS is very low. Taken together, general genetic screening for patients presenting with symptoms suggesting FTLD cannot be recommended at this point. So far, testing for mutations in *PGRN* and *MAPT* may be plausible for FTLD patients with a positive family history. Most importantly, it is essential to obtain a thorough family history by asking the relatives or caregivers during several visits for family members that showed signs of personality changes or language impairment, as well as signs of movement disorders. The clinical subtype may also hint at a candidate gene. So far, patients with familial bvFTLD may contain mutations in the *MAPT* or *PGRN* genes, patients with PNFA in the *PGRN* gene. For SD and FTLD-MND, genetic screening cannot be recommended.

In sporadic cases, *PGRN* mutations may be found, but here again, genetic screening will not be of great value.

Despite a great effort to find genetic risk factors for FTLD, none has been surely identified so far. At the moment, not all gene mutations have been identified in patients with familial FTLD.

Gene	Location	Protein	Clinical Phenotype	Families	Mutations
MAPT	17q21.1	Microtubule associated protein tau	bvFTLD, FTDP	134	44
PGRN	17q21.31	Progranulin	bvFTLD, PNFA, CBD	231	69
VCP	9p13.3	Valosin-containing protein	IBMPFD	41	17
CHM2B	3p11.2	Charged multivesicular Body Protein 2B	bvFTLD with movement deficits	5	4
TARDBP	1p36.2	TAR DNA-binding protein of 43 kDa (TDP-43)	bvFTLD, FTLD-ALS	92	34
Not determined (C9ORF72)	Linkage to chromosome 9p13.2-21.3	Not determined (*C9ORF72:* uncharacterized)	bvFTLD, FTLD-ALS		

Table 2.

4. Neuropathology

The pathological hallmark of FTLD is the presence of intracellular protein aggregates. These inclusions are immunoreactive for ubiquitin. In the last couple of years it has become clear that FTLD encompasses a vast spectrum of neuropathological features. The protein tau was the first protein identified as the main component of intraneuronal inclusions in around 40 % of cases with FTLD. For over a decade other associated disease proteins in cases positive for ubiquitin but negative for tau could not be identified. Subsequently, these cases were termed FTLD-U. Then in 2006 and 2009, TDP-43 and FUS were identified to be the main components in many ubiquitin-positive, tau-negative inclusions, and the terms FTLD-TDP and FTLD-FUS were introduced, respectively. Up to date, the associated protein in most cases has been identified, with the exemption of cases with *CHMP2B* mutations.

In other pathological cases with FTLD, no clear pathology could be identified and was termed „dementia lacking distinctive histology" (DLDH). DLDH may be very rare, and it has been suggested that lack of sensitivity for ubiquitin immunostaining may account for the failure to find specific pathology (Mackenzie, Shi et al. 2006).

In the following section, an overview over the three key disease associated proteins, namely tau, TDP-43, and FUS, will be given.

4.1 Tau

Tau is physiological localized to the axon in order to stabilize microtubules, filaments of the cytoskeleton apparatus (Goedert, Wischik et al. 1988). Tau is a phosphoprotein with high numbers of serine and threonine residues; thereby tau serves as a substrate by many kinases. Tau is crucial for the neuronal metabolism including signal transduction and

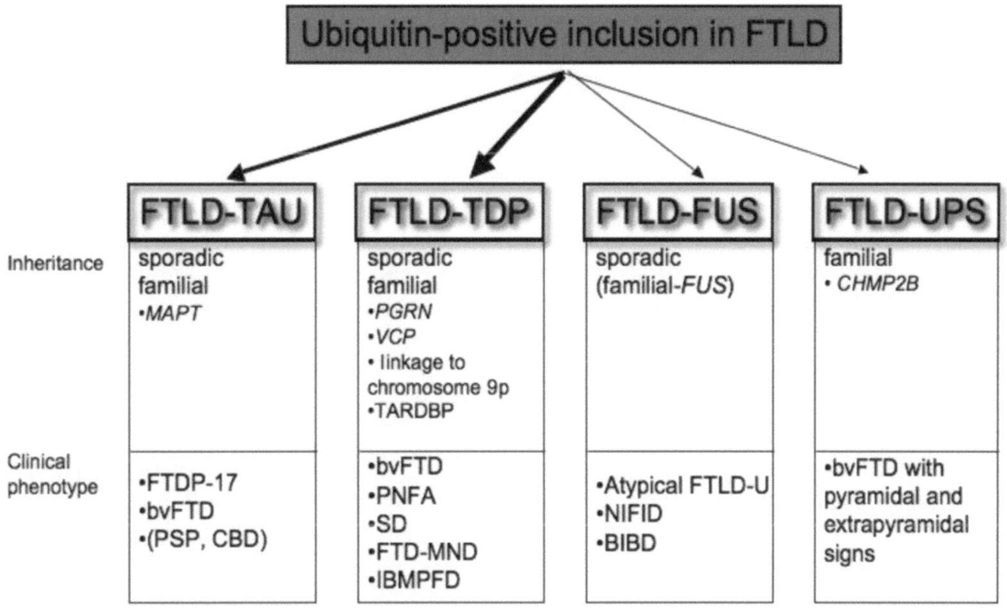

intracellular transport as well as neuronal plasticity. Six isoforms of tau are known and are generated by alternative mRNA splicing. The isoforms differ in the number of amino acids in the protein chain, the presence of three (3R tau type) or four (4R tau type) domains responsible for binding to microtubules, and one or two inserts containing from 29 to 58 amino acids. The isoforms are modified posttranslational by hyperphosphorylation, glycation, or oxidation, which can change the protein's properties and disturb its normal function.

Under pathological conditions, tau becomes posttranslational modified through enhanced phosphorylation at its serine and threonine residues as well as at additional sites. Hyperphosphorylated tau then dissociates from microtubules, causing them to depolymerize. Tau then is deposited in aggregates and can now also be found in dendrites. Hyperphosphorylated inclusions can be found in the soma and neurites of neurons (neurofibrillar tangles), as well as in astroglia ("astrocytic plaque"), and oligodendrocytes ("coiled bodies"). In glia, tau can be found predominantly in its 4R isoform. One common hypothesis is that soluble rather than insoluble tau is neurotoxic.

Tau inclusions can be found within frontal and temporal cortex, as well as hippocampus and subcortical neurons, but also sometimes in midbrain, brainstem, cerebellum, and spinal cord.

Mutations have been identified in the *MAPT* gene, leading mainly to a clinical phenotype of FTLD with parkinsonism.

PSP and CBD are considered a tauopathy as well and are thought to be within the clinical, genetical, and pathological spectrum of FTLD. Here also, tau aggregates can be found within glial cells.

4.2 TDP-43

TDP-43 is highly conserved, abundantly expressed protein in neurons and glia, and predominantly localized to the nucleus (Buratti, Dork et al. 2001; Wang, Wang et al. 2004).

TDP-43 is involved in transcription and splicing regulation (Buratti and Baralle 2008; Lagier-Tourenne, Polymenidou et al. 2010). In addition, TDP-43 may have an effect on microRNA biogenesis, apoptosis, stabilisation of mRNA, and cell division (Strong, Volkening et al. 2007; Buratti and Baralle 2008). The protein TDP-43 is encoded by the gene *TARDBP* located on chromosome 1p36.2. *TARDBP* contains 5 coding and one non-coding exon. TDP-43 is composed of 414 amino acids and has a molecular weight of 43 kDa. TDP-43 consists of two RNA-recognition motif domains, and a Gly-rich C-terminal site for binding to single-stranded DNA, RNA, and protein. In addition it possesses a nuclear localization signal and a nuclear export signal, so TDP-43 shuttles between the nucleus and cytoplasm (Buratti, Dork et al. 2001; Wang, Wang et al. 2004; Buratti, Brindisi et al. 2005; Ayala, Misteli et al. 2008; Winton, Igaz et al. 2008). Transient redistribution from the nucleus to the cytoplasm following neuronal injury indicates that TDP-43 is involved in repair mechanisms (Sato, Takeuchi et al. 2009). TDP-43 may regulate neuronal plasticity and maintenance of dendritic integrity (Wang, Wu et al. 2008; Lu, Ferris et al. 2009).

In FTLD, TDP-43 undergoes post-translational modifications, i.e., hyperphosphorylation, ubiquitination, and N-terminal truncation (Neumann, Sampathu et al. 2006; Hasegawa, Arai et al. 2008; Igaz, Kwong et al. 2008). In FTLD, staining against TDP-43 localized to the cytoplasm and neurites in the frontotemporal cortex and the dentate granule cells of the hippocampus. TDP-43 positive inclusion bodies are not restricted to neurons, but were identified in glia as well (Mackenzie, Baborie et al. 2006; Sampathu, Neumann et al. 2006).

Nevertheless, TDP-43 can be distinguished according to their subcellular location and proportion into four patterns (Mackenzie, Baborie et al. 2006; Sampathu, Neumann et al. 2006; Mackenzie, Neumann et al. 2011). Here, the harmonized classification system for FTLD-TDP pathology is used (Mackenzie, Neumann et al. 2011).

Type A presents mainly cases with bvFTLD and PNFA; TDP-43 is highly expressed in neuronal cytoplasmic inclusions and dystrophic neurites in cortical layer 2. Type A represents all cases with *PGRN* mutations. Type B is associated with bvFTLD and FTLD-ALS, and TDP-43 is mainly located in cytoplasmic inclusions. Type C presents with SD and with TDP-43 in dystrophic neurites. Type D is found only in patients with *VCP* mutations with high neuronal intranuclear TDP-43 inclusions.

The pathogenesis of TDP-43 proteinopathy is unclear. The subcellular redistribution of TDP-43 from the nucleus into the cytoplasm in neurons with inclusion bodies suggests a loss-of function mechanism. This is supported by *in vitro* studies in human cell lines, in which knock-down of TDP-43 induced impaired neurite outgrowth and increased cell death (Ayala, Misteli et al. 2008; Iguchi, Katsuno et al. 2009).

It is noteworthy that TDP-43 can present with each clinical subtype, i.e., bvFTLD, SD, and PNFA. TDP-43 proteinopathies can be found associated with genetic mutations in *GRN, linkage to chromosome 9p*, and *VCP*.

Other disorders with TDP-43 pathology were reported in Perry Syndrome (Wider, Dickson et al. 2009), Guamanian ALS-parkinsonism-dementia complex (Hasegawa, Arai et al. 2007), but also in some cases of Alzheimer's disease and dementia with Lewy bodies (Arai, Mackenzie et al. 200; Higashi, Iseki et al. 2007). TDP-43 has not been described in inclusion bodies in Parkinson's disease so far.

4.3 FUS

In 2009, FUS (fused in sarcoma) protein was identified in cases of ubiquitin-positive, tau-negative and TDP-43 negative cases (Neumann, Rademakers et al. 2009). Up to 10% of

FTLD- ubiqutin positive, tau and TDP-43 negative cases are immunoreactive for FUS (Mackenzie, Neumann et al. 2011).

Neuropathological subtypes of FTLD-TDP (Mackenzie, Neumann et al. 2011)		
Classification	**Pathology**	**Disease association**
Type A	**Abundant NCI and DN** Variable NII	bvFTLD, PNFA *PGRN* mutations
Type B	**Few NCI and DN**	bvFTLD, FTLD-ALS with linkage to chromosome 9p
Type C	**Abundant DN, few NCI**	SD, bvFTLD
Type D	**Abundant NII** Abundant DN, few NCI	IBMPFD with *VCP* mutations
NCI - neuronalcytoplasmic inclusions DN - dystrophic neurites NII - neuronal intranuclear inclusions		

Table 3.

FUS protein is comprised of 526 amino acids, ubiquitously expressed, and is located to the nucleus and cytoplasm (Andersson, Stahlberg et al. 2008). Its precise function is scarcely deciphered but it may be involved in cell proliferation, transcription regulation such as regulation of RNA splicing, and RNA and microRNA processing (Lagier-Tourenne, Polymenidou et al. 2010). FUS was originally discovered as a part of the fusion oncogenes in human cancers (Law, Cann et al. 2006). It contains an RNA recognition motif, a zinc finger motif and possesses a non-classical nuclear localization signal at its C-terminus (Law, Cann et al. 2006; Zakaryan and Gehring 2006).
Pathologically, FUS positive inclusions are found in neuronal and glial cells. Albeit to a lesser degree, like TDP-43 there is redistribution from the nucleus to the cytoplasm. No disease-associated modifications of this protein like truncation, phosphorylation have yet been identified.
Cases with FTLD-FUS on neuropathological examination show a more or less characteristic clinical phenotype. Patients had an early-onset bvFTLD, and showed motor symptoms including mild rigidity and/or intermittent hyperkinesias. FUS pathology is abundant in the frontal and temporal lobe, as well as hippocampus and maybe in the striatum and brainstem (Neumann, Rademakers et al. 2009; Neumann, Roeber et al. 2009). Most cases show inclusions in the lower motor neuron, despite missing clinical features of motor neuron disease. FUS show intranuclear inclusions with vermiform filaments that can be found in dentate granule cells (Neumann, Rademakers et al. 2009; Neumann, Roeber et al. 2009).
On neuroimaging studies, caudate atrophy may be indicator of FTLD-FUS, since the volume is smaller than in patients with FTLD-tau and FTLD-TDP (Josephs, Whitwell et al.).
Neuronal intermediate filament inclusion disease (NIFID) is characterized microscopically by neuronal inclusions for all class IV intermedate filaments like α-internexin and FUS (Neumann, Roeber et al. 2009). FUS pathology is also seen in cases with BIBD (Munoz, Neumann et al. 2009).

4.4 Summary

FTLD is characterized by focal atrophy of the frontal and/or temporal lobes with relative sparing of the parietal and occipital. Neuronal loss is mainly observed within layer 2.

Abnormal protein aggregates are located mainly in the cytoplasm. These inclusions stain positive ubiquitin. Tau, TDP-43, or FUS were identified as the ubiquitinated pathological protein in most cases. However, some ubiquitin-positive, tau-negative, TDP-43-negative and FUS-negative cases are still open and are termed FTLD-UPS. Some of these cases carry a CHMP2B mutation, but the pathological protein is not yet identified.

Tau, TDP-43, and FUS all undergo post-translational modification, but the exact toxic species has not been identified.

5. References

Andersson, M. K., A. Stahlberg, et al. (2008). "The multifunctional FUS, EWS and TAF15 proto-oncoproteins show cell type-specific expression patterns and involvement in cell spreading and stress response." *BMC Cell Biol* 9: 37.

Arai, T., I. R. Mackenzie, et al. (2009). "Phosphorylated TDP-43 in Alzheimer's disease and dementia with Lewy bodies." *Acta Neuropathol* 117(2): 125-36.

Ayala, Y. M., T. Misteli, et al. (2008). "TDP-43 regulates retinoblastoma protein phosphorylation through the repression of cyclin-dependent kinase 6 expression." *Proc Natl Acad Sci U S A* 105(10): 3785-9.

Badadani, M., A. Nalbandian, et al. (2010). "VCP associated inclusion body myopathy and paget disease of bone knock-in mouse model exhibits tissue pathology typical of human disease." *PLoS One* 5(10).

Baker, M., I. R. Mackenzie, et al. (2006). "Mutations in progranulin cause tau-negative frontotemporal dementia linked to chromosome 17." *Nature* 442(7105): 916-9.

Behrens, M. I., O. Mukherjee, et al. (2007). "Neuropathologic heterogeneity in HDDD1: a familial frontotemporal lobar degeneration with ubiquitin-positive inclusions and progranulin mutation." *Alzheimer Dis Assoc Disord* 21(1): 1-7.

Belly, A., G. Bodon, et al. (2010). "CHMP2B mutants linked to frontotemporal dementia impair maturation of dendritic spines." *J Cell Sci* 123(Pt 17): 2943-54.

Benajiba, L., I. Le Ber, et al. (2009). "TARDBP mutations in motoneuron disease with frontotemporal lobar degeneration." *Ann Neurol* 65(4): 470-3.

Benussi, L., G. Binetti, et al. (2008). "A novel deletion in progranulin gene is associated with FTDP-17 and CBS." *Neurobiol Aging* 29(3): 427-35.

Bersano, A., R. Del Bo, et al. (2009). "Inclusion body myopathy and frontotemporal dementia caused by a novel VCP mutation." *Neurobiol Aging* 30(5): 752-8.

Boeve, B. F. and M. Hutton (2008). "Refining frontotemporal dementia with parkinsonism linked to chromosome 17: introducing FTDP-17 (MAPT) and FTDP-17 (PGRN)." *Arch Neurol* 65(4): 460-4.

Borghero, G., G. Floris, et al. (2011). "A patient carrying a homozygous p.A382T TARDBP missense mutation shows a syndrome including ALS, extrapyramidal symptoms, and FTD." *Neurobiol Aging*. DOI:10.1016/j.neurobiolaging.2011.06.009

Borroni, B., S. Archetti, et al. (2008). "Progranulin genetic variations in frontotemporal lobar degeneration: evidence for low mutation frequency in an Italian clinical series." *Neurogenetics* 9(3): 197-205.

Borroni, B., C. Bonvicini, et al. (2009). "Mutation within TARDBP leads to frontotemporal dementia without motor neuron disease." *Hum Mutat* 30(11): E974-83.

Bronner, I. F., P. Rizzu, et al. (2007). "Progranulin mutations in Dutch familial frontotemporal lobar degeneration." *Eur J Hum Genet* 15(3): 369-74.

Bruni, A. C., P. Momeni, et al. (2007). "Heterogeneity within a large kindred with frontotemporal dementia: a novel progranulin mutation." *Neurology* 69(2): 140-7.

Buratti, E. and F. E. Baralle (2008). "Multiple roles of TDP-43 in gene expression, splicing regulation, and human disease." *Front Biosci* 13: 867-78.

Buratti, E., A. Brindisi, et al. (2005). "TDP-43 binds heterogeneous nuclear ribonucleoprotein A/B through its C-terminal tail: an important region for the inhibition of cystic fibrosis transmembrane conductance regulator exon 9 splicing." *J Biol Chem* 280(45): 37572-84.

Buratti, E., T. Dork, et al. (2001). "Nuclear factor TDP-43 and SR proteins promote in vitro and in vivo CFTR exon 9 skipping." *Embo J* 20(7): 1774-84.

Cairns, N. J., M. Grossman, et al. (2004). "Clinical and neuropathologic variation in neuronal intermediate filament inclusion disease." *Neurology* 63(8): 1376-84.

Cairns, N. J., M. Neumann, et al. (2007). "TDP-43 in familial and sporadic frontotemporal lobar degeneration with ubiquitin inclusions." *Am J Pathol* 171(1): 227-40.

Cannon, A., M. Baker, et al. (2006). "CHMP2B mutations are not a common cause of frontotemporal lobar degeneration." *Neurosci Lett* 398(1-2): 83-4.

Capell, A., S. Liebscher, et al. (2011). "Rescue of progranulin deficiency associated with frontotemporal lobar degeneration by alkalizing reagents and inhibition of vacuolar ATPase." *J Neurosci* 31(5): 1885-94.

Chow, T. W., A. Graff-Guerrero, et al. (2011). "Open-label study of the short-term effects of memantine on FDG-PET in frontotemporal dementia." *Neuropsychiatr Dis Treat* 7: 415-24.

Chow, T. W. and M. F. Mendez (2002). "Goals in symptomatic pharmacologic management of frontotemporal lobar degeneration." *Am J Alzheimers Dis Other Demen* 17(5): 267-72.

Chow, T. W., B. L. Miller, et al. (1999). "Inheritance of frontotemporal dementia." *Arch Neurol* 56(7): 817-22.

Cruts, M., I. Gijselinck, et al. (2006). "Null mutations in progranulin cause ubiquitin-positive frontotemporal dementia linked to chromosome 17q21." *Nature* 442(7105): 920-4.

Cruts, M., S. Kumar-Singh, et al. (2006). "Progranulin mutations in ubiquitin-positive frontotemporal dementia linked to chromosome 17q21." *Curr Alzheimer Res* 3(5): 485-91.

Custer, S. K., M. Neumann, et al. (2010). "Transgenic mice expressing mutant forms VCP/p97 recapitulate the full spectrum of IBMPFD including degeneration in muscle, brain and bone." *Hum Mol Genet* 19(9): 1741-55.

Deakin, J. B., S. Rahman, et al. (2004). "Paroxetine does not improve symptoms and impairs cognition in frontotemporal dementia: a double-blind randomized controlled trial." *Psychopharmacology (Berl)* 172(4): 400-8.

Dejesus-Hernandez, M., I. R. Mackenzie, et al. (2011). "Expanded GGGGCC Hexanucleotide Repeat in Noncoding Region of C9ORF72 Causes Chromosome 9p-Linked FTD and ALS." *Neuron*.

Di Fabio, R., A. Tessa, et al. (2010). "Familial frontotemporal dementia with parkinsonism associated with the progranulin c.C1021T (p.Q341X) mutation." *Parkinsonism Relat Disord* 16(7): 484-5.

Diehl-Schmid, J., H. Forstl, et al. (2008). "A 6-month, open-label study of memantine in patients with frontotemporal dementia." *Int J Geriatr Psychiatry* 23(7): 754-9.

Diehl-Schmid, J., T. Grimmer, et al. (2007). "Decline of cerebral glucose metabolism in frontotemporal dementia: a longitudinal 18F-FDG-PET-study." *Neurobiol Aging* 28(1): 42-50.

Djamshidian, A., J. Schaefer, et al. (2009). "A novel mutation in the VCP gene (G157R) in a German family with inclusion-body myopathy with Paget disease of bone and frontotemporal dementia." *Muscle Nerve* 39(3): 389-91.

Ferrari, R., D. Kapogiannis, et al. (2010). "Novel Missense Mutation in Charged Multivesicular Body Protein 2B in a Patient With Frontotemporal Dementia." *Alzheimer Dis Assoc Disord.* DOI: 10.1097/WAD.0b013e3181df20c7

Finch, N., M. Baker, et al. (2009). "Plasma progranulin levels predict progranulin mutation status in frontotemporal dementia patients and asymptomatic family members." *Brain* 132(Pt 3): 583-91.

Franceschi, M., D. Anchisi, et al. (2005). "Glucose metabolism and serotonin receptors in the frontotemporal lobe degeneration." *Ann Neurol* 57(2): 216-25.

Frings, L., I. Mader, et al. (2011). "Quantifying change in individual subjects affected by frontotemporal lobar degeneration using automated longitudinal MRI volumetry." *Hum Brain Mapp.* DOI: 10.1002/hbm.21304

Gabryelewicz, T., M. Masellis, et al. (2010). "Intra-familial clinical heterogeneity due to FTLD-U with TDP-43 proteinopathy caused by a novel deletion in progranulin gene (PGRN)." *J Alzheimers Dis* 22(4): 1123-33.

Gass, J., A. Cannon, et al. (2006). "Mutations in progranulin are a major cause of ubiquitin-positive frontotemporal lobar degeneration." *Hum Mol Genet* 15(20): 2988-3001.

Ghetti, B., S. Spina, et al. (2008). "In vivo and postmortem clinicoanatomical correlations in frontotemporal dementia and parkinsonism linked to chromosome 17." *Neurodegener Dis* 5(3-4): 215-7.

Ghidoni, R., L. Benussi, et al. (2008). "Low plasma progranulin levels predict progranulin mutations in frontotemporal lobar degeneration." *Neurology* 71(16): 1235-9.

Gidaro, T., A. Modoni, et al. (2008). "An Italian family with inclusion-body myopathy and frontotemporal dementia due to mutation in the VCP gene." *Muscle Nerve* 37(1): 111-4.

Gijselinck, I., S. Engelborghs, et al. (2010). "Identification of 2 Loci at chromosomes 9 and 14 in a multiplex family with frontotemporal lobar degeneration and amyotrophic lateral sclerosis." *Arch Neurol* 67(5): 606-16.

Gijselinck, I., J. van der Zee, et al. (2008). "Progranulin locus deletion in frontotemporal dementia." *Hum Mutat* 29(1): 53-8.

Gitcho, M. and R. H. Baloh (2008). "TDP-43 A315T mutation in familial motor neuron disease." *Ann Neurol.*

Gitcho, M. A., E. H. Bigio, et al. (2009). "TARDBP 3'-UTR variant in autopsy-confirmed frontotemporal lobar degeneration with TDP-43 proteinopathy." *Acta Neuropathol* 118(5): 633-45.

Gitcho, M. A., J. Strider, et al. (2009). "VCP mutations causing frontotemporal lobar degeneration disrupt localization of TDP-43 and induce cell death." *J Biol Chem* 284(18): 12384-98.

Goedert, M., C. M. Wischik, et al. (1988). "Cloning and sequencing of the cDNA encoding a core protein of the paired helical filament of Alzheimer disease: identification as the microtubule-associated protein tau." *Proc Natl Acad Sci U S A* 85(11): 4051-5.

Goldman, J. S., J. M. Farmer, et al. (2005). "Comparison of family histories in FTLD subtypes and related tauopathies." *Neurology* 65(11): 1817-9.

Grimmer, T., J. Diehl, et al. (2004). "Region-specific decline of cerebral glucose metabolism in patients with frontotemporal dementia: a prospective 18F-FDG-PET study." *Dement Geriatr Cogn Disord* 18(1): 32-6.

Gydesen, S., J. M. Brown, et al. (2002). "Chromosome 3 linked frontotemporal dementia (FTD-3)." *Neurology* 59(10): 1585-94.

Hasegawa, M., T. Arai, et al. (2007). "TDP-43 is deposited in the Guam parkinsonism-dementia complex brains." *Brain* 130(Pt 5): 1386-94.

Hasegawa, M., T. Arai, et al. (2008). "Phosphorylated TDP-43 in frontotemporal lobar degeneration and amyotrophic lateral sclerosis." *Ann Neurol* 64(1): 60-70.

Haubenberger, D., R. E. Bittner, et al. (2005). "Inclusion body myopathy and Paget disease is linked to a novel mutation in the VCP gene." *Neurology* 65(8): 1304-5.

Higashi, S., E. Iseki, et al. (2007). "Concurrence of TDP-43, tau and alpha-synuclein pathology in brains of Alzheimer's disease and dementia with Lewy bodies." *Brain Res* 1184: 284-94.

Hodges, J. R., R. Davies, et al. (2003). "Survival in frontotemporal dementia." *Neurology* 61(3): 349-54.

Hodges, J. R., J. Mitchell, et al. (2010). "Semantic dementia: demography, familial factors and survival in a consecutive series of 100 cases." *Brain* 133(Pt 1): 300-6.

Hodges, J. R., K. Patterson, et al. (1999). "The differentiation of semantic dementia and frontal lobe dementia (temporal and frontal variants of frontotemporal dementia) from early Alzheimer's disease: a comparative neuropsychological study." *Neuropsychology* 13(1): 31-40.

Huey, E. D., J. Grafman, et al. (2006). "Characteristics of frontotemporal dementia patients with a Progranulin mutation." *Ann Neurol* 60(3): 374-80.

Huey, E. D., K. T. Putnam, et al. (2006). "A systematic review of neurotransmitter deficits and treatments in frontotemporal dementia." *Neurology* 66(1): 17-22.

Hutchinson, A. D. and J. L. Mathias (2007). "Neuropsychological deficits in frontotemporal dementia and Alzheimer's disease: a meta-analytic review." *J Neurol Neurosurg Psychiatry* 78(9): 917-28.

Hutton, M., C. L. Lendon, et al. (1998). "Association of missense and 5'-splice-site mutations in tau with the inherited dementia FTDP-17." *Nature* 393(6686): 702-5.

Igaz, L. M., L. K. Kwong, et al. (2008). "Enrichment of C-terminal fragments in TAR DNA-binding protein-43 cytoplasmic inclusions in brain but not in spinal cord of frontotemporal lobar degeneration and amyotrophic lateral sclerosis." *Am J Pathol* 173(1): 182-94.

Iguchi, Y., M. Katsuno, et al. (2009). "TDP-43 depletion induces neuronal cell damage through dysregulation of Rho family GTPases." *J Biol Chem* 284(33): 22059-66.

Jendroska, K., M. N. Rossor, et al. (1995). "Morphological overlap between corticobasal degeneration and Pick's disease: a clinicopathological report." *Mov Disord* 10(1): 111-4.

Josephs, K. A., Z. Ahmed, et al. (2007). "Neuropathologic features of frontotemporal lobar degeneration with ubiquitin-positive inclusions with progranulin gene (PGRN) mutations." *J Neuropathol Exp Neurol* 66(2): 142-51.

Josephs, K. A., J. L. Holton, et al. (2003). "Neurofilament inclusion body disease: a new proteinopathy?" *Brain* 126(Pt 10): 2291-303.

Josephs, K. A., R. C. Petersen, et al. (2006). "Clinicopathologic analysis of frontotemporal and corticobasal degenerations and PSP." *Neurology* 66(1): 41-8.

Josephs, K. A., J. L. Whitwell, et al. (2010). "Caudate atrophy on MRI is a characteristic feature of FTLD-FUS." *Eur J Neurol* 17(7): 969-75.

Ju, J. S., R. A. Fuentealba, et al. (2009). "Valosin-containing protein (VCP) is required for autophagy and is disrupted in VCP disease." *J Cell Biol* 187(6): 875-88.

Kabashi, E. (2008). "TARDBP mutations in individuals with sporadic and familial amyotrophic lateral sclerosis." *Nat Genet.*

Kabashi, E., L. Lin, et al. (2010). "Gain and loss of function of ALS-related mutations of TARDBP (TDP-43) cause motor deficits in vivo." *Hum Mol Genet* 19(4): 671-83.

Kavirajan, H. (2009). "Memantine: a comprehensive review of safety and efficacy." *Expert Opin Drug Saf* 8(1): 89-109.

Kertesz, A., D. Morlog, et al. (2008). "Galantamine in frontotemporal dementia and primary progressive aphasia." *Dement Geriatr Cogn Disord* 25(2): 178-85.

Kertesz, A. and D. Munoz (2004). "Relationship between frontotemporal dementia and corticobasal degeneration/progressive supranuclear palsy." *Dement Geriatr Cogn Disord* 17(4): 282-6.

Kimonis, V. E., E. Fulchiero, et al. (2008). "VCP disease associated with myopathy, Paget disease of bone and frontotemporal dementia: review of a unique disorder." *Biochim Biophys Acta* 1782(12): 744-8.

Kovacs, G. G., J. R. Murrell, et al. (2009). "TARDBP variation associated with frontotemporal dementia, supranuclear gaze palsy, and chorea." *Mov Disord* 24(12): 1843-7.

Kwiatkowski, T. J., Jr., D. A. Bosco, et al. (2009). "Mutations in the FUS/TLS gene on chromosome 16 cause familial amyotrophic lateral sclerosis." *Science* 323(5918): 1205-8.

Laaksovirta, H., T. Peuralinna, et al. (2010). "Chromosome 9p21 in amyotrophic lateral sclerosis in Finland: a genome-wide association study." *Lancet Neurol* 9(10): 978-85.

Lagier-Tourenne, C., M. Polymenidou, et al. (2010). "TDP-43 and FUS/TLS: emerging roles in RNA processing and neurodegeneration." *Hum Mol Genet* 19(R1): R46-64.

Lang, A. E., C. Bergeron, et al. (1994). "Parietal Pick's disease mimicking cortical-basal ganglionic degeneration." *Neurology* 44(8): 1436-40.

Law, W. J., K. L. Cann, et al. (2006). "TLS, EWS and TAF15: a model for transcriptional integration of gene expression." *Brief Funct Genomic Proteomic* 5(1): 8-14.

Le Ber, I., A. Camuzat, et al. (2009). "Chromosome 9p-linked families with frontotemporal dementia associated with motor neuron disease." *Neurology* 72(19): 1669-76.

Le Ber, I., A. Camuzat, et al. (2008). "Phenotype variability in progranulin mutation carriers: a clinical, neuropsychological, imaging and genetic study." *Brain* 131(Pt 3): 732-46.

Le Ber, I., J. van der Zee, et al. (2007). "Progranulin null mutations in both sporadic and familial frontotemporal dementia." *Hum Mutat* 28(9): 846-55.

Lebert, F., W. Stekke, et al. (2004). "Frontotemporal dementia: a randomised, controlled trial with trazodone." *Dement Geriatr Cogn Disord* 17(4): 355-9.

Litvan, I. (2001). "Therapy and management of frontal lobe dementia patients." *Neurology* 56(11 Suppl 4): S41-5.

Lopez de Munain, A., A. Alzualde, et al. (2008). "Mutations in progranulin gene: clinical, pathological, and ribonucleic acid expression findings." *Biol Psychiatry* 63(10): 946-52.

Lu, Y., J. Ferris, et al. (2009). "Frontotemporal dementia and amyotrophic lateral sclerosis-associated disease protein TDP-43 promotes dendritic branching." *Mol Brain* 2: 30.

Luty, A. A., J. B. Kwok, et al. (2008). "Pedigree with frontotemporal lobar degeneration--motor neuron disease and Tar DNA binding protein-43 positive neuropathology: genetic linkage to chromosome 9." *BMC Neurol* 8: 32.

Mackenzie, I. R., A. Baborie, et al. (2006). "Heterogeneity of ubiquitin pathology in frontotemporal lobar degeneration: classification and relation to clinical phenotype." *Acta Neuropathol* 112(5): 539-49.

Mackenzie, I. R., M. Baker, et al. (2006). "The neuropathology of frontotemporal lobar degeneration caused by mutations in the progranulin gene." *Brain* 129(Pt 11): 3081-90.
Mackenzie, I. R., M. Neumann, et al. (2011). "A harmonized classification system for FTLD-TDP pathology." *Acta Neuropathol* 122(1): 111-3.
Mackenzie, I. R., M. Neumann, et al. (2011). "Nomenclature and nosology for neuropathologic subtypes of frontotemporal lobar degeneration: an update." *Acta Neuropathol* 119(1): 1-4.
Mackenzie, I. R., J. Shi, et al. (2006). "Dementia lacking distinctive histology (DLDH) revisited." *Acta Neuropathol* 112(5): 551-9.
Mendez, M. F., J. S. Shapira, et al. (2007). "Preliminary findings: behavioral worsening on donepezil in patients with frontotemporal dementia." *Am J Geriatr Psychiatry* 15(1): 84-7.
Mendez, M. F., J. S. Shapira, et al. (2007). "Accuracy of the clinical evaluation for frontotemporal dementia." *Arch Neurol* 64(6): 830-5.
Mesulam, M., N. Johnson, et al. (2007). "Progranulin mutations in primary progressive aphasia: the PPA1 and PPA3 families." *Arch Neurol* 64(1): 43-7.
Mesulam, M. M. (2001). "Primary progressive aphasia." *Ann Neurol* 49(4): 425-32.
Mitsuyama, Y. and T. Inoue (2009). "Clinical entity of frontotemporal dementia with motor neuron disease." *Neuropathology* 29(6): 649-54.
Moretti, R., P. Torre, et al. (2004). "Rivastigmine in frontotemporal dementia: an open-label study." *Drugs Aging* 21(14): 931-7.
Moretti, R., P. Torre, et al. (2002). "Effects of selegiline on fronto-temporal dementia: a neuropsychological evaluation." *Int J Geriatr Psychiatry* 17(4): 391-2.
Moretti, R., P. Torre, et al. (2003). "Frontotemporal dementia: paroxetine as a possible treatment of behavior symptoms. A randomized, controlled, open 14-month study." *Eur Neurol* 49(1): 13-9.
Morita, M., A. Al-Chalabi, et al. (2006). "A locus on chromosome 9p confers susceptibility to ALS and frontotemporal dementia." *Neurology* 66(6): 839-44.
Mosconi, L., W. H. Tsui, et al. (2008). "Multicenter standardized 18F-FDG PET diagnosis of mild cognitive impairment, Alzheimer's disease, and other dementias." *J Nucl Med* 49(3): 390-8.
Munoz, D. G., M. Neumann, et al. (2009). "FUS pathology in basophilic inclusion body disease." *Acta Neuropathol* 118(5): 617-27.
Neary, D., J. Snowden, et al. (2005). "Frontotemporal dementia." *Lancet Neurol* 4(11): 771-80.
Neary, D., J. S. Snowden, et al. (1998). "Frontotemporal lobar degeneration: a consensus on clinical diagnostic criteria." *Neurology* 51(6): 1546-54.
Neumann, M., I. R. Mackenzie, et al. (2007). "TDP-43 in the ubiquitin pathology of frontotemporal dementia with VCP gene mutations." *J Neuropathol Exp Neurol* 66(2): 152-7.
Neumann, M., R. Rademakers, et al. (2009). "A new subtype of frontotemporal lobar degeneration with FUS pathology." *Brain* 132(Pt 11): 2922-31.
Neumann, M., S. Roeber, et al. (2009). "Abundant FUS-immunoreactive pathology in neuronal intermediate filament inclusion disease." *Acta Neuropathol* 118(5): 605-16.
Neumann, M., D. M. Sampathu, et al. (2006). "Ubiquitinated TDP-43 in frontotemporal lobar degeneration and amyotrophic lateral sclerosis." *Science* 314(5796): 130-3.
Perry, R. J. and B. L. Miller (2001). "Behavior and treatment in frontotemporal dementia." *Neurology* 56(11 Suppl 4): S46-51.

Pick, A. (1892). "Ueber die Beziehungen der senilen Hirnatrophie zur Aphasie." *Prager Medizinische Wochenschrift* 17: 165-167.

Pick, A. (1906). "Über einen weiteren Symptomenkomplex im Rahmen der Dementia senilis, bedingt durch umschriebene stärkere Hirnatrophie (gemischte Apraxie)." *Monatsschr. Neurol. Psychiat.* 19: 97-108.

Pickering-Brown, S. M., M. Baker, et al. (2006). "Mutations in progranulin explain atypical phenotypes with variants in MAPT." *Brain* 129(Pt 11): 3124-6.

Pickering-Brown, S. M., S. Rollinson, et al. (2008). "Frequency and clinical characteristics of progranulin mutation carriers in the Manchester frontotemporal lobar degeneration cohort: comparison with patients with MAPT and no known mutations." *Brain* 131(Pt 3): 721-31.

Pijnenburg, Y. A., E. L. Sampson, et al. (2003). "Vulnerability to neuroleptic side effects in frontotemporal lobar degeneration." *Int J Geriatr Psychiatry* 18(1): 67-72.

Poorkaj, P., T. D. Bird, et al. (1998). "Tau is a candidate gene for chromosome 17 frontotemporal dementia." *Ann Neurol* 43(6): 815-25.

Procter, A. W., M. Qurne, et al. (1999). "Neurochemical features of frontotemporal dementia." *Dement Geriatr Cogn Disord* 10 Suppl 1: 80-4.

Renton, A. E., E. Majounie, et al. (2011). "A Hexanucleotide Repeat Expansion in C9ORF72 Is the Cause of Chromosome 9p21-Linked ALS-FTD." *Neuron.*

Ringholz, G. M., S. H. Appel, et al. (2005). "Prevalence and patterns of cognitive impairment in sporadic ALS." *Neurology* 65(4): 586-90.

Ritson, G. P., S. K. Custer, et al. (2010). "TDP-43 mediates degeneration in a novel Drosophila model of disease caused by mutations in VCP/p97." *J Neurosci* 30(22): 7729-39.

Rohrer, J. D., R. Guerreiro, et al. (2009). "The heritability and genetics of frontotemporal lobar degeneration." *Neurology* 73(18): 1451-6.

Rollinson, S., S. Mead, et al. (2011). "Frontotemporal lobar degeneration genome wide association study replication confirms a risk locus shared with amyotrophic lateral sclerosis." *Neurobiol Aging* 32(4): 758 e1-7.

Rosso, S. M., L. Donker Kaat, et al. (2003). "Frontotemporal dementia in The Netherlands: patient characteristics and prevalence estimates from a population-based study." *Brain* 126(Pt 9): 2016-22.

Sampathu, D. M., M. Neumann, et al. (2006). "Pathological heterogeneity of frontotemporal lobar degeneration with ubiquitin-positive inclusions delineated by ubiquitin immunohistochemistry and novel monoclonal antibodies." *Am J Pathol* 169(4): 1343-52.

Sato, T., S. Takeuchi, et al. (2009). "Axonal ligation induces transient redistribution of TDP-43 in brainstem motor neurons." *Neuroscience* 164(4): 1565-78.

Schlachetzki, J. C., K. Schmidtke, et al. (2009). "Frequency of progranulin mutations in a German cohort of 79 frontotemporal dementia patients." *J Neurol* 256(12): 2043-51.

Schroder, R., G. D. Watts, et al. (2005). "Mutant valosin-containing protein causes a novel type of frontotemporal dementia." *Ann Neurol* 57(3): 457-61.

Schumacher, A., P. Friedrich, et al. (2009). "No association of common VCP variants with sporadic frontotemporal dementia." *Neurobiol Aging* 30(2): 333-5.

Seelaar, H., W. Kamphorst, et al. (2008). "Distinct genetic forms of frontotemporal dementia." *Neurology* 71(16): 1220-6.

Shatunov, A., K. Mok, et al. (2010). "Chromosome 9p21 in sporadic amyotrophic lateral sclerosis in the UK and seven other countries: a genome-wide association study." *Lancet Neurol* 9(10): 986-94.

Skibinski, G., N. J. Parkinson, et al. (2005). "Mutations in the endosomal ESCRTIII-complex subunit CHMP2B in frontotemporal dementia." *Nat Genet* 37(8): 806-8.

Sleegers, K., N. Brouwers, et al. (2009). "Serum biomarker for progranulin-associated frontotemporal lobar degeneration." *Ann Neurol* 65(5): 603-9.

Snowden, J., D. Neary, et al. (2007). "Frontotemporal lobar degeneration: clinical and pathological relationships." *Acta Neuropathol* 114(1): 31-8.

Snowden, J. S., D. Bathgate, et al. (2001). "Distinct behavioural profiles in frontotemporal dementia and semantic dementia." *J Neurol Neurosurg Psychiatry* 70(3): 323-32.

Snowden, J. S., S. M. Pickering-Brown, et al. (2006). "Progranulin gene mutations associated with frontotemporal dementia and progressive non-fluent aphasia." *Brain* 129(Pt 11): 3091-102.

Spillantini, M. G., R. A. Crowther, et al. (1998). "Tau pathology in two Dutch families with mutations in the microtubule-binding region of tau." *Am J Pathol* 153(5): 1359-63.

Spina, S., J. R. Murrell, et al. (2007). "Corticobasal syndrome associated with the A9D Progranulin mutation." *J Neuropathol Exp Neurol* 66(10): 892-900.

Sreedharan, J. (2008). "TDP-43 mutations in familial and sporadic amyotrophic lateral sclerosis." *Science.*

Stevens, M., C. M. van Duijn, et al. (1998). "Familial aggregation in frontotemporal dementia." *Neurology* 50(6): 1541-5.

Strong, M. J., K. Volkening, et al. (2007). "TDP43 is a human low molecular weight neurofilament (hNFL) mRNA-binding protein." *Mol Cell Neurosci* 35(2): 320-7.

Swanberg, M. M. (2007). "Memantine for behavioral disturbances in frontotemporal dementia: a case series." *Alzheimer Dis Assoc Disord* 21(2): 164-6.

Swartz, J. R., B. L. Miller, et al. (1997). "Frontotemporal dementia: treatment response to serotonin selective reuptake inhibitors." *J Clin Psychiatry* 58(5): 212-6.

Urwin, H., A. Authier, et al. (2010). "Disruption of endocytic trafficking in frontotemporal dementia with CHMP2B mutations." *Hum Mol Genet* 19(11): 2228-38.

Valdmanis, P. N., N. Dupre, et al. (2007). "Three families with amyotrophic lateral sclerosis and frontotemporal dementia with evidence of linkage to chromosome 9p." *Arch Neurol* 64(2): 240-5.

van der Zee, J., D. Pirici, et al. (2009). "Clinical heterogeneity in 3 unrelated families linked to VCP p.Arg159His." *Neurology* 73(8): 626-32.

van der Zee, J., H. Urwin, et al. (2008). "CHMP2B C-truncating mutations in frontotemporal lobar degeneration are associated with an aberrant endosomal phenotype in vitro." *Hum Mol Genet* 17(2): 313-22.

van Es, M. A., J. H. Veldink, et al. (2009). "Genome-wide association study identifies 19p13.3 (UNC13A) and 9p21.2 as susceptibility loci for sporadic amyotrophic lateral sclerosis." *Nat Genet* 41(10): 1083-7.

Van Langenhove, T., J. van der Zee, et al. (2010). "Genetic contribution of FUS to frontotemporal lobar degeneration." *Neurology* 74(5): 366-71.

van Swieten, J. C., M. Stevens, et al. (1999). "Phenotypic variation in hereditary frontotemporal dementia with tau mutations." *Ann Neurol* 46(4): 617-26.

Vance, C., A. Al-Chalabi, et al. (2006). "Familial amyotrophic lateral sclerosis with frontotemporal dementia is linked to a locus on chromosome 9p13.2-21.3." *Brain* 129(Pt 4): 868-76.

Vance, C., B. Rogelj, et al. (2009). "Mutations in FUS, an RNA processing protein, cause familial amyotrophic lateral sclerosis type 6." *Science* 323(5918): 1208-11.

Vossel, K. A. and B. L. Miller (2008). "New approaches to the treatment of frontotemporal lobar degeneration." *Curr Opin Neurol* 21(6): 708-16.

Walker, A. J., S. Meares, et al. (2005). "The differentiation of mild frontotemporal dementia from Alzheimer's disease and healthy aging by neuropsychological tests." *Int Psychogeriatr* 17(1): 57-68.

Wang, H. Y., I. F. Wang, et al. (2004). "Structural diversity and functional implications of the eukaryotic TDP gene family." *Genomics* 83(1): 130-9.

Wang, I. F., L. S. Wu, et al. (2008). "TDP-43, the signature protein of FTLD-U, is a neuronal activity-responsive factor." *J Neurochem* 105(3): 797-806.

Watts, G. D., D. Thomasova, et al. (2007). "Novel VCP mutations in inclusion body myopathy associated with Paget disease of bone and frontotemporal dementia." *Clin Genet* 72(5): 420-6.

Watts, G. D., J. Wymer, et al. (2004). "Inclusion body myopathy associated with Paget disease of bone and frontotemporal dementia is caused by mutant valosin-containing protein." *Nat Genet* 36(4): 377-81.

Whitwell, J. L., S. D. Weigand, et al. (2011). "Trajectories of brain and hippocampal atrophy in FTD with mutations in MAPT or GRN." *Neurology* 77(4): 393-8.

Wider, C., D. W. Dickson, et al. (2009). "Pallidonigral TDP-43 pathology in Perry syndrome." *Parkinsonism Relat Disord* 15(4): 281-6.

Winton, M. J., L. M. Igaz, et al. (2008). "Disturbance of nuclear and cytoplasmic TAR DNA-binding protein (TDP-43) induces disease-like redistribution, sequestration, and aggregate formation." *J Biol Chem* 283(19): 13302-9.

Wittenberg, D., K. L. Possin, et al. (2008). "The early neuropsychological and behavioral characteristics of frontotemporal dementia." *Neuropsychol Rev* 18(1): 91-102.

Yang, Y. and H. P. Schmitt (2001). "Frontotemporal dementia: evidence for impairment of ascending serotoninergic but not noradrenergic innervation. Immunocytochemical and quantitative study using a graph method." *Acta Neuropathol* 101(3): 256-70.

Zakaryan, R. P. and H. Gehring (2006). "Identification and characterization of the nuclear localization/retention signal in the EWS proto-oncoprotein." *J Mol Biol* 363(1): 27-38.

11

From Protein Tangles to Genetic Variants: The Central Role of Tau in Neurodegenerative Disease

Heike Julia Wobst and Richard Wade-Martins
Department of Physiology, Anatomy and Genetics and Oxford Parkinson's Disease Centre, University of Oxford
United Kingdom

1. Introduction

Since the first description in 1907 of intracellular tangles in degenerating neurons in the brain of a woman who had suffered from progressive dementia by Alois Alzheimer, research in the microtubule-associated protein tau (MAPT or tau), the major component of these intracellular deposits, and its involvement in neurodegenerative processes, has undergone a shift in paradigm. Originally regarded by many scientists as a second string player in Alzheimer's disease, it is now becoming increasingly clear that tau plays a crucial role in many neurodegenerative diseases. The discovery of neurofibrillary tangles in other progressive nervous system disorders - now commonly referred to as tauopathies - as well as the more recent association of *MAPT* genetic variants with Parkinson's disease have contributed to this heightened interest. In this chapter, we will review the developments of tau research from the beginnings to recent advances. We will focus on the increasing evidence implicating tau as a major player in neurodegeneration as well as on efforts to establish and optimize animal models of tauopathy to understand the molecular basis of this group of neurodegenerative diseases. In the final chapter section we will look forward and summarize the potential strategies for therapeutic strategies targeting tau for the treatment of tauopathic neurodegenerative diseases.

2. Tau protein

2.1 Tau structure and function

Tau proteins are low molecular weight polypeptides that are encoded by the gene *MAPT* (microtubule-associated protein tau) on chromosome 17q21. The *MAPT* gene spans ~135kb of genomic DNA and comprises 16 exons (Fig. 1). Alternative splicing of exons 2, 3 and 10 gives rise to six tau isoforms in the adult human central nervous system. Exons 6 and 8 are never found in mRNA transcripts in humans. Exon 4a is expressed in the form of high molecular weight tau in the peripheral nervous system, but never in the brain. Exon 0 is part of the promoter and while transcribed, is not translated (Buee et al., 2000). *MAPT* is primarily expressed in the central nervous system, and predominantly found in the axonal part of neurons. However, tau is expressed in glial cells as well. Trace amounts of *MAPT* transcripts have been found and described in peripheral organs including testes, kidneys and heart (Buee et al., 2000).

The six tau isoforms found in the adult human CNS range from 352 to 441 amino acids in length and 45 - 65 kDa in molecular weight. The different isoforms have been found to be differentially expressed during development. While in the foetal human central nervous system only the shortest tau isoform is expressed, all six alternatively spliced isoforms are found in the adult human brain (Goedert et al., 1989). Furthermore, it is conceivable that the different tau splicing variants are expressed in distinct spatial patterns throughout the adult CNS, with different isoforms being predominant in different neuronal subpopulations.

Structurally, tau proteins are characterised by a C-terminal microtubule-binding domain, which is composed of repeats of highly conserved tubulin-binding motifs (Fig 1). The isoforms differ in their number of tubulin-binding repeats; inclusion of exon 10 (10^+) gives rise to isoforms with 4 repeats (4R), exclusion leads to isoforms with 3 repeats (3R). The N-terminal projection domain is characterised by the absence (2^-3^-) or presence of either one (2^+3^- or 2^-3^+) or two (2^+3^+) 29 amino-acid-long inserts generated by alternative splicing of exons 2 and 3, as well as by a proline-rich region (Andreadis et al., 1992).

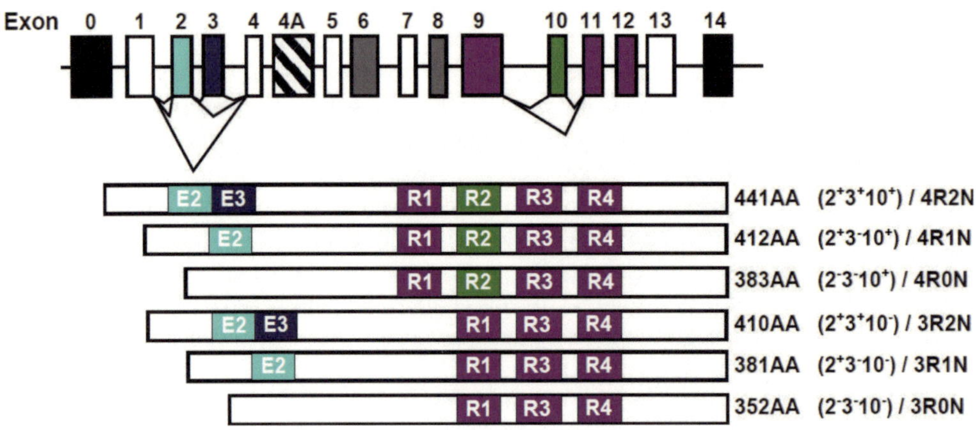

Fig. 1. Human *MAPT* gene and the six human adult isoforms in the CNS derived through alternative splicing. The *MAPT* gene encodes 16 exons, of which three (4A, 6 and 8) are not present in any of the six mature isoforms found in the human CNS. Exon 0 is part of the promoter region. Alternative splicing of exons 2, 3 and 10 gives rise to six tau isoforms. The isoforms differ by the number of tubulin-binding motifs in the MT-binding domain (R1-R4) as well as the absence or presence of either one or two 29-amino acid long motifs in the N-terminal domain (E2, E3)

2.2 Tau structure and function

The primary function of tau is the stabilisation of microtubules and the promotion of microtubule polymerisation, by binding to microtubules via the C-terminal MT-binding domain (Cleveland et al., 1977; Weingarten et al., 1975). It has been shown that 4R tau isoforms are more efficient promoters of tubulin polymerisation than 3R isoforms, hinting at different functions of the different isoforms (Goedert & Jakes, 1990). Through their polymerisation and stabilisation of microtubules, tau proteins thus have a pivotal role in maintaining the appropriate neuron morphology. Since the microtubule network provides the railroad of the cellular transport machinery, tau is also implicated in axonal transport and thus in function and viability of neurons.

Aside from the stabilisation and polymerisation of microtubules, several studies have suggested tau to have a number of other functions in the cell: Tau proteins bind to spectrin and actin filaments, thereby possibly interconnecting different cytoskeletal elements (Carlier et al., 1984; Griffith & Pollard, 1982). Furthermore, it has been proposed that tau interacts with the neural plasma membrane, thus contributing to the development of cell polarity, and with mitochondria, enabling the interaction of the organelles with microtubules (Brandt et al., 1995; Jancsik et al., 1989). Tau proteins are also believed to have a direct role in regulating the function of motor proteins, as it has been shown that tau inhibits activity of both kinesin and dynamin (Dixit et al., 2008). While tau is predominantly found in axons in the cytosol, nuclear localisation of the protein has also been described. Recently, it has been shown that nuclear tau interacts with neuronal DNA and protects DNA integrity against mild heat-stress induced damage (Sultan et al., 2011). Furthermore, tau interacts with non-receptor tyrosine kinases such as fyn via its N-terminal projection domain (Lee et al., 1998). Through this interaction tau has been shown to sequester and relocate fyn, a kinase known to modulate NMDA receptor function (Ittner et al., 2010). Thus, tau is also involved in tyrosine kinase-mediated signal transduction processes.

2.3 Tau phosphorylation

Promoting microtubule polymerisation and maintaining microtubule stability are the main functions of tau proteins. These functions are regulated by post-translational modifications. The most common posttranslational modification of tau is the phosphorylation of serine, threonine and tyrosine residues. The longest tau isoform harbours 85 putative phosphorylation sites, most of which are serine residues (Martin et al., 2011). Phosphorylation of tau decreases the binding affinity to microtubules, thus reducing microtubule assembly and stability (Biernat et al., 1993; Bramblett et al., 1993). Non-physiologically phosphorylated or hyperphosphorylated tau species have been found in all known tauopathies and it has been shown that the accumulation of abnormally phosphorylated tau precedes the formation of tau tangles (Bancher et al., 1989), indicating that dysregulation of the phosphorylation status of tau might be an early event in tau misfolding and subsequent formation of tangles. The phosphorylation status of tau proteins is dynamically regulated through a balance between kinase and phosphatase function. Disruption of this balance is believed to be at least partly responsible for the onset of tauopathies such as Alzheimer's disease. Three classes of kinases have been shown to be involved in the phosphorylation of tau proteins: proline-directed protein kinases (PDPKs, including GSK3β and Cdk5), non-PDPKs (such as PKA and CamKII) and tyrosine-specific protein kinases (Martin et al., 2011). Besides overactivation of kinases inhibition of protein phosphatases is thought to contribute to abnormal phosphorylation of tau. It has been shown that protein phosphatase 2A (PP2A), a ubiquitously expressed serine/threonine phosphatase, is involved in the regulation of the phosphorylation status of tau (Drewes et al., 1993; Gong et al., 2000). Investigation of brains of Alzheimer's disease patients has revealed a 50% decrease in PP2A activity compared to control brains (Gong et al., 1993).

Besides phosphorylation, several other forms of posttranslational modifications of tau have been described; among these are truncation, o-glycosylation, nitration, ubiquitination and glycation. Truncated and non-physiologically o-glycosylated forms of tau have been found in Alzheimer's disease brains, but not in control brains (Martin et al., 2011), indicating that tau function is tightly regulated by posttranslational modifications and that aberrant modifications might at least be partly responsible for the formation of neurofibrillary tangles and the onset of neurodegeneration.

2.4 Tau aggregation

Neurofibrillary tangles (NFTs) are intracellular aggregates composed of hyperphosphorylated tau. These intracellular deposits are the defining hallmark of all tauopathies, such as Alzheimer's disease, FTDP-17 and Pick's disease. Ultrastructurally, tangles are composed of paired helical filaments (PHFs) and less prevalent straight filaments. PHFs are composed of two strands of hyperphosphorylated tau filament twisted around each other with a periodicity of 80 nm whereas straight filaments do not show this periodicity (Crowther, 1991).

Many neurodegenerative diseases, such as Alzheimer's disease, Parkinson's disease or Creutzfeld-Jacob's disease share a common denominator: The initial misfolding and subsequent aggregation of specific proteins into highly organised and mostly thread-like structures termed amyloid. While many proteins with a propensity to self-aggregation are natively unfolded, they do not share an obvious sequence identity, suggesting that the ability to form amyloid structures is an inherent property of polypeptide chains (Chiti & Dobson, 2006). A recent physicochemical definition classifies amyloid as polymerised proteins forming a cross-β structure (Fandrich, 2007). According to this definition, NFTs classify as amyloid structures, as there is strong evidence that tau fibrils display cross-β structure both *in vitro* and *in vivo* (Berriman et al., 2003). *In vitro* aggregation of tau into filament structures has been shown to be dependent on a hexapeptide motif in the third repeat of the MT-binding domain (von Bergen et al., 2000).

Kinetic studies have shown that the aggregation of amyloid fibrils from polypeptides such as Aβ peptide and α-synuclein occurs through nucleation-dependent polymerisation, a chemical reaction characterised by an initial lag phase, an exponential growth phase and a steady-state phase (Harper & Lansbury, 1997). The same reaction scheme has been shown to apply to aggregation of tau *in vitro* (Friedhoff et al., 1998), indicating that similar mechanistic principles underlie the formation of PHFs as well as the formation of Aβ plaques and α-synuclein deposits. However, in contrast to aggregating polypeptides such as Aβ and α-synuclein, tau proteins do not exhibit stretches of hydrophobicity and a propensity to form cross-β structures. Instead, tau is a hydrophilic protein with high solubility and a random coil conformation, structural characteristics that are unfavourable for aggregation. It is not fully understood how the initial transition of tau protein from random coil structure to aggregation-prone state with increased β-sheet content occurs in tauopathies. As discussed in section 2.3, tau hyperphosphorylation is believed to play a crucial role in the early events of NFT formation. Furthermore, point mutations of tau found in patients suffering from FTDP-17, a rare genetic tauopathy, lead to increased aggregation propensity. Truncation of the protein, most notably by caspase cleavage, is also indicated as an early event in tau aggregation (Gamblin et al., 2003).

2.5 Mechanisms of tau-mediated neurodegeneration

The precise mechanism by which aggregation of tau into neurofibrillary tangles induces neurodegeneration remains unclear. Neuronal cell death could result either from a loss of tau protein function or from a toxic gain of function - or most probably, from a combination of both mechanisms. Modulation of cytoskeleton stability and dynamics is of crucial importance in maintaining proper cell morphology, intracellular transport and viability. In the loss-of-function model, hyperphosphorylated tau is detached from the microtubules and instead aggregates into fibrillary structures, thereby leading to a destabilisation of microtubules and thus compromised cell integrity. Furthermore, loss of tau function could compromise axonal transport. Transport of vesicles, mRNA and organelles is driven by motor proteins that use the microtubules as a railroad across the axons and requires a finely regulated balance between stability and plasticity of microtubules. However, the validity of the tau loss-of-function model has been somewhat questioned by the fact that tau knockout mice appear phenotypically normal, probably due to compensatory mechanisms by other microtubule-associated proteins (Dawson et al., 2001; Harada et al., 1994).

Amyloid aggregates such as Aβ and α-synuclein oligomers and fibrils have been widely shown to be toxic *in vitro* and *in vivo*. Together with the fact that the number of NFTs in Alzheimer's disease correlates with the degree of cognitive impairment (Arriagada et al., 1992) this suggests that tau aggregates are likely to be directly neurotoxic. The toxicity of tau aggregates has been shown in several cell culture models (Bandyopadhyay et al., 2007; Khlistunova et al., 2006). Intracellular NFTs could be toxic due to their large size, thereby disrupting cell function and axonal transport. Furthermore, tangles might sequester more tau proteins, thereby exacerbating the loss-of-function effects, or other proteins important for cell viability (Ballatore et al., 2007). However, as with Aβ and α-synuclein aggregates, recent studies suggest that the most toxic species might not be the end stage NFTs, but early oligomeric aggregation intermediates (Kayed & Jackson, 2009; Maeda et al., 2007). A mouse model of tauopathy was discovered to exhibit synapse loss and microgliosis that preceded the formation of NFTs (Yoshiyama et al., 2007). A more recent study showed that caspase activation precedes NFT formation in another mouse tauopathy model (de Calignon et al., 2010). Furthermore, subcortical stereotactic injection of tau oligomers into wild-type mice leads to memory impairment and synaptic dysfunction (Lasagna-Reeves et al., 2011).

The loss-of function and gain-of-function models of tau-mediated neurodegeneration are not exclusive, and it is likely that neuronal impairment and cell death are the result of both mechanisms. However, while much progress has been made into elucidating these mechanisms, the link between tau misfolding and aggregation on the one hand and neurodegeneration on the other hand remains largely elusive.

3. From tangles to gene

3.1 Alzheimer's disease and the beginnings of tau research

In 1907, Alois Alzheimer, a German psychiatrist and neuropathologist, published his historic case report "*Über eine eigenartige Erkrankung der Hirnrinde*" (about a peculiar disease of the cerebral cortex). In this report, Alzheimer described the case of a 51-old woman suffering from progressive memory loss, personality changes and impaired language ability. Less than five years after the onset of disease, the woman died and Alzheimer performed post-mortem analysis of her brain. Using the silver staining method by Bielschowsky, the psychiatrist was able to detect two pathological features in the patient's brain: a "peculiar matter in the cortex" as well as "tangled bundles" of fibrils on the insides of neuronal cells (Strassnig & Ganguli, 2005). However, almost 80 years elapsed before the molecular compositions of these two deposits were discovered: While the extracellular plaques found in the cortex are composed of Aβ peptide, the intracellular tangled bundles, now known as neurofibrillary tangles (NFTs), primarily consist of tau protein (Grundke-Iqbal et al., 1986; Masters et al., 1985). This progressive disorder of the central nervous system would eventually be given the name Alzheimer's disease (AD). To date, Alzheimer's disease is the most common neurodegenerative disorder worldwide, with almost 27 million people affected in 2006, and case numbers expected to quadruple by 2050 (Brookmeyer et al., 2007).

According to the widely accepted amyloid cascade hypothesis, overproduction and aggregation of amyloid-β (Aβ) is the central trigger in the pathogenesis of AD. Aβ peptides are 40 or 42 amino acid-long cleavage products of the transmembrane protein APP, whose function remains unknown to this day. In the amyloid cascade hypothesis, aggregation of tau proteins into NFTs is considered a secondary downstream event, triggered by Aβ aggregation. This view is supported by genetic evidence, which shows linkage of mutations in APP with FAD, whereas no genetic link between *MAPT* and Alzheimer's disease has been described so far. Furthermore, it has been shown that overproduction of Aβ induces increased tau phosphorylation and that cerebral injection of Aβ fibrils exacerbates the formation of tangles in a tau transgenic mouse model (Gotz et al., 2001b; Wang et al., 2006).

The evidence supporting the amyloid cascade hypothesis was so great that some scientists were sceptical whether tau pathology in AD played a role in pathogenesis or whether the observed neurofibrillary tangles represented a mere epiphenomenon of the disease. Several studies, however, have implicated an important role of tau in Alzheimer's disease pathogenesis. It has been shown that the number of NFTs, but not of plaques, can be correlated with severity of the disease (Arriagada et al., 1992). Furthermore, experiments have suggested that tau is required for Aβ-induced toxicity, as cultured hippocampal cells from a tau knockout mouse are not susceptible to Aβ-induced neurodegeneration, and for Aβ-induced impairment of hippocampal long-term potentiation (Rapoport et al., 2002; Shipton et al., 2011). These results corroborate the amyloid hypothesis, placing tau as a downstream player of amyloid-β in AD, while at the same time underlining the central role of the microtubule-binding proteins.

The last 25 years since the identification of tau as the major component of PHFs have not only led to a new understanding of the importance of tau in Alzheimer's disease. In fact, it is becoming increasingly clear that tau is a major player in many neurodegenerative diseases. Three discoveries have paved the way for this shift of paradigm: 1) A group of sporadic neurodegenerative diseases exist displaying tau tangle pathology in the absence of Aβ plaques, such as corticobasal degeneration and progressive supranuclear palsy. All diseases exhibiting tau pathology including AD are now collectively referred to as *tauopathies* (Table 1). 2) Mutations in the *MAPT* gene are associated with a familial neurodegenerative tauopathy termed frontotemporal dementia with parkinsonism linked to chromosome 17 (FTDP-17). 3) Association studies have pulled out *MAPT* as an important risk factor in Parkinson's disease, the second most prevalent neurodegenerative disease worldwide. In the following sections, we will discuss these findings in more detail.

3.2 Sporadic tauopathies

While Alzheimer's disease is characterised by the presence of both tau deposits and amyloid plaques, several other tauopathies have been described with tau pathology in the absence of other forms of fibrillary deposits (Table 1). Three such neurodegenerative disorders are corticobasal degeneration, progressive supranuclear palsy and Pick's disease. Due to their neuropathological and phenotypical overlaps, these diseases are now grouped as frontotemporal dementias.

Progressive supranuclear palsy (PSP) is a rare neurodegenerative disorder with a prevalence of ca. 6 per 100,000. Clinically, cases of PSP typically present with levodopa-unresponsive parkinsonism with prominent postural instability, supranuclear gaze palsy, speech difficulties, depression and mild dementia. The affected brain regions are typically neurons and glial cells in the basal ganglia (most notably globus pallidus and substantia nigra), diencephalon, brain stem and spinal cord. The fibrillary inclusions found in PSP brains predominantly consist of 4R isoforms in the form of straight filaments (Dickson et al., 2007). This is in stark contrast to AD, where NFTs are composed of equimolar ratios of 3R and 4R isoforms in the form of paired helical filaments.

Tauopathies
Alzheimer' disease *(a)*
Amyotrophic lateral sclerosis/parkinsonism-dementia complex *(b)*
Argyrophilic grain dementia *(b)*
Creutzfeld-Jacob disease *(a)*
Dementia pugilistica *(a)*
Diffuse neurofibrillary tangles with calcification *(b)*
Down's syndrome *(a)*
Frontotemporal dementia with parkinsonism linked to chromosome 17 *(b)*
Gerstmann-Sträussler-Scheinker disease *(a)*
Hallervorden-Spatz disease *(c)*
Multiple system atrophy *(c)*
Niemann-Pick disease, type C
Pick's disease *(b)*
Postencephalitic parkinsonism
Prion protein cerebral amyloid angiopathy *(a)*
Progressive subcortical gliosis *(b)*
Progressive supranuclear palsy *(b)*
Subacute sclerosing panencephalitis
Tangle-only/tangle-predominant dementia *(b)*

Table 1. Neurodegenerative tauopathies. (a) Tauopathies with amyloid deposits, (b) neurofibrillary lesions most predominant, (c) tauopathies with predominant synuclein-positive lesions

Another sporadic tauopathy that predominantly shows 4R pathology is corticobasal degeneration (CBD), but in contrast to PSP, NFTs are primarily composed of twisted filaments. The cardinal symptoms are similar to those of PSP, but typically include cortical features such as myoclonus and lack vertical gaze palsy. Whereas in PSP the affected brain regions are predominantly hindbrain structures, forebrain regions including the cerebral cortex show atropy in CBD (Kouri et al., 2011; Mahapatra et al., 2004). Due to their overlapping pathology and symptoms, there is a widespread opinion that PSP and CBD might in fact represent two different ends of a disease spectrum that is caused by the accumulation of 4R tau isoforms.

In contrast to both CBD and PSP, Pick's disease is classified as a 3R tauopathy. The disease stems from frontotemporal lobar and limbic atrophy and histologically is characterised by the appearance of deposits called Pick bodies. The symptoms correspond to a cognitive phenotype, with progressive dementia and personality changes such as obsessive-compulsive disorder, apathy and frontal disinhibition. A motor phenotype is usually absent (Buee et al., 2000; Mahapatra et al., 2004).

3.3 Frontotemporal dementia with parkinsonism linked to chromosome 17

Frontotemporal dementias (FTD) are a heterogeneous group of neurodegenerative diseases characterised by progressive dementia due to atrophy of the frontal and temporal lobes. FTD is one of the most common forms of dementia besides Alzheimer's disease. While the majority of cases are thought to occur sporadically, familial cases of the disease were described as far back as 1939 (Gasparini et al., 2007). In 1994, a familial case of dementia with parkinsonism was described. The disease was termed disinhibition-dementia-parkinsonism-amyotrophy complex and was linked to a locus on chromosome 17q21-22 (Wilhelmsen et al., 1994). Subsequently, other families with hereditary frontotemporal dementia-parkinsonism syndromes were also assigned this locus (Baker et al., 1997; Froelich et al., 1997). In 1996, the term frontotemporal dementia with parkinsonism linked to chromosome 17 (FTDP-17) was coined to describe the two major symptoms associated with the rare familial disease (Foster et al., 1997). As it was already known at that time that the *MAPT* gene was located on chromosome 17q21 and that the product of this gene, tau protein, was associated with AD, another neurodegenerative dementia, it was speculated that aberrations in the *MAPT* gene could be associated with FTDP-17. In 1998, the first mutations in the *MAPT* gene were identified in association with FTDP-17 (Hutton et al., 1998; Poorkaj et al., 1998; Spillantini et al., 1998), providing the ultimate demonstration of a causative role of tau in the onset of neurodegeneration. To date, 41 *MAPT* mutations in over 100 families have been described.

FTDP-17 is a very rare neurodegenerative disease transmitted in an autosomal-dominant inheritance pattern and showing high penetrance (>95%). The age of onset of the disease is usually between 25 - 65 years of age and the duration from the onset of the first symptoms to death varies between 3 - 10 years (Boeve & Hutton, 2008). The mutation R406W is an exception, as it is associated with a slower disease progression (van Swieten et al., 1999). The symptoms associated with FTDP-17 are various. Patients usually present either a dementia predominant or a parkinsonism predominant phenotype. The range of symptoms associated can be grouped into three categories: personality changes, motor function impairment and cognitive decline. The list of changes in personality of affected individuals is long and includes disinhibition, apathy, aggressive behaviour, obsessive-compulsive behaviour, hyper-religiosity, bluntness and hyperorality. Paranoia and hallucinations can lead to an initial misdiagnosis as a psychiatric disorder. Cognitive dysfunctions are manifested as memory impairment, loss of orientation and judgement and language difficulties progressing to mutism. The cardinal symptoms associated with parkinsonism are rigidity, bradykinesia, postural instability and resting tremor, though the latter symptom is frequently absent. In contrast to Parkinson's disease, motor symptoms do not or only slightly improve with levodopa treatment (Basun et al., 1997; Wilhelmsen et al., 1994; Wszolek et al., 2006). Histologically, FTDP-17 is characterised by atrophy of the frontal and temporal lobes, and sometimes subcortical nuclei, amygdala and brainstem, with gliosis and spongiosis. Tau deposits can appear in neurons or in neurons and glial cells. The morphology of these deposits can vary considerable depending on patient and mutation and can appear either as neurofibrillary tangles, Pick bodies or diffuse (Tsuboi, 2006).

3.4 *MAPT* mutations in FTDP-17

Mutations in the *MAPT* gene encompass intronic mutations and missense, deletion and silent mutations in the coding regions (Table 2). The majority of mutations known to cause FTDP-17 are found in the latter category. The effects of mutations can be grouped into two categories: mutations that alter the alternative splicing of primary tau mRNA transcripts or/and have an effect on tau protein. The majority of mutations affect either the mRNA or the protein level, but a few mutations exert their effects on both splicing and protein function. The type of effect seen depends both on the location and the type of mutation. The most common mutations are the missense mutation P301L, which has been observed in 25 families, and the intronic mutation +16, described in 22 families (Rademakers et al., 2004).

All coding region mutations exert their effects on the physicochemical properties of tau protein. The majority of mutations cluster in exons 9 - 12, the microtubule-binding domain, especially in the alternatively spliced exon 10. The only known mutations outside the microtubule-binding domain have been found in exons 1 (R5H and R5L) and 13 (G389R, R406W and T427M). While most mutations in these exons as well as exons 9, 11 and 12 affect all tau isoforms, only 4R tau is affected by mutations in exon 10 (Gasparini et al., 2007). The primary mechanism by which missense and deletion mutations in the coding regions alter the properties of tau protein is by decreasing affinity for microtubules. This can be shown by an *in vitro* assay monitoring microtubule assembly (Hong et al., 1998). Exceptions are the S305N mutation in exon 10 and Q336R in exon 12, which have been shown to increase microtubule assembly (Hasegawa et al., 1999; Pickering-Brown et al., 2004). Reduced affinity of tau for microtubule-binding sites could lead to a destabilisation of microtubules and, as a result, impaired neuron morphology, axonal transport and neurotransmitter release. Furthermore, a low binding affinity could result in a net increase of free soluble tau, thereby reaching the critical concentration required to trigger a nucleation-dependent polymerisation reaction. Besides their effect on microtubule binding, some mutations in the coding regions result in an increased propensity to heparin or arachidonic acid-induced self-aggregation *in vitro*. Some mutations have an effect on specific tau isoforms only. Mutations in exon 10 such as ΔK280, N296H, P301S and P301L, can only increase aggregation of 4R tau. The missense mutation I260V in exon 9 has the same effect, while K257T only increases tau fibril formation in 3R isoforms (Grover et al., 2003; Rizzini et al., 2000).

All intronic mutations described so far lie in the introns 9 and 10, surrounding the alternatively spliced exon 10. These intronic mutations as well as several coding region mutations, most of them found in exon 10, have an effect on alternative splicing of exon 10, thereby shifting the ratio of 3R to 4R tau. In the healthy adult human CNS, the ratio of 3R to 4R tau is approximately equimolar (Hong et al., 1998). Most intronic mutations as well many of the coding region mutations in exon 10 lead to an increase of exon 10 inclusion, thereby shifting the ratio of tau isoforms towards 4R (Table 2). The deletion ΔK280 as well as the intronic +19 mutation are exceptions, as they have been shown to decrease exon 10 splicing-in *in vitro* (D'Souza et al., 1999; Stanford et al., 2003). The fact that an imbalance in the ratio between 3R and 4R isoforms is sufficient to cause neurodegeneration suggests that maintaining this ratio is important for maintaining normal CNS function. The reason why a

Region	Mutation	Exon 10 inclusion	Microtubule assembly	Tau filament formation
Exon 1	R5H	no effect	↓	↑
Exon 1	R5L	no effect	↓	↑
Exon 9	K257T	no effect	↓	3R ↑
Exon 9	I260V	no effect	4R ↓	4R ↑
Exon 9	L266V	↑	↓	4R ↑
Exon 9	G272V	ND	↓	↑
Exon 10	N279K	↑	no effect	ND
Exon 10	ΔK280	↓	4R ↓	4R ↑
Exon 10	L284L	↑	no effect	no effect
Exon 10	ΔN296	↑	4R ↓	4R ↑
Exon 10	N296H	↑	4R ↓	4R ↑
Exon 10	N296N	↑	no effect	no effect
Exon 10	P301L	no effect	4R ↓	4R ↑
Exon 10	P301S	no effect	4R ↓	4R ↑
Exon 10	G303V	↑	ND	ND
Exon 10	S305N	↑	4R ↑	ND
Exon 10	S305S	↑	no effect	no effect
Exon 11	L315R	ND	↓	no effect
Exon 11	K317M	ND	ND	ND
Exon 11	S320F	ND	↓	ND
Exon 12	G335V	ND	↓	↑
Exon 12	Q336R	ND	↑	↑
Exon 12	V337M	ND	↓	↑
Exon 12	E342V	↑	ND	ND
Exon 12	S352L	ND	↓	↑
Exon 12	S356T	ND	ND	ND
Exon 12	K369I	ND	↓	altered
Exon 13	G389R	ND	↓	ND
Exon 13	R406W	ND	↓	conflicting
Exon 13	T427M	ND	ND	ND
Intron 9	IVS9-10	↑	no effect	no effect
Intron 10	ISV10+3	↑	no effect	no effect
Intron 10	ISV10+11	↑	no effect	no effect
Intron 10	ISV10+12	↑	no effect	no effect
Intron 10	ISV10+13	↑	no effect	no effect
Intron 10	ISV10+14	↑	no effect	no effect
Intron 10	ISV10+16	↑	no effect	no effect
Intron 10	ISV10+19	↓	no effect	no effect

Table 2. *MAPT* mutations found in FTDP-17 and their effects on exon 10 inclusion, microtubule assembly and tau filament formation. ↑ = increased, ↓ = decreased, ND = not determined

shift of isoform ratio has such detrimental effects remains unclear. Tau containing four repeats has been shown to have a greater affinity towards microtubules and promote a faster assembly of microtubules than 3R isoforms (Goedert & Jakes, 1990). Furthermore, *in vitro* studies have indicated that 4R tau is more effective at microtubule stabilisation than 3R tau, by decreasing both the rate and the overall length of shortening of microtubules (Panda et al., 2003). These results suggest that an equimolar ratio of three- and four-repeat tau might be needed to maintain a balance between microtubule stability and plasticity and thereby ensure proper neuron function and morphology. Furthermore, it is conceivable that an overproduction of 4R tau leads to an increased concentration of unbound 4R tau in the cytosol, thereby facilitating the formation of four-repeat containing tau aggregates. However, this proposed model possibly requires the existence of two different binding sites on microtubules for 3R and 4R isoforms (Goode et al., 2000). Tau aggregation assays *in vitro* have furthermore shown that 3R tau isoforms directly inhibit the assembly of 4R tau into filaments, suggesting that restoring an equimolar tau isoform ratio might have therapeutic implications in tauopathies (Adams et al., 2010).

The alternative splicing of exon 10 is regulated by mRNA splice sites as well as by both exonic and intronic regulatory sequences. Alterations of the splice site and regulatory sequences are responsible for dysregulated inclusion of exon 10 in the intronic and several coding region mutations. Like most alternatively spliced exons, exon 10 contains a weak 5′ splice site, leading to a weak interaction with the U1 snRNP. This site is strengthened by the coding region mutations S305N/S and the intronic mutation +3, which results in increased exon 10 splicing (Hutton et al., 1998; Spillantini et al., 1998; Stanford et al., 2000). Notably, a large part of exon 10 is directly involved in splicing regulation, as it harbours several exonic splicing enhancers and a silencer. Exon splicing enhancers are elements that increase the inclusion of an alternatively spliced exon, while an exon splicing silencer decreases inclusion. Likewise, intronic sequences that increase or decrease splicing are termed intron splicing enhancers or silencers (D'Souza & Schellenberg, 2005). Three exon splice enhancer (a SC35-like enhancer, a polypurine enhancer PPE and a AC-rich element ACE) are located at the 5' end of exon 10, followed by an exon splicing silencer element and another ESE at the 3' end of the exon (D'Souza & Schellenberg, 2005). While the mutation N279K strengthens the PPE, thereby increasing exon 10 inclusion, the opposite result is achieved through the lysine deletion at position 280. The silent mutation L284L has been shown to lie close to and affect the ACE enhancer (D'Souza et al., 1999; D'Souza & Schellenberg, 2005). The mutations N296H and N296N are thought to enhance exon 10 inclusion by converting a silencer to an enhancer sequence (D'Souza & Schellenberg, 2000).

The regulation of exon 10 splicing through intronic sequences is explained by two alternative models: The stem-loop theory proposes that a secondary stem loop structure blocks binding of U1 snRNP to the 5' splice site. The intronic mutations +10, +11, +12, +13, +14 and +16 disrupt the stem loop in this model, thereby increasing exon 10 splicing (Gasparini et al., 2007; Hutton et al., 1998; Spillantini et al., 1998). The alternative linear sequence theory suggests that three sequences in the intron following exon 10 modulate splicing: an intron splicing silencer and an intron splicing modulator, which are located downstream of the 5' splicing site. In this model, protein regulators bind to these sites; silencing of splicing via the splicing silencer element is counterbalanced by a splicing modulator. Mutations in the intron are thought to disrupt the interactions of the splicing silencer element with its bound factors. The +19 mutation is an exception, as it lies within the intron splicing modulator sequence and disrupts its repression of the splicing silencer (D'Souza et al., 1999; D'Souza & Schellenberg, 2000).

Several coding region mutations (L266V, ΔK280, ΔN296, N296H and S305N) exert their effects both on the mRNA splicing and on the protein level. The deletion mutations as well as the missense mutations L266V and N296H decrease microtubule assembly *in vitro*, while S305N leads to an enhanced assembly (D'Souza et al., 1999; Hasegawa et al., 1999; Hogg et al., 2003; Yoshida et al., 2002). All these mutations enhance inclusion of exon 10, except ΔK280. While this mutation might result in an increased production of 3R tau, it also strongly decreases the affinity for microtubules and enhances tau polymerisation *in vitro* (D'Souza et al., 1999).

In conclusion, mutations in the tau gene lead to a pathological aggregation of tau protein through several mechanisms: 1) by decreasing the affinity of tau for microtubules, 2) by enhancing self-aggregation of tau into fibrils and 3) by altering the ratio of 3R and 4R isoforms on the mRNA level. Most mutations exert their effects through more than one of these mechanisms and a few mutations have been shown to affect tau on all three levels.

Establishing phenotype-genotype relationships for *MAPT* mutations has proven to be difficult. Patients harbouring the same mutation, even within the same family, can present with very different clinical symptoms. Assessment of nine patients harbouring the P301S mutation showed a frontotemporal dementia predominant phenotype in three, and a parkinsonism predominant phenotype in six individuals (Baba et al., 2007). The missense mutation N279K on the other hand results in similar parkinsonism-predominant clinical symptoms with dementia even between affected individuals with different ethnic backgrounds (Arima et al., 2000; Delisle et al., 1999; Soliveri et al., 2003). The variability in clinical phenotypes of patients harbouring the same mutation might be the result of environmental factors, interaction with other genes or the interaction between tau mutation and tau haplotype. In contrast to the clinical phenotype, mutations and their locations can be correlated to the type of tau tangle pathology, isoform distribution and affected cell types. Missense and deletion mutations in exon 10 and intronic mutations in the down-stream intron result in tau pathology with a twisted ribbon morphology that affect both neuronal and glial cells. The deposits are predominantly - or in the case of exon 10 coding region mutations solely - composed of 4R isoforms. Mutations in coding regions outside of exon 10 present neuronal tau pathology with glial cells unaffected. The tau inclusions are formed by filaments that are composed of both 3R and 4R isoforms and that resemble the PHFs and SFs found in Alzheimer's disease or show twisted ribbon morphology (Gasparini et al., 2007; Goedert, 2005). However, the mutation K257T in exon 9 leads to the deposition of tangles predominantly composed of 3R tau species (Rizzini et al., 2000).

3.5 Tau as a genetic risk factor for neurodegenerative diseases

Even before the description of the first *MAPT* mutations in familial cases of frontotemporal dementia, an association between progressive supranuclear palsy and the *MAPT* gene was identified: A dinucleotide TG repeat allele termed A0 in intron 9 was shown to be overrepresented in patients with PSP compared to healthy controls (Conrad et al., 1997). Subsequently, genetic analysis revealed eight single nucleotide polymorphisms in exons 1, 2, 3 and 9 that were in complete linkage disequilibrium with each other and the A0 allele (Baker et al., 1999). This region of disequilibrium spans the entire *MAPT* locus and the resulting two haplotypes are termed H1 and H2. In addition to the eight SNPs, a 238 bp deletion in intron 9 was found to be inherited as part of the H2 haplotype. This deletion is now frequently used for haplotype assessment in *MAPT* association studies. The most common allele H1 and genotype H1/H1 were shown to be significantly overrepresented in PSP compared to healthy controls (Baker et al., 1999). In Caucasians, the frequency of the H1 haplotype is about 78% in healthy controls compared to ca 94% in PSP. The genotype H2/H2 seems to be protective against PSP, as no cases with that genotype were described. Interestingly, the H2 haplotype is only found in Caucasians and is absent in Asian and Native American populations (Evans et al., 2004).

Subsequently, the H1 haplotype was further expanded to include the promoter region of *MAPT* and now spans a region of ~1.8Mb in complete linkage disequilibrium (de Silva et al., 2001; Pittman et al., 2004). This extended haplotype contains several genes in addition to *MAPT*, including *CRHR1* (corticotrophin-releasing hormone receptor 1), *NSF* (N-ethylmaleimide sensitive factor), *IMP5* (intramembrane protease 5), *WNT3* and *STH* (saitohin), a gene nested in the intron 9 of *MAPT* (Conrad et al., 2002; Pittman et al., 2004). A ~900kb segment of the H2 haplotype including *MAPT* has been found to be inverted in respect to H1. Subsequently, the H1 haplotype was further divided into sub-haplotypes with SNPs that show variation only in the H1 haplotype and the association of these sub-haplotypes with PSP and CBD was investigated. One subhaplotype, termed H1c, was shown to be highly associated with PSP and CBD in case-control cohorts (Pittman et al., 2005).

Shortly after the association between the H1 haplotype and PSP was discovered, association studies showed that H1 was also overrepresented in the sporadic tauopathy CBD (Di Maria et al., 2000; Houlden et al., 2001). Many other association studies have been performed to investigate a possible association between *MAPT* haplotypes and other sporadic tauopathies, most notably Alzheimer's disease. However, genetic analyses showed no association between AD and *MAPT* (Abraham et al., 2009; Baker et al., 2000; Mukherjee et al., 2007). Conversely, studies showed a significant association of the *MAPT* locus with amyotrophic lateral sclerosis and parkinsonism dementia complex of Guam (ALS-G-PDC-G) (Poorkaj et al., 2001; Sundar et al., 2007).

The mechanisms underlying the association of the H1 haplotype with sporadic tauopathies is not completely clear. It has been shown that while total mRNA transcript levels are comparable between H1 and H2 haplotype carriers, the H1 haplotype expresses significantly higher levels of exon 10-containing mRNA compared to H2 in the globus pallidus and frontal cortex, two brain regions affected by neurodegeneration in tauopathy (Caffrey et al., 2006), suggesting that a subtle increase of 10^{+} transcripts confers an increased susceptibility to neurodegeneration. Furthermore, post-mortem analysis of H1/H2 heterozygous brain tissue revealed that the neuroprotective haplotype H2 expresses significantly higher levels of transcripts containing exons 2 and 3 ($2^{+}3^{+}$) in comparison to H1 (Caffrey et al., 2008).

In recent years, gene and genome-wide association studies have been performed to investigate an association between *MAPT* and Parkinson's disease (PD). Several studies have shown an overrepresentation of the H1 haplotype in PD compared to controls (Healy et al., 2004; Simon-Sanchez et al., 2009). The association of tau with sporadic PD is puzzling insofar as it is a neurodegenerative disease that is not classified as a tauopathy due to the absence of NFTs in the majority of patients. The role of tau in the disease pathogenesis of PD is unknown. However, FTDP-17, CBD and PSP are parkinsonism-plus-syndromes, showing a motor phenotype that overlaps with PD. In rare instances, localisation of tau in Lewy bodies, the defining pathological hallmark of PD, has been described (Arima et al., 1999). Furthermore, it has been shown that tau binds α-synuclein and that α-synuclein stimulates protein kinase A to phosphorylate tau protein (Jensen et al., 1999). *In vitro* aggregation assays have shown that co-incubation of tau and α-synuclein promotes the aggregation of both protein species (Giasson et al., 2003). A recent association study confirmed the genetic link between *MAPT* and PD and showed a significantly higher expression of 4R tau in PD brains compared to controls (Tobin et al., 2008). While the mechanism by which tau influences PD pathogenesis remains unclear, tau protein has emerged as the central player in many neurodegenerative diseases. The assumption that tau protein or at least some of its isoforms might be involved in modulating the detrimental effects of α-synuclein is thus not far-fetched.

4. Animal models of tauopathy

The discovery that mutations in tau are sufficient to cause neurodegeneration prompted an increased desire to understand the functional relationship between tau, tangles and cell death in the CNS. For this purpose, transgenic animals have been created to model the histopathological and clinical phenotypes observed in tauopathies.

4.1 Mouse models expressing one wild-type tau isoform

The first transgenic mouse models of human tauopathy were generated before *MAPT* mutations were shown to cause the rare familial neurodegenerative disorder FTDP-17. Thus, early models were created by introducing cDNA under the regulation of different promoters into the mouse genome to overexpress human wild-type tau (Gotz et al., 1995; Ishihara et al., 1999). In the first published model, the longest human tau isoform was expressed under the control of the Thy-1 promoter (Gotz et al., 1995). The resulting mouse showed localisation of human tau in neuron soma, axons and dendrites. While NFTs were not present, tau was found to be phosphorylated at sites that were previously shown to be hyperphosphorylated in AD. Other models expressing single tau isoforms under the control of different promoters soon followed. Characterisation of a mouse expressing the shortest human tau isoform driven by the mouse prion protein promoter (MoPrP) revealed insoluble hyperphosphorylated tau and argyrophilic intraneuronal inclusions at a young age, which matured into PHFs in old mice. These mice also showed signs of axonal degeneration (Ishihara et al., 1999; Ishihara et al., 2001). This mouse model was remarkable insofar as it was the first transgenic rodent to display an age-dependent accumulation of hyperphosphorylated tau and assembly into *bona fide* fibrillary tau deposits as well as axonal degeneration. However, while being a valuable effort to elucidate the mechanisms of neurofibrillary tangle formation and tau-mediated neurodegeneration, wild-type transgenic mouse models of tauopathy generated by placing tau cDNA under the control of high-expression promoters presented several shortcomings: 1.) Formation of neurofibrillary tangles was rarely observed and only at an advanced age. Furthermore, NFT localisation and axon degeneration was not necessarily reflecting human tauopathies, as the tangles were detected in abundance in spinal cord neurons (Ishihara et al., 2001). 2.) The phenotype of the mouse models was heavily dependent on the promoter chosen to drive expression. 3.) The models allowed only expression of one tau isoform, whereas six isoforms are found in the adult human CNS. 4.) Confounding effects caused by the co-existence of both human and murine tau could not be excluded. Subsequent mouse models of tauopathy were thus designed to address all of these concerns.

4.2 Mouse models expressing one mutant tau isoform

After the discovery of *MAPT* mutations and their causative role in familial neurodegenerative disease and findings that mere overexpression of tau did not yield a phenotype that accurately resembled the neuropathological and behavioural changes found in human tauopathies, efforts were focused on generating mouse models expressing mutant human tau. As with the wild-type tau models, animals were created by inserting cDNA constructs under the control of a suitable promoter into the mouse genome, resulting in the expression of one mutant tau isoform harbouring mutations found in FTDP-17. Since most *MAPT* mutations are found in the exons encoding the microtubule-binding domain, most notably exon 10, research has also been focused on transgenic mouse models harbouring mutations in this domain. In 2000, the first mutant tau mouse model (termed JNPL3) was reported. The animals expressed the 4R tau isoform lacking the two N-terminal domains (2-3-10^{+}) with the missense mutation P301L, the most common observed coding region mutation in FTDP-17, under the mouse prion promoter (Lewis et al., 2000). Neurofibrillary tangles were observed in the diencephalon, brain stem, cerebellar nuclei and spinal cord and an even wider distribution of pre-tangle tau species was observed. Areas with high NFT load displayed gliosis. The spinal cord motor neurons showed axonal degeneration, leading to a progressive motor deficit. The widespread pathology was especially remarkable as the expression level of the transcript was low in comparison to previously described wild-type models, indicating that tau mutations confer great pathogenicity to the protein (Lewis et al., 2000).

In another study, mice harbouring the P301L mutation in the longest tau isoform under the regulation of the promoter Thy1.2 were compared to mice expressing the wild-type longest human isoform at comparable expression levels (Terwel et al., 2005). While the wild-type tau mice lived a normal lifespan, they displayed axonopathy in the brain and spinal cord and a severe motor phenotype in beam walk and accelerated rotarod tests starting at a young age (6-8 weeks). No tau aggregates were observed in these mice. The P301L mutant transgenic mice on the other hand developed NFTs from about 6 months onwards, but showed no axonopathy and only minor motor function impairment; however, all mice died before the age of 13 months (Terwel et al., 2005). These two mouse lines thus gave an early indication that NFTs might not be the toxic, disease-causing tau species but that formation of late-stage tangles and axonal degeneration and cell death might be distinct, albeit overlapping, events.

Comparison of the two described P301L tau mouse models again highlights that choice of promoter and expressed tau isoform has a significant influence on the phenotype of the resulting transgenic animal. As the missense mutation P301L is the most common mutation, many other cDNA-based mutant mouse models have been created (Gotz et al., 2001a; Higuchi et al., 2005; Murakami et al., 2006). Apart from the P301L mutation, two other FTDP-17 mutations in exon 10 have been used to create classic cDNA models, the missense mutations N279K and P301S (Allen et al., 2002; Taniguchi et al., 2005). The N279K mutation was shown to cause hyperactivity and cognitive deficits in the absence of discernible NFTs, suggesting, as other studies before, that formation of NFTs might be a late event and that pre-NFT tau species might cause the behavioural phenotype (Taniguchi et al., 2005). The 4R P301S model (driven by the Thy1 promoter) on the other hand displayed abundant tau filaments, most notably in the brain stem and spinal cord, but also the hippocampus and cortex. At 5 - 6 months the animals developed paraparesis and widespread brain and spinal cord degeneration (Allen et al., 2002).

Outside of exon 10, research has focused on coding region mutations in exon 9 (G272V), exon 11 (V337M), exon 12 (K369I) and exon 13 (R406W). The G272V model presented filament formation in oligodendrocytes, a rare instant of glial tau pathology, although the animals did not develop any overt neurological deficits (Gotz et al., 2001c). The mutation V337M in a 4R tau isoform, under the regulation of the PDGF-β promoter, led to the formation of filamentous tau aggregates and neurodegeneration in the hippocampus. The behavioural phenotype was characterised by an inability to experience a state of fear in response to environmental stimuli (Tanemura et al., 2002). Another mouse model was based on the K369I mutation in exon 12, controlled by the murine Thy1.2 promoter. The mice exhibited a progressive histopathology with an age-dependent increase in tau inclusions as well as an early-onset motor phenotype characterised by the classical parkinsonism signs tremor, bradykinesia, postural instability and gait abnormalities, possibly due to the transgene being expressed in the substantia nigra (Ittner et al., 2008).

Several mouse lines have been created harbouring 4R human tau with the R406W mutation in exon 13 (Ikeda et al., 2005; Tatebayashi et al., 2002; Zhang et al., 2004). All models developed age-dependent neuronal accumulation of hyperphosphorylated tau and NFTs composed of straight, not paired helical, filaments. Mutant tau expressed under the control of the hamster prion promoter led to formation of tau inclusions in the hippocampus, amygdala, neocortex, cerebellum and spinal cord and the transgenic animals developed motor impairment and progressive memory loss (Ikeda et al., 2005). Expression of R406W tau under the mouse prion promoter showed a similar pattern of NFT-like pathology excepting the amygdala; however, no behavioural analysis was reported (Zhang et al., 2004). Interestingly, in mouse models expression of tau under regulation of the forebrain-specific CaMKII promoter, tau was barely detected in the spinal cord, resembling human expression, where tau gene expression is weak in the spinal cord. The transgenic mice showed memory impairment, but no motor deficit, mirroring the human condition, in which R406W is associated with an AD-like phenotype. This result is probably due to the low expression of tau in spinal cord neurons, which excludes a confounding effect of the behavioural phenotype due to neurogenic muscle atrophy (Tatebayashi et al., 2002).

The use of cDNA-based transgenes harbouring tau mutations found in FTDP-17 marked an important step in creating a model that resembles human condition. The mutant models overwhelmingly showed accumulation of hyperphosphorylated tau and formation on NFT-like inclusions. Furthermore, several lines were behaviourally characterised and displayed motor or cognitive deficits or both. The use of these mouse models gave an early indication that NFTs as the final stage of tau aggregate formation might not be the tau species responsible for neurodegeneration and associated memory deficits. However, the models still had several drawbacks, most notably the variability of the resulting phenotype depending on the promoter chosen and the fact that only a single isoform was expressed.

4.3 Other cDNA-based mouse models

Following the generation of mouse models expressing tau with mutations found in FTDP-17, several transgenic lines were created expressing human tau harbouring two tau mutations (G272V+P301S; K257T+P301S) or three mutations (G272V+P301L+R406W) (Lim et al., 2001; Rosenmann et al., 2008; Schindowski et al., 2006). Especially noteworthy is the K257T+P301S mutant model by Rosenmann et al., as transgene expression in this mouse line is driven by a rat genomic tau promoter, which shares 75% sequence similarity with the mouse tau promoter (Rosenmann et al., 2008). The resulting mice displayed formation of neurofibrillary tangles in hippocampus, cortex and brain stem. The animals showed spatial memory deficits, signs of anxiety (assessed as excessive defecation) and impaired *in vivo* LTP but no overt motor phenotype.

Other models were created using transgenes driven by inducible promoters. The advantage of these animals over models with constitutive promoters is that the expression of the transgene can be switched on and off. Ramsden et al. created a mouse expressing 4R tau with the mutation P301L under the control of the forebrain-specific CaMKII promoter (Ramsden et al., 2005). This promoter was controlled by the tet-operon response element, which suppresses expression in response to doxocycline. The resulting animal developed age-dependent progression of tau pathology with NFT formation in the neocortex and later in hippocampus and limbic structures. Forebrain atrophy and prominent loss of neurons in the neocortex and hippocampus was accompanied by impairment of spatial memory (Ramsden et al., 2005). Suppression of transgene expression by doxocycline at a young age (2.5 months) halted the progression of tangle pathology in comaprison to untreated animals, though tangle numbers were not reduced. However, the progression of tau pathology became independent of transgene expression at 4 months of age (Santacruz et al., 2005). Long-term suppression of tau expression (4 - 4.5 months) was shown to protect against neuronal loss and brain atrophy. Administration of doxocycline even after 4 months of age, when NFT-progression became independent of tau transgene expression, significantly improved spatial memory (Santacruz et al., 2005). These highly significant results proved earlier speculations that the mechanisms that lead to NFT formation and those that lead to cell death and memory loss are at least partly uncoupled.

While mutations in tau are associated with FTDP-17, there has never been any link between tau mutations and Alzheimer's disease. However, models of AD with mutations found in patients with early-onset AD were overwhelmingly unsucessful in triggering tau pathology. Thus, transgenic models wich combine *APP* and *MAPT* mutations have been created to achieve the reproduction of both neuropathological hallmarks and to better understand the relationship between tau and Aβ in AD. Perhaps the most well-known model of AD was created by Oddo et al., a triple transgenic model (3xTg-AD) harbouring the *MAPT* mutation P301L but also two mutations associated with AD, M146V in *PS1* and the Swedish mutation in *APP* (a double mutation KM670/671NL). The resulting mouse developed both plaque and tangle pathology as well as deficits in LTP (Oddo et al., 2003b). Furthermore, plaque development preceded tangle pathology in these mice, a finding that is consistent with and supporting of the amyloid hypothesis (Oddo et al., 2003a).

4.4 Genomic DNA mouse models

While the introduction of *MAPT* mutations associated with FTDP-17 led to a significant improvement in the capacity of the mouse models to produce NFT pathology and degeneration more closely reflecting the situation in human disease, some of the basic drawbacks remained, such as the dependency of the phenotype displayed by the animals on the promoter chosen, and the restriction to expression of one tau isoform. However, in 2000 Duff et al. introduced a genomic *MAPT* mouse model (Duff et al., 2000). In this model, the whole genomic human *MAPT* locus including its endogenous promoter were introduced into the mouse genome using the PAC transgene technology. The resulting mouse expressed all six human tau isoforms. However, no tangle pathology was observed and mice did not show hindlimb-clasping or spinal cord abnormalities, as often shown by cDNA-based models of tauopathy (Duff et al., 2000). However, as the results might have been confounded by the presence of endogenous mouse tau protein, another genomic *MAPT* mouse model was created by Ansdorfer et al., in which the original mouse created by Duff et al. was backcrossed onto an endogenous mouse *MAPT* knockout background (Andorfer et al., 2003). The animals displayed hyperphosphorylated tau and NFT formation as well as changes in neuronal morphology and a decrease in cortical thickness due to extensive cell death (Andorfer et al., 2005; Andorfer et al., 2003).

4.5 Other models of tauopathy

While rodent models are often the species of choice to reproduce the molecular and cellular pathology of neurodegenerative diseases, the use of models from other branches of the phylogenetic tree can be advantageous. *Caenorhabditis elegans, Drosophila melanogaster* and the zebrafish *Danio rerio* are easily genetically manipulated, have a short generation time, low maintenance costs and can be used for high-throughput screening experiments. Tauopathy models of all of these species have been created displaying key features of tauopathic neurodegenerative disease.

Neuronal expression of wild-type or mutant (P301L and V337M) 4R human tau in a model of *C.elegans* results in a decreased life-span, uncoordinated movement, accumulation of insoluble and phosphorylated tau species with a phosphorylation pattern similar to the pattern of hyperphosphorylation observed in AD and FTDP-17 in humans, progressive axonal degeneration and neuronal loss as well as defective presynaptic cholinergic transmission. While both the wild-type and the mutant transgene resulted in a phenotype, expression of mutant tau led to a more pronounced deterioration (Kraemer et al., 2003).

A study using *Drosophila* models of tauopathy expressing wild-type or mutant (R406W) human tau showed a shortened life-span, vacuolisation, degeneration of cortical cells and phosphorylation of tau at sites found abnormally phosphorylated in tauopathies, but no formation of NFTs (Wittmann et al., 2001). The phenotype was more pronounced in flies expressing mutant tau. Expression of mutant tau in photoreceptor cells triggered an abnormal rough eye phenotype (Wittmann et al., 2001). Co-expression of wild-type human tau and *shaggy*, the *Drosophila* homolog of GSK-3β, however, led to the formation of NFTs in another study, and exacerbated the neurodegenerative phenotype (Jackson et al., 2002).

In a very elegant and sophisticated approach, Paquet et al. generated transgenic zebrafish larvae expressing fluorescently-labelled P301L mutant human tau, allowing *in vivo* imaging of neuronal cell death (Paquet et al., 2009). The model showed tau phosphorylation and tangle formation, neuronal cell death, abnormal motor neuron morphology as well as behavioural deficits. The phenotype occurred rapidly within the first few days of embryonic development, even though zebrafish have a life-span comparable to that of mice under laboratory conditions, marking a big advantage over classic rodent models, which only develop a phenotype after months or even years (Paquet et al., 2009).

5. Outlook

Almost 20 years ago the amyloid hypothesis of Alzheimer's disease was put forward; overwhelming evidence indicates Aβ, the proteolytic cleavage product of APP, as the culprit protein in disease initiation. In the amyloid hypothesis, aggregation of tau into NFTs is a downstream event and for years it was doubted whether tau played any role in disease etiopathology. Since then, however, several lines of evidence have shown that while tau misfolding and aggregation is in all probability not causative of AD, the protein is a fundamental factor in the disease cascade. The findings that tau deposits are found in other neurodegenerative diseases in the absence of amyloid plaques and that mutations in tau are sufficient to cause a familial neurodegenerative dementia and parkinsonism syndrome have added to the heightened interest in tau and its role in neurodegenerative processes.

The association of tau haplotype variants with an increased risk of idiopathic Parkinson's disease have put tau and its encoding gene *MAPT* in the centre of neurodegenerative pathways. Thus, tau is implicated in the two most common neurodegenerative diseases worldwide, Alzheimer's disease and Parkinson's disease, as well as several other rare disorders such as PSP, CBD, FTDP-17, Pick's disease and ALS-G/PDC-G. The association of NFTs with several neurodegenerative diseases, collectively referred to as tauopathies (PD not being classified as a tauopathy, as NFTs are usually, though not necessarily, absent), has highlighted the need for transgenic models of tau-mediated neurodegenerative disease.

The first mouse models of tauopathy were created before mutations in *MAPT* were found to cause FTDP-17 and were based on overexpression of either 3R or 4R human wild-type tau. While these models reproduced some key features of tauopathies such as hyperphosphorylation of tau as well as motor deficits, discernible NFT formation was usually not observed or at an advanced age only. However, this changed with the generation of mouse models expressing mutant human tau. Mice harbouring mutations in the tau transgene found to cause FTDP-17 in humans show age-dependent formation of NFTs in neuronal and in some instances glial cells. However, several studies indicate that the appearance of NFTs is independent of axonal degeneration, neuronal cell death and motor and cognitive deficits. This is especially surprising as the number of NFTs in the brains of Alzheimer's disease patients correlates well with severity of disease. It is now widely believed that NFTs represent late-stage pathology of tauopathies that might in fact be neuroprotective and that pre-tangle tau species are responsible for tau-mediated neurodegeneration. Further studies are required to shed light onto the role of NFTs in degeneration and cell death.

Early mouse models of tauopathy were limited in their capacity to accurately represent human condition. Most notably, the created animals were cDNA-based models. This approach allowed only expression of one tau isoform, which was heavily dependent on the promoter chosen. Furthermore, in most models tau was heavily expressed in spinal cord neurons, which does not reflect human disease; the associated degeneration and cell death is very likely to be responsible for the regularly observed motor phenotype, whereas the motor deficit in human tauopathies is not caused by degeneration of spinal cord neurons. Those shortcomings were addressed in genomic models of tauopathy, which express all tau isoforms under the regulation of the human endogenous tau promoter. However, only two genomic tau mouse lines have been created so far, expressing wild-type human tau isoforms. In a next step, genomic rodent models of tauopathy with mutant tau will hopefully lead to an improved understanding of the mechanisms underlying tau-mediated neurodegeneration, and accurately represent all key features of human tauopathy in terms of isoform ratios, affected brain areas and cell types and associated motor and cognitive deficits. Other models of tauopathy such as *Drosopila melanogaster* or *Danio rerio* can assist in the investigation of disease mechanisms, as they have been shown to reproduce several aspects of human tauopathic disease in a very short timespan, enabling for example high-throughput screening of potential intervention strategies. This will be especially important as the central role of tau in neurodegenerative processes has led to a heightened interest in tau as a potential therapeutic target, most notably in AD.

Several therapeutic strategies are being investigated for the treatment of tauopathies. Paclitaxel, a microtubule-stabilising agent, has been shown to reverse axonal transport deficits and ameliorate a motor phenotype in a mouse model of tauopathy (Zhang et al., 2005), possibly by rescuing the loss of microtubule integrity caused by tau loss of function. Hyperphosphorylation of tau is considered to be an early event in disease pathogenesis, and inhibition of kinases responsible for tau phosphorylation, notably GSK-3β, which has also been implicated in the processing of APP, is under intense investigation, with several studies in advanced clinical stages. Lithium, which has been shown to inhibit GSK-3β activity and is used for the treatment of bipolar disorder, resulted in lower levels of tau phosphorylation and reduced load of aggregated tau and axonal degeneration in the JNPL3 mouse model (Noble et al., 2005). Furthermore, treatment of a mouse model of AD with a thiadiazolidinone compound reduced tau phosphorylation, decreased amyloid deposition (possibly through decreased processing of APP), protected against neuronal cell death and prevented memory deficits (Sereno et al., 2009).

Transgenic tau mouse models have implicated that NFTs are not the aggregate species responsible for axonal degeneration and cell death, but that earlier aggregation intermediates might be the neurotoxic species. Inhibition of the aggregation pathway or redirection of aggregated species into monomers or off-pathway, non-toxic aggregates could help decrease the load of neurotoxic tau species. Screening of small molecule aggregation inhibitors can be performed in high-throughput fashion *in vitro* by monitoring heparin-induced assembly of tau proteins into well-defined filaments. Several classes of small molecules have been shown to inhibit tau aggregation *in vitro* (Ballatore et al., 2010; Bulic et al., 2009). One of the first compounds found to inhibit tau fibril assembly was the phenothiazine methylene blue (Wischik et al., 1996). A concluded phase II clinical study showed significant efficacy of methylene blue to arrest disease progression in mild and moderate AD (Wischik et al., 2008). Originally believed to exert its effect by inhibition of tau aggregation, studies now suggest that the compound also improves mitochondrial function, which has been shown to be impaired in AD brains (Atamna et al., 2008). Furthermore, a decrease of tau levels might prove a therapeutic strategy in neurodegenerative tauopathies. Cytosolic proteins can be degraded either by the ubiquitin-proteasome system (UPS) or by lysosomal degradation. Hsp90 is a molecular chaperone, whose function is the assistance of protein folding and stabilisation against UPS-mediated degradation. Inhibition of Hsp90 has been shown to decrease levels of phosphorylated tau and to facilitate the elimination of aggregated tau through degradation via the UPS (Dickey et al., 2007; Luo et al., 2007).

These findings illustrate the manifold mechanisms through which tau-targeted therapeutic strategies can slow or possibly reverse disease progression in tauopathies. While most of therapeutic intervention strategies targeting tau are investigated for the treatment of Alzheimer's disease, it is very likely that they would also be effective in other tauopathies such as PSP, CBD and FTDP-17. In order to further investigate the molecular principles underlying these therapeutic strategies it will be vital to improve animal models of tauopathies that reproduce the key aspects of this class of neurodegenerative diseases. As the numbers of AD cases is expected to rise sharply in the next decades, tau as a central player in neurodegeneration is and will be at the forefront of research into neurodegenerative mechanisms and therapeutic intervention strategies.

6. Acknowledgements

H.J.W. is funded by a University College War Memorial Scholarship and the Medical Research Council. Work in our laboratory in this area has been funded by the Wellcome Trust, CurePSP, Alzheimer's Research UK and the Monument Trust Discovery Award.

7. References

Abraham, R., Sims, R., Carroll, L., Hollingworth, P., O'Donovan, M. C., et al. (2009). An association study of common variation at the MAPT locus with late-onset Alzheimer's disease. *Am J Med Genet B Neuropsychiatr Genet* 150B(8): 1152-5.

Adams, S. J., DeTure, M. A., McBride, M., Dickson, D. W. & Petrucelli, L. (2010). Three repeat isoforms of tau inhibit assembly of four repeat tau filaments. *PLoS One* 5(5): e10810.

Allen, B., Ingram, E., Takao, M., Smith, M. J., Jakes, R., et al. (2002). Abundant tau filaments and nonapoptotic neurodegeneration in transgenic mice expressing human P301S tau protein. *J Neurosci* 22(21): 9340-51.

Andorfer, C., Acker, C. M., Kress, Y., Hof, P. R., Duff, K., et al. (2005). Cell-cycle reentry and cell death in transgenic mice expressing nonmutant human tau isoforms. *J Neurosci* 25(22): 5446-54.

Andorfer, C., Kress, Y., Espinoza, M., de Silva, R., Tucker, K. L., et al. (2003). Hyperphosphorylation and aggregation of tau in mice expressing normal human tau isoforms. *J Neurochem* 86(3): 582-90.

Andreadis, A., Brown, W. M. & Kosik, K. S. (1992). Structure and novel exons of the human tau gene. *Biochemistry* 31(43): 10626-33.

Arima, K., Hirai, S., Sunohara, N., Aoto, K., Izumiyama, Y., et al. (1999). Cellular co-localization of phosphorylated tau- and NACP/alpha-synuclein-epitopes in lewy bodies in sporadic Parkinson's disease and in dementia with Lewy bodies. *Brain Res* 843(1-2): 53-61.

Arima, K., Kowalska, A., Hasegawa, M., Mukoyama, M., Watanabe, R., et al. (2000). Two brothers with frontotemporal dementia and parkinsonism with an N279K mutation of the tau gene. *Neurology* 54(9): 1787-95.

Arriagada, P. V., Growdon, J. H., Hedley-Whyte, E. T. & Hyman, B. T. (1992). Neurofibrillary tangles but not senile plaques parallel duration and severity of Alzheimer's disease. *Neurology* 42(3 Pt 1): 631-9.

Atamna, H., Nguyen, A., Schultz, C., Boyle, K., Newberry, J., et al. (2008). Methylene blue delays cellular senescence and enhances key mitochondrial biochemical pathways. *FASEB J* 22(3): 703-12.

Baba, Y., Baker, M. C., Le Ber, I., Brice, A., Maeck, L., et al. (2007). Clinical and genetic features of families with frontotemporal dementia and parkinsonism linked to chromosome 17 with a P301S tau mutation. *J Neural Transm* 114(7): 947-50.

Baker, M., Graff-Radford, D., Wavrant DeVrieze, F., Graff-Radford, N., Petersen, R. C., et al. (2000). No association between TAU haplotype and Alzheimer's disease in population or clinic based series or in familial disease. *Neurosci Lett* 285(2): 147-9.

Baker, M., Kwok, J. B., Kucera, S., Crook, R., Farrer, M., et al. (1997). Localization of frontotemporal dementia with parkinsonism in an Australian kindred to chromosome 17q21-22. *Ann Neurol* 42(5): 794-8.

Baker, M., Litvan, I., Houlden, H., Adamson, J., Dickson, D., et al. (1999). Association of an extended haplotype in the tau gene with progressive supranuclear palsy. *Hum Mol Genet* 8(4): 711-5.

Ballatore, C., Brunden, K. R., Piscitelli, F., James, M. J., Crowe, A., et al. (2010). Discovery of brain-penetrant, orally bioavailable aminothienopyridazine inhibitors of tau aggregation. *J Med Chem* 53(9): 3739-47.

Ballatore, C., Lee, V. M. & Trojanowski, J. Q. (2007). Tau-mediated neurodegeneration in Alzheimer's disease and related disorders. *Nat Rev Neurosci* 8(9): 663-72.

Bancher, C., Brunner, C., Lassmann, H., Budka, H., Jellinger, K., et al. (1989). Accumulation of abnormally phosphorylated tau precedes the formation of neurofibrillary tangles in Alzheimer's disease. *Brain Res* 477(1-2): 90-9.

Bandyopadhyay, B., Li, G., Yin, H. & Kuret, J. (2007). Tau aggregation and toxicity in a cell culture model of tauopathy. *J Biol Chem* 282(22): 16454-64.

Basun, H., Almkvist, O., Axelman, K., Brun, A., Campbell, T. A., et al. (1997). Clinical characteristics of a chromosome 17-linked rapidly progressive familial frontotemporal dementia. *Arch Neurol* 54(5): 539-44.

Berriman, J., Serpell, L. C., Oberg, K. A., Fink, A. L., Goedert, M., et al. (2003). Tau filaments from human brain and from in vitro assembly of recombinant protein show cross-beta structure. *Proc Natl Acad Sci U S A* 100(15): 9034-8.

Biernat, J., Gustke, N., Drewes, G., Mandelkow, E. M. & Mandelkow, E. (1993). Phosphorylation of Ser262 strongly reduces binding of tau to microtubules: distinction between PHF-like immunoreactivity and microtubule binding. *Neuron* 11(1): 153-63.

Boeve, B. F. & Hutton, M. (2008). Refining frontotemporal dementia with parkinsonism linked to chromosome 17: introducing FTDP-17 (MAPT) and FTDP-17 (PGRN). *Arch Neurol* 65(4): 460-4.

Bramblett, G. T., Goedert, M., Jakes, R., Merrick, S. E., Trojanowski, J. Q., et al. (1993). Abnormal tau phosphorylation at Ser396 in Alzheimer's disease recapitulates development and contributes to reduced microtubule binding. *Neuron* 10(6): 1089-99.

Brandt, R., Leger, J. & Lee, G. (1995). Interaction of tau with the neural plasma membrane mediated by tau's amino-terminal projection domain. *J Cell Biol* 131(5): 1327-40.

Brookmeyer, R., Johnson, E., Ziegler-Graham, K. & Arrighi, H. M. (2007). Forecasting the global burden of Alzheimer's disease. *Alzheimers Dement* 3(3): 186-91.

Buee, L., Bussiere, T., Buee-Scherrer, V., Delacourte, A. & Hof, P. R. (2000). Tau protein isoforms, phosphorylation and role in neurodegenerative disorders. *Brain Res Brain Res Rev* 33(1): 95-130.

Bulic, B., Pickhardt, M., Schmidt, B., Mandelkow, E. M., Waldmann, H., et al. (2009). Development of tau aggregation inhibitors for Alzheimer's disease. *Angew Chem Int Ed Engl* 48(10): 1740-52.

Caffrey, T. M., Joachim, C., Paracchini, S., Esiri, M. M. & Wade-Martins, R. (2006). Haplotype-specific expression of exon 10 at the human MAPT locus. *Hum Mol Genet* 15(24): 3529-37.

Caffrey, T. M., Joachim, C. & Wade-Martins, R. (2008). Haplotype-specific expression of the N-terminal exons 2 and 3 at the human MAPT locus. *Neurobiol Aging* 29(12): 1923-9.

Carlier, M. F., Simon, C., Cassoly, R. & Pradel, L. A. (1984). Interaction between microtubule-associated protein tau and spectrin. *Biochimie* 66(4): 305-11.

Chiti, F. & Dobson, C. M. (2006). Protein misfolding, functional amyloid, and human disease. *Annu Rev Biochem* 75: 333-66.

Cleveland, D. W., Hwo, S. Y. & Kirschner, M. W. (1977). Purification of tau, a microtubule-associated protein that induces assembly of microtubules from purified tubulin. *J Mol Biol* 116(2): 207-25.

Conrad, C., Andreadis, A., Trojanowski, J. Q., Dickson, D. W., Kang, D., et al. (1997). Genetic evidence for the involvement of tau in progressive supranuclear palsy. *Ann Neurol* 41(2): 277-81.

Conrad, C., Vianna, C., Freeman, M. & Davies, P. (2002). A polymorphic gene nested within an intron of the tau gene: implications for Alzheimer's disease. *Proc Natl Acad Sci U S A* 99(11): 7751-6.

Crowther, R. A. (1991). Straight and paired helical filaments in Alzheimer disease have a common structural unit. *Proc Natl Acad Sci U S A* 88(6): 2288-92.

D'Souza, I., Poorkaj, P., Hong, M., Nochlin, D., Lee, V. M., et al. (1999). Missense and silent tau gene mutations cause frontotemporal dementia with parkinsonism-chromosome 17 type, by affecting multiple alternative RNA splicing regulatory elements. *Proc Natl Acad Sci U S A* 96(10): 5598-603.

D'Souza, I. & Schellenberg, G. D. (2000). Determinants of 4-repeat tau expression. Coordination between enhancing and inhibitory splicing sequences for exon 10 inclusion. *J Biol Chem* 275(23): 17700-9.

D'Souza, I. & Schellenberg, G. D. (2005). Regulation of tau isoform expression and dementia. *Biochim Biophys Acta* 1739(2-3): 104-15.

Dawson, H. N., Ferreira, A., Eyster, M. V., Ghoshal, N., Binder, L. I., et al. (2001). Inhibition of neuronal maturation in primary hippocampal neurons from tau deficient mice. *J Cell Sci* 114(Pt 6): 1179-87.

de Calignon, A., Fox, L. M., Pitstick, R., Carlson, G. A., Bacskai, B. J., et al. (2010). Caspase activation precedes and leads to tangles. *Nature* 464(7292): 1201-4.

de Silva, R., Weiler, M., Morris, H. R., Martin, E. R., Wood, N. W., et al. (2001). Strong association of a novel Tau promoter haplotype in progressive supranuclear palsy. *Neurosci Lett* 311(3): 145-8.

Delisle, M. B., Murrell, J. R., Richardson, R., Trofatter, J. A., Rascol, O., et al. (1999). A mutation at codon 279 (N279K) in exon 10 of the Tau gene causes a tauopathy with dementia and supranuclear palsy. *Acta Neuropathol* 98(1): 62-77.

Di Maria, E., Tabaton, M., Vigo, T., Abbruzzese, G., Bellone, E., et al. (2000). Corticobasal degeneration shares a common genetic background with progressive supranuclear palsy. *Ann Neurol* 47(3): 374-7.

Dickey, C. A., Kamal, A., Lundgren, K., Klosak, N., Bailey, R. M., et al. (2007). The high-affinity HSP90-CHIP complex recognizes and selectively degrades phosphorylated tau client proteins. *J Clin Invest* 117(3): 648-58.

Dickson, D. W., Rademakers, R. & Hutton, M. L. (2007). Progressive supranuclear palsy: pathology and genetics. *Brain Pathol* 17(1): 74-82.

Dixit, R., Ross, J. L., Goldman, Y. E. & Holzbaur, E. L. (2008). Differential regulation of dynein and kinesin motor proteins by tau. *Science* 319(5866): 1086-9.

Drewes, G., Mandelkow, E. M., Baumann, K., Goris, J., Merlevede, W., et al. (1993). Dephosphorylation of tau protein and Alzheimer paired helical filaments by calcineurin and phosphatase-2A. *FEBS Lett* 336(3): 425-32.

Duff, K., Knight, H., Refolo, L. M., Sanders, S., Yu, X., et al. (2000). Characterization of pathology in transgenic mice over-expressing human genomic and cDNA tau transgenes. *Neurobiol Dis* 7(2): 87-98.

Evans, W., Fung, H. C., Steele, J., Eerola, J., Tienari, P., et al. (2004). The tau H2 haplotype is almost exclusively Caucasian in origin. *Neurosci Lett* 369(3): 183-5.

Fandrich, M. (2007). On the structural definition of amyloid fibrils and other polypeptide aggregates. *Cell Mol Life Sci* 64(16): 2066-78.

Foster, N. L., Wilhelmsen, K., Sima, A. A., Jones, M. Z., D'Amato, C. J., et al. (1997). Frontotemporal dementia and parkinsonism linked to chromosome 17: a consensus conference. Conference Participants. *Ann Neurol* 41(6): 706-15.

Friedhoff, P., von Bergen, M., Mandelkow, E. M., Davies, P. & Mandelkow, E. (1998). A nucleated assembly mechanism of Alzheimer paired helical filaments. *Proc Natl Acad Sci U S A* 95(26): 15712-7.

Froelich, S., Basun, H., Forsell, C., Lilius, L., Axelman, K., et al. (1997). Mapping of a disease locus for familial rapidly progressive frontotemporal dementia to chromosome 17q12-21. *Am J Med Genet* 74(4): 380-5.

Gamblin, T. C., Chen, F., Zambrano, A., Abraha, A., Lagalwar, S., et al. (2003). Caspase cleavage of tau: linking amyloid and neurofibrillary tangles in Alzheimer's disease. *Proc Natl Acad Sci U S A* 100(17): 10032-7.

Gasparini, L., Terni, B. & Spillantini, M. G. (2007). Frontotemporal dementia with tau pathology. *Neurodegener Dis* 4(2-3): 236-53.

Giasson, B. I., Forman, M. S., Higuchi, M., Golbe, L. I., Graves, C. L., et al. (2003). Initiation and synergistic fibrillization of tau and alpha-synuclein. *Science* 300(5619): 636-40.

Goedert, M. (2005). Tau gene mutations and their effects. *Mov Disord* 20 Suppl 12: S45-52.

Goedert, M. & Jakes, R. (1990). Expression of separate isoforms of human tau protein: correlation with the tau pattern in brain and effects on tubulin polymerization. *EMBO J* 9(13): 4225-30.

Goedert, M., Spillantini, M. G., Jakes, R., Rutherford, D. & Crowther, R. A. (1989). Multiple isoforms of human microtubule-associated protein tau: sequences and localization in neurofibrillary tangles of Alzheimer's disease. *Neuron* 3(4): 519-26.

Gong, C. X., Lidsky, T., Wegiel, J., Zuck, L., Grundke-Iqbal, I., et al. (2000). Phosphorylation of microtubule-associated protein tau is regulated by protein phosphatase 2A in mammalian brain. Implications for neurofibrillary degeneration in Alzheimer's disease. *J Biol Chem* 275(8): 5535-44.

Gong, C. X., Singh, T. J., Grundke-Iqbal, I. & Iqbal, K. (1993). Phosphoprotein phosphatase activities in Alzheimer disease brain. *J Neurochem* 61(3): 921-7.

Goode, B. L., Chau, M., Denis, P. E. & Feinstein, S. C. (2000). Structural and functional differences between 3-repeat and 4-repeat tau isoforms. Implications for normal tau function and the onset of neurodegenetative disease. *J Biol Chem* 275(49): 38182-9.

Gotz, J., Chen, F., Barmettler, R. & Nitsch, R. M. (2001a). Tau filament formation in transgenic mice expressing P301L tau. *J Biol Chem* 276(1): 529-34.

Gotz, J., Chen, F., van Dorpe, J. & Nitsch, R. M. (2001b). Formation of neurofibrillary tangles in P301l tau transgenic mice induced by Abeta 42 fibrils. *Science* 293(5534): 1491-5.

Gotz, J., Probst, A., Spillantini, M. G., Schafer, T., Jakes, R., et al. (1995). Somatodendritic localization and hyperphosphorylation of tau protein in transgenic mice expressing the longest human brain tau isoform. *EMBO J* 14(7): 1304-13.

Gotz, J., Tolnay, M., Barmettler, R., Chen, F., Probst, A., et al. (2001c). Oligodendroglial tau filament formation in transgenic mice expressing G272V tau. *Eur J Neurosci* 13(11): 2131-40.

Griffith, L. M. & Pollard, T. D. (1982). The interaction of actin filaments with microtubules and microtubule-associated proteins. *J Biol Chem* 257(15): 9143-51.

Grover, A., England, E., Baker, M., Sahara, N., Adamson, J., et al. (2003). A novel tau mutation in exon 9 (1260V) causes a four-repeat tauopathy. *Exp Neurol* 184(1): 131-40.

Grundke-Iqbal, I., Iqbal, K., Quinlan, M., Tung, Y. C., Zaidi, M. S., et al. (1986). Microtubule-associated protein tau. A component of Alzheimer paired helical filaments. *J Biol Chem* 261(13): 6084-9.

Harada, A., Oguchi, K., Okabe, S., Kuno, J., Terada, S., et al. (1994). Altered microtubule organization in small-calibre axons of mice lacking tau protein. *Nature* 369(6480): 488-91.

Harper, J. D. & Lansbury, P. T., Jr. (1997). Models of amyloid seeding in Alzheimer's disease and scrapie: mechanistic truths and physiological consequences of the time-dependent solubility of amyloid proteins. *Annu Rev Biochem* 66: 385-407.

Hasegawa, M., Smith, M. J., Iijima, M., Tabira, T. & Goedert, M. (1999). FTDP-17 mutations N279K and S305N in tau produce increased splicing of exon 10. *FEBS Lett* 443(2): 93-6.

Healy, D. G., Abou-Sleiman, P. M., Lees, A. J., Casas, J. P., Quinn, N., et al. (2004). Tau gene and Parkinson's disease: a case-control study and meta-analysis. *J Neurol Neurosurg Psychiatry* 75(7): 962-5.

Higuchi, M., Zhang, B., Forman, M. S., Yoshiyama, Y., Trojanowski, J. Q., et al. (2005). Axonal degeneration induced by targeted expression of mutant human tau in oligodendrocytes of transgenic mice that model glial tauopathies. *J Neurosci* 25(41): 9434-43.

Hogg, M., Grujic, Z. M., Baker, M., Demirci, S., Guillozet, A. L., et al. (2003). The L266V tau mutation is associated with frontotemporal dementia and Pick-like 3R and 4R tauopathy. *Acta Neuropathol* 106(4): 323-36.

Hong, M., Zhukareva, V., Vogelsberg-Ragaglia, V., Wszolek, Z., Reed, L., et al. (1998). Mutation-specific functional impairments in distinct tau isoforms of hereditary FTDP-17. *Science* 282(5395): 1914-7.

Houlden, H., Baker, M., Morris, H. R., MacDonald, N., Pickering-Brown, S., et al. (2001). Corticobasal degeneration and progressive supranuclear palsy share a common tau haplotype. *Neurology* 56(12): 1702-6.

Hutton, M., Lendon, C. L., Rizzu, P., Baker, M., Froelich, S., et al. (1998). Association of missense and 5'-splice-site mutations in tau with the inherited dementia FTDP-17. *Nature* 393(6686): 702-5.

Ikeda, M., Shoji, M., Kawarai, T., Kawarabayashi, T., Matsubara, E., et al. (2005). Accumulation of filamentous tau in the cerebral cortex of human tau R406W transgenic mice. *Am J Pathol* 166(2): 521-31.

Ishihara, T., Hong, M., Zhang, B., Nakagawa, Y., Lee, M. K., et al. (1999). Age-dependent emergence and progression of a tauopathy in transgenic mice overexpressing the shortest human tau isoform. *Neuron* 24(3): 751-62.

Ishihara, T., Zhang, B., Higuchi, M., Yoshiyama, Y., Trojanowski, J. Q., et al. (2001). Age-dependent induction of congophilic neurofibrillary tau inclusions in tau transgenic mice. *Am J Pathol* 158(2): 555-62.

Ittner, L. M., Fath, T., Ke, Y. D., Bi, M., van Eersel, J., et al. (2008). Parkinsonism and impaired axonal transport in a mouse model of frontotemporal dementia. *Proc Natl Acad Sci U S A* 105(41): 15997-6002.

Ittner, L. M., Ke, Y. D., Delerue, F., Bi, M., Gladbach, A., et al. (2010). Dendritic function of tau mediates amyloid-beta toxicity in Alzheimer's disease mouse models. *Cell* 142(3): 387-97.

Jackson, G. R., Wiedau-Pazos, M., Sang, T. K., Wagle, N., Brown, C. A., et al. (2002). Human wild-type tau interacts with wingless pathway components and produces neurofibrillary pathology in Drosophila. *Neuron* 34(4): 509-19.

Jancsik, V., Filliol, D., Felter, S. & Rendon, A. (1989). Binding of microtubule-associated proteins (MAPs) to rat brain mitochondria: a comparative study of the binding of MAP2, its microtubule-binding and projection domains, and tau proteins. *Cell Motil Cytoskeleton* 14(3): 372-81.

Jensen, P. H., Hager, H., Nielsen, M. S., Hojrup, P., Gliemann, J., et al. (1999). alpha-synuclein binds to Tau and stimulates the protein kinase A-catalyzed tau phosphorylation of serine residues 262 and 356. *J Biol Chem* 274(36): 25481-9.

Kayed, R. & Jackson, G. R. (2009). Prefilament tau species as potential targets for immunotherapy for Alzheimer disease and related disorders. *Curr Opin Immunol* 21(3): 359-63.

Khlistunova, I., Biernat, J., Wang, Y., Pickhardt, M., von Bergen, M., et al. (2006). Inducible expression of Tau repeat domain in cell models of tauopathy: aggregation is toxic to cells but can be reversed by inhibitor drugs. *J Biol Chem* 281(2): 1205-14.

Kouri, N., Whitwell, J. L., Josephs, K. A., Rademakers, R. & Dickson, D. W. (2011). Corticobasal degeneration: a pathologically distinct 4R tauopathy. *Nat Rev Neurol* 7(5): 263-72.

Kraemer, B. C., Zhang, B., Leverenz, J. B., Thomas, J. H., Trojanowski, J. Q., et al. (2003). Neurodegeneration and defective neurotransmission in a Caenorhabditis elegans model of tauopathy. *Proc Natl Acad Sci U S A* 100(17): 9980-5.

Lasagna-Reeves, C. A., Castillo-Carranza, D. L., Sengupta, U., Clos, A. L., Jackson, G. R., et al. (2011). Tau oligomers impair memory and induce synaptic and mitochondrial dysfunction in wild-type mice. *Mol Neurodegener* 6: 39.

Lee, G., Newman, S. T., Gard, D. L., Band, H. & Panchamoorthy, G. (1998). Tau interacts with src-family non-receptor tyrosine kinases. *J Cell Sci* 111 (Pt 21): 3167-77.

Lewis, J., McGowan, E., Rockwood, J., Melrose, H., Nacharaju, P., et al. (2000). Neurofibrillary tangles, amyotrophy and progressive motor disturbance in mice expressing mutant (P301L) tau protein. *Nat Genet* 25(4): 402-5.

Lim, F., Hernandez, F., Lucas, J. J., Gomez-Ramos, P., Moran, M. A., et al. (2001). FTDP-17 mutations in tau transgenic mice provoke lysosomal abnormalities and Tau filaments in forebrain. *Mol Cell Neurosci* 18(6): 702-14.

Luo, W., Dou, F., Rodina, A., Chip, S., Kim, J., et al. (2007). Roles of heat-shock protein 90 in maintaining and facilitating the neurodegenerative phenotype in tauopathies. *Proc Natl Acad Sci U S A* 104(22): 9511-6.

Maeda, S., Sahara, N., Saito, Y., Murayama, M., Yoshiike, Y., et al. (2007). Granular tau oligomers as intermediates of tau filaments. *Biochemistry* 46(12): 3856-61.

Mahapatra, R. K., Edwards, M. J., Schott, J. M. & Bhatia, K. P. (2004). Corticobasal degeneration. *Lancet Neurol* 3(12): 736-43.

Martin, L., Latypova, X. & Terro, F. (2011). Post-translational modifications of tau protein: implications for Alzheimer's disease. *Neurochem Int* 58(4): 458-71.

Masters, C. L., Simms, G., Weinman, N. A., Multhaup, G., McDonald, B. L., et al. (1985). Amyloid plaque core protein in Alzheimer disease and Down syndrome. *Proc Natl Acad Sci U S A* 82(12): 4245-9.

Mukherjee, O., Kauwe, J. S., Mayo, K., Morris, J. C. & Goate, A. M. (2007). Haplotype-based association analysis of the MAPT locus in late onset Alzheimer's disease. *BMC Genet* 8: 3.

Murakami, T., Paitel, E., Kawarabayashi, T., Ikeda, M., Chishti, M. A., et al. (2006). Cortical neuronal and glial pathology in TgTauP301L transgenic mice: neuronal degeneration, memory disturbance, and phenotypic variation. *Am J Pathol* 169(4): 1365-75.

Noble, W., Planel, E., Zehr, C., Olm, V., Meyerson, J., et al. (2005). Inhibition of glycogen synthase kinase-3 by lithium correlates with reduced tauopathy and degeneration in vivo. *Proc Natl Acad Sci U S A* 102(19): 6990-5.

Oddo, S., Caccamo, A., Kitazawa, M., Tseng, B. P. & LaFerla, F. M. (2003a). Amyloid deposition precedes tangle formation in a triple transgenic model of Alzheimer's disease. *Neurobiol Aging* 24(8): 1063-70.

Oddo, S., Caccamo, A., Shepherd, J. D., Murphy, M. P., Golde, T. E., et al. (2003b). Triple-transgenic model of Alzheimer's disease with plaques and tangles: intracellular Abeta and synaptic dysfunction. *Neuron* 39(3): 409-21.

Panda, D., Samuel, J. C., Massie, M., Feinstein, S. C. & Wilson, L. (2003). Differential regulation of microtubule dynamics by three- and four-repeat tau: implications for the onset of neurodegenerative disease. *Proc Natl Acad Sci U S A* 100(16): 9548-53.

Paquet, D., Bhat, R., Sydow, A., Mandelkow, E. M., Berg, S., et al. (2009). A zebrafish model of tauopathy allows in vivo imaging of neuronal cell death and drug evaluation. *J Clin Invest* 119(5): 1382-95.

Pickering-Brown, S. M., Baker, M., Nonaka, T., Ikeda, K., Sharma, S., et al. (2004). Frontotemporal dementia with Pick-type histology associated with Q336R mutation in the tau gene. *Brain* 127(Pt 6): 1415-26.

Pittman, A. M., Myers, A. J., Abou-Sleiman, P., Fung, H. C., Kaleem, M., et al. (2005). Linkage disequilibrium fine mapping and haplotype association analysis of the tau gene in progressive supranuclear palsy and corticobasal degeneration. *J Med Genet* 42(11): 837-46.

Pittman, A. M., Myers, A. J., Duckworth, J., Bryden, L., Hanson, M., et al. (2004). The structure of the tau haplotype in controls and in progressive supranuclear palsy. *Hum Mol Genet* 13(12): 1267-74.

Poorkaj, P., Bird, T. D., Wijsman, E., Nemens, E., Garruto, R. M., et al. (1998). Tau is a candidate gene for chromosome 17 frontotemporal dementia. *Ann Neurol* 43(6): 815-25.

Poorkaj, P., Tsuang, D., Wijsman, E., Steinbart, E., Garruto, R. M., et al. (2001). TAU as a susceptibility gene for amyotropic lateral sclerosis-parkinsonism dementia complex of Guam. *Arch Neurol* 58(11): 1871-8.

Rademakers, R., Cruts, M. & van Broeckhoven, C. (2004). The role of tau (MAPT) in frontotemporal dementia and related tauopathies. *Hum Mutat* 24(4): 277-95.

Ramsden, M., Kotilinek, L., Forster, C., Paulson, J., McGowan, E., et al. (2005). Age-dependent neurofibrillary tangle formation, neuron loss, and memory impairment in a mouse model of human tauopathy (P301L). *J Neurosci* 25(46): 10637-47.

Rapoport, M., Dawson, H. N., Binder, L. I., Vitek, M. P. & Ferreira, A. (2002). Tau is essential to beta -amyloid-induced neurotoxicity. *Proc Natl Acad Sci U S A* 99(9): 6364-9.

Rizzini, C., Goedert, M., Hodges, J. R., Smith, M. J., Jakes, R., et al. (2000). Tau gene mutation K257T causes a tauopathy similar to Pick's disease. *J Neuropathol Exp Neurol* 59(11): 990-1001.

Rosenmann, H., Grigoriadis, N., Eldar-Levy, H., Avital, A., Rozenstein, L., et al. (2008). A novel transgenic mouse expressing double mutant tau driven by its natural promoter exhibits tauopathy characteristics. *Exp Neurol* 212(1): 71-84.

Santacruz, K., Lewis, J., Spires, T., Paulson, J., Kotilinek, L., et al. (2005). Tau suppression in a neurodegenerative mouse model improves memory function. *Science* 309(5733): 476-81.

Schindowski, K., Bretteville, A., Leroy, K., Begard, S., Brion, J. P., et al. (2006). Alzheimer's disease-like tau neuropathology leads to memory deficits and loss of functional synapses in a novel mutated tau transgenic mouse without any motor deficits. *Am J Pathol* 169(2): 599-616.

Sereno, L., Coma, M., Rodriguez, M., Sanchez-Ferrer, P., Sanchez, M. B., et al. (2009). A novel GSK-3beta inhibitor reduces Alzheimer's pathology and rescues neuronal loss in vivo. *Neurobiol Dis* 35(3): 359-67.

Shipton, O. A., Leitz, J. R., Dworzak, J., Acton, C. E., Tunbridge, E. M., et al. (2011). Tau protein is required for amyloid {beta}-induced impairment of hippocampal long-term potentiation. *J Neurosci* 31(5): 1688-92.

Simon-Sanchez, J., Schulte, C., Bras, J. M., Sharma, M., Gibbs, J. R., et al. (2009). Genome-wide association study reveals genetic risk underlying Parkinson's disease. *Nat Genet* 41(12): 1308-12.

Soliveri, P., Rossi, G., Monza, D., Tagliavini, F., Piacentini, S., et al. (2003). A case of dementia parkinsonism resembling progressive supranuclear palsy due to mutation in the tau protein gene. *Arch Neurol* 60(10): 1454-6.

Spillantini, M. G., Murrell, J. R., Goedert, M., Farlow, M. R., Klug, A., et al. (1998). Mutation in the tau gene in familial multiple system tauopathy with presenile dementia. *Proc Natl Acad Sci U S A* 95(13): 7737-41.

Stanford, P. M., Halliday, G. M., Brooks, W. S., Kwok, J. B., Storey, C. E., et al. (2000). Progressive supranuclear palsy pathology caused by a novel silent mutation in exon 10 of the tau gene: expansion of the disease phenotype caused by tau gene mutations. *Brain* 123 (Pt 5): 880-93.

Stanford, P. M., Shepherd, C. E., Halliday, G. M., Brooks, W. S., Schofield, P. W., et al. (2003). Mutations in the tau gene that cause an increase in three repeat tau and frontotemporal dementia. *Brain* 126(Pt 4): 814-26.

Strassnig, M. & Ganguli, M. (2005). About a peculiar disease of the cerebral cortex: Alzheimer's original case revisited. *Psychiatry (Edgmont)* 2(9): 30-3.

Sultan, A., Nesslany, F., Violet, M., Begard, S., Loyens, A., et al. (2011). Nuclear tau, a key player in neuronal DNA protection. *J Biol Chem* 286(6): 4566-75.

Sundar, P. D., Yu, C. E., Sieh, W., Steinbart, E., Garruto, R. M., et al. (2007). Two sites in the MAPT region confer genetic risk for Guam ALS/PDC and dementia. *Hum Mol Genet* 16(3): 295-306.

Tanemura, K., Murayama, M., Akagi, T., Hashikawa, T., Tominaga, T., et al. (2002). Neurodegeneration with tau accumulation in a transgenic mouse expressing V337M human tau. *J Neurosci* 22(1): 133-41.

Taniguchi, T., Doe, N., Matsuyama, S., Kitamura, Y., Mori, H., et al. (2005). Transgenic mice expressing mutant (N279K) human tau show mutation dependent cognitive deficits without neurofibrillary tangle formation. *FEBS Lett* 579(25): 5704-12.

Tatebayashi, Y., Miyasaka, T., Chui, D. H., Akagi, T., Mishima, K., et al. (2002). Tau filament formation and associative memory deficit in aged mice expressing mutant (R406W) human tau. *Proc Natl Acad Sci U S A* 99(21): 13896-901.

Terwel, D., Lasrado, R., Snauwaert, J., Vandeweert, E., Van Haesendonck, C., et al. (2005). Changed conformation of mutant Tau-P301L underlies the moribund tauopathy, absent in progressive, nonlethal axonopathy of Tau-4R/2N transgenic mice. *J Biol Chem* 280(5): 3963-73.

Tobin, J. E., Latourelle, J. C., Lew, M. F., Klein, C., Suchowersky, O., et al. (2008). Haplotypes and gene expression implicate the MAPT region for Parkinson disease: the GenePD Study. *Neurology* 71(1): 28-34.

Tsuboi, Y. (2006). Neuropathology of familial tauopathy. *Neuropathology* 26(5): 471-4.

van Swieten, J. C., Stevens, M., Rosso, S. M., Rizzu, P., Joosse, M., et al. (1999). Phenotypic variation in hereditary frontotemporal dementia with tau mutations. *Ann Neurol* 46(4): 617-26.

von Bergen, M., Friedhoff, P., Biernat, J., Heberle, J., Mandelkow, E. M., et al. (2000). Assembly of tau protein into Alzheimer paired helical filaments depends on a local sequence motif ((306)VQIVYK(311)) forming beta structure. *Proc Natl Acad Sci U S A* 97(10): 5129-34.

Wang, Z. F., Li, H. L., Li, X. C., Zhang, Q., Tian, Q., et al. (2006). Effects of endogenous beta-amyloid overproduction on tau phosphorylation in cell culture. *J Neurochem* 98(4): 1167-75.

Weingarten, M. D., Lockwood, A. H., Hwo, S. Y. & Kirschner, M. W. (1975). A protein factor essential for microtubule assembly. *Proc Natl Acad Sci U S A* 72(5): 1858-62.

Wilhelmsen, K. C., Lynch, T., Pavlou, E., Higgins, M. & Nygaard, T. G. (1994). Localization of disinhibition-dementia-parkinsonism-amyotrophy complex to 17q21-22. *Am J Hum Genet* 55(6): 1159-65.

Wischik, C. M., Bentham, P., Wischik, D. J. & Seng, K. M. (2008). O3-04-07: Tau aggregation inhibitor (TAI) therapy with rember(TM) arrests disease progression in mild and moderate Alzheimer's disease over 50 weeks. *Alzheimer's and Dementia* 4(4, Supplement 1): T167-T167.

Wischik, C. M., Edwards, P. C., Lai, R. Y., Roth, M. & Harrington, C. R. (1996). Selective inhibition of Alzheimer disease-like tau aggregation by phenothiazines. *Proc Natl Acad Sci U S A* 93(20): 11213-8.

Wittmann, C. W., Wszolek, M. F., Shulman, J. M., Salvaterra, P. M., Lewis, J., et al. (2001). Tauopathy in Drosophila: neurodegeneration without neurofibrillary tangles. *Science* 293(5530): 711-4.

Wszolek, Z. K., Tsuboi, Y., Ghetti, B., Pickering-Brown, S., Baba, Y., et al. (2006). Frontotemporal dementia and parkinsonism linked to chromosome 17 (FTDP-17). *Orphanet J Rare Dis* 1: 30.

Yoshida, H., Crowther, R. A. & Goedert, M. (2002). Functional effects of tau gene mutations deltaN296 and N296H. *J Neurochem* 80(3): 548-51.

Yoshiyama, Y., Higuchi, M., Zhang, B., Huang, S. M., Iwata, N., et al. (2007). Synapse loss and microglial activation precede tangles in a P301S tauopathy mouse model. *Neuron* 53(3): 337-51.

Zhang, B., Higuchi, M., Yoshiyama, Y., Ishihara, T., Forman, M. S., et al. (2004). Retarded axonal transport of R406W mutant tau in transgenic mice with a neurodegenerative tauopathy. *J Neurosci* 24(19): 4657-67.

Zhang, B., Maiti, A., Shively, S., Lakhani, F., McDonald-Jones, G., et al. (2005). Microtubule-binding drugs offset tau sequestration by stabilizing microtubules and reversing fast axonal transport deficits in a tauopathy model. *Proc Natl Acad Sci U S A* 102(1): 227-31.

Part 2

Parkinson's Disease

12

Gut Hormones Restrict Neurodegeneration in Parkinson's Disease

Jacqueline Bayliss, Romana Stark,
Alex Reichenbach and Zane B. Andrews
Department of Physiology
Monash University
Australia

1. Introduction

Parkinson's disease is the most common neurodegenerative movement disorder and the second most common neurological disorder behind Alzheimer's disease in today's society. It is a progressive disorder that affects more than 1% of people older than 60. Cardinal features of Parkinson's disease include motor dysfunction such as rigidity, resting tremor, postural instability and bradykinesia. These debilitating symptoms manifest due to the massive loss of dopamine in the striatum, the nerve terminal region of dopamine neurons are located in the substantia nigra pars compacta (SNpc). This anatomical circuit is known as the nigrostriatal pathway and plays a critical role in fine tuning motor functions.

At present there are only a few known monogenic mutations accelerating the onset of Parkinson's disease, therefore most cases are considered sporadic and develop as a complex polygenic interaction with age and environment. Although the pathogenesis of Parkinson's disease is largely unknown, mitochondrial dysfunction, oxidative stress, intracellular protein accumulation (Lewy Bodies containing α-synuclein) and abnormal protein degradation all play a key role in disease progression. Because loss of dopamine in the striatum causes motor dysfunction in Parkinson's disease, dopamine supplementation can be used to alleviate motor symptoms but this is only a temporary solution as the efficacy diminishes with age and as the disease progresses. There are no known therapies that halt or reduce the progression of the disease, largely because the cause of Parkinson's disease remains enigmatic.

Parkinson's disease also causes symptoms in other parts of the nervous system. Constipation and gastrointestinal (GI) problems are often some of the earliest symptoms, well before the presence of dopamine dysfunction, and post mortem studies in Parkinson's disease patients identified protein accumulation in the enteric nervous system of the GI tract [1]. This 'Braak's hypothesis' suggests protein accumulation in enteric neurons spreads in a retrograde manner to the brain through the dorsal motor nucleus of the vagus and triggers Parkinson's disease. Braak observed in post mortem tissue that patients with pre-symptomatic Parkinson's disease had protein aggregation in the peripheral nervous system but not the central nervous system [1]. Protein aggregation ascended into the central nervous system and correlated with the development of motor dysfunction. This observation shows that the topographic ascending lesion pattern resembles a falling row of dominos and prompts the question; does Parkinson's disease originate outside the central nervous system?

Recent evidence supports the hypothesis that GI abnormalities, which precede central nervous system changes, trigger Parkinson's disease. For example, mice expressing mutant α-synuclein in gut enteric neurons exhibited extensive GI dysfunction followed by motor abnormalities [2]. Moreover, low doses of rotenone, a compound found in pesticides that causes Parkinson's-like conditions, produced GI disturbances and enteric neuronal α-synuclein aggregates in rats before neuronal protein aggregation [3, 4]. These studies, taken together with the early GI disturbances in humans, clearly implicate the GI system in the pathogenesis of Parkinson's disease.

The stomach and intestines comprise the GI 'digestive' system, which produces a number of hormones to aid energy metabolism, digestion and nutrient uptake into the circulation. Despite the fact that evidence suggests GI dysfunction triggers Parkinson's disease, little is known about gastrointestinal hormones in Parkinson's disease. This chapter examines how gut hormones influence the nigrostriatal dopamine system.

2. Ghrelin

Ghrelin is best known as a key modulator of energy homeostasis, with critical roles in appetite, adipocyte metabolism and glucose homeostasis [5-7]. These effects are mediated by ghrelin activating the growth hormone secretagogue receptor (GHSR)[8], a seven-transmembrane G-protein-coupled receptor [9] expressed in the brain, heart, lung, pancreas, intestine and adipose tissue [8, 10].

Pro-ghrelin mRNA is highly expressed in the stomach but is also found in the duodenum, jejunum, ileum, colon and pancreas [8]. Pro-ghrelin is acylated in the stomach by ghrelin o-acyltransferase (GOAT) with a medium-chain fatty acid (usually n-octanoic acid) added to serine-3 [11, 12]. Once ghrelin is acylated, it is transported to the golgi apparatus where it is cleaved to form 28 amino-acid mature ghrelin [13]. Both acyl and des-acyl ghrelin are secreted from the stomach into the circulation via the gastric vein [14] with des-acyl ghrelin being dominant in the blood [14].

Within the brain, abundant GHSR expression is found not only in the hypothalamus, reflecting the importance in energy metabolism, but also in many regions outside the hypothalamus [15]. Indeed, the substantia nigra pars compacta (SNpc) houses significant GHSR expression and the GHSR co-localizes with tyrosine hydroxylase (TH) (a dopaminergic marker) neurons, suggesting that ghrelin may play an important functional role in this nucleus. We showed recently that ghrelin binds to dopamine neurons in the SNpc and elicits action potential firing in identified dopamine neurons [16]. Moreover ghrelin increases TH expression (an enzyme involved in dopamine biosynthesis) in the midbrain, and increased dopamine turnover in the dorsal striatum - the innervation site of nerve terminals from dopamine cells in the SNpc [16]. Ghrelin also activates neighbouring dopamine neurons in the ventral tegmental area (VTA) and increases dopamine turnover in the ventral striatum [17], also known as the nucleus accumbens - the innervation site of nerve terminals from dopamine neurons in the VTA. Thus, ghrelin regulates dopamine neuronal function in the SNpc in a manner that suggests a neuroprotective effect against dopaminergic degeneration, as seen in Parkinson's disease.

We used transgenic mice models to show that ghrelin prevents neurodegeneration in SNpc dopamine neurons. For example, using the mitochondrial toxin MPTP, which selective kills dopamine neurons in the SNpc, we demonstrated that ghrelin knockout mice displayed greater SNpc dopamine cell loss and greater dopamine loss in the striatum. GHSR knockout mice also showed a greater dopamine cell loss in the SNpc and dopamine concentration in the striatum. However, re-expression of the GHSR on dopamine neurons only, using a cre/lox method, completely prevents the greater loss of dopamine neurons in the SNpc and dopamine concentration in the striatum [17]. These results conclusively demonstrate that ghrelin signaling in the SNpc, via the GHSR, restricts SNpc dopamine cell degeneration in mouse models of Parkinson's disease.

Moreover, i.p. ghrelin injection restricts dopamine cell loss in the SNpc and dopamine loss in the striatum *in vivo* [16, 18, 19], providing proof-of-principle data that ghrelin treatment to humans may alleviate symptoms of Parkinson's disease and prevent the development/progression of Parkinson's disease. Ghrelin reduces apoptosis *in vivo* and *in vitro* and attenuates MPTP-induced caspase 3 activity by regulating Bcl-2 and Bax [18, 20]. Bcl-2 and Bax are mitochondrial apoptotic signaling molecules suggesting that ghrelin exerts an influence on mitochondrial function. Ghrelin also reduced microglial activation in the SNpc after MPTP-induced dopamine cell death [19], which participates in the pathogenesis of Parkinson's disease. A recent study shows that apoptosis in degenerating cells produces a caspase-dependent signal that activates microglia [21], therefore it remains unknown as to whether the microglial activation is a direct effect of ghrelin or an indirect effect of greater caspase-mediated apoptotic cell death. However, studies show that ghrelin reduces pro-inflammatory markers such as tumor necrosis factor-α and interleukin 1β [19], produces anti-inflammatory effects in the periphery [22-24] and in a central hemorrhage model of brain damage [25]. These studies indicate that ghrelin probably has at least some direct effect on microglial activation but also an indirect effect via caspase-mediated signaling [21].

The neuroprotective effects of ghrelin involve enhanced mitochondrial function in SNpc dopamine neurons. For example, ghrelin treatment maintains mitochondrial biogenesis in dopamine neurons after MPTP-induced degeneration [16]. Uncoupling protein-2 (UCP2) is the key mitochondrial target through which ghrelin prevents degeneration. Ghrelin injections restrict dopamine neuronal degeneration after MPTP treatment in UCP2 wild type but not UCP2 knockout mice, highlighting the critical importance of UCP2 to prevent degeneration [16]. The neuroprotective effects of ghrelin on MPTP-induced nigrostriatal dopamine dysfunction included UCP2-dependent mitochondrial respiration, suppression of ROS production and mitochondrial biogenesis [16]. The critical role of UCP2 is supported by previous studies demonstrating that UCP2 is critical for nigrostriatal dopamine function [26] and protects against MPTP-induced degeneration [27-29].

Ghrelin is a hormone that is most well studied for its role in food intake and body weight regulation [6, 7]. Within the hypothalamus ghrelin initiates food intake by activating NPY neurons in the arcuate nucleus [5]. Activation of the ghrelin receptor (GHSR) increases AMPK activity, mitochondrial biogenesis and respiration, and drives food intake [30]. Furthermore, inhibition of AMPK prevents the ability of ghrelin to increase food intake [31]. AMPK is an integrator of cellular energy status and responds to metabolic stress by promoting pathways that favor energy production (fatty acid oxidation, glucose uptake) over energy (ATP) consumption [32]. AMPK activation also promotes mitochondrial biogenesis and function in peripheral and neuronal tissues [33-36], and because of this, we hypothesized that ghrelin mediates neuroprotection in the SNpc by increasing AMPK activity. Indeed, we recently demonstrated that increasing AMPK in the brain prevents MPTP-induced neurodegeneration [37]. We used a dietary approach to chronically activate

AMPK by feeding mice a normal chow diet containing 1% guanidinopropionic acid (GPA) before examining SNpc TH neurodegeneration in a mouse model of Parkinson's disease. GPA is a creatine analogue that inhibits creatine kinase activity, reduces intracellular phosphate levels and thereby robustly increases AMPK activity [33, 38]. Further, GPA stimulates AMPK-dependent mitochondrial biogenesis [35] through increased PGC1 alpha in muscle tissue [39]. In this study we showed that orally administered GPA protects SNpc TH neurons by directly increasing AMPK activity in these neurons. We used design-based stereology to show that GPA regulates TH cell number, cell volume and mitochondrial number and morphology within SNpc TH neurons while decreasing degeneration. In particular, GPA prevented a MPTP-induced decrease of TH cell number in the SNpc and partially retained dopamine levels in the striatum. We speculate that elevated AMPK activity confers the neuroprotective effects of GPA by regulating mitochondrial biogenesis and function. Robust pAMPK staining in TH neurons with and without MPTP indicates that GPA directly enhances AMPK function in SNpc TH neurons. The ability of GPA to activate AMPK in the brain is consistent with previous reports showing that GPA increases AMPK activity in peripheral tissues, such as muscle [33, 35, 40, 41]. Because ghrelin activates AMPK in the hypothalamus to drive food intake and AMPK activity in dopamine neurons reduces degeneration [42], we hypothesize that ghrelin prevents degeneration by increasing AMPK activity in the SNpc. This hypothesis requires further experimental proof.

It is interesting to note that calorie restriction (i.e. negative energy balance) increases plasma ghrelin and calorie restriction has profound beneficial effects on lifespan, neuroprotection, cognition and mood [43-51]. Cultured cells treated with serum from calorie-restricted rats display mitochondrial biogenesis, enhanced bioenergetic capacity and reduced ROS production [52]. These results suggest that the effects of calorie restriction are mediated by a humeral factor affecting mitochondrial metabolism. Indeed, ghrelin levels are increased during calorie restriction in mice, rats and humans [53-57] and ghrelin improved mitochondrial function by regulating ROS, respiration [16, 30], enzyme activity [58] and gene expression [59]. Therefore, ghrelin may underpin many of the enhanced neuronal functions during calorie restriction including neuroprotection [60]. While this hypothesis still needs experimental proof, recent studies support this concept. For example, calorie restriction did not produce a normal anti-anxiety effect in GHSR knockout mice [56] and GOAT knockout mice, which have no acyl ghrelin, were unable to maintain blood glucose levels during calorie restriction. These results show that ghrelin mediates anti-anxiety and glucose homeostasis in calorie restricted mice. Based on this, we hypothesized that ghrelin will mediate the neuroprotective effects of calorie restriction in MPTP mouse models of Parkinson's disease.

In contrast to calorie restriction, plasma ghrelin levels are decreased in obesity in mice and humans [61-63]. Recent evidence also associates obesity with Parkinson's disease in humans [64-66] and obesity is predicted to decrease lifespan in the future [67]. Indeed, obesity increases the susceptibility to MPTP-induced nigrostriatal dysfunction [68], causes reactive gliosis and exacerbates chemically-induced neurodegeneration [69]. Given that ghrelin protects against degeneration in mouse models of Parkinson's disease, we hypothesized that lower ghrelin levels in obesity contribute to dopamine degeneration in the SNpc [16].

The animal studies described above highlight the promise for ghrelin therapy in human Parkinson's disease patients. In Parkinson's disease, patients show delayed gastric emptying and other gastrointestinal symptoms [70, 71], which may be related to disturbed ghrelin secretion in Parkinson's disease, as ghrelin affects gastroprotection and gut motility [72-75].

In order to determine ghrelin levels in Parkinson's disease patients, Unger et al. measured postprandial ghrelin in 20 healthy controls and 39 Parkinson's disease patients. Their results show that Parkinson's disease patients had significantly reduced postprandial acyl ghrelin levels relative to controls [76]. An additional study also showed that Parkinson's disease patients exhibit a paradoxical relationship between BMI and ghrelin concentrations. In normal people, high plasma ghrelin correlates with low BMI, however Parkinson's disease patients show that the lower the BMI, the lower the plasma ghrelin concentration [77]. These two studies clearly demonstrate that Parkinson's disease patients have impaired ghrelin secretion and highlight a potential therapeutic application for ghrelin in Parkinson's disease. Indeed, ghrelin is a unique hormone with potentially diverse therapeutic applications in Parkinson's disease. First, ghrelin could improve gastrointestinal dysfunction in Parkinson's disease. Second, ghrelin could prevent further nigral degeneration by acting directly on dopamine cells in the SNpc. Third, because weight loss is a common symptom of Parkinson's disease, exogenous ghrelin could help maintain normal energy homeostasis by promoting appetite and weight gain. Fourth, depression is a common symptom of Parkinson's disease and ghrelin positively affects mood and reduces anxiety [56]. Fifth, Parkinson's disease patients occasionally display learning and memory deficits and ghrelin enhances learning and memory by activating synaptic plasticity in the hippocampus [78]. These observations strongly suggest ghrelin has multiple beneficial effects on Parkinson's disease patients and no predictable side effects. Future studies should test the clinical efficacy of ghrelin treatment in Parkinson's disease patients, especially since many patients experience uncontrolled weight loss and impaired appetite regulation. This highlights the therapeutic potential of ghrelin in Parkinson's disease patients to maintain appetite and energy balance, and prevent further degeneration.

3. Glucagon like peptide 1 (GLP1)

GLP1 is a hormone produced by the proglucagon gene expressed in L cells predominantly in the lower gut (distal intestine and colon) but it is also found at lower levels in the pancreas and brain. Other proglucagon products include glucagon, glicentin, glucagon like peptide 2 and oxyntomodulin. GLP1 is a well-known satiety signal that is released into the bloodstream in response to ingested nutrients, such as fats and sugars. GLP1 inhibits food intake in several species including humans and is also a promising target to restrict diabetes since it accentuates glucose-dependent insulin release, inhibits glucagon and increases pancreatic β-cell growth [79]. GLP1 acts on the GLP1R, which is expressed in the gut, pancreas, brainstem, hypothalamus, thalamus, hippocampus and vagal afferent nerves [80-82]. The presence of the GLP1R in the brain indicates that GLP1 could have effects on neuronal function. Indeed, activation of the GLP1R promotes cell survival and plasticity including enhanced learning, protection from apoptotic cell death and from oxidative insults [83-89]. In contrast, treatment with GLP1R antagonists or studies with GLP1R knockout mice all demonstrate impaired synaptic plasticity as well as impaired learning, cognition and memory [85, 87]. These observations directly suggest that GLP1 has neuroprotective effects. For example, both central and peripheral GLP1 enhances synaptic plasticity in mice [87] and the GLP1 agonist exendin-4 increases neurogenesis in the hypothalamus [90] and stimulates both neurons and glia from neural progenitor cells in vitro and in vivo [91]. Moreover exendin-4 activates human neuronal cell differentiation and proliferation [92, 93] in vitro. Clearly, the ability to increase neurogenesis implicates GLP1 as

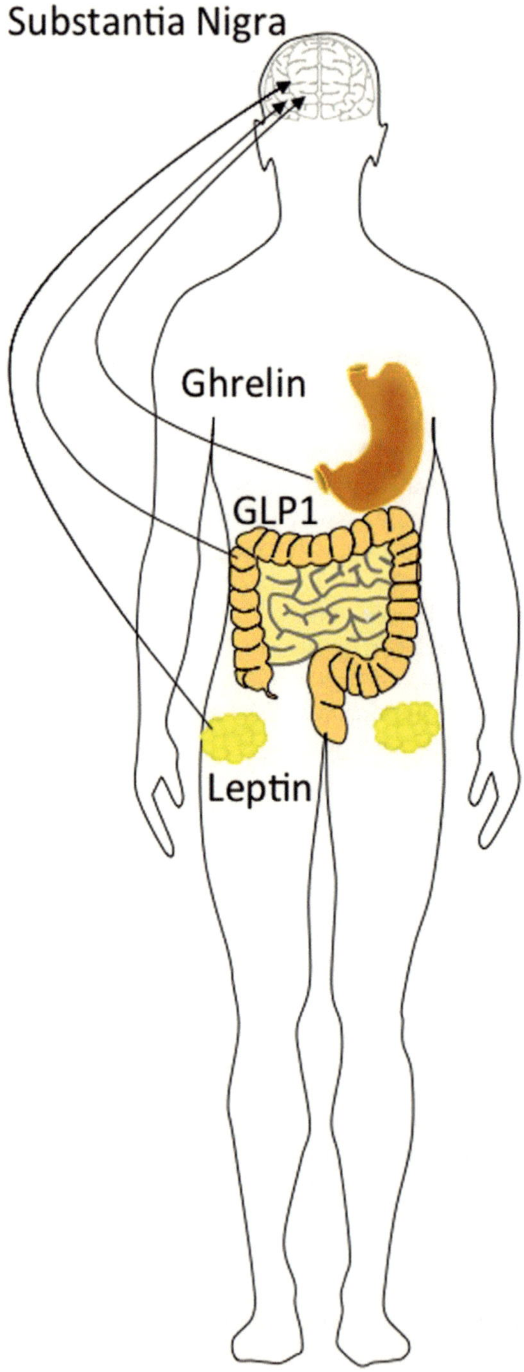

Fig. 1. Metabolic hormones directly target dopamine neurons in the substantia nigra. Ghrelin, glucagon-like peptide 1 (GLP1) and leptin receptors are all present in the substantia nigra suggesting a direct action of these hormones on dopamine neuronal function

a potential therapeutic agent that combats degeneration and facilitates regeneration in neurological disorders such as Parkinson's disease.

Recent animal studies show that GLP1 is an excellent therapeutic target to treat Parkinson's disease. For example, exendin-4 treatment for 2 weeks reduces amphetamine-induced circling behavior in 6-OHDA lesioned rats and reduced TH cell death in the SNpc [91]. The GLP1-induced neuroprotection was ascribed to neurogenesis in the subventricular zone and an increase in neural stem cells in the medial striatum. Harkavyi et al, also found similar results using two different Parkinson's disease models [94]. Exendin-4 reduced circling behavior in both 6-OHDA and lipopolysaccharide (LPS) models of Parkinson's disease. Consistent with these behavioural experiments, exendin-4 attenuated striatal dopamine loss and TH cell loss in the SNpc [94]. This study underscores the therapeutic potential of GLP1, as it showed that exendin arrests degeneration even after established nigral lesions. Li et al, detected GLP1R mRNA in both primary cortical neurons and ventral mesencephalic dopamine neurons [95]. Both GLP1 and exendin-4 prevent hypoxia and 6-OHDA-induced cell death in cells from GLP1R wild type but not GLP1R knockout mice. *In vivo*, exendin-4 protected dopamine neurons against degeneration, preserved dopamine levels and improved motor function in the MPTP mouse model of Parkinson's disease [95]. In order to characterize the neuroprotective properties of GLP1, Li et al overexpressed GLP1R in human neuroblastoma SH-SY5Y cells. Both Exendin-4 and GLP stimulated cell proliferation and cell viability by 2-fold after 24 hours and prevented hypoxia and 6-OHDA-induced cell death [93]. Exendin-4 and GLP1 ameliorated caspase 3 activity, decreased pro-apoptotic Bax and increase anti-apoptotic Bcl-2 proteins. Protein kinase A and PI3K pathways mediated the neuroprotective functions of GLP1R signaling although MAPK also played a minor role [93].

Exendin-4 has strong anti-inflammatory properties and GLP1 inhibits LPS-induced cytokine release [96, 97] and the anti-inflammatory effect of GLP1 could be mediated by promoting adipokines that target the brain to reduce neuroinflammation and improve neuroprotection [98] or by a direct effect as glia (and neurons) express the GLP1R [96]. Indeed, Kim et al, illustrated that systemic exendin-4 injection restricted the loss of dopamine neurons in the SNpc and dopamine fibers in the striatum by deactivating microglia in these regions [99]. Microglia are well described to exacerbate degeneration [21] by increasing pro-inflammatory cytokines, thus reduced microglial activation by exendin-4 in the nigrostriatal pathway suppresses degeneration. These studies highlighted above demonstrate the utility of activating GLP1R to treat Parkinson's disease. Indeed, research shows that activating GLP1R restricts degeneration not only in Parkinson's disease but also in models of Alzheimer's disease [100] and stroke [95]. The GLP1R agonist, exendin-4, provides the most attractive therapeutic potential as it has a much longer half-life than GLP1 itself (hours vs. minutes). Given that GLP1R activation with exendin-4 in animal studies provides significant neuroprotection in different models of Parkinson's disease, future studies are required to translate these findings into a clinical application. The ability of GLP1R activation to increase neurogenesis may provide long lasting protection against ongoing degeneration in Parkinson's disease patients. However, GLP1 suppresses food intake and this is an unwanted side effect in Parkinson's disease patients. Future studies need to address and circumvent these issues.

4. Leptin

Although leptin is predominantly secreted from adipose tissue and is not a gut hormone, it is pertinent to add a section on leptin and Parkinson's disease, as leptin is also an important

Figure 2

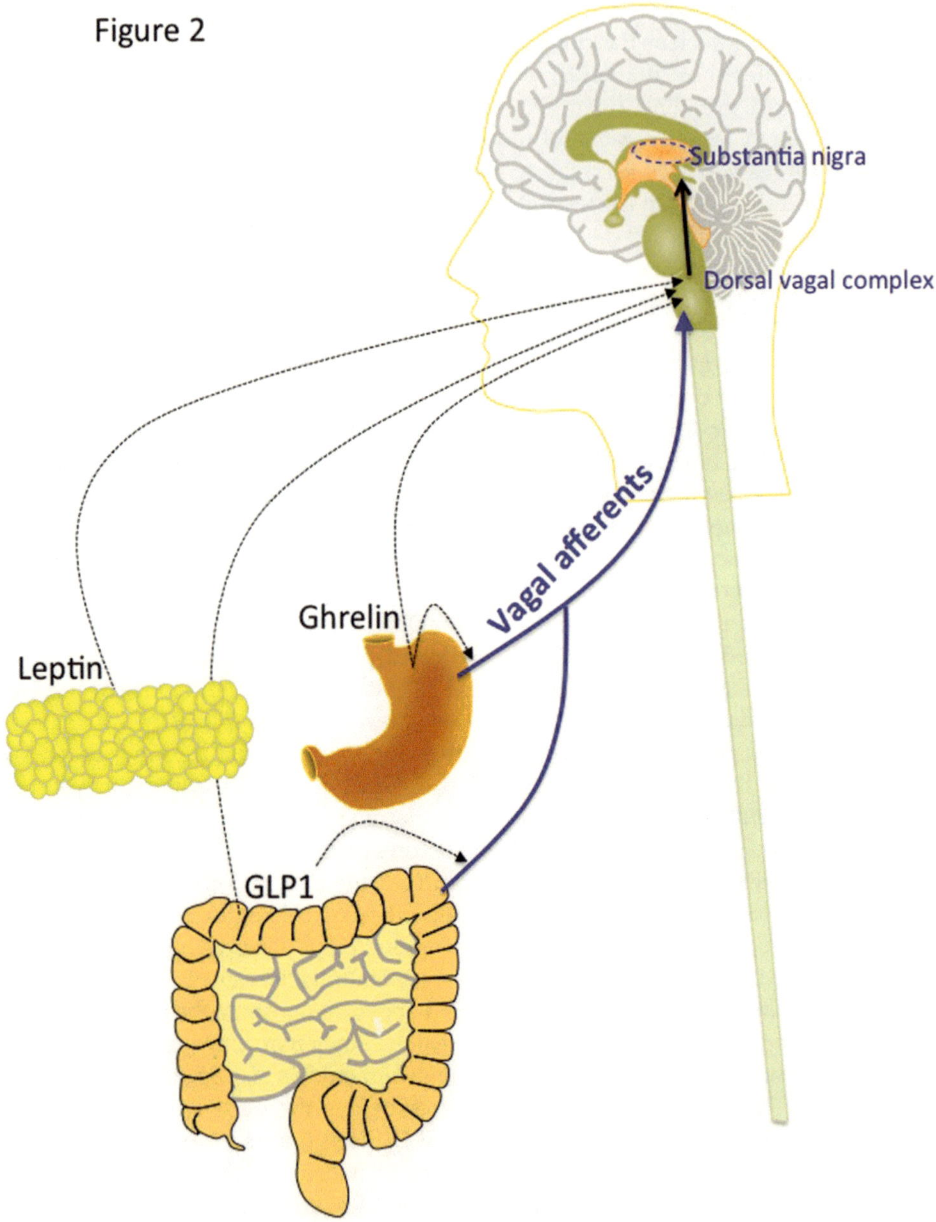

Fig. 2. Metabolic hormones indirectly target substantia nigra neurons through the brainstem. Ghrelin, glucagon-like peptide 1 and leptin receptors are present in the dorsal vagal complex. Vagal afferents from the stomach and intestines are also present in the dorsal vagal complex. Braak's hypothesis states that dopamine dysfunction is a product of retrograde degeneration from the gut (stomach/intestines), through the brainstem (dorsal vagal complex). Ghrelin and GLP1 may promote healthy gut function and thereby restrict retrograde degeneration. This circuit highlights the complicated and integrated manner in which metabolic hormones directly and indirectly regulate higher brain function

metabolic hormone. Leptin is best known for the hypothalamic regulation of energy homeostasis, including suppressing appetite and increasing energy expenditure [101]. However, significant leptin receptor expression exists outside the hypothalamus including in midbrain dopamine neurons [102] relevant to Parkinson's disease. The first indication that leptin plays a neuroprotective role came from in vitro studies. Lu et al showed that leptin prevents MPP+-induced cell death in SH-SY5Y cells through the phosphatidylinositol 3 kinase (PI3K) pathway but not the STAT3 or MAPK pathway [103]. Leptin also protects the nigrostriatal dopaminergic system from 6-hydroxydopamine (6-OHDA) induced degeneration *in vivo* [104]. 6-OHDA treatment caused a significant loss of dopamine neurons in the SNpc and dopamine concentration in the striatum that was reversed with leptin pretreatment. The 6-OHDA model offers an additional advantage over the MPTP mouse model as it allows a quantifiable measure of motor dysfunction. These studies showed that leptin decreased apomorphine-induced asymmetrical rotations contralateral to the side of 6-OHDA injections. Leptin pretreatment attenuated key apoptotic markers such as activated caspase 9 and activated caspase 3, DNA fragmentation and cytochrome C release. ERK1/2 phosphorylation mediated the anti-apoptotic effects of leptin by recruiting pCREB in cultured dopamine neurons. pCREB is an important transcription factor in dopamine neurons that induces neuroprotection by increasing BDNF expression and leptin increased BDNF in this study.

There are conflicting reports about plasma leptin concentrations in Parkinson's disease patients. Fiszer et al reported patients with weight loss had reduced plasma leptin concentrations [77] whereas Aziz et al observed no difference in the total levels of leptin or diurnal variation [105]. These results indicate that unintended weight loss in Parkinson's disease patients is unlikely to be due to abnormal serum leptin concentrations. Current human studies have only measured plasma leptin in relation to weight loss, future studies should also examine the effect on disease progression, as animal studies highlighted above suggest that leptin may have neuroprotective effects on SNpc dopamine neurons.

5. Conclusion

Gastrointestinal dysfunction, such as constipation, is a common symptom of Parkinson's disease that is observed well before any motor dysfunction caused by dopaminergic degeneration in the nigrostriatal pathway. Recent evidence suggests that Parkinson's disease may even start in the gastrointestinal tract. According to the 'Braak's' hypothesis, protein aggregation in enteric neurons spreads in a retrograde manner to the brain through the dorsal motor nucleus of the vagus and triggers Parkinson's disease [1]. In support of this theory, mutant α-synuclein in gut enteric neurons caused gastrointestinal (GI) dysfunction followed by motor abnormalities [2] and rotenone treatment, a compound found in pesticides that causes Parkinson's-like conditions, caused enteric neuronal α-synuclein accumulation and GI dysfunction in rats before neuronal protein aggregation [3, 4]. These studies, taken together with the early GI disturbances in humans, clearly implicate the GI system in the pathogenesis of Parkinson's disease. This chapter highlights recent work on two important gut hormones, ghrelin and GLP1, that also regulate nigrostriatal dopamine function. It is interesting to note that both hormones influence gut function, neuronal metabolism, appetite and peripheral energy metabolism, suggesting a novel link between neurodegeneration and energy metabolism. Future studies are required to translate promising results in animal studies into clinical therapies.

6. Acknowledgements

This work was supported by a Monash Fellowship, Monash University, Australia, an Australia Research Council Future Fellowship and NHMRC grants (NHMRC 546131, 1011274) to ZBA.

7. References

[1] Braak H, Rub U, Gai WP, Del Tredici K. Idiopathic Parkinson's disease: possible routes by which vulnerable neuronal types may be subject to neuroinvasion by an unknown pathogen. J Neural Transm. 2003 May;110(5):517-36.

[2] Kuo YM, Li Z, Jiao Y, Gaborit N, Pani AK, Orrison BM, et al. Extensive enteric nervous system abnormalities in mice transgenic for artificial chromosomes containing Parkinson disease-associated alpha-synuclein gene mutations precede central nervous system changes. Hum Mol Genet. 2010 May 1;19(9):1633-50.

[3] Drolet RE, Cannon JR, Montero L, Greenamyre JT. Chronic rotenone exposure reproduces Parkinson's disease gastrointestinal neuropathology. Neurobiol Dis. 2009 Oct;36(1):96-102.

[4] Pan-Montojo F, Anichtchik O, Dening Y, Knels L, Pursche S, Jung R, et al. Progression of Parkinson's disease pathology is reproduced by intragastric administration of rotenone in mice. PLoS One. 2010;5(1):e8762.

[5] Andrews ZB. Central mechanisms involved in the orexigenic actions of ghrelin. Peptides. 2011 May 17.

[6] Briggs DI, Andrews ZB. A Recent Update on the Role of Ghrelin in Glucose Homeostasis. Curr Diabetes Rev. 2011 May 4.

[7] Briggs DI, Andrews ZB. Metabolic status regulates ghrelin function on energy homeostasis. Neuroendocrinology. 2011;93(1):48-57.

[8] Kojima M, Hosoda H, Date Y, Nakazato M, Matsuo H, Kangawa K. Ghrelin is a growth-hormone-releasing acylated peptide from stomach. Nature. 1999 Dec 9;402(6762):656-60.

[9] Howard AD, Feighner SD, Cully DF, Arena JP, Liberator PA, Rosenblum CI, et al. A receptor in pituitary and hypothalamus that functions in growth hormone release. Science. 1996 Aug 16;273(5277):974-7.

[10] Guan XM, Yu H, Palyha OC, McKee KK, Feighner SD, Sirinathsinghji DJ, et al. Distribution of mRNA encoding the growth hormone secretagogue receptor in brain and peripheral tissues. Brain Res Mol Brain Res. 1997 Aug;48(1):23-9.

[11] Yang J, Brown MS, Liang G, Grishin NV, Goldstein JL. Identification of the acyltransferase that octanoylates ghrelin, an appetite-stimulating peptide hormone. Cell. 2008 Feb 8;132(3):387-96.

[12] Gutierrez JA, Solenberg PJ, Perkins DR, Willency JA, Knierman MD, Jin Z, et al. Ghrelin octanoylation mediated by an orphan lipid transferase. Proc Natl Acad Sci U S A. 2008 Apr 29;105(17):6320-5.

[13] Zhu X, Cao Y, Voogd K, Steiner DF. On the processing of proghrelin to ghrelin. J Biol Chem. 2006 Dec 15;281(50):38867-70.

[14] Murakami N, Hayashida T, Kuroiwa T, Nakahara K, Ida T, Mondal MS, et al. Role for central ghrelin in food intake and secretion profile of stomach ghrelin in rats. J Endocrinol. 2002 Aug;174(2):283-8.

[15] Zigman JM, Jones JE, Lee CE, Saper CB, Elmquist JK. Expression of ghrelin receptor mRNA in the rat and the mouse brain. J Comp Neurol. 2006 Jan 20;494(3):528-48.
[16] Andrews ZB, Erion D, Beiler R, Liu ZW, Abizaid A, Zigman J, et al. Ghrelin promotes and protects nigrostriatal dopamine function via a UCP2-dependent mitochondrial mechanism. J Neurosci. 2009 Nov 11;29(45):14057 65.
[17] Abizaid A, Liu ZW, Andrews ZB, Shanabrough M, Borok E, Elsworth JD, et al. Ghrelin modulates the activity and synaptic input organization of midbrain dopamine neurons while promoting appetite. J Clin Invest. 2006 Dec;116(12):3229-39.
[18] Jiang H, Li LJ, Wang J, Xie JX. Ghrelin antagonizes MPTP-induced neurotoxicity to the dopaminergic neurons in mouse substantia nigra. Exp Neurol. 2008 Aug;212(2):532-7.
[19] Moon M, Kim HG, Hwang L, Seo JH, Kim S, Hwang S, et al. Neuroprotective effect of ghrelin in the 1-methyl-4-phenyl-1,2,3,6-tetrahydropyridine mouse model of Parkinson's disease by blocking microglial activation. Neurotox Res. 2009 May;15(4):332-47.
[20] Dong J, Song N, Xie J, Jiang H. Ghrelin antagonized 1-methyl-4-phenylpyridinium (MPP(+))-induced apoptosis in MES23.5 cells. J Mol Neurosci. 2009 Feb;37(2):182-9.
[21] Burguillos MA, Deierborg T, Kavanagh E, Persson A, Hajji N, Garcia-Quintanilla A, et al. Caspase signalling controls microglia activation and neurotoxicity. Nature. 2011 Apr 21;472(7343):319-24.
[22] Huang CX, Yuan MJ, Huang H, Wu G, Liu Y, Yu SB, et al. Ghrelin inhibits post-infarct myocardial remodeling and improves cardiac function through anti-inflammation effect. Peptides. 2009 Dec;30(12):2286-91.
[23] Chow KB, Cheng CH, Wise H. Anti-inflammatory activity of ghrelin in human carotid artery cells. Inflammation. 2009 Dec;32(6):402-9.
[24] Theil MM, Miyake S, Mizuno M, Tomi C, Croxford JL, Hosoda H, et al. Suppression of experimental autoimmune encephalomyelitis by ghrelin. J Immunol. 2009 Aug 15;183(4):2859-66.
[25] Ersahin M, Toklu HZ, Erzik C, Cetinel S, Bangir D, Ogunc AV, et al. The Anti-Inflammatory and Neuroprotective Effects of Ghrelin in Subarachnoid Hemorrhage-Induced Oxidative Brain Damage in Rats. J Neurotrauma. 2010 Mar 5;27(6):1143-55.
[26] Andrews ZB, Rivera A, Elsworth JD, Roth RH, Agnati L, Gago B, et al. Uncoupling protein-2 promotes nigrostriatal dopamine neuronal function. European Journal of Neuroscience. 2006;24(1):32-6.
[27] Andrews ZB, Diano S, Horvath TL. Mitochondrial uncoupling proteins in the CNS: in support of function and survival. Nature Reviews Neuroscience. 2005;6(11):829-40.
[28] Andrews ZB, Horvath B, Barnstable CJ, Elsworth J, Yang L, Beal MF, et al. Uncoupling protein-2 is critical for nigral dopamine cell survival in a mouse model of Parkinson's disease.[erratum appears in J Neurosci. 2005 Feb 23;25(8):table of contents]. Journal of Neuroscience. 2005;25(1):184-91.
[29] Conti B, Sugama S, Lucero J, Winsky-Sommerer R, Wirz SA, Maher P, et al. Uncoupling protein 2 protects dopaminergic neurons from acute 1,2,3,6-methyl-phenyl-tetrahydropyridine toxicity. J Neurochem. 2005 Apr;93(2):493-501.

[30] Andrews ZB, Liu ZW, Walllingford N, Erion DM, Borok E, Friedman JM, et al. UCP2 mediates ghrelin's action on NPY/AgRP neurons by lowering free radicals. Nature. 2008 Jul 30;454(7206):846-51.

[31] Lopez M, Lage R, Saha AK, Perez-Tilve D, Vazquez MJ, Varela L, et al. Hypothalamic fatty acid metabolism mediates the orexigenic action of ghrelin. Cell Metab. 2008 May;7(5):389-99.

[32] Steinberg GR, Kemp BE. AMPK in Health and Disease. Physiol Rev. 2009 Jul;89(3):1025-78.

[33] Bergeron R, Ren JM, Cadman KS, Moore IK, Perret P, Pypaert M, et al. Chronic activation of AMP kinase results in NRF-1 activation and mitochondrial biogenesis. Am J Physiol Endocrinol Metab. 2001 Dec;281(6):E1340-6.

[34] Jager S, Handschin C, St-Pierre J, Spiegelman BM. AMP-activated protein kinase (AMPK) action in skeletal muscle via direct phosphorylation of PGC-1alpha. Proc Natl Acad Sci U S A. 2007 Jul 17;104(29):12017-22.

[35] Zong H, Ren JM, Young LH, Pypaert M, Mu J, Birnbaum MJ, et al. AMP kinase is required for mitochondrial biogenesis in skeletal muscle in response to chronic energy deprivation. Proc Natl Acad Sci U S A. 2002 Dec 10;99(25):15983-7.

[36] Dasgupta B, Milbrandt J. Resveratrol stimulates AMP kinase activity in neurons. Proc Natl Acad Sci U S A. 2007 Apr 24;104(17):7217-22.

[37] Horvath TL, Erion DM, Elsworth JD, Roth RH, Shulman GI, Andrews ZB. GPA protects the nigrostriatal dopamine system by enhancing mitochondrial function. Neurobiol Dis. 2011 Mar 13.

[38] Reznick RM, Shulman GI. The role of AMP-activated protein kinase in mitochondrial biogenesis. J Physiol. 2006 Jul 1;574(Pt 1):33-9.

[39] Williams DB, Sutherland LN, Bomhof MR, Basaraba SA, Thrush AB, Dyck DJ, et al. Muscle-specific differences in the response of mitochondrial proteins to beta-GPA feeding: an evaluation of potential mechanisms. Am J Physiol Endocrinol Metab. 2009 Jun;296(6):E1400-8.

[40] Reznick RM, Zong H, Li J, Morino K, Moore IK, Yu HJ, et al. Aging-associated reductions in AMP-activated protein kinase activity and mitochondrial biogenesis. Cell Metab. 2007 Feb;5(2):151-6.

[41] Chaturvedi RK, Adhihetty P, Shukla S, Hennessy T, Calingasan N, Yang L, et al. Impaired PGC-1alpha function in muscle in Huntington's disease. Hum Mol Genet. 2009 Aug 15;18(16):3048-65.

[42] Horvath TL, Diano S, Tschop M. Ghrelin in hypothalamic regulation of energy balance. Curr Top Med Chem. 2003;3(8):921-7.

[43] Colman RJ, Anderson RM, Johnson SC, Kastman EK, Kosmatka KJ, Beasley TM, et al. Caloric restriction delays disease onset and mortality in rhesus monkeys. Science. 2009 Jul 10;325(5937):201-4.

[44] Maswood N, Young J, Tilmont E, Zhang Z, Gash DM, Gerhardt GA, et al. Caloric restriction increases neurotrophic factor levels and attenuates neurochemical and behavioral deficits in a primate model of Parkinson's disease. Proc Natl Acad Sci U S A. 2004 Dec 28;101(52):18171-6.

[45] Contestabile A. Benefits of caloric restriction on brain aging and related pathological States: understanding mechanisms to devise novel therapies. Curr Med Chem. 2009;16(3):350-61.

[46] Komatsu T, Chiba T, Yamaza H, Yamashita K, Shimada A, Hoshiyama Y, et al. Manipulation of caloric content but not diet composition, attenuates the deficit in learning and memory of senescence-accelerated mouse strain P8. Exp Gerontol. 2008 Apr;43(4):339-46.
[47] Carter CS, Leeuwenburgh C, Daniels M, Foster TC. Influence of calorie restriction on measures of age-related cognitive decline: role of increased physical activity. J Gerontol A Biol Sci Med Sci. 2009 Aug;64(8):850-9.
[48] Halagappa VK, Guo Z, Pearson M, Matsuoka Y, Cutler RG, Laferla FM, et al. Intermittent fasting and caloric restriction ameliorate age-related behavioral deficits in the triple-transgenic mouse model of Alzheimer's disease. Neurobiol Dis. 2007 Apr;26(1):212-20.
[49] Abbott JD, Kent S, Levay EA, Tucker RV, Penman J, Tammer AH, et al. The effects of calorie restriction olfactory cues on conspecific anxiety-like behaviour. Behav Brain Res. 2009 Aug 12;201(2):305-10.
[50] Mantis JG, Fritz CL, Marsh J, Heinrichs SC, Seyfried TN. Improvement in motor and exploratory behavior in Rett syndrome mice with restricted ketogenic and standard diets. Epilepsy Behav. 2009 Jun;15(2):133-41.
[51] Levay EA, Govic A, Penman J, Paolini AG, Kent S. Effects of adult-onset calorie restriction on anxiety-like behavior in rats. Physiol Behav. 2007 Dec 5;92(5):889-96.
[52] Lopez-Lluch G, Hunt N, Jones B, Zhu M, Jamieson H, Hilmer S, et al. Calorie restriction induces mitochondrial biogenesis and bioenergetic efficiency. Proc Natl Acad Sci U S A. 2006 Feb 7;103(6):1768-73.
[53] Yukawa M, Cummings DE, Matthys CC, Callahan HS, Frayo RS, Spiekerman CF, et al. Effect of aging on the response of ghrelin to acute weight loss. J Am Geriatr Soc. 2006 Apr;54(4):648-53.
[54] Redman LM, Veldhuis JD, Rood J, Smith SR, Williamson D, Ravussin E. The effect of caloric restriction interventions on growth hormone secretion in nonobese men and women. Aging Cell. 2010 Feb;9(1):32-9.
[55] Barazzoni R, Zanetti M, Stebel M, Biolo G, Cattin L, Guarnieri G. Hyperleptinemia prevents increased plasma ghrelin concentration during short-term moderate caloric restriction in rats. Gastroenterology. 2003 May;124(5):1188-92.
[56] Lutter M, Sakata I, Osborne-Lawrence S, Rovinsky SA, Anderson JG, Jung S, et al. The orexigenic hormone ghrelin defends against depressive symptoms of chronic stress. Nat Neurosci. 2008 Jul;11(7):752-3.
[57] Zhao TJ, Liang G, Li RL, Xie X, Sleeman MW, Murphy AJ, et al. Ghrelin O-acyltransferase (GOAT) is essential for growth hormone-mediated survival of calorie-restricted mice. Proc Natl Acad Sci U S A. 2010 Apr 20;107(16):7467-72.
[58] Barazzoni R, Zhu X, Deboer M, Datta R, Culler MD, Zanetti M, et al. Combined effects of ghrelin and higher food intake enhance skeletal muscle mitochondrial oxidative capacity and AKT phosphorylation in rats with chronic kidney disease. Kidney Int. 2010 Jan;77(1):23-8.
[59] Barazzoni R, Bosutti A, Stebel M, Cattin MR, Roder E, Visintin L, et al. Ghrelin regulates mitochondrial-lipid metabolism gene expression and tissue fat distribution in liver and skeletal muscle. Am J Physiol Endocrinol Metab. 2005 Jan;288(1):E228-35.
[60] Andrews ZB. The extra-hypothalamic actions of ghrelin on neuronal function. Trends Neurosci. 2011 Jan;34(1):31-40.

[61] Briggs DI, Enriori PJ, Lemus MB, Cowley MA, Andrews ZB. Diet-induced obesity causes ghrelin resistance in arcuate NPY/AgRP neurons. Endocrinology. 2010;151(10):4745-55.
[62] Briggs DI, Lemus MB, Kua E, Andrews ZB. Diet-induced obesity attenuates fasting-induced hyperphagia. J Neuroendocrinol. 2011 Apr 25.
[63] Tschop M, Weyer C, Tataranni PA, Devanarayan V, Ravussin E, Heiman ML. Circulating ghrelin levels are decreased in human obesity. Diabetes. 2001 Apr;50(4):707-9.
[64] Abbott RD, Ross GW, White LR, Nelson JS, Masaki KH, Tanner CM, et al. Midlife adiposity and the future risk of Parkinson's disease. Neurology. 2002 Oct 8;59(7):1051-7.
[65] Hu G, Jousilahti P, Bidel S, Antikainen R, Tuomilehto J. Type 2 diabetes and the risk of Parkinson's disease. Diabetes Care. 2007 Apr;30(4):842-7.
[66] Hu G, Jousilahti P, Nissinen A, Antikainen R, Kivipelto M, Tuomilehto J. Body mass index and the risk of Parkinson disease. Neurology. 2006 Dec 12;67(11):1955-9.
[67] Olshansky SJ, Passaro DJ, Hershow RC, Layden J, Carnes BA, Brody J, et al. A potential decline in life expectancy in the United States in the 21st century. N Engl J Med. 2005 Mar 17;352(11):1138-45.
[68] Choi JY, Jang EH, Park CS, Kang JH. Enhanced susceptibility to 1-methyl-4-phenyl-1,2,3,6-tetrahydropyridine neurotoxicity in high-fat diet-induced obesity. Free Radic Biol Med. 2005 Mar 15;38(6):806-16.
[69] Sriram K, Benkovic SA, Miller DB, O'Callaghan JP. Obesity exacerbates chemically induced neurodegeneration. Neuroscience. 2002;115(4):1335-46.
[70] Goetze O, Wieczorek J, Mueller T, Przuntek H, Schmidt WE, Woitalla D. Impaired gastric emptying of a solid test meal in patients with Parkinson's disease using 13C-sodium octanoate breath test. Neurosci Lett. 2005 Mar 3;375(3):170-3.
[71] Unger MM, Hattemer K, Moller JC, Schmittinger K, Mankel K, Eggert K, et al. Real-time visualization of altered gastric motility by magnetic resonance imaging in patients with Parkinson's disease. Mov Disord. 2010 Apr 15;25(5):623-8.
[72] Brzozowski T, Konturek PC, Konturek SJ, Kwiecien S, Drozdowicz D, Bielanski W, et al. Exogenous and endogenous ghrelin in gastroprotection against stress-induced gastric damage. Regulatory peptides. 2004 Aug 15;120(1-3):39-51.
[73] Brzozowski T, Konturek PC, Sliwowski Z, Drozdowicz D, Kwiecien S, Pawlik M, et al. Neural aspects of ghrelin-induced gastroprotection against mucosal injury induced by noxious agents. Journal of physiology and pharmacology : an official journal of the Polish Physiological Society. 2006 Nov;57 Suppl 6:63-76.
[74] Shimizu Y, Chang EC, Shafton AD, Ferens DM, Sanger GJ, Witherington J, et al. Evidence that stimulation of ghrelin receptors in the spinal cord initiates propulsive activity in the colon of the rat. J Physiol. 2006 Oct 1;576(Pt 1):329-38.
[75] Shafton AD, Sanger GJ, Witherington J, Brown JD, Muir A, Butler S, et al. Oral administration of a centrally acting ghrelin receptor agonist to conscious rats triggers defecation. Neurogastroenterol Motil. 2009 Jan;21(1):71-7.
[76] Unger MM, Moller JC, Mankel K, Eggert KM, Bohne K, Bodden M, et al. Postprandial ghrelin response is reduced in patients with Parkinson's disease and idiopathic REM sleep behaviour disorder: a peripheral biomarker for early Parkinson's disease? J Neurol. 2010 Dec 24.

[77] Fiszer U, Michalowska M, Baranowska B, Wolinska-Witort E, Jeske W, Jethon M, et al. Leptin and ghrelin concentrations and weight loss in Parkinson's disease. Acta Neurol Scand. 2009 Dec 17.
[78] Diano S, Farr SA, Benoit SC, McNay EC, da Silva I, Horvath B, et al. Ghrelin controls hippocampal spine synapse density and memory performance. Nature Neuroscience. 2006;9(3):381-8.
[79] Drucker DJ. The biology of incretin hormones. Cell metabolism. 2006 Mar;3(3):153-65.
[80] Drucker DJ. Enhancing the action of incretin hormones: a new whey forward? Endocrinology. 2006 Jul;147(7):3171-2.
[81] Turton MD, O'Shea D, Gunn I, Beak SA, Edwards CM, Meeran K, et al. A role for glucagon-like peptide-1 in the central regulation of feeding. Nature. 1996 Jan 4;379(6560):69-72.
[82] Campos RV, Lee YC, Drucker DJ. Divergent tissue-specific and developmental expression of receptors for glucagon and glucagon-like peptide-1 in the mouse. Endocrinology. 1994 May;134(5):2156-64.
[83] Cabou C, Campistron G, Marsollier N, Leloup C, Cruciani-Guglielmacci C, Penicaud L, et al. Brain glucagon-like peptide-1 regulates arterial blood flow, heart rate, and insulin sensitivity. Diabetes. 2008 Oct;57(10):2577-87.
[84] Drucker DJ. Glucagon-like peptides: regulators of cell proliferation, differentiation, and apoptosis. Molecular endocrinology. 2003 Feb;17(2):161-71.
[85] During MJ, Cao L, Zuzga DS, Francis JS, Fitzsimons HL, Jiao X, et al. Glucagon-like peptide-1 receptor is involved in learning and neuroprotection. Nat Med. 2003 Sep;9(9):1173-9.
[86] Greig NH, Mattson MP, Perry T, Chan SL, Giordano T, Sambamurti K, et al. New therapeutic strategies and drug candidates for neurodegenerative diseases: p53 and TNF-alpha inhibitors, and GLP-1 receptor agonists. Annals of the New York Academy of Sciences. 2004 Dec;1035:290-315.
[87] McClean PL, Gault VA, Harriott P, Holscher C. Glucagon-like peptide-1 analogues enhance synaptic plasticity in the brain: a link between diabetes and Alzheimer's disease. Eur J Pharmacol. 2010 Mar 25;630(1-3):158-62.
[88] Perry TA, Greig NH. A new Alzheimer's disease interventive strategy: GLP-1. Curr Drug Targets. 2004 Aug;5(6):565-71.
[89] Stoffers DA, Kieffer TJ, Hussain MA, Drucker DJ, Bonner-Weir S, Habener JF, et al. Insulinotropic glucagon-like peptide 1 agonists stimulate expression of homeodomain protein IDX-1 and increase islet size in mouse pancreas. Diabetes. 2000 May;49(5):741-8.
[90] Belsham DD, Fick LJ, Dalvi PS, Centeno ML, Chalmers JA, Lee PK, et al. Ciliary neurotrophic factor recruitment of glucagon-like peptide-1 mediates neurogenesis, allowing immortalization of adult murine hypothalamic neurons. The FASEB journal : official publication of the Federation of American Societies for Experimental Biology. 2009 Dec;23(12):4256-65.
[91] Bertilsson G, Patrone C, Zachrisson O, Andersson A, Dannaeus K, Heidrich J, et al. Peptide hormone exendin-4 stimulates subventricular zone neurogenesis in the adult rodent brain and induces recovery in an animal model of Parkinson's disease. J Neurosci Res. 2008 Feb 1;86(2):326-38.

[92] Luciani P, Deledda C, Benvenuti S, Cellai I, Squecco R, Monici M, et al. Differentiating effects of the glucagon-like peptide-1 analogue exendin-4 in a human neuronal cell model. Cell Mol Life Sci. 2010 Nov;67(21):3711-23.

[93] Li Y, Tweedie D, Mattson MP, Holloway HW, Greig NH. Enhancing the GLP-1 receptor signaling pathway leads to proliferation and neuroprotection in human neuroblastoma cells. J Neurochem. 2010 Jun;113(6):1621-31.

[94] Harkavyi A, Abuirmeileh A, Lever R, Kingsbury AE, Biggs CS, Whitton PS. Glucagon-like peptide 1 receptor stimulation reverses key deficits in distinct rodent models of Parkinson's disease. J Neuroinflammation. 2008;5:19.

[95] Li Y, Perry T, Kindy MS, Harvey BK, Tweedie D, Holloway HW, et al. GLP-1 receptor stimulation preserves primary cortical and dopaminergic neurons in cellular and rodent models of stroke and Parkinsonism. Proceedings of the National Academy of Sciences of the United States of America. 2009 Jan 27;106(4):1285-90.

[96] Iwai T, Ito S, Tanimitsu K, Udagawa S, Oka J. Glucagon-like peptide-1 inhibits LPS-induced IL-1beta production in cultured rat astrocytes. Neurosci Res. 2006 Aug;55(4):352-60.

[97] Li Y, Cao X, Li LX, Brubaker PL, Edlund H, Drucker DJ. beta-Cell Pdx1 expression is essential for the glucoregulatory, proliferative, and cytoprotective actions of glucagon-like peptide-1. Diabetes. 2005 Feb;54(2):482-91.

[98] Kim Chung le T, Hosaka T, Yoshida M, Harada N, Sakaue H, Sakai T, et al. Exendin-4, a GLP-1 receptor agonist, directly induces adiponectin expression through protein kinase A pathway and prevents inflammatory adipokine expression. Biochem Biophys Res Commun. 2009 Dec 18;390(3):613-8.

[99] Kim S, Moon M, Park S. Exendin-4 protects dopaminergic neurons by inhibition of microglial activation and matrix metalloproteinase-3 expression in an animal model of Parkinson's disease. J Endocrinol. 2009 Sep;202(3):431-9.

[100] Qin Z, Sun Z, Huang J, Hu Y, Wu Z, Mei B. Mutated recombinant human glucagon-like peptide-1 protects SH-SY5Y cells from apoptosis induced by amyloid-beta peptide (1-42). Neurosci Lett. 2008 Oct 31;444(3):217-21.

[101] Gautron L, Elmquist JK. Sixteen years and counting: an update on leptin in energy balance. The Journal of clinical investigation. 2011 Jun 1;121(6):2087-93.

[102] Hommel JD, Trinko R, Sears RM, Georgescu D, Liu ZW, Gao XB, et al. Leptin receptor signaling in midbrain dopamine neurons regulates feeding. Neuron. 2006 Sep 21;51(6):801-10.

[103] Lu J, Park CS, Lee SK, Shin DW, Kang JH. Leptin inhibits 1-methyl-4-phenylpyridinium-induced cell death in SH-SY5Y cells. Neurosci Lett. 2006 Oct 30;407(3):240-3.

[104] Weng Z, Signore AP, Gao Y, Wang S, Zhang F, Hastings T, et al. Leptin protects against 6-hydroxydopamine-induced dopaminergic cell death via mitogen-activated protein kinase signaling. J Biol Chem. 2007 Nov 23;282(47):34479-91.

[105] Aziz NA, Pijl H, Frolich M, Roelfsema F, Roos RA. Leptin, adiponectin, and resistin secretion and diurnal rhythmicity are unaltered in Parkinson's disease. Mov Disord. 2011 Mar;26(4):760-1.

13

Grape Secondary Metabolites – Benefits for Human Health

Teodora Dzhambazova, Violeta Kondakova,
Ivan Tsvetkov and Rossitza Batchvarova
AgroBioInstitute,
Bulgaria

1. Introduction

Grapevine is one of the ancient crops linked with human history during the evolutionary development of man. The fruits and wine have taken part in daily life and ancient ceremonies of our predecessors and currently grapevine is one of the most widely cultivated fruit crop in the world. It is consumed fresh, dry or as beverage but the most popular consumption form in the world is wine. Recent decades researchers found another reason to praise grape products: its beneficial effect on health. In the late Eighties grape and wine have been in the spotlight because of the finding of so called 'French Paradox' that linked moderate red wine consumption to a lower incidence of cardiovascular disease. As an addition, epidemiological studies demonstrated the beneficial effect of moderate wine intake on the neurodegenerative process (Marambaud et al., 2005). These findings gave boost to numerous studies of grape and wine effects on health, revealing evidences about the protective effect of grape compounds against cancer and age-related disorders, such as certain neurological diseases and metabolic disorders. Moreover, scientists proved that some compounds of grape are implicated in important biological functions in the body such as antioxidant defense system, immunological regulation and anti-inflammatory processes. The main question is what makes grape so useful and healthy?

The answer is found in the fruit and wine constituents, i.e. grape secondary metabolites. The secondary metabolites are exclusively produced by plants and represent more than 30 000 different substances that give individual properties of plant species and define them as healthy, healing or even poisonous. Grape is rich in secondary metabolites which makes this fruit crop so popular among the scientific society. Different research groups have undertaken the study of grape metabolomics and revealed the rich profile of grape and wine, including polyphenols such as resveratrol, caffeic acid, catechin, quercetin etc., all of which present highly bioactive substances. In recent years the analyses of grape composition and its effect on human health led to the conclusion that resveratrol is one of the key grape substances responsible for the preventive and therapeutic abilities of wine. Recent study of Iriti et al. (2006) discovered another key substance in grape - melatonin, which is considered for one of the most powerful antioxidants involved in various physiological functions in human body (Srinivasan et al., 2006). It is noteworthy that the health promoting effects of grape and wine are due to the secondary metabolites presented in them.

2. Resveratrol

Resveratrol is one of the polyphenol substances which are considered to have antioxidant activities and to extend life (Lagouge et al., 2006). Resveratrol is a stilbene which is produced naturally by more than 70 plant species as a defensive reaction against pathogens or under stress conditions (UV radiation). As far as resveratrol is a phytoalexin it is produced in plants during the process of a long-term resistance to a certain pathogens or abiotic stress and it is reported that in grapes resveratrol provides a resistance to fungal diseases (LeBlanc, 2006). Resveratrol is soluble in fats and exists in two isomeric forms: cis and trans. Both forms could be bound to a glucose molecule so that resveratrol also occurs naturally as glucoside in grapes which is known as piceid.

Resveratrol is naturally occurring in grapevines where it is almost exclusively synthesized in berry skins, but in muscadine grapes it is found also in seeds (LeBlanc, 2006). The content of this substance in red grapes is higher than in white ones. Total resveratrol content in 100 g red grapes varies between 0.15 mg and 0.78 mg. It is estimated that fresh grape skins contain between 50 and 100 μg resveratrol per gram wet weight (Baliga et al., 2005). The levels of resveratrol in grape are influenced by grape cultivar, its geographic origin and exposure to a fungal disease or other stress conditions. It is found that during the process of winemaking this substance could increase its content depending on fermentation time during which the wine spends in contact with the grape skins. Therefore, the content of resveratrol in white wines is considerably lower since this wine is made after removing the grape skins. In contrary red wine is fermented with the grape skins allowing the wine to absorb more quantity of resveratrol. Some reports suggest that during the winemaking process resveratrol glucosides (piceids) convert to resveratrol and thus the higher concentration of the substance in wine in comparison of that found in fresh grape juice is explained (LeBlanc, 2006).

Recently, scientists are interested in biological activity of phytoalexins and their effect on human health. According to data concerning incidences of coronary heart disease collected from World Health Organization (WHO) in the period of 80s-90s last century, it is reported that French people suffer less from this disease despite having a diet relatively rich in saturated fats and this fact is known as a French paradox (LeBlanc, 2006). Different research groups were investigating the reason for French paradox and why French people have less incidences of coronary heart disease in comparison with Americans although the fact that French consume daily in average more saturated fats (15,6% of total energy intake) than American people (11,3% of total energy intake) (Elmadfa & Kornsteiner, 2009). It has been suggested that the high consumption of red wine in France is a primary factor for the French paradox. The data suggest that wine consumption reduces coronary heart diseases much more than other alcohol beverages and therefore the presence of other wine components different from alcohol provide higher prevention of heart diseases. An increased interest in wine bioactive compounds gave a boost in research of resveratrol and its effect on human health.

2.1 Resveratrol and its cardioprotective effect

The occurrence of the French paradox boosted the researchers to analyze the effect of resveratrol on people with a known predisposition to cardiovascular heart disease. A recent study of Sacanella et al. (2007) reported that 2 glasses of 100 ml red wine per day for 4 weeks is resulting in a greater reduction of inflammatory biomarkers, cellular adhesion molecules

and monocyte adhesion to endothelium, which is not found for the white wine. Resveratrol is a key constituent of red wine which has variety of activities associated with its cardioprotective effect. This assertion is well-founded with the results from Hung's research showing that synthesized and purified trans-resveratrol is effective to prevent reperfusion-induced arrhythmias and mortality in rats (Hung et al., 2000). It is considered that the protective mechanism of resveratrol is due to its activity as intracellular antioxidant, anti-inflammatory agent, and due to its ability to induce angiogenesis and expression of nitric oxide synthase (Bhat et al., 2001) as well to block low-density lipoprotein (LDL) peroxidation and increase the levels of high-density lipoprotein (HDL) (Petrovski et al., 2011). In the study conducted by Klinge et al. (2008) are analyzed the signaling pathways and molecular mechanisms by which resveratrol in concentrations compatible with oral consumption (nanomolar concentrations) is activating the protection against coronary heart diseases and is improving the function of endothelium of blood vessels. It is found that nanomolar concentration of this compound is enough to stimulate rapidly nitric oxide production in endothelial cells by increasing the interaction between estrogen receptor α-Src and calveolin-1, which is one of the components of signaling pathway of resveratrol's protective action. As far as inflammation plays a key role in atherosclerosis, resveratrol can attenuate the condition through its anti-inflammatory effect, which involves inhibition of the synthesis of pro-inflammatory compounds such as prostaglandin E_2 and interleukin-6 (Petrovski et al., 2011). Another cardioprotective mechanism of resveratrol is its ability to inhibit platelet aggregation, thus preventing formation of thrombi (Petrovski et al., 2011).
Another important side of resveratrol's heart protective effect is its participation in so called 'preconditioning' which is known to be one of the most powerful technique for promoting a cardioprotection (Das et al., 1993; Sato et al., 2000). The preconditioning includes several short cycles of reversible ischemia, each followed by another short duration of reperfusion. The process of preconditioning-mediated cardioprotection makes the heart resistant to subsequent lethal ischemic injury (Das & Maulik, 2006). Preconditioning induces the expression of some heat shock proteins and endogenous antioxidant enzymes such as superoxide dismutase and also enhances the signal transduction by activating the survival signals and inhibiting the death ones. Resent study of Das & Maulik (2006) reported that resveratrol may act as a phytopharmacological preconditioning agent by activation of signaling pathways of preconditioning. These pathways include activation of adenosine A_1 and A_3 receptors, multiple kinases, K_{ATP} mitochondrial ATP-sensitive potassium channel and nitric oxide production - all of them are important factors with crucial role in preconditioning-mediated cardioprotection (Das & Maulik, 2006; Petrovski et al., 2011). Resveratrol provides cardioprotection by improving postischemic recovery and reducing the size of myocardial infarct and cardiomyocyte apoptosis (Das & Maulik, 2006). However, the mechanisms of enhancing the heart endogenous defense are not completely clear and more studies are necessary for better understanding of these signaling pathways.

2.2 Resveratrol and its therapeutic potential in neurological disorders

In addition to the cardioprotective effect of resveratrol, recent data suggest that this phytoalexine has protective and therapeutic potential against certain neurological disorders. Neurodegenerative diseases are one of the significant challenges of medicine and involve malfunction or progressive loss of structure of neurons and even cell death. Although the profound research in this area, so far the mechanisms of diseases pathologies are poorly understood. Many of these diseases are heritable and caused by genetic mutations. Other causes of such disorders include toxins, chemicals and certain medical conditions such as alcoholism or stroke. With the research progress it has been hypothesized that the oxidative stress and damage caused by reactive oxygen species (ROS) play a major role in neurodegeneration (Pallàs et al., 2009). The oxidative stress is induced by imbalance between production and detoxification of ROS leading to damage of all cell components, including DNA, proteins, lipids and even neuronal messengers. This could lead to irreversible damage of neuron structure and function, thus contributing to the pathogenesis of neurodegeneration. Other toxic reactions that cause neurodegeneration involve inflammation and dysfunction of mitochondrial activity (Ramassamy, 2006). As far as resveratrol is reported to have a strong antioxidant and anti-inflammatory activity its beneficial properties could be used in the treatment and prevention of neurodegenerative diseases. Epidemiological studies have shown that the moderate red wine consumption is correlated with a significant reduction of Alzheimer's disease and dementia (Marambaud et al., 2005; Orgogozo et al., 1997). Furthermore, *in vivo* studies with animals demonstrate the protective effect of resveratrol in models of neurotoxicity (Virgili & Contestabile, 2000). These results gave boost of studying the molecular targets of resveratrol as a potential phytoceutical in neurological diseases. The most common neurodegenerative disorders include Alzheimer's, Parkinson's and Huntington's diseases.

2.2.1 Alzheimer's disease (AD)

AD is the most common form of dementia, which is associated with senile plaques caused by aggregation of β-amyloid peptide (βAP). It has been shown that intra- and extra-cellular βAP is responsible for the initiation of synaptic malfunctions and occurrence of AD-symptoms (Wirths et al., 2004). Yu and colleagues (2006) reported that βAPs can cause massive neuronal cell loss by inducing apoptosis. It is suggested that βAPs trigger the apoptosis by interaction with various neuronal receptors and free radical production that activate different cell-death-signalling pathways (Yuan & Yankner, 2000). Valerio et al. (2006) found that the activation of protein complex NF-kB in microglia plays a crucial role in βAP-induced neuronal cell death. This signaling pathway can be modulated and significantly reduced by inhibition of the degradation of cytoplasmatic protein IkB that acts as an inhibitor of NF-kB. That very pathway is reported to be a target of resveratrol, where the grape compound inhibits the degradation of IkB thus showing neuroprotective and therapeutic effect (Pallàs et al., 2009).

In a study Marambaud et al. (2005) investigated whether resveratrol is modulating the levels of βAPs in the neocortex and hippocampus of brains damaged from AD. The *in vitro* research reports that the βAP levels were significantly decreased in cells treated with resveratrol. Further *in vitro* experiments demonstrate that the polyphenol promotes intracellular degradation of βAPs without increasing the total protease activity (Marambaud et al., 2005).

Another possible therapeutic mechanism of resveratrol is its similarity with the effects of calorie restriction. In the survey of Pallàs et al. (2009) are discussed studies, which demonstrated that short-term calorie restriction is associated with reduction of βAP-plaques in transgenic mouse models of AD. It is suggested that the dietary regime promotes processing of the amyloid precursor protein via pathway that does not result in βAPs. This is possible when the processing is made by α-secretase cleavage instead of β- and γ-secretases. As far as resveratrol mimics the calorie restriction pathways, it can be hypothesized that it reduces the βAPs using the same pathway (Pallàs et al., 2009).

Moreover, βAPs induce apoptosis via production of reactive oxygen species, which can be scavenged by the strong anti-oxidation effect of resveratrol (Jang et al., 2007). These data prove that resveratrol stimulates the clearance of senile plaques and prevents from the neurotoxic effect of βAPs, thus having a neuroprotective effect.

Inflammation, being associated with the development of AD, is another target of resveratrol. The anti-inflammatory properties of resveratrol have a beneficial effect on prevention and treatment of neurodegenerative process.

2.2.2 Parkinson's disease (PD)

PD is another neurodegenerative disorder that is characterized by a selective death of dopamine-producing cells in the substantia nigra (Gao et al., 2002). As contributing factors to the disease, mitochondrial dysfunction, inflammation, oxidative stress and apoptosis appear to have a major role in the development and progression of PD. Recent studies showed that resveratrol has neuroprotective function against the deleterious effect of 6-hydroxydopamine (6-OHDA) in rat models of PD (Jin et al., 2008; Khan et al., 2010). The conducted trials revealed that resveratrol suppresses the expression of pro-inflammatory cytokines (TNF-α) and enzymes (COX-2), which play a key role in the inflammatory process that is related with the progression of neurodegenerative diseases. Jin et al. (2008) demonstrated that the overexpression of COX-2 and TNF-α mRNA is involved in the pathogenesis of PD and resveratrol can be used to reduce the levels of these proteins, resulting in improvement of pathological lesions in substantia nigra neurons in rat models of PD. These results confirm the beneficial effect of resveratrol in the treatment of PD.

2.2.3 Huntington's disease (HD)

HD is a neurodegenerative genetic disorder caused by a mutation of the gene coding Huntingtin protein. The mutation results in synthesis of a different form of the protein that forms aggregates with neurotoxic effect leading to degeneration of specific brain areas. The mutant protein damages mitochondria in the affected neurons, causing dysfunction and death of the cells. One of the experimental models of HD is the utilization of the neurotoxin 3-nitropropionic acid on rodents. One of the major mechanisms of toxin action is the induction of mitochondrial dysfunction via oxidative stress. Several studies reported the protection activity of resveratrol against this neurotoxin and suggested that it was its antioxidant properties that are responsible for the prevention of the functional effect of the toxin (Binienda et al., 2010; Kumar et al., 2006). Furthermore, some authors reported that the beneficial effect of resveratrol is through activation of SIRT1 (Howitz et al., 2003; Lagouge et al., 2006). However, Pallos et al. (2008), working with Drosophila model of HD, demonstrated that resveratrol has a neuroprotective effect in a dose-dependent manner but through mechanisms that are independent of Sir2 activation (the human ortholog is SIRT1).

Another research demonstrates that the phenolic constituents of red wine can inhibit the harmful effect of oxidative stress as a result of nitric oxide production (Bastianetto et al., 2000), which is neurodegenerative event with damages relevant to those occurring during chronic inflammation, cerebral ischemia or excitotoxicity. The *in vitro* study showed that resveratrol is capable of protecting and rescuing rat's hypothalamic cells against nitric oxide - induced toxicity (Bastianetto et al., 2000).

Hence, the results from the above mentioned studies lead to the conclusion that the red wine polyphenol constitute, resveratrol, possesses a therapeutic potential and has a beneficial effect for the prevention of age-related neurodegenerative disorders. The data about the antioxidant activities of resveratrol support the hypothesis of beneficial effects of moderate daily red wine consumption against the occurrence of neuropathological diseases of chronic or acute nature. Presented studies confirm the neuroprotective value of resveratrol and its ability to rescue neuron cells but yet the exact mechanisms and pathways of its action remain not fully revealed and further studies are needed.

2.3 Resveratrol and its longevity and anti-ageing properties

Ageing processes are determined by metabolic disorders which occur with the age increasing. Metabolic disorders are tightly linked to compromised mitochondrial functions (Petersen et al., 2003) as a result of reduced expression of genes controlling mitochondrial biogenesis in humans and animals (Lagouge et al., 2006). Numerous studies revealed that the gene PGC-1α (peroxisome proliferator-activated receptor γ co-activator) has a crucial role in mitochondrial activity (Wu et al., 1999), skeletal muscle fiber-type switching (Puigserver & Spiegelman, 2003), controlling of adaptive thermogenesis (Puigserver et al., 1998) and together with SIRT1 gene promotes the adaptation to caloric restriction (Rodgers et al., 2005). SIRT1 gene encodes a member of sirtuin family of proteins and interacts with PGC-1α, taking part in regulation of longevity, apoptosis and DNA repair (Sinclair, 2005). Recent studies showed that resveratrol significantly increases the SIRT1 activity through allosteric interaction (Howitz et al., 2003). In the *in vivo* animal studies conducted by Lagouge et al. (2006) is demonstrated that resveratrol impacts on the regulation of energy homeostasis by inducing mitochondrial activity through increasing SIRT1 activity and thus modulating PGC-1α functions. In series of experiments is demonstrated that the intake of resveratrol 200 or 400 mg/kg/day has a beneficial effect on body weight by inducing a resistance to weight gain and enhances the adaptive thermogenesis by increasing the cold tolerance (Lagouge et al., 2006). Resveratrol treatment induces mitochondrial morphological changes in muscles and brown adipose tissue such as enlarging of mitochondrial structures and increasing presence of cristae and thus the polyphenol has a beneficial influence on the energy homeostasis and reduces the weight gaining in conditions of high fat diet.

As far as resveratrol changes the morphological structure of mitochondria in muscles, this substance enhances the enzymatic activity of organelles and induces the muscle fiber-type switching resulting in increased resistance to muscle fatigue (Booth et al., 2002). All these data lead to the conclusion that resveratrol enhances mitochondrial activity resulting in suppression of ageing symptoms by increasing of fatty acid oxidation, amelioration of fat burning, maintaining of energy homeostasis and induction of muscle fatigue resistance.

Besides its anti-ageing properties, there are evidences that resveratrol works as a longevity agent. In year 2003 the team of David Sinclair reported that resveratrol increases cell survival by stimulating SIRT1-dependent deacetylation of p53 tumor suppressor (Howitz et al., 2003). Nevertheless, some studies with yeast (Kaeberlein et al., 2004) and nematode *Caenorhabditis elegans* (Guarente & Picard, 2005) questioned the involvement of sirtuin in lifespan extension leaving this assertion quite controversial (Markus & Morris, 2008). These results suggest that the wide effects of resveratrol are not always a result of sirtuin activation. In the recent review of Markus & Morris (2008) is revealed that resveratrol is also involved in sirtuin-independent pathway which is central to the control of lifespan. In this pathway the target of resveratrol is PI3K (phosphoinositide 3-kinase) which implicates the polyphenol in insulin-like signaling pathway for activating of mitochondrial biogenesis (Frojdo et al., 2007).

The reports that resveratrol has positive effect on lifespan extension in mice prompt to more extensive research of *in vivo* resveratrol's effects in mammals (Baur et al., 2006; Lagouge et al., 2006). The findings of the French (Lagouge et al., 2006) and American (Baur et al., 2006) research groups are promising for therapeutic properties of resveratrol in human metabolic disorders.

3. Melatonin

Melatonin (N-acetyl-5-methoxytryptamine) is an indoleamine, a naturally occurring compound found in animals, plants and microbes. In human body melatonin plays an important role for regulation of sleep-wake cycles, induction of immune system, sexual development and vascular tone (Iriti et al., 2006).

For a long time it was thought that melatonin is a neurohormone exclusively synthesized in vertebrates, but in recent years it was found that this substance is presented in plants, bacteria, algae, fungi and invertebrates (Iriti & Faoro 2006). Few years ago, Iriti et al. (2006) discovered melatonin in different grape cultivars, which gave a boost of series of studies concerning the presence and biosynthesis of this compound in grape and wine (Guerrero et al., 2008; Mercolini et al., 2008). Melatonin content in grape is reported to range from 5 to 96 pg/g, while in wine the content was found to vary from 50-80 pg/ml (Spanish wines) to 400-500 pg/ml (Italian wines) with higher content in red wines (Iriti et al., 2010). It was reported that the human serum concentration of melatonin significantly increases 1 hour after intake of 100 ml red wine (Guerrero et al., 2008), resulting in increased plasma antioxidant capacity. These results show that the effect of this neurohormone in humans could be modulated by moderate administration of wine. Recent studies are directed to melatonin treatment of cancer, immune disorders, cardiovascular diseases, depression, circadian rhythm sleep disorders and sexual dysfunction. Therefore, the reported presence of melatonin in grape and wine gives an additional support to the hypothesis about the beneficial health effects of moderate wine consumption.

3.1 Antioxidant properties of melatonin

Melatonin is a pervasive substance whose powerful antioxidant property is particularly directed to a protection of nuclear and mitochondrial DNA by scavenging OH, O_2^-, H_2O_2, NO and inhibition of lipid peroxidation. Reiter et al. (2003) reported melatonin to be an efficient scavenger of free radicals in mitochondria, which are a major source of reactive species in the cell. Moreover, the authors reported that melatonin suppresses the apoptotic signals originating in mitochondria, thus diminishing disorders that are related to mitochondrial dysfunction - brain damages, age-related disease, etc. It was found that melatonin is effective against brain damages caused by release of free radicals containing oxygen atom (Tütüncüler et al., 2005) and also can reduce the brain damages caused by some types of Parkinson's disease. The antioxidant effect of melatonin provides a protection from neurodegeneration as well as from the mutagenic and carcinogenic actions of free radicals and thus, melatonin contributes enhancing of longevity (Oaknin-Bendahan et al., 1995).

Other evidence concerning the strong antioxidative properties of melatonin is its positive effect for successful treatment for septic shock in newborns, which is discussed by Reiter et al. (2003). As far as the excessive free radical generation is considered to be one of the causes for sepsis the authors attributed the beneficial actions of melatonin to its antioxidant properties. Moreover, in this review the authors presented numerous evidences about the positive effect of melatonin in treatment of a variety of conditions associated with elevated oxidative stress in newborns, children and adults (Reiter et al., 2003).

So far, the obtained information from numerous studies, some of which are above mentioned, leads to the conclusion that melatonin acts on multiple ways for reduction of oxidative stress, i.e. direct scavenge of free radicals and reactive species, stimulation of antioxidative enzymes, stimulation of mitochondrial function, synergy with classic antioxidants, etc. The powerful direct and indirect antioxidant actions of melatonin, proved by *in vitro* and clinical tests, are promising for prevention and treatment of disease states that involve damage caused by free radicals.

3.2 Melatonin effects on nervous system

As far as melatonin in mammals plays a role of neurohormone, it is obviously that it is involved in various function associated with nervous system. It has a key role in regulation of circadian rhythm that coordinates sleep-wake cycle and takes part in modulation of mood and behavior. Since melatonin (exogenous and endogenous) possesses the ability to pass the blood-brain barrier it has a direct effect on brain. Moreover, it is reported that melatonin from edible plants binds to melatonin receptors in mammalian brain and exerts its biological activity (Iriti et al., 2010). Melatonin has a broad range of action, which is not limited only to the regulation of circadian rhythm. Findings from mice and rat trials have shown that melatonin receptors appear to play important role in mechanisms of learning and memory (Larson et al., 2006) as well as that melatonin facilitates short-term memory (Argyriou et al., 1998). The study conducted by Baydas and co-workers (2002) suggested that the beneficial effect of melatonin on memory and learning processes could be due to its involvement in structural remodeling of synaptic connections during these processes. In another study is demonstrated the powerful antioxidant effect of melatonin in ethanol-treated rats where melatonin prevents lipid peroxidation in brain resulting from chronic ethanol exposure (Gönenç et al., 2005).

The melatonin acts through three main mechanisms, namely receptor-mediated, protein-mediated and non-receptor-mediated. The receptor-mediated activity of melatonin involves membrane (MT_1 and MT_2) and nuclear receptors (RORα and RZRβ) and is responsible for the immune system and upregulation of antioxidant enzymes (Srinivasan et al., 2006). The non-receptor-madiated action of melatonin involves its antioxidant properties as a direct scavenger of reactive species.

Interestingly, melatonin secretion decreases with ageing, which was suggested to be associated with the manifestation of age-related neurodegenerative diseases (Srinivasan et al., 2006). Moreover, it is reported a significant reduction of melatonin secretion in people with dementia in comparison with nondemented controls (Papolla et al., 1997), thus, suggesting exogenous melatonin to be extensively explored as a therapeutic and preventive agent in neurodegenerative diseases.

3.2.1 Alzheimer's disease (AD)

It has been reported by many researchers that the melatonin levels are much lower in AD patients in comparison with the hormone levels detected in aged matched controls (Skene & Swaab, 2003). Another finding indicated one of the melatonin receptors (MT_2) to mediate the melatonin effects in human hippocampus - a mechanism that appear to be impaired in AD patients (Savaskan et al., 2005). The study of Savaskan et al. (2005) is the first immunohistochemical assay that identifies the exact cellular distribution of MT_2 in human

hippocampus and proves the altered expression and cellular loss of this receptor in AD patients. All these data prove the importance of melatonin and its targets for the neurological processes and suggest its beneficial effect for treatment of AD.
As far as deposition of cerebral βAPs is a primary hallmark of AD, the effect of melatonin against the neurotoxic properties of βAPs is examined. It was found that melatonin prevents death of cultured neuronal cells caused by exposure to βAPs (Pappolla et al., 1997). As an addition, the oxidative stress, along with the neurotoxicity of βAPs, is proposed to play a significant role in the pathogenesis of AD lesions. Pappolla et al. (1992) first presented evidences that proof the role of oxidative damage in the development and progression of AD. These finding was confirmed by recent trial with transgenic mouse models of AD (Feng et al., 2006). Both, oxidative stress and deposition of βAPs, were found to be related with damage and severe modifications of brain lipids, proteins and DNA and to trigger apoptosis in AD brain (Feng et al., 2006). The authors summarize that these neuronal alterations in certain regions of AD brains are indicated by some pro-apoptotic markers such as increased levels of Par-4 (proapoptotic protein), elevated expression of Bax (apoptosis-effector gene) and upregulated caspases (enzymes, main executors of apoptosis). In this study the authors demonstrated that in transgenic mouse models of AD the early melatonin supplement prevents the abnormal upregulation of pro-apoptotic markers, thus inhibiting the consequential initiation of apoptotic cascade (Feng et al., 2006). However, melatonin fails in reducing βAPs-plaques and expressing antioxidant activity in old transgenic mouse models with already established AD (Quinn et al., 2005), thus limiting the therapeutic properties of exogenous melatonin only to the early stages of the disease. Nevertheless, the demonstrated neuroprotective effect of melatonin supplement in the early stage of AD (Feng et al., 2006) is promising for the prevention of AD development. Even though melatonin cannot inhibit the AD progression when it is in advanced stage, it shows to be useful in symptomatic treatment concerning sleep disturbance, sundowning etc. (Srinivasan et al., 2006).

3.2.2 Parkinson's disease (PD) and Huntington's disease (HD)

Several studies demonstrated the neuroprotective effect of melatonin in experimental models of PD. The protective effect is suggested to be complex due to the multiple targets involved in the melatonin action against oxidative stress, which is reviewed by Srinivasan (2002) and Srinivasan et al. (2005). However, some studies, summarized in the profound review of Srinivasan et al. (2006), reported about adverse effect of melatonin leading to aggravation of motor deficit in animal models of PD. The presence of such contradictory results concerning melatonin action in PD models calls for more profound studies in this area.
A large body of evidence supports the thesis that mitochondrial dysfunction and defects in brain energy metabolism trigger HD. Thus, the oxidative stress, excitotoxicity and apoptosis play crucial role in the pathogenesis of HD. Therefore, the powerful anti-oxidant property of melatonin is proposed to have beneficial effect in HD patients. The experimental animal models of the disease use neurotoxins, quinolinic acid or 3-nitropropionic acid, to mimic mitochondrial dysfunction. When the effect of melatonin is tested in both models, the results showed prevention of oxidative stress damage and cell death in the quinolinic acid-model (Southgate et al., 1998) and protection of brain structures after induced oxidative stress in 3-nitropropionic acid-models (Túnez et al., 2004). These results confirm the neuroprotective ability of melatonin against induced oxidative stress, but more experiments are needed to elucidate the melatonin effect on the other key factors of the disease - excitotoxicity and apoptosis.

Although various experimental models of AD, PD and HD prove the ability of exogenous melatonin to counteract diseases progression, the exact direct and indirect pleiotropic mechanisms of hormone actions are not completely revealed. Since central nervous system is highly susceptible to oxidative stress, it is suggested that the beneficial effect of melatonin is mostly due to its powerful antioxidant activity exerted at various levels. However, the research work in this area should be continued in order to elucidate the therapeutic potential of exogenous melatonin in neurodegenerative disorders.
All these data suggest that melatonin is an important substance associated with numerous health benefits. Recent results proved that melatonin presented in plant foods preserves its bioavailability and suggest that it may counteract numerous disease conditions, including age-related and neurological disorders, carcinogenesis, cardiovascular diseases and diabetes (Iriti et al., 2010). It is noteworthy that grape and wine appear to be a rich source of melatonin and interestingly, it is found that melatonin level in grape could be increased by agrochemical treatments, while its level in wine may be modulated during the indoleamine synthesis by yeasts during the fermentation process of winemaking (Iriti et al., 2006). The presence of melatonin in these products gives new evidence for the healthpromoting effect of grape and wine.
Grape and wine are rich in phytoceuticals but it is still little known about their beneficial effects on human health. Thus, metabolomics offers an opportunity for revealing the properties of a large number of plant secondary metabolites and for better understanding of their phytoceutical effects on humans.

4. Conclusions

So far, metabolite analyses of grape showed its rich content of secondary metabolites, which are highly beneficial for human health. This brief presenting of evidences about the beneficial effects of resveratrol and melatonin reveal only a little part of the effectiveness of grape secondary metabolites. The above reported data about very few grape secondary metabolites (resveratrol and melatonin) proved their biological potential as natural antioxidants, therapeutic agents for numerous pathological disorders and demonstrated the significance of grape and wine compounds. These natural substances showed an enormous promise for utilization as phytoceuticals for prevention and treatment of diseases (cancer, cardiovascular diseases, neurodegenerative disorders and others) which are so common for our society. However, it is still not completely clear which of the cellular mechanisms and signaling pathways are involved or activated by these phytoceuticals in the processes of disease prevention and therefore more detailed research in this area is necessary.

5. References

Argyriou, A.; Prast, H. & Philippu, A. (1998). Melatonin facilitates short-term memory. *European Journal of Pharmacology,* Vol.349, No2-3, pp. 159-162

Baliga, M.S.; Meleth, S. & Katiyar, S.K. (2005). Growth inhibitory and antimetastatic effect of green tea polyphenols on metastasis-specific mouse mammary carcinoma 4T1 cells in vitro and in vivo systems. *Clinical Cancer Research,* Vol.11, pp. 1918-1927

Bastianetto, S.; Zheng, W.-H. & Quirion, R. (2000). Neuroprotective abilities of resveratrol and other red wine constituents against oxide-related toxicity in cultured hippocampal neurons. *British Journal of Pharmacology,* Vol.131, No4, pp. 711-720

Baur, J.A.; Pearson, K.J.; Price, N.L.;Jamieson, H.A.; Lerin, C.; Karla, A.; Prabhu, V.V.; Allard, J.S.; Lopez-Lluch, G.; Lewis, K.; Pistell, P.J.; Poosala, S.; Becker, K.G.; Boss, O.; Gwinn, D.; Wang, M.; Ramaswamy, S.; Fishbein, K.W.; Spencer, R.G.; Lakatta, E.G.; Le Couteur, D.; Shaw, R.J.; Navas, P.; Puigserver, P.; Ingram, D.K.; de Cabo, R. & Sinclair, D.A. (2006). Resveratrol improves health and survival of mice on a high-calorie diet. *Nature,* Vol.444, (November 2006), pp. 337-342

Baydas, G.; Nedzvetsky, V.S.; Nerush, P.A.; Kirichenko, S.V.; Demechenko, H.M. & Reiter, R.J. (2002). A novel role for melatonin: regulation of the expression of cell adhesion molecules in the rat hippocampus and cortex. *Neuroscience Letters*, Vol.326, pp. 109-112

Bhat, K.P.; Kosmeder, J.W. & Pezzuto, J.M. (2001). Biological effects of resveratrol. *Antioxidants & Redox Signaling*, Vol.3, No6, (December 2001), pp. 1041-1064

Binienda, Z.K.; Beaudoin, M.A.; Gough, B.; Ali, S.F. & Virmani, A. (2010). Assessment of 3-nitropropionic acid-evoked peripheral neuropathy in rats: Neuroprotective effects of acetyl-L-carnitine and resveratrol. *Neuroscience Letters,* Vol.480, pp. 117-121

Booth, F.W.; Chakravarthy, M.V. & Spangenburg, E.E. (2002). Exercise and gene expression: physiological regulation of the human genome through physical activity. *The Journal of Physiology,* Vol.543, pp. 399-411

Das, D.K.; Engelman, R.M. & Kimura, Y. (1993). Molecular adaptation of cellular defenses following preconditioning of the heart by repeated ischemia. *Cardiovascular Research,* Vol.27, pp. 578-584

Das, D.K. & Maulik, N. (2006). Resveratrol in cardioprotection: A therapeutic promis of alternative medicine. *Molecular Interventions,* Vol.6, No1, pp. 36-47

Elmadfa, I. & Kornsteiner, M. (2009). Dietary Fat Intake - A Global Perspective. *Annals of Nutrition & Metabolism,* Vol. 54 (suppl 1), pp. 8-14

Feng, Z.; Qin, C.; Chang, Y. & Zhang, J.-T. (2006). Early melatonin supplementation alleviates oxidative stress in a transgenic mouse model of Alzheimer's disease. *Free Radical Biology & Medicine,* Vol. 40, pp. 101-109

Frojdo, S.; Cozzone, D.; Vidal, H. & Pirola, L. (2007). Resveratrol is a class IA phosphoinositide 3-kinase inhibitor. *Biochemical Journal,* Vol. 406, pp. 511-518

Gao, H.M.; Jiang, J.; Wilson, B.; Zhang, W.; Hong, J.S. & Liu, B. (2002). Microglial activation-mediated delayed and progressive degeneration of rat nigral dopaminergic neurons: relevance to Parkinson's disease. *Journal of Neurochemistry,* Vol. 81, No. 6, pp. 1285-1297

Gönenç, S.; Uysal, N.; Açikgöz, O.; Kayatekin, B.M.; Sönmez, A.; Kiray, M.; Aksu, İ.; Güleçer, B.; Topçu, A. & Şemin, İ. (2005). Effects of melatonin on oxydative stress and spatial memory impairment induced by acute ethanol treatment in rats. *Physiological Research,* Vol. 54, pp. 341-348

Guarente, L. & Picard, F. (2005). Calorie restriction – the SIR2 connection. *Cell,* Vol. 120, pp. 473-482

Guerrero, J.M.; Martínez-Cruz, F. & Elorza, F.L. (2008). Significant amount of melatonin in red wine: its consumption increases blood melatonin levels in humans. *Food Chemistry,* doi: 10.1016/j.foodchem.2008.02.007

Howitz, K.T.; Bitterman, K.J.; Cohen, H.Y.; Lamming, D.W.; Lavu, S.; Wood, J.G.; Zipkin, R.E.; Chung, P.; Kisielewski, A.; Zhang, L.L.; Scherer, B. & Sinclair, D.A. (2003). Small molecule activators of sirtuins extend Saccharomyces cerevisiae lifespan. *Nature,* Vol. 425, pp. 191-196

Hung, L.-M.; Chen, J.-K.; Huang, S.-S.; Lee, R.-S. & Su, M.-J. (2000). Cardioprotective effect of resveratrol, a natural antioxidant derived from grapes. *Cardiovascular Research,* Vol. 47, pp. 549-555

Iriti, M. & Faoro, F. (2006). Grape phytochemicals: a bouquet of old and new nutraceuticals for human health. *Medical Hypotheses,* Vol. 67, pp. 833-838

Iriti, M.; Rossoni, M. & Farao, F. (2006). Melatonin content in grape: myth or panacea? *Journal of the Science of Food & Agriculture,* Vol. 86, No. 10, pp. 1432-1438

Iriti, M.; Varoni, E.M. & Vitalini, S. (2010). Melatonin in traditional Mediterranean diets. Journal of Pineal Research, Vol. 49, No. 2, pp. 101-105

Jang, M.H.; Piao, X.L.; Kim, H.Y.; Cho, E.J.; Baek, S.H.; Kwon, S.W. & Park, J.H. (2007). Resveratrol oligomers from Vitis amurensis attenuate beta-amyloid-induced oxidative stress in PC12 cells. *Biological Pharmaceutical Bulletin,* Vol. 30, pp. 1130-1134

Jin, F.; Wu, Q.; Lu, Y.-F.; Gong, Q.-H. & Shi, J.-S. (2008). Neuroprotective effect of resveratrol on 6-OHDA-induced Parkinson's disease in rats. *European Journal of Pharmacology,* Vol. 600, No. 1-3, pp. 78-82

Kaeberlein, M.; Kirkland, K.T.; Fields, S. & Kennedy, B.K. (2004). Sir2-independent life span extension by calorie restriction in yeast. *PLoS Biology,* Vol. 2, No. 9, pp. 1381-1387

Khan, M.M.; Ahmad, A.; Ishrat, T.; Khan, M.B.; Hoda, M.N.; Khuwaja, G.; Raza, S.S.; Khan, A.; Javed, H.; Vaibhav, K. & Islam, F. (2010). Resveratrol attenuates 6-hydroxydopamine oxidative damage and dopamine depletion in rat model of Parkinson's disease. *Brain Research,* Vol. 1328, pp. 139-151

Klinge, C.M.; Wickramasinghe, N.S.; Ivanova, M.M. & Dougherty, S.M. (2008). Resveratrol stimulates nitric oxide production by increasing estrogen receptor and phosphorylation in human umbilical vein endothelial cells. *The FASEB Journal,* Vol. 22, pp. 2185-2197

Kumar, P.; Padi, S.S.W.; Naidu, P.S. & Kumar, A. (2006). Effect of resveratrol on 3-nitropropionic acid-induced biochemical and behavioural changes: possible neuroprotective mechanisms. *Behavioural Pharmacology,* Vol. 17, pp. 485-492

Lagouge, M.; Argmann, C.; Gerhart-Hines, Z.; Meziane, H.; Lerin, C.; Daussin, F.; Messadeg, N.; Milne, J.; Lambert, P.; Elliott, P.; Geny, B.; Laakso, M.; Puigserver, P. & Auwerx, J. (2006). Resveratrol Improves Mitochondrial Function and Protects against Metabolic Disease by Activating SIRT1 and PGC-1α. *Cell,* Vol. 127, No. 6, pp. 1109-1122

Larson, J.; Jessen, R.E.; Uz, T.; Arslan, A.D.; Kurtuncu, M.; Imbesi, M. & Manev, H. (2006). Impaired hippocampal long-term potentiation in melatonin MT_2 receptor-deficient mice. *Neuroscience Letters,* Vol. 393, No. 1, pp. 23-26

LeBlanc, M.R. (2006). Cultivar, Juice Extraction, Ultra Violet Irradiation and Storage Influence the Stilbene Content of Muscadine Grapes (Vitis Rotundifolia Michx.). Dissertation, Louisiana State University

Marambaud, P.; Zhao, H. & Davies, P. (2005). Resveratrol Promotes Clearance of Alzheimer's Disease Amyloid-β Peptides. *Journal of Biological Chemistry,* Vol. 280, No. 45, pp. 37377-37382

Mercolini, L.; Saracino, M.A.; Bugamelli, F.; Ferranti, A.; Malaguti, M.; Hrelia, S. & Raggi, M.A. (2008). HPLC-F analysis of melatonin and resveratrol isomers in wine using a SPE procedure. Journal of Separation Science, Vol. 31, No. 6-7, pp. 1007-1014

Markus, M. & Morris, B.J. (2008). Resveratrol in prevention and treatment of common clinical conditions of aging. *Clinical Interventions in Aging,* Vol. 3, No. 2, pp. 331-339

Oaknin-Bendahan, S.; Anis, Y.; Nir, I. & Zisapel, N. (1995). Effects of long-term administration of melatonin and a putative antagonist on the ageing rat. *NeuroReport,* Vol. 6, No. 5, pp. 785-788

Orgogozo, J.M.; Dartigues, J.F.; Lafont, S.; Letenneur, L.; Commenges, D.; Salamon, R.; Renaud, S. & Breteler, M.B. (1997). Wine consumption and dementia in the elderly:

a prospective community study in the Bordeaux area. *Revue Neurologique*, Vol. 153, No. 3, pp. 185-192

Pallàs, M.; Casadesús, G.; Smith, M.A.; Coto-Montes, A.; Pelegri, C.; Vilaplana, J. & Camins, A. (2009). Resveratrol and neurodegenerative diseases: Activation of SIRT1 as the potential pathway towards neuroprotection. *Current Neurovascular Research*, Vol. 6, pp. 70-81

Pallos, J.; Bodai, L.; Lukacsovich, T.; Purcell, J.M.; Steffan, J.S.; Thompson, L.M. & Marsh, J.L. (2008). Inhibition of specific HDACs and sirtuins suppresses pathogenesis in a Drosophila model of Huntington's disease. *Human Molecular Genetics*, Vol. 17, No. 23, pp. 3767-3775

Pappolla, M.A.; Omar, R.A.; Kim, R.S. & Robakis, N.K. (1992). Immunohistochemical evidence of oxidative stress in Alzheimer's disease. *The American Journal of Pathology*, Vol. 140, No. 3, pp. 621-628

Pappolla, M.A.; Sos, M.; Omar, R.A.; Bick, R.J.; Hickson-Bick, D.L.M.; Reiter, R.J.; Efthimiopoulos, S. & Robakis, N.K. (1997). Melatonin prevents death of neuroblastoma cells exposed to the Alzheimer amyloid peptide. The *Journal of Neuroscience*, Vol. 17, No. 5, pp. 1683-1690

Petersen, K.F.; Befroy, D.; Dufour, S.; Dziura, J.; Ariyan, C.; Rothman, D.L.; DiPietro, L.; Cline, G.W. & Shulman, G.I. (2003). Mitochondrial dysfunction in the elderly: possible role in insulin resistance. *Science*, Vol. 300, No. 5622, pp. 1140-1142

Petrovski, G.; Gurusamy, N. & Das, D.K. (2011). Resveratrol in cardiovascular health and disease. *Annals of the NY academy of sciences*, Vol. 1215, pp. 22-33

Puigserver, P. & Spiegelman, B.M. (2003). Peroxisome proliferator-activated receptor-gamma coactivator 1 alpha (PGC-1 alpha): transcriptional coactivator and metabolic regulator. *Endocrine Reviews*, Vol. 24, No. 1, pp. 78-90

Puigserver, P.; Wu, Z.; Park, C.W.; Graves, R.; Wright, M. & Spiegelman, B.M. (1998). A cold-inducible coactivator of nuclear receptors linked to adaptive thermogenesis. *Cell*, Vol. 92, No. 6, pp. 829-839

Quinn, J.; Kulhanek, D.; Nowlin, J.; Jones, R.; Pratico, D.; Rokach, J. & Stackman, R. (2005). Chronic melatonin therapy fails to alter amyloid burden or oxidative damage in old Tg2576 mice: implications for clinical trials. *Brain Research*, Vol. 1037, No. 1-2, pp. 209-213

Ramassamy, C. (2006). Emerging role of polyphenolic compounds in the treatment of neurodegenerative diseases: A review of their intracellular targets. *European Journal of Pharmacology*, Vol. 545, pp. 51-64

Reiter, R.J.; Tan, D.; Mayo, J.C.; Sainz, R.M., Leon, J. & Czarnocki, Z. (2003). Melatonin as an antioxidant: biochemical mechanisms and pathophysiological implications in humans. *Acta Biochimica Polonica*, Vol. 50, No. 4, pp. 1129-1146

Rodgers, J.T.; Lerin, C.; Haas, W.; Gygi, S.P.; Spiegelman, B.M. & Puigserver P. (2005). Nutrient control of glucose homeostasis through a complex of PGC-1alpha and SIRT1. *Nature*, Vol. 434, pp. 113-118

Sacanella, E.; Vazquez-Agell, M.; Mena, M.P.; Antúnez, E.; Fernández-Solá, J.; Nicolás, J.M.; Lamuela-Raventós, R.M.; Ros, E. & Estruch, R. (2007). Down-regulation of adhesion molecules and other inflammatory biomarkers after moderate wine consumption in healthy women: a randomized trial. *The American Journal of Clinical Nutrition*, Vol. 86, No. 5, pp. 1463-1469

Sato, M.; Cordis, G.A.; Maulik, N. & Das, D.K. (2000). SAPKs regulation of ischemic preconditioning. *American Journal of Physiology-Heart & Circulatory Physiology*, Vol. 279, No. 3, pp. H901-H907

Savaskan, E.; Ayoub, M.A.; Ravid, R.; Angeloni, D.; Fraschini, F.; Meier, F.; Eckert, A.; Müller-Spahn, F. & Jockers, R. (2005). Reduced hippocampal MT_2 melatonin receptor expression in Alzheimer's disease. *Journal of Pineal Research*, Vol. 38, pp. 10-16

Sinclair, D.A. (2005). Toward a unified theory of caloric restriction and longevity regulation. *Mechanisms of Ageing & Development*, Vol. 126, pp. 987-1002

Skene, D.J. & Swaab, D.F. (2003). Melatonin rhythmicity: effect of age and Alzheimer's disease. *Experimental Gerontology*, Vol. 38, pp. 199-206

Southgate, G.S., Daya, S. & Potgieter, B. (1998). Melatonin plays a protective role in quinolinic acid-induced neurotoxicity in the rat hippocampus. *Journal of Chemical Neuroanatomy*, Vol. 14, No. 3-4, pp. 151-156

Srinivasan, V. (2002). Melatonn oxidative stress and neurodegenerative diseases. *Indian Journal of Experimental Biology*, Vol. 40, pp. 668-679

Srinivasan, V.; Pandi-Perumal, S.R.; Cardinali, D.P.; Poeggeler, B. & Hardeland, R. (2006). Melatonin in Alzheimer's disease and other neurodegenerative disorders, In: *Behavioral and Brain Fnctions 2, doi: 10.1186/1744-9081-2-15*, 20.06.2011, Available from http://www.behavioralandbrainfunctions.com/content/2/1/15

Srinivasan, V.; Pandi-Perumal, S.R.; Maestroni, G.J.M.; Esquifino, A.I.; Hardeland, R. & Cardinali, D.P. (2005). Role of melatonin in neurodegenerative diseases. *Neurotoxicity Research*, Vol. 7, No. 4, pp. 293-318

Túnez, I.; Montilla, P.; Muñoz, M. del C. ; Feijóo, M. & Salcedo, M. (2004). Protective effect of melatonin on 3-nitropropionic acid-induced oxidative stress in synaptosomes in an animal model of Huntington's disease. *Journal of Pineal Research*, Vol. 37, No. 4, pp. 252-256

Tütüncüler, F.; Eskiocak, S.; Basaran, U.N.; Ekuklu, G.; Ayvaz, S. & Vatansever, U. (2005). The protective role of melatonin in experimental in experimental hypoxic brain damage. *Pediatrics International*, Vol. 47, No. 4, pp. 434-439

Valerio, A.; Boroni, F.; Benarese, M.; Sarnico, I.; Ghisi, V.; Bresciani, L.G.; Ferrario, M.; Borsani, G.; Spano, P. & Pizzi, M. (2006). NF-kappaB pathway: A target for preventing beta-amyloid (Abeta)-induced neuronal damage and Abeta42 production. *European Journal of Neuroscience*, Vol. 23, pp. 1711-1720

Virgili, M. & Contestabile, A. (2000). Partial neuroprotection of in vivo excitotoxic brain damage by chronic administration of the red wine antioxidant agent, trans-resveratrol in rats. *Neuroscience Letters*, Vol. 281, pp. 123-126

Wirths, O.; Multhaup, G. & Bayer, T.A. (2004). A modified beta-amyloid hypothesis: intraneuronal accumulation of the beta-amyloid peptide- the first step of a fatal cascade. *Journal of Neurochemistry*, Vol. 91, pp. 513-520

Wu, Z.; Puigserver, P.; Andersson, U.; Zhang, C.; Adelmant, G.; Mootha, V.; Troy, A.; Cinti, S.; Lowell, B.; Scarpulla, R. & Spiegelman, B.M. (1999). Mechanisms controlling mitochondrial biogenesis and respiration through the thermogenic coactivator PGC-1. *Cell*, Vol. 98, No. 1, pp. 115-124

Yu, M.-S.; Suen, K.-C.; Kwok, N.-S.; So, K.-F.; Hugon, J. & Chang R.C.-C. (2006). Beta-amyloid peptides induces neuronal apoptosis via a mechanism independent of unfolded protein responses. *Apoptosis*, Vol. 11, No. 5, pp. 687-700

Yuan, J. & Yankner, B.A. (2000). Apoptosis in the neuvous system. *Nature*, Vol. 407, pp. 802-809

Part 3

Prion Diseases

14

Computational Studies of the Structural Stability of Rabbit Prion Protein Compared to Human and Mouse Prion Proteins

Jiapu Zhang
Centre in Informatics and Applied Optimization & Graduate School of Sciences, Informatics Technology and Engineering, University of Ballarat, Mount Helen, VIC 3353 Australia

1. Introduction

Prion diseases are invariably fatal and highly infectious neurodegenerative diseases affecting humans and animals. The neurodegenerative diseases such as Creutzfeldt-Jakob disease, variant Creutzfeldt-Jakob diseases, Gerstmann-Str*ä*ussler-Scheinker syndrome, Fatal Familial Insomnia, Kuru in humans, scrapie in sheep, bovine spongiform encephalopathy (or 'mad-cow' disease) and chronic wasting disease in cattle belong to prion diseases. By now there have not been some effective therapeutic approaches to treat all these prion diseases. In 2008, canine mammals including dogs (canis familials) were the first time academically reported to be resistant to prion diseases Polymenidoua et al. (2008). Rabbits are the mammalian species known to be resistant to infection from prion diseases from other species Vorberg et al. (2003). Horses were reported to be resistant to prion diseases too Perez et al. (2010). By now all the NMR structures of dog, rabbit and horse prion proteins had been released into protein data bank respectively in 2005, 2007 and 2010 Lysek et al. (2005); Perez et al. (2010); Wen et al. (2010a). Thus, at this moment it is very worth studying the NMR molecular structures of horse, dog and rabbit prion proteins to obtain insights into their immunity prion diseases.

The author found that dog and horse prion proteins have stable molecular dynamical structures whether under neutral or low pH environments, but rabbit prion protein has stable molecular dynamical structures only under neutral pH environment. Under low pH environment, the stable α-helical molecular structures of rabbit prion protein collapse into β-sheet structures. This article focuses the studies on rabbit prion protein (within its C-terminal NMR, X-ray and Homology molecular structured region $RaPrP^C$ (120-230)), compared with human and mouse prion proteins ($HuPrP^C$ (125-228) and $MoPrP^C$ (124-226) respectively). The author finds that some salt bridges contribute to the structural stability of rabbit prion protein under neutral pH environment.

As we all know, the disease infectious prions PrP^{Sc} are rich in β-sheets (about 43% β-sheet) Griffith (1967) and the normal cellular prions PrP^C are predominant in α-helices (42% α-helix, 3% β-sheet) Pan et al. (1993). Prion diseases are believed caused by the conversion of normal PrP^C to abnormally folded PrP^{Sc}, and prion diseases are so-called protein 'structural conformational' diseases. Thus, we may study the molecular structures of prion proteins to obtain some insights of prion diseases. Human prion diseases include the Creutzfeldt-Jakob disease, variant Creutzfeldt-Jakob diseases, Gerstmann-Sträussler-Scheinker syndrome, Fatal Familial Insomnia, and Kuru. The NMR solution structure of the human prion protein (1QLX.pdb) was released into the PDB bank (www.pdb.org) in 1999 and last modified in 2009 Zahn et al. (2000). Mice are popular experimental laboratory animals and the NMR structure of mouse prion protein (1AG2.pdb) was released into the PDB bank in 1997 and last modified in 2009 Riek et al. (1996). Rabbits, dogs and horses were reported to be resistant to prion diseases Perez et al. (2010); Polymenidoua et al. (2008); Vorberg et al. (2003) and by the end of 2010 their NMR structures (2FJ3.pdb, 1XYK.pdb, and 2KU4.pdb respectively) were completed to release into the PDB bank Lysek et al. (2005); Perez et al. (2010); Wen et al. (2010a). The X-ray structure of rabbit prion protein (3O79.pdb) was released into PDB bank in 2010 too Khan et al. (2010). At this moment it is very worth studying these molecular structures of horse, dog, rabbit, human and mouse prion proteins to reveal some secrets of prion diseases. The author found that dog and horse prion proteins have stable molecular dynamical structures whether under neutral or low pH environments Zhang and Liu (2011); Zhang (2011a), but rabbit prion protein has stable molecular dynamical structures only under neutral pH environment Zhang (2010); Zhang and Liu (2011); Zhang (2011a;b). Under low pH environment, among all the prion proteins above-mentioned only for the rabbit prion protein, its stable α-helical molecular structures collapse into β-sheet structures Zhang (2010); Zhang and Liu (2011); Zhang (2011a;b). The conversion of disease PrP^{Sc} from normal PrP^C is just involving 'conformational change' from predominantly α-helical protein to one rich in β-sheet structure. This article specially focuses on the rabbit prion protein to obtain some insights into the immunity of rabbits to prion diseases.

For the rabbit prion protein, we have its NMR and X-ray structures (2FJ3.pdb and 3O79.pdb respectively). Early in 2004, Epa Zhang et al. (2006) made molecular modeling of a homology structure (denoted 6EPA.pdb) for rabbit prion protein $RaPrP^C$(120-229), which was constructed using the NMR structure of the human prion protein (1QLX.pdb) as the template. Besides all these structures of rabbit prion protein, the knowledge on their conformational evolution/dynamics is considered essential to understand rabbit prion and the molecular modeling (MM) and molecular dynamics (MD) approach takes advantage beyond the experimental limit. In Section 2, this article first briefly reviews the main MD results of the homology MM structure Zhang et al. (2006) at 500 K and of the wild-type NMR structure at 450 K Zhang (2011b), compared with the MD of the wild-type NMR structures of human ($HuPrP^C$ (125-228), 1QLX.pdb) and mouse ($MoPrP^C$ (124-226), 1AG2.pdb) prion proteins. Section 3 will present the wild-type NMR rabbit, human and mouse MD comparisons at 350 K. Because the X-ray structure 3O79.pdb was produced differently from the NMR structure 2FJ3.pdb and the Homology structure 6EPA.pdb, we will not do their MD comparisons; however, in Section 4, we will give detailed sequence and structure alignment analysis of all these three rabbit prion structures compared with human and mouse wild-type structures. Section 5 gives some concluding remarks on rabbit prion protein and prion diseases.

2. MD reviews on the 500 K homology rabbit prion protein and the 450 K NMR rabbit prion protein

2.1 The homology rabbit prion protein at 500 K Zhang et al. (2006)

Zhang et al. Zhang et al. (2006) studied the MD of $RaPrP^C$(120-229) homology structure (6EPA.pdb). The MD simulations used Amber 8 Case et al. (2004) PMEMD program, with explicit water at different temperatures and pH values. The simulation conditions are listed in Table 1 of Zhang et al. (2006). The RMSD (root mean square deviation) and radius of gyration results are shown in Fig.s 2-3 of Zhang et al. (2006), where we may see that rabbit prion protein has more stable structural dynamical behavior compared to the human and mouse prion proteins at 500 K under neutral pH environment. This is also shown in Fig. 4 of Zhang et al. (2006) of snapshots for human, mouse and rabbit prion proteins at 5ns, 10ns, 15ns, 20ns, 25ns, and 30ns respectively. Fig. 4 of Zhang et al. (2006) shows that the helices of HuPrP and MoPrP were unfolded but RaPrP still keeps the helical structures at 500 K under neutral pH environment. The performance of RaPrP also shows that 500 K is a not a very bad temperature chosen for theoretical research for RaPrP. Under low pH environment at 500 K, these helical structures of RaPrP were unfolded. One of the reasons of the rabbit prion protein unfolding is due to the remove of the salt bridges such as N177-R163 (Fig. 5 of Zhang et al. (2006)). We may see in Fig. 5 of Zhang et al. (2006) the salt bridge / hydrogen bond between Arginine 163 and Aspartic acid 177 is conserved through a large part of the simulations and contributes to the protein stability of rabbit prion protein structure. Simulations at low pH value, where this salt bridge is absent, show RMSD and radius of gyration values for the rabbit prion protein to be of the same magnitude as the human and mouse prion proteins.

2.2 The NMR rabbit prion protein at 450 K Zhang (2011b)

Zhang Zhang (2011b) did the MD studies on the NMR rabbit prion protein $RaPrP^C$(124-228) (2FJ3.pdb) at 450 K under both neutral and low pH environments for the simulations of 20 ns. Zhang Zhang (2011b) found that "the secondary structures under low pH environment at 450 K have great differences between rabbit prion protein and human and mouse prion proteins: the α-helices of rabbit prion protein were completely unfolded and began to turn into β-sheets but those of human and mouse prion proteins were not changed very much. These results indicate the C-terminal region of $RaPrP^C$ has lower thermostability than that of $HuPrP^C$ and $MoPrP^C$. Under the low pH environment, the salt bridges such as D177-R163, D201-R155 were removed (thus the free energies of the salt bridges changed the thermostability) so that the structure nearby the central helices 1Ű3 was changed for rabbit prion protein" Zhang (2011b). The author continued his MD simulations for another 10 ns. The secondary structures for the MD simulations of 30 ns (Fig. 1) shows the same conclusion as that of Zhang (2011b).

We may say that the salt bridges such as D177-R163, N201-R155 contribute to the structural stability of wild-type rabbit prion protein (Fig. 1). At 450 K, whether in neutral or in low pH environments, the α-helical secondary structures of dog prion protein have not changed for the long 30 ns' simulations Zhang and Liu (2011); at 350 K, horse prion protein has the same molecular structural dynamics Zhang (2011a) during the 30 ns' long simulations.

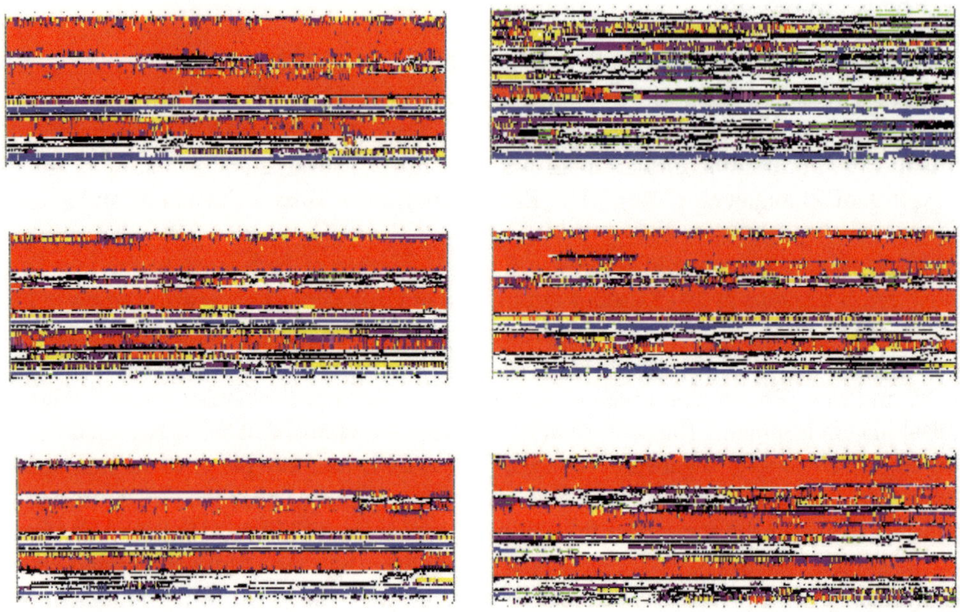

Fig. 1. Secondary structures of rabbit, human and mouse prion proteins (from up to down) at 450 K under neutral and low (from left to right) pH environments (red: α-helix, pink: π-helix, yellow: 3_{10}-helix, green: β-bridge, blue: β-sheet, purple: Turn, Black: Bend; x-axis: time (0-30 ns), y-axis: residue numbers).

3. 350 K

350 K might be a practical temperature for some experimental laboratory works. Zhang Zhang (2011c) did MD simulations for wild-type rabbit, dog and horse prion NMR structures at 350 K. The findings of 350 K are: "dog and horse prion proteins have stable molecular structures whether under neutral or low pH environments. Rabbit prion protein has been found having stable molecular structures under neutral pH environment, but without structural stability under low pH environment. Under low pH environment, the salt bridges such as D177-R163 were broken and caused the collapse of the stable α-helical molecular structures". Here the MD simulations are done for wild-type human and mouse prion proteins in the use of the same Materials and Methods as in Zhang (2011c).

Seeing Fig. 2, we know that at 350 K human and mouse prion proteins have stable molecular structures whether under neutral or low pH environments.

Clearly the following salt bridges play an important role to the NMR structural stability of rabbit prion protein: (1) GLU210-ARG207-GLU206-LYS203 (99.78%, 88.85%, 82.74%, H3-H3), GLU210-HIS176 (74.31%, H3-H2), GLU206-HIS176 (57.10%, H3-H2), ARG207-HIS176 (0.52%, H3-H2), ASP177-ARG163 (19.54%, H2-S2); (2) ARG150-ASP146-ARG147-ASP143 (91.38%, 100%, 86.43%, H1-H1), HIS139-ARG150 (50.96%), HIS139-ASP146 (92.62%); (3) ASP201-ARG155 (10.07%, H3-H1), ASP201-ARG150 (2.61%, H3-H1), ASP201-ARG147

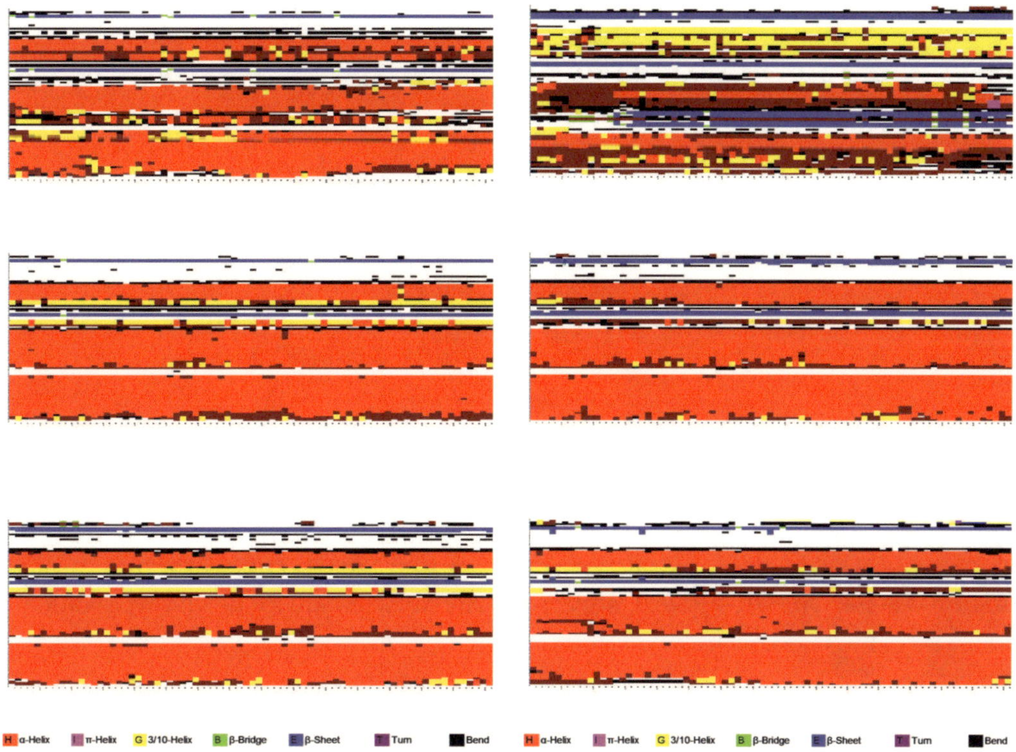

Fig. 2. Secondary structures of rabbit, human and mouse prion proteins (from up to down) at 350 K under neutral to low pH environments (from left to right) (X-axis: 0 ns - 30 ns (from left to right), Y-axis: residue numbers 124 - 228 / 125 - 228 / 124 - 226 (from up to down)).

(0.01%, H3-H1), ASP201-HIS186 (0.50%, H3-H2); and(4) ARG155-ASP201 (10.07%, H1-H3), TYR156-HIS186 (H1-H2, 71.69%), ARG155-GLU151 (20.70%, H1-H1), ARG155-GLU195 (0.06%), where H1, H2, H3 denote the α-helix 1, 2, 3 respectively, S1, S2 denote the β-strand 1 and 2 respectively, and '%' denotes the percentage during the whole simulation of 30 ns. Compared with human, mouse, dog and horse NMR prion proteins, rabbit NMR prion protein has some special salt bridges which contribute to its structural stability at 350 K during the simulation of 30 ns (Fig. 3) (human, mouse, dog and horse NMR prion proteins have not these salt bridges).

4. Alignment analyses

We make the sequence alignment of PrP from horse, dog, rabbit, human and mouse protein (Fig. 4).

In Fig. 4, "*" means that the residues in that column are identical in all sequences in the alignment, ":" means that conserved substitutions have been observed, "." means that semi-conserved substitutions are observed, the RED color takes place at small (small+ hydrophobic (incl.aromatic-Y)) residues, the BLUE color takes place at acidic residues, the MAGENTA color takes place at Basic-H residues,GREEN color takes place at

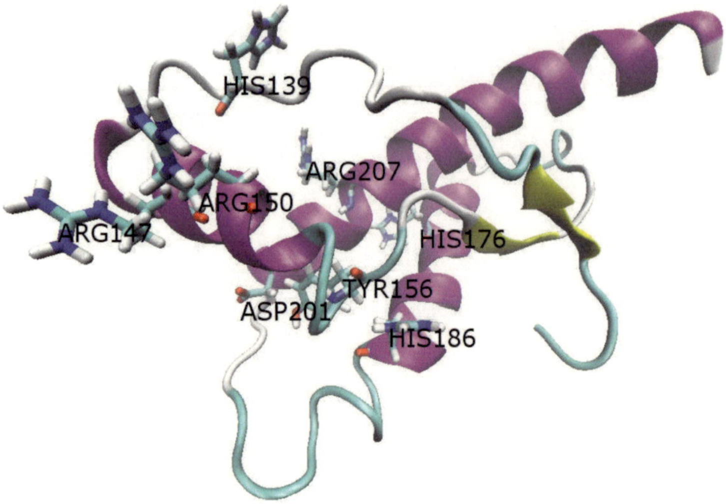

Fig. 3. Some special salt bridges ARG207-HIS176, TYR156-HIS186, HIS139-ARG150, ASP201-ARG147, ASP201-ARG150, ASP201-HIS186, ARG155-GLU151 of wild-type NMR rabbit prion protein at 350 K.

Hydroxyl+sulfhydryl+amine+G residues, and Grey color takes place at unusual amino/imino acids etc.. For the structural domain, in Fig. 4 we can see some special residues listed in Table 1 for horse, dog, human and mouse prion proteins, which might contribute to characters of each structure respectively. Rabbits differ from horses, dogs, humans and mice at: S173 (N174

Horse	S167 (others are D), Y222 (others are S), Q226 (others are Y), V241 (others are I), F245 (others are S)
Dog	L129 (others are M), S165 (others are P), N170 (others are S), S173 (others are N), V244 (others are I)
Human	I138 (immunities are L), S143 (others are N), H155 (others are Y), M166 (others are V), I183 (immunities are V), E219 (others are Q), S230 (immunities are A)
Mouse	I183 (immunities are V), V215 (others are I), D217 (others are Q), S230 (immunities are A)

Table 1. Alignment analysis of special residues for HoPrP, DoPrP, HuPrP, and MoPrP.

for horse, T174 for dogs, N174 for humans and mice), Q219 (K220 for horses and humans, R220 for dogs and mice), A224 (F225 for horses, Y225 for dogs, humans and mice), L232 (I233 for dogs, V233 for horse, humans and mice), and G228 (others are S229). For rabbits, at positions 89 and 97 the residues are special from all others (G89 (others are N90), S97 (others are N98)). These special residues are illuminated in Fig. 5. Some recent researches are focusing on the loop between $\beta2$ and $\alpha2$, i.e. PrP(164-171) Apostol et al. (2011); Fernandez-Funez et al. (2011); Khan et al. (2010); Perez et al. (2010); Wen et al. (2010a;b); we may see in Fig. 5 that the immune animals horses, dogs and rabbits have some residues in this loop different from humans and mice.

Lastly, we illuminate the figure (Fig. 6) of rabbit prion protein, including the homology, NMR and X-ray structures (6EPA.pdb, 2FJ3.pdb, and 3O79.pdb respectively). We superpose the homology structure onto the NMR structure and find the RMSD value is 3.2031669 angstroms.

```
CLUSTAL 2.1 multiple sequence alignment

                 901234567890123456789012345678901234567890 12345678901234567890123456
HorsePrP         MVKSHVGGWILVLFVATWSDVGLCKKRPKPGG-WNTGGSRYPGQGSPGGNRYPPQGGGGW 59
DogPrP           MVKSHIGSWILVLFVAMWSDVGLCKKRPKPGGGWNTGGSRYPGQGSPGGNRYPPQGGGGW 60
RabbitPrP        --MAHLGYWMLLLFVATWSDVGLCKKRPKPGGGWNTGGSRYPGQSSPGGNRYPPQGGG-W 57
HumanPrP         --MANLGCWMLVLFVATWSDLGLCKKRPKPGG-WNTGGSRYPGQGSPGGNRYPPQGGGGW 57
MousePrP         --MANLGYWLLALFVTMWTDVGLCKKRPKPGG-WNTGGSRYPGQGSPGGNRYPPQGG-TW 56
                   :::* *:* ***: *:*:*********** ***********.************  *

                 89012345678901234567890123456789012345 678901234567890123456
HorsePrP         GQPHGGGWGQPHGGGWGQPHGGGWGQPHGGGGWGQGG-SHGQWNKPSKPKTNMKHVAGAA 118
DogPrP           GQPHGGGWGQPHGGGWGQPHGGGWGQPHGGGGWGQGG-THSQWNKPSKPKTNMKHVAGAA 119
RabbitPrP        GQPHGGGWGQPHGGGWGQPHGGGWGQPHGGG-WGQGG-THNQWGKPSKPKTSMKHVAGAA 115
HumanPrP         GQPHGGGWGQPHGGGWGQPHGGGWGQPHGGG-WGQGGGTHSQWNKPSKPKTNMKHMAGAA 116
MousePrP         GQPHGGGWGQPHGGSWGQPHGGSWGQPHGGG-WGQGGGTHNQWNKPSKPKTNLKHVAGAA 115
                 **************.*******.******** ***** :*.**.*******.:**:****

                 119        130       140       150       160       170
                 789012345678901234567890123456789012345678901234567890123456
HorsePrP         AAGAVVGGLGGYMLGSAMSRPLIHFGNDYEDRYYRENMYRYPNQVYYRPVSEYSNQNNFV 178
DogPrP           AAGAVVGGLGGYLLGSAMSRPLIHFGNDCEDRYYRENMYRYPNQVYYRSVDQYNNQSTFV 179
RabbitPrP        AAGAVVGGLGGYMLGSAMSRPLIHFGNDYEDRYYRENMYRYPNQVYYRPVDQYSNQNSFV 175 -1
HumanPrP         AAGAVVGGLGGYMLGSAMSRPIIHFGSDYEDRYYRENMHRYPNQVYYRPMDEYSNQNNFV 176
MousePrP         AAGAVVGGLGGYMLGSAMSRPMIHFGNDWEDRYYRENMYRYPNQVYYRPVDQYSNQNNFV 175
                 ************:********:****.* *********:*********.:.:*.**..**

                  180       190       200       210       220        231
                 7890123456789012345678901234567890123456789012345667 8901234
HorsePrP         HDCVNITVKQHTVTTTTKGENFTETDVKIMERVVEQMCITQYQKEYEAFQQ--RGASVVL 236
DogPrP           HDCVNITVKQHTVTTT-KGENFTETDIKMMERVVEQMCITQYQRESEAYYQ--RGASVIL 236
RabbitPrP        HDCVNITVKQHTVTTTTKGENFTETDIKIMERVVEQMCITQYQQESQAAYQ--RAAGVLL 233 -1
HumanPrP         HDCVNITIKQHTVTTTTKGENFTETDVKMMERVVEQMCITQYERESQAYYQ--RGSSMVL 234
MousePrP         HDCVNITIKQHTVTTTTKGENFTETDVKMMERVVEQMCVTQYQKESQAYYDGRRSSSTVL 235
                 *******:******** *********:*:*********:***::* :*  :  *.:. :*

                 5678901234567890123
HorsePrP         FSSPPVVLLIFFLIFLIVG 255
DogPrP           FSSPPVILLVSFLIFLIVG 255
RabbitPrP        FSSPPVILLISFLIFLIVG 252
HumanPrP         FSSPPVILLISFLIFLIVG 253
MousePrP         FSSPPVILLISFLIFLIVG 254
                 ******:**: ********
```

Fig. 4. Horse, dog, rabbit, human and mouse prion protein sequence alignment.

Similarly, we superpose the X-ray structure onto the NMR structure and we get their RMSD value is 2.7918559 angstroms. This implies the homology structure 6EPA.pdb made in 2004 by Epa Zhang et al. (2006) is as effective as the X-ray structure 3O79.pdb released recently on date 2010-11-24 (last modified on 2011-02-02).

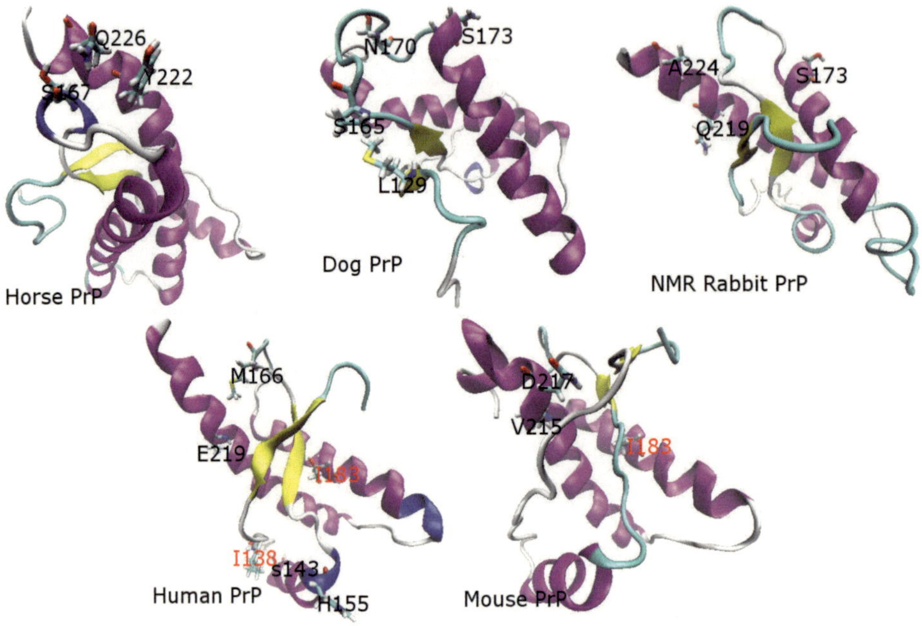

Fig. 5. Special residues owned only by HoPrP, DoPrP, RaPrP, HuPrP, and MoPrP respectively.

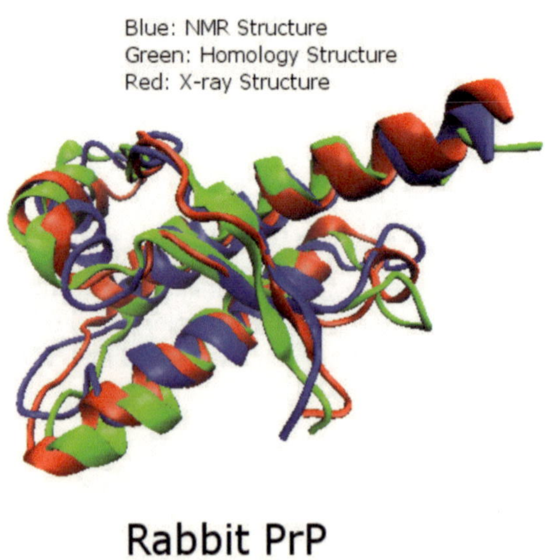

Fig. 6. Rabbit prion protein NMR, homology and X-ray structures (2FJ3.pdb, 6EPA.pdb, and 3O79.pdb).

5. Conclusion

To really reveal the secrets of prion diseases is very hard. Prion proteins have two regions: unstructured region and structured region. Rabbits, horses, and dogs were reported having immunity to prion diseases. Fortunately, by the end of 2010 all the NMR molecular structures of rabbit, horse, and dog prion proteins had been released into PDB bank already; for rabbit prion protein, its X-ray structure was also released into PDB bank in the end of 2010. Prion diseases are 'structural conformational' diseases. This paper timely presents a clue to reveal some secrets in the view of the dynamics of prion molecular structures. MD results of the author nearly in the passing 10 years show to us a common conclusion: under low pH environment at many levels of temperatures with different starting MD velocities, rabbit prion protein always unfolds its α-helical structures into β-sheet structures. Prion diseases are just caused by the conversion from predominant α-helices of PrP^C into rich β-sheets of PrP^{Sc}. Hence, we should furthermore study rabbits, horses and dogs, compared with humans and mice in order to reveal some secrets of prion diseases; for us, it is a long shot but certainly worth pursuing.

6. Acknowledgments

This research is supported by a Victorian Life Sciences Computation Initiative (http://www.vlsci.org.au) grant number VR0063 on its Peak Computing Facility at the University of Melbourne, an initiative of the Victorian Government. The author appreciates kind invitations and acceptance of this paper from the INTECH Open Access Publisher.

7. References

Apostol M.I., Wiltzius J.J.W., Sawaya M.R., Cascio D., Eisenberg D., 2011. Atomic structures suggest determinants of transmission barriers in mammalian prion disease. Biochem. 50, 2456–2463.

Case D.A., Darden T.A., Cheatham T.E., Simmerling III C.L., Wang J., Duke R.E., Luo R., Merz K.M., Wang B., Pearlman D.A., Crowley M., Brozell S., Tsui V., Gohlke H., Mongan J., Hornak V., Cui G., Beroza P., Schafmeister C., Caldwell J.W., Ross W.S., Kollman P.A., 2004. AMBER 8, University of California, San Francisco.

Fernandez-Funez P., Zhang Y., Sanchez-Garcia J., Jensen K., Zou W.Q., Rincon-Limas D.E., 2011. Pulling rabbits to reveal the secrets of the prion protein. Commun. Integr. Biol. 4(3), 262-266.

Griffith J.S., 1967. Self-replication and scrapie. Nature 215, 1043—1044.

Khan M.Q., Sweeting B., Mulligan V.K., Arslan P.E., Cashman N.R., Pai E.F., Chakrabartty A., 2010. Prion disease susceptibility is affected by beta-structure folding propensity and local side-chain interactions in PrP. Proc. Natl. Acad. Sci. USA 107: 19808-19813.

Lysek D.A., Schorn C., Nivon L.G., Esteve-Moya V., Christen B., Calzolai L., von Schroetter C., Fiorito F., Herrmann T., Guntert P., Wuthrich K., 2005. Prion protein NMR structures of cats, dogs, pigs, and sheep. Proc. Natl. Acad. Sci. USA 102, 640-645.

Nisbet R.M., Harrison C.F., Lawson V.A., Masters C.L., Cappai R., Hill A.F., 2010. Residues surrounding the glycosylphosphatidylinositol anchor attachment site of PrP modulate prion infection: insight from the resistance of rabbits to prion disease. J. Virol. 84 (13), 6678–6686.

Pan K.M., Baldwin M., Nguyen J., Gasset M., Serban A., Groth D., Mehlhorn I., Huang Z.W., Fletterick R., Cohenu F.E., Prusiner S.B., 1993. Conversion of alpha-helices into beta-sheets features in the formation of the scrapie prion proteins. Proc. Natl. Acad. Sci. USA 90(23), 10962-10966.

Perez D.R., Damberger F.F., Wuthrich K., 2010. Horse prion protein NMR structure and comparisons with related variants of the mouse prion protein. J. Mol. Biol. 400(2), 121-128.

Polymenidoua M., Trusheimb H., Stallmacha L., Moosa R., Julius J.A., Mielea G., Lenzbauerb C., Aguzzia A., 2008. Canine MDCK cell lines are refractory to infection with human and mouse prions. Vaccine 26(21), 2601-2614.

Riek R., Hornemann S., Wider G., Billeter M., Glockshuber R., Wuthrich K., 1996. NMR structure of the mouse prion protein domain PrP(121-321). Nature 382, 180-182.

Tabrett C.A., Harrison C.F., Sshmidt B., Bellingham S.A., Hardy T., Sanejouand Y.H., Hill A.F., Hogg P.J., 2010. Changing the solvent accessibility of the prion protein disulfide bond markedly influences its trafficking and effect on cell function. Biochem. J. 428, 169–182.

Vorberg I., Martin H.G., Eberhard P., Suzette A.P., 2003. Multiple amino acid residues within the rabbit prion protein inhibit formation of its abnormal isoform. J. Virol. 77, 2003–2009.

Wen Y., Li J., Yao W., Xiong M., Hong J., Peng Y., Xiao G., Lin D.H., 2010. Unique structural characteristics of the rabbit prion protein. J. Biol. Chem.285: 31682-31693.

Wen Y., Li J., Xiong M.Q., Peng Y., Yao W.M., Hong J., Lin D.H., 2010. Solution structure and dynamics of the I214V mutant of the rabbit prion protein. PLoS ONE 5(10), e13273.

Zahn R., Liu A., Luhrs T., Riek R., Von Schroetter C., Garcia F.L., Billeter M., Calzolai L., Wider G. Wuthrich K., 2000. NMR solution structure of the human prion protein. Proc. Natl. Acad. Sci. USA 97(1), 145-150.

Zhang J.P., 2010. Studies on the structural stability of rabbit prion probed by molecular dynamics simulations of its wild-type and mutants. J. Theor. Biol. 264(1), 119—122.

Zhang J.P., Liu D.D.W., 2011. Molecular dynamics studies on the structural stability of wild-type dog prion protein. J. Biomol. Struct. Dyn. 28(6), 861-869.

Zhang J.P., 2011. The structural stability of wild-type horse prion protein. J. Biomol. Struct. Dyn., in press.

Zhang J.P., 2011. Comparison studies of the structural stability of rabbit prion protein with human and mouse prion proteins. J. Theor. Biol. 269(1), 88—95.

Zhang J.P., 2011. The nature of the infectious agents: PrP models of resistant species to prion diseases (dog, rabbit and horses). Book Chapter In: Prions and Prion Diseases: New Developments (J.M. Verdier Eds.), NOVA Publishers, 2011. arXiv:1106.4628v1.

Zhang J.P., Varghese J.N., Epa V.C., 2006. Studies on the conformational stability of the rabbit prion protein. CSIRO Preventative Health National Research Flagship Science Retreat, Aitken Hill, Melbourne, 12—15 September 2006, Poster in Excellence (last document of webpage http://sites.google.com/site/jiapuzhang/).

15

The Effects of Trimethylamine N-Oxide on the Structural Stability of Prion Protein

Barbara Yang, Kuen-Hua You,
Shing-Chuen Wang, Hau-Ren Chen and Cheng-I Lee
Department of Life Science, National Chung Cheng University
Taiwan,
ROC

1. Introduction

Transmissible spongiform encephalopathies (TSEs) are diseases that affect the central nervous system in both humans and animals. TSEs can be ascribed to conformational conversion of prion protein (PrP). "Prion" stands for "proteinaceous infectious particle", which was discovered in the disease-transmitting material of infectious brain tissues and named by Prusiner (Prusiner 1982). The normal, cellular form of PrP (PrP^C) is a α-helix-rich glycoprotein attached to the outer cell surface by a glycophosphatidyl inositol linkage. The biological role of PrP^C remains ambiguous. Since Cu^{2+} is unique among divalent metal ions in its ability to bind to PrP^C in the octarepeat region (four copies of the repeat ProHisGlyGlyGlyTrpGlyGln) in the N-terminal domain (Whittal et al. 2000), the prion protein has been suggested to play a role in maintaining cellular copper concentration and signal transduction (Brown et al. 1998; Mouillet-Richard et al. 2000). PrP^C is non-infectious, whereas the abnormal and infectious, Scrapie isoform of PrP (PrP^{Sc}) has been considered to be the major infectious component of the genetic, sporadic and transmissible fatal neuro degenerative prion diseases that affect both human and animals (Prusiner 1998). PrP^{Sc} is rich in β-sheet structures and it has a pronounced tendency to misfold and to subsequently aggregate into highly stable and insoluble amyloid plaques. This PrP^{Sc} plagess are resistant to digestion by proteinase K, whereas PrP^C is sensitive to digestion by proteinase K (Prusiner 1998). PrP^{Sc} is responsible for many diseases in humans, including Kuru, Gerstmann-Sträussler-Scheinker disease (GSS), fatal familial insomnia (FFI), Creutzfeldt-Jakob disease (CJD) and the BSE-related, variant Creutzfeldt-Jakob disease (vCJD) (Horwich & Weissman 1997; Prusiner 1997; Will et al. 1996). The infectious nature of these fatal diseases differ from other infectious diseases in that the pathogen is a proteinaceous particle rather than typical pathogens, such as viruses, bacteria and fungi. Therefore, a "protein-only" hypothesis has been proposed (Griffith 1967; Prusiner 1998). A protein designated as "protein X" has been proposed to be involved in structural conversion of PrP^C into PrP^{Sc} (Telling et al. 1995) in the protein-only model. After decades of study on prion proteins, protein X has not been identified. Thus, the mechanism of how PrP^C is converted into PrP^{Sc} remains ambiguous.

The structure of prion proteins has been studied in human (Calzolai & Zahn 2003; Donne et al. 1997; Zahn et al. 2000), hamster (James et al. 1997) and mouse sequences (Gossert et al.

2005; Riek et al. 1996). The structure of truncated mouse PrP (121-231) has been solved and reveals a α-helical protein containing 52% of α-helical and 3% of β-sheet structures (PDB code: 1AG2, (Riek et al. 1996)). Furthermore, NMR structure of hamster prion 90-231 reveals a flexible N-terminus and a structured C-terminal fragment (125-228) containing 43% of α-helical and 6% of β-sheet structures (PDB code: 1B10, (James et al. 1997)). The high flexibility of the N-terminus was confirmed in recombinant full-length hamster prion protein PrP 29-231 (Donne et al. 1997). The representative NMR structure of mouse prion is shown in Figure 1.

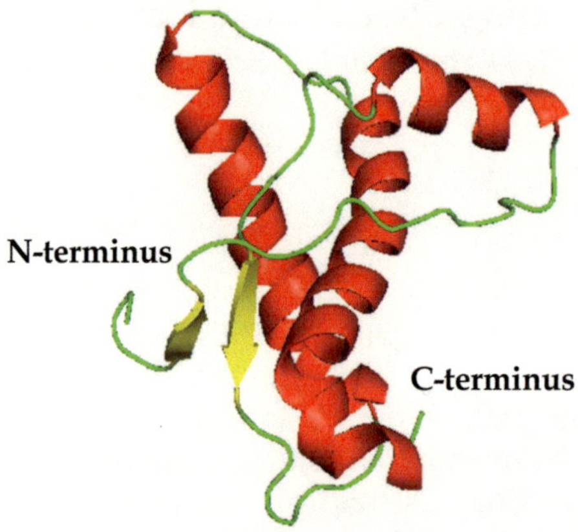

Fig. 1. The NMR structure of mouse prion protein (PDB code: 1AG2, (Riek et al. 1996)). The α-helical structures are represented by red ribbons, and the antiparallel β-sheet structure is colored in yellow. This figure was produced using the PyMol graphic package

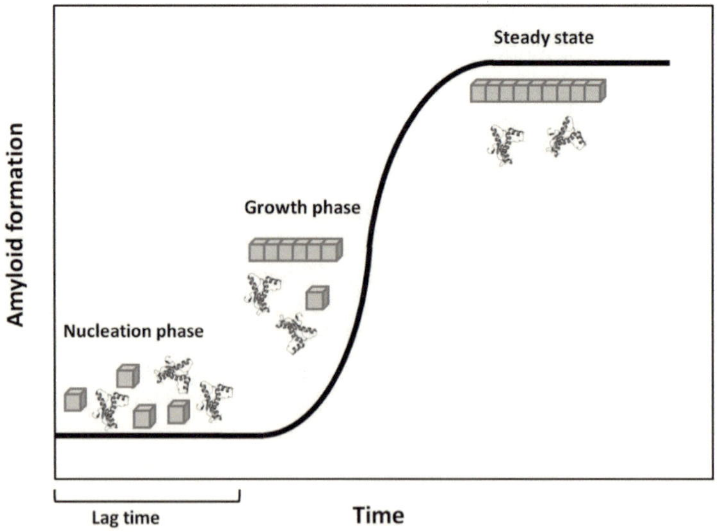

Fig. 2. Representative curve of nuclei-dependent polymerization model for amyloid formation

The formation of amyloid fibrils can be described by the polymerization model (Tsong & Baldwin 1972) illustrated in Figure 2. In this nucleation-dependent polymerization model, the conversion of proteins into nuclei that subsequently serve as seeds for amyloid fibrils is the rate-limiting step. Therefore, amyloid formation has a lag phase in which nucleation from protein monomers takes place. The spectroscopic signal for detecting amyloid fibrils is very weak during this nucleation phase, but the signal will enhance significantly during the fast polymerization catalyzed by the nuclei in the growth phase. Finally, the signal remains constant at a steady stateas that the ordered amyloid fibrils and protein monomers are at equilibrium.

In previous studies of recombinant PrP, a partially folded intermediate of PrP 90-231 has been suggested (Apetri et al. 2004; Kuwata et al. 2002; Nicholson et al. 2002). These partially unfolded states can potentially initiate amyloid formation (Abedini & Raleigh 2009; Chiti & Dobson 2009). Consequently, extensive works on the interaction of samll molecules and PrP have been conducted in order to find pharmacological chaperones that can stabilize the structure of PrP^{C} (Nicoll et al. 2010). Chemical chaperones is an important target in the developments of therapies for prion disease. In the study of protein folding, osmolyte is a well-know factor that acts as a chemical chaperone to assist proteins to fold. Furthermore, cellular osmolarity can be changed by the ion-transportations. An increase in intracellular osmolarity caused by ion-transoprtation resulting astrocyte dysfunction in neurological disorders has been reviewed (Seifert et al. 2006). Therefore, it is essential to study osmolytes that affect folding of prion proteins. The chemical structure of the osmolyte trimethylamine N-oxide (TMAO) is illustrated in Figure 3 that TMAO is a zwitterionic compound at neutral pH, but is positively charged below pH 4.7 (Lin & Timasheff 1994). TMAO is a well known protective osmolyte that can increase structural stability of proteins against chemical or temperature-induced denaturation (Baskakov et al. 1998; Bolen & Baskakov 2001; Celinski & Scholtz 2002; Gursky 1999; Qu et al. 1998). TMAO has an extraordinary ability to force thermodynamically unstable proteins to fold (Baskakov & Bolen 1998). In contrast, TMAO destabilizes proteins at low pH (Singh et al. 2005).

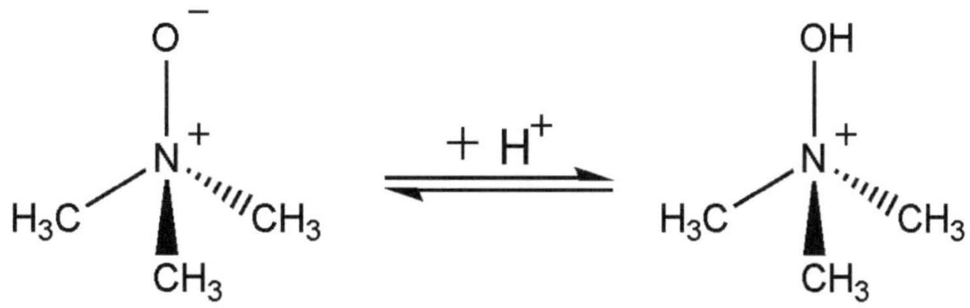

Fig. 3. Chemical structure of zwitterionic TMAO in equilibrium with its cationic form

A previous study by Tatzel and co-workers indicated that TMAO and the organic solvent dimethylsulfoxide (DMSO) prevent scrapie formation *in vitro* (Tatzelt et al. 1996). This study suggests a potential stratagy for preventing PrP^{Sc} by stabilizing the conformation of PrP^{C}. In contrast, later studies indicated that TMAO destabilized the α-helical conformation of full-length human prion at neutral pH at high temperature (Nandi et al. 2006) and human prion proteins at low pH (Granata et al. 2006). The structure of α-helix-rich prion protein is destabilized and the prion protein is converted to β-sheet structured oligomeric species (Nandi et al. 2006).

In this study, we examined the effect of TMAO on conformational stability in full-length mouse prion proteins (MoPrPs) and their structural conversion to amyloid fibrils. A possible mechanism of TMAO on fibril formation is proposed based on the nucleation-dependent polymerization model.

2. Materials and methods

We characterized TMAO-induced structural change in MoPrP by circular dichroism spectroscopy and 8-anilino-1-naphthalenesulfonic acid (ANS)-binding fluorescence assay, and compared the effect of TMAO on the formation of amyloid fibrils by thioflavin T (ThT) binding assay and transmission electron microscopy (TEM).
Chemicals used in this work were purchased from Sigma Chemcial Co. (St. Louis, Missouri, USA), and used without further purification.

2.1 Protein expression and purification

Plasmid pET101 encoding mouse prion (23-231) was transformed into competent *E. coli* BL21 (DE3) and expressed in the form of inclusion bodies. The protein was purified on a Ni-sepharose column according to a previously described procedure (Bocharova et al. 2005). The purity of the isolated protein was confirmed by SDS-PAGE. The correct native conformation, containing mainly α-helical structures, was confirmed by circular dichroism spectroscopy.

2.2 Far-UV circular dichroism spectroscopy

Far-UV circular dichroism spectra of mouse prion was recorded with a J-815 (Jasco, Japan) spectropolarimeter equipped with a Peltier temperatue control system (model PTC 423). For measurements in the far-UV region, a quartz cell with a path length of 0.1 cm was used in nitrogen atmosphere. For protein samples, the concentration of MoPrP was kept constant at 10 μM in 10 mM 2-(*N*-morpholino)ethanesulfonic acid (MES, pH 6.0). Far-UV circular dichroism spectra between 200 and 250 nm were recorded. An accumulation of five scans with a scan speed of 50 nm per minute was performed at 20 °C. The thermal-induced denaturation of proteins was conducted by heating protein solutions at the rate of 1 °C/min, and measuring the molar ellipticity at 222 nm every 0.5 °C. The reading of molar ellipticity at 222 nm in accordance with temperature change was normalized for further analysis. The data were analyzed with Origin 6.0 from OriginLab (Northampton, Massachusetts, USA).

2.3 ANS fluorescence assay

ANS solution was added into 10 μM of TMAO-incubated MoPrP in 10 mM MES (pH 6.0) to a final concentration of 100 μM. For each sample, two fluorescence emission spectra were collected by a F-4500 fluorometer (Hitachi, Japan) with excitation either at 295 nm or 385 nm, respectively.

2.4 Fibril formation

Fibril conversion was conducted at 20 μM protein in the solution containing 2 M guanidine hydrochloride (GdnHCl) and 50 mM MES (pH 6) at 37 °C as described in a previous study on mouse prion fibrils (Bocharova et al. 2005). At the end of the experiments, the fibril samples were dialyzed against 20 mM sodium acetate (pH 5.5) for further experiments.

2.5 ThT fluorescence assay of fibril conversion

Aliquots withdrawn during the time course of incubation at 37 °C were diluted into 5 mM sodium acetate buffer (pH 5.5) to a final sample concentration of 0.5 μM. ThT solution was added to a final concentration of 10 μM. For each sample, two emission spectra were collected by a F-4500 fluorometer (Hitachi, Japan) equipped with a 150 W Xenon lamp. The fluorescence spectra were recorded from 470 to 550 nm with excitation wavelength of 450 nm. The maximum fluorescence emission at 482 nm was determined. The reported fluorescence readings were average values for two measurements.

2.6 TEM

The aliquotes of mouse prion fibril samples were stained with 2% tungsten phosphoric acid onto carbon-coated 200-mesh copper grids. The samples were adsorbed onto copper grids for 30 sec and subsequently washed with PBS and mQH_2O. The samples were air-dried before imaging. The TEM images were collected by a H-7100 TEM (Hitachi, Japan). The analysis of fibril length and width was carried out on WICF ImageJ software (National Institutes of Health).

3. Results and discussion

We characterized the effect of the osmolyte TMAO on the structure of MoPrP by far-UV circular dichroism spectroscopy and ANS-binding fluorescence assay. Furthermore, we tested the effect of TMAO on amyloid fibril formation. The prion fibrils grown at different concentrations of TMAO were analyzed by TEM.

3.1 Secondary structure and protein stability

We collected far-UV circular dichroism spectra for MoPrP at pH 6.0 at 20 °C. As shown in Figure 4, MoPrP has the typical feature of α-helical conformation as indicated by the circular dichroic signals at 208 nm and 222 nm. In prior investigations of TMAO and its effects on MoPrP structure, circular dichroism spectra of MoPrP in 2 M TMAO were recorded every hour. These spectra collected within 6 hours are very similar (data not shown). Since the extension of incubation does not affect the structural features of MoPrP, the following spectroscopic experiments were conducted without prolonged incubation.

3.1.1 TMAO causes unfolding and destabilizes MoPrP

We investigated the addition of TMAO in the range of 0.5 ~ 2 M and its effect on MoPrP using circular dichroism spectroscopy. The results are presented in Figure 4A. Osmolyte TMAO exhibits substantial interference below 205 nm. Therefore, the interfering circular dichroic signal was removed from the plot. In the absence of TMAO, MoPrP has clear circular dichroic feature of α-helical conformation at 208 and 222 nm. After addition of 0.5 M and 1.0 M TMAO, the circular dichroic signal indicative of α-helix structure at 208 nm decreased slightly, while the signal at 222 nm remained generally unchanged. Significantly, addition of 1.5 M and 2.0 M weakens the entire α-helical conformation. The unfolding of α-helical structure has been reported with similar work performed at low pH (Granata et al. 2006). Consistently, the significant unfolding of prion proteins is carried out at > 1.0 M TMAO as illustrated in Figure 4B. Differently, the dichroic signal at 208 nm is affected by TMAO more severely than that at 222 nm. The dichroic signal at 208 nm dominants the dichroic curve of α-helix in the absence of TMAO, but this signal is largely weakened by the addition of TMAO. The dichroic curve of TMAO-affected partially folded α-helical structure observed in this work is not identical to the curves observed in the similar work performed at high temperature (Nandi et al. 2006). These results indicated that TMAO affect the structure of prion proteins differently under different conditions. At neutral pH, TMAO is zwitterionic, but it becomes cationic at low pH. Full-length prion protein includes polybasic N-terminal region 23-30 which is essential for effective folding into the native cellular conformation (Ostapchenko et al. 2008). Therefore, the differentiation of TMAO-induced conformational change at different pH values can be partially, if not all, ascribed to the interaction between TMAO and the polybasic N-terminal region.

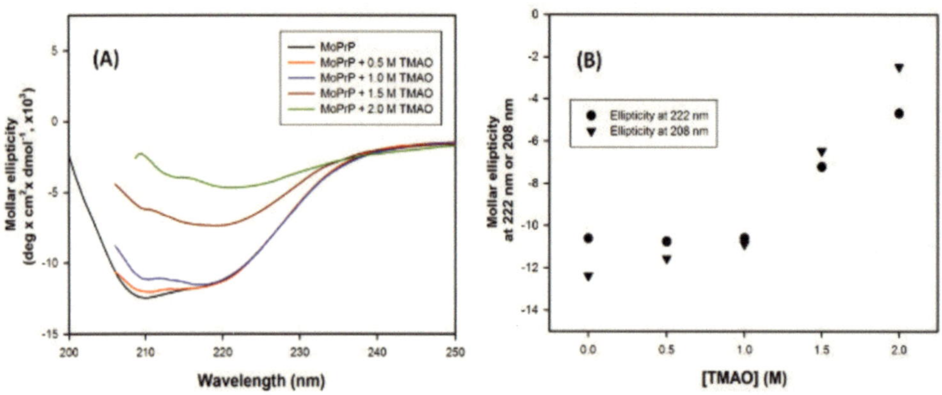

Fig. 4. (A) Far-UV circular dichroism spectra of 10 μM MoPrP measured after the addition of TMAO. (B) Comparison of mollar ellipticity at 222 nm and 208 nm in various concentration of TMAO

TMAO is known to increase the melting temperature of various proteins (Arakawa & Timasheff 1985). Therefore, in addition to the conformation change, the structural stability of MoPrP in the presence of TMAO was examined with thermal-induced denaturation monitored by the molar ellipticity at 222 nm. The molar ellipticity was normalized to represent the fraction of unfolded proteins as presented in Figure 5.

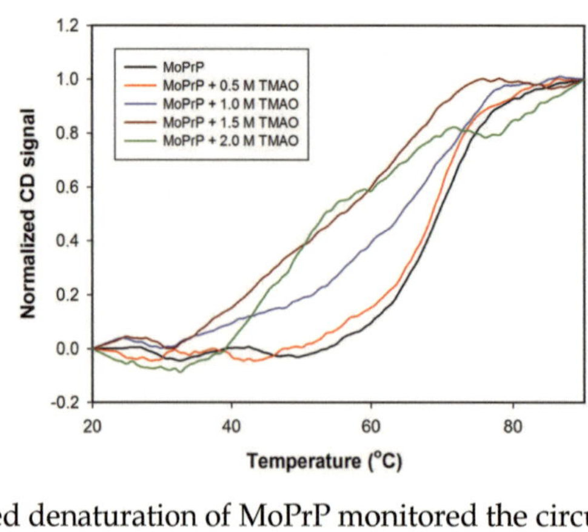

Fig. 5. Thermal-induced denaturation of MoPrP monitored the circular dichroic signal at 222 nm

The curves of heat-induced denaturation can be described by a cooperative two-state model of denaturation in which proteins are transited between natively folded states and denatured unfolded states. By monitoring the circular dichroic signal at 222 nm, the natively folded MoPrP has the minimum intensity, whereas fully unfolded proteins has the maximum readings. These denaturation curves can be analyzed based on the Gibbs-Helmholtz equation:

$$\Delta G_U^\circ(T) = \Delta H^\circ(T_m)(1-\frac{T}{T_m}) - \Delta G_p^\circ[(T_m - T) + T\ln(\frac{T}{T_m})] \quad (1)$$

Based on the above equation, the melting temperature (T_m) of MoPrP can be determine. In the absence of TMAO, the T_m of MoPrP is 68.63 °C. Addition of 0.5 M TMAO does not affect the thermal-denaturation curve significantly, as the T_m value was calculated to be 68.19 °C. In the presence of 1.0 ~ 1.5 M TMAO, the thermal-denaturation curve shifted toward low temperature significantly, as MoPrP starts to denature at ~32 °C. In contrast to the denaturation curve collected in the absence of TMAO, the thermal-denaturation curves of MoPrP treated with ≥ 1.0 M TMAO are not typical of cooperative two-state unfolding. These curves implies that TMAO changes the unfolding pathway, and that more intermediates are present at high concentration of TMAO.

3.2 TMAO-induced conformational change within the native state

The hydrophobic dye ANS has been widely used to detect the conformational changes in proteins, as ANS preferentially binds to hydrophobic protein surfaces. The binding of ANS to hydrophobic area causes significant increase in the fluorescence emission of ANS. Therefore, we detected ANS fluorescence emission upon excitation at at 385 nm to detect the change of hydrophobicity of MoPrP as presented in Figure 6. Clearly, ANS-bound MoPrP emits fluorescence at 470 nm and 495 nm upon excitation at 385 nm which indicates the presence of two distinct ANS-binding pockets. Addition of 0.5 M TMAO weakens the fluorescence emission of ANS slightly, but addition of 1.0 ~ 2.0 M TMAO substantially increased ANS fluorescence. The increase of ANS emission at 470 nm is more pronounced than the fluorescence at 495 nm. It indicates that the hydrophobicity represents by 470 nm is more sensitive to TMAO than the other one at 495 nm. Overall, this result indicates that TMAO increases hydrophobic surface at two distinct sites in MoPrP.

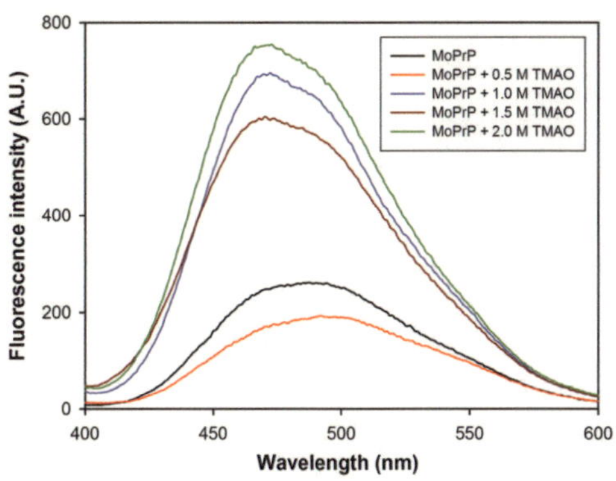

Fig. 6. Fluorescence of ANS in the absence and in the presence of TMAO upon excitation at 385 nm

In addition to the change of hydrophobicity in MoPrP, we detected ANS fluorescence emission upon excitation at 295 nm to study the TMAO-induced conformational change. Excitation at 295 nm excites tryptophan (Trp) and ANS at the same time, but this excitation causes the energy transfer from Trp (donor) in the N-terminus to ANS (acceptor). As the energy transfer efficiency (E) is determined by the distance of donor-acceptor (r) in the relation of $E \alpha r^{-6}$, the fluorescence spectra with excitation at 295 nm provide the distance information between Trp and ANS-bound residues. As illustrated in Figure 7, in the absence of TMAO, MoPrP has fluorescence emission at 350 nm and 485 nm arising from Trp and ANS-binding, respectively. Upon the addition of TMAO, the energy in Trp transfers to MoPrP-bound ANS efficiently that the signal of Trp at 350 nm is completely abolished, and the fluorescence of ANS is significantly enhanced. The fluorescence spectra of ANS in the presence of TMAO illustrate a strong peak at 408 nm, a medium, broad peak at ~460 nm and a weak, broad peak at ~490 nm overlapped with the broad peak at 460 nm. The fluorescence at 490 nm is a typical emission of ANS-binding as observed in Figure 6. This weak signal at 490 nm could be ascribed to MoPrP-bound ANS molecules that do not accept energy from Trp efficiently. As the addition of TMAO causes the peaks at 408 nm and at 460 nm to increase at different degrees, it is predicted that there are two distinct hydrophobic pockets near the N-terminal region but away from Trp with different distances.

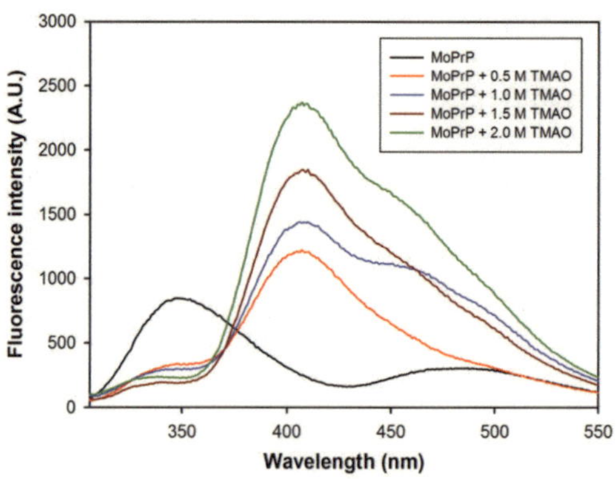

Fig. 7. Fluorescence of ANS in the absence and in the presence of TMAO upon excitation at 295 nm

3.2 Fibril conversion in TMAO

Partially unfolded MoPrP can potentially initiate formation of amyloid fibrils (Abedini & Raleigh 2009; Chiti & Dobson 2009). In 2 M GdnHCl, MoPrP is about half folded and is readily converted into amyloid fibrils (Breydo et al. 2005). Formation of amyloid fibrils can be monitored by ThT-binding fluorescence because the fluorescence of ThT is greatly enhanced when ThT binds to β-sheet rich structures, which are the main structures found in the amyloid fibrils (LeVine 1999). Therefore, the intensity of ThT-binding fluorescence represents the amount of amyloid fibrils converted from protein monomers in the absence of TMAO. As illustrated in Figure 8, the kinetics of fibril conversion shows sigmoidal curves. The MoPrP starts to form amyloid fibrils after 6 hours of incubation as monitored by ThT-binding fluorescence. The prion fibrils grow rapidly such that the maximum ThT fluorescence reached ~400 after 8 hours of amyloid fibril conversion. In the presence of 0.5

or 1.0 M of TMAO, the amyloid fibrils grow very well such that the maximum values of ThT fluorescence are higher in comparison to those in the absence of TMAO. When the concentration of TMAO is increased to 1.5 M and above, MoPrP rarely converts to amyloid fibrils as indicated by low ThT-binding fluorescence.

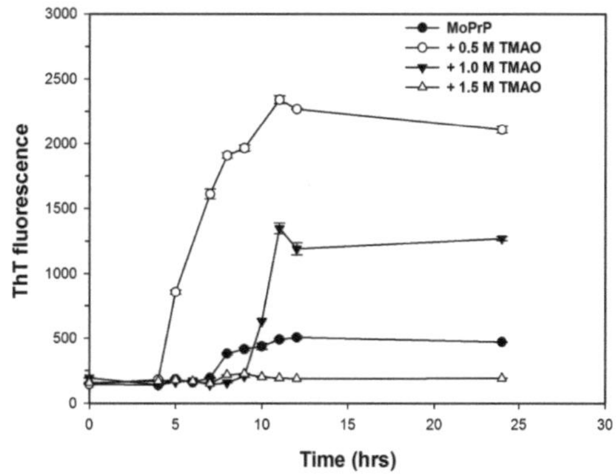

Fig. 8. Kinetic traces for amyloid fibril formation from MoPrP monitored by ThT-binding fluorescence in the presence of 2 M GdnHCl and various concentrations of TMAO at pH 6.0 at 37 °C. The fluorescence readings were average values of two measurements

The quantity of prion fibrils judged by the maximum ThT fluorescence in the presence of TMAO is presented in Figure 9A. Clearly, addition of 0.5 and 1.0 M TMAO promotes amyloid formation as the reading of ThT-fluorescence is greatly enhanced in comparison to that in the absence of TMAO. In contrast, when the concentration of TMAO was increased further, the fibril conversion was inhibited. It is interesting to observe enhancement of fibril conversion by TMAO at ≤ 1.0 M. This result is consistent with previous work performed on α-synuclein that 1.0 M TMAO yields large amount of fibril whereas 2.0 and 3.0 M of TMAO inhibits the fibril formation (Uversky et al. 2001).

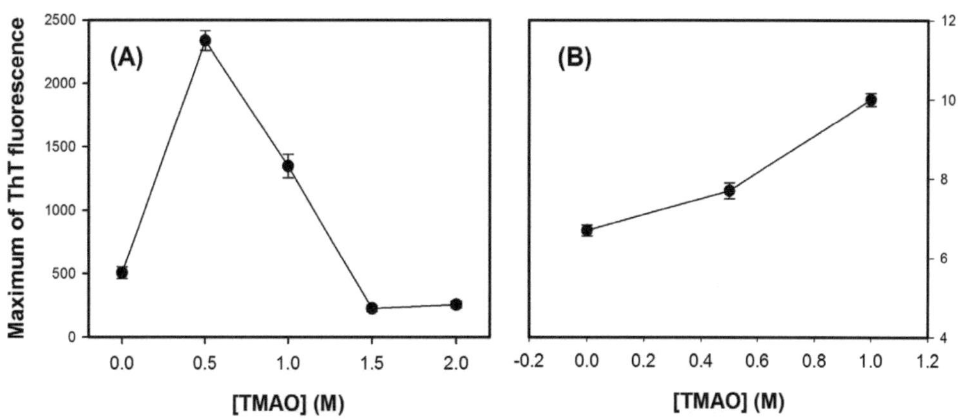

Fig. 9. (A)The quantity of amyloid fibrils converted from MoPrP monitored by the maximum of ThT-binding fluorescence measured two times, and (B) the calculated lag phase of fibril conversion in the absence and in the presence of TMAO

The formation of amyloid fibrils in the presence of 0 ~ 1.5 M TMAO follows the nucleation-dependent polymerization model as illustrated in Figure 2. According to this nucleation-dependent polymerization model, the lag phase of amyloid formation from MoPrP can be determined by fitting the time-dependent changes in the ThT fluorescence (F) over time (t) of the reaction as shown in the following equation (Bocharova et al. 2005):

$$F = F_0 + \frac{\Delta F}{1+\exp[k(t_m - t)]} \tag{2}$$

Where F_0 is the minimum level of ThT fluorescence during the lag phase, ΔF is the difference of ThT fluorescence between the maximum level (steady state) and the minimum level (lag phase), k is the rate constant of fibril growth (h^{-1}), and t_m is the observed time at the midpoint of transition. The lag time (t_l) of fibril formation can be calculated as:

$$t_l = t_m - \frac{2}{k} \tag{3}$$

According to these two equations, the lag time for fibril formation in the presence of 0, 0.5 and 1.0 M TMAO was determined as presented in Figure 9B. Previous work on fibril conversion from α-synuclein in the presence of TMAO reported acceleration of amyloid formation in a wide range of TMAO concentration (1.0 ~ 3.0 M) due to osmolyte-induced stabilization of the partially folded intermediate (Uversky et al. 2001). Similarly, TMAO stabilizes some partially folded intermediates. However, these partially folded intermediates slightly disfavour the nucleation reaction resulting in slight extension of the nucleation phase and also the following growth phase.

3.3 Morphology of prion fibrils grown with TMAO

Variation of conditions for fibril formation from the identical protein can yield different morphology. For example, Makarava and Baskakov have observed curved and straight fibrils from the same mouse prion protein and identical solvent conditions but different in the shaking speed (Makarava & Baskakov 2008). Therefore, we investigated the morphology of mouse prion fibrils by electron microscopy. In our experiment, for mature mouse prion fibrils grown in 2 M GdnHCl, the length is mostly longer than 500 nm, and the width is about 20 nm as illustrated in Figure 10.

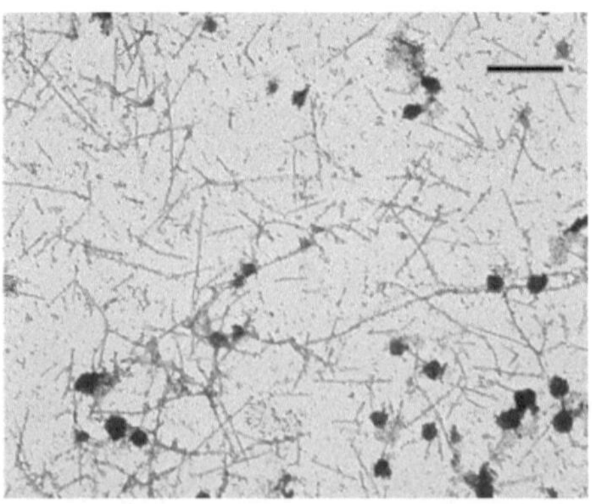

Fig. 10. TEM image of mature prion fibrils grown in 2 M GdnHCl at pH 6.0 at 37 °C. The scale bar represents 500 nm

The growth phase of fibril conversion in the absence of TMAO is very short, whereas this elongation process takes longer in the addition of TMAO. To compare the morphology of prion fibrils during elongation in the absence and in the presence of TMAO, we collected TEM images of fibril samples in the middle point of growth phase. As illustrated in Figure 11, the prion fibrils grown in the absence of TMAO are long and straight, whereas fibrils converted in the presence of TMAO look like short rods.

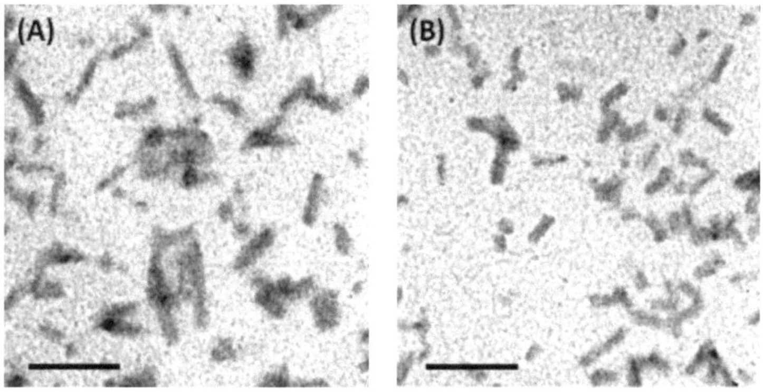

Fig. 11. TEM images of mouse prion fibrils at the middle point of growth phase (A) in the absence of TMAO and (B) in the presence of 1.0 M TMAO. The scale bar represents 200 nm

Oligomers, protofibrils and mature fibrils involved in the formation of amyloid fibrils are typically distinguished by the length and width of the fibrils. Therefore, we statistically compared the length and the width of prion fibrils converted in the absence and in the presence of 0.5 M and 1.0 M TMAO. As illustrated in Figure 12A, in the absence of TMAO, the fibril length is populated in two groups including one normal distribution between 60 ~ 180 nm and an elongation at > 180 nm. Prion fibrils with the addition of 0.5 M TMAO are normally distributed between 20 ~ 160 nm and the most populated length is 80 ~ 120 nm. Increasing TMAO to 1.0 M shortens the prion fibrils, so that the fibril length ranges from 20 to 140 nm with the most populated length being 40 ~ 60 nm. The average length of prion fibrils is 144 nm in the absence of TMAO. Addition of TMAO shortens the average length of prion fibrils to 92 and 61 nm in the presence of 0.5 M and 1.0 M, respectively. In contrast to the fibril length, the width of prion fibrils is similar as illustrated in Figure 12B, and the average of the width is 19 nm regardless the presence of TMAO.

The structural effect of osmolyte TMAO on prion proteins and fibril conversion has been investigated extensively in this work. At pH 6.0, 20 °C, the α-helical conformation of MoPrP is unfolded by TMAO. When the concentration of TMAO is low at ≤ 1.0 M, the degree of unfolding is small and the fibril conversion takes place on the mostly folded α-helical structures. In contrast to low concentration of TMAO, high concentration of TMAO at >1.0 M largely unfolds the α-helix and this unfolding inhibits amyloid formation completely. In other words, low concentration of TMAO decellarates the prion nucleation represented by lag phase in nucleation-dependent polymerization model, whereas TMAO enhances the growth of prion fibrils. This contrast effect indicates that the structural requirement of prion proteins in nucleation and in fibril elongation is different. The importance of partial unfolding of prion in amyloid formation has been suggested (Apetri et al. 2004; Kuwata et al. 2002; Nicholson et al. 2002). The structure of partially folded prion protein that initiates amyloid formation remains unclear. Our recent computational simulation proposed that the

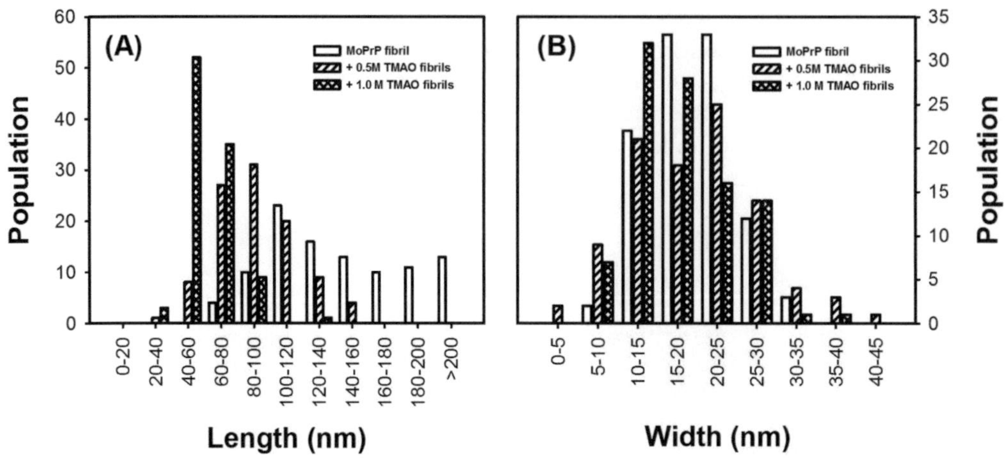

Fig. 12. Histrogram of length and width of prion fibrils measured on 100 fibrils in the absence and in the presence of 0.5 M and 1.0 M TMAO

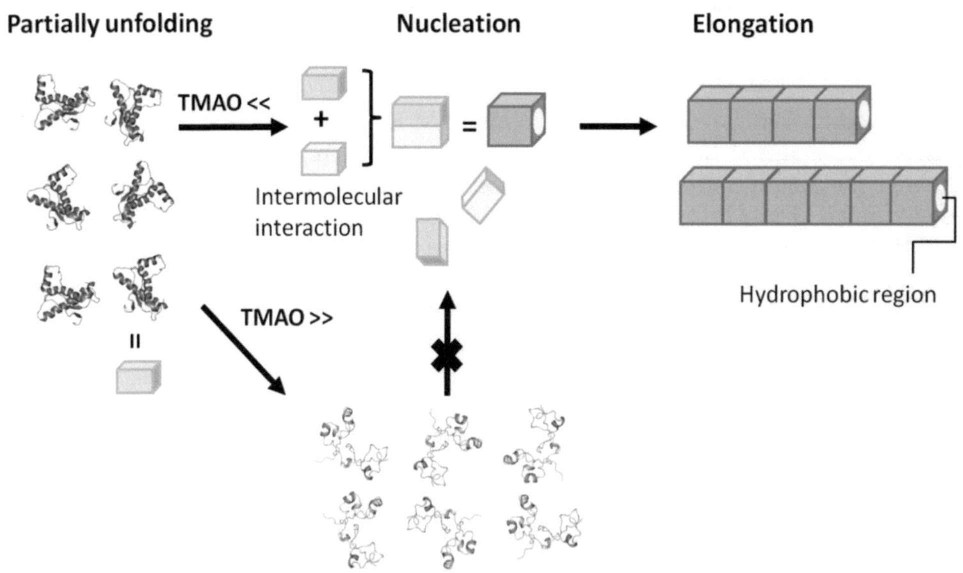

Fig. 13. A scheme illustrating the proposed effect of TMAO based on nucleation-dependent polymerization model

denatured state of prion protein is partially folded with α-helical conformation (Lee & Chang 2010). In prion nucleation, high α-helical conformation is preferred and intermolecular β-sheet interactions occur between prion monomers (Lee et al. 2010). This interaction of intermolecular β-sheets is most likely the initiation of nucleation. This intermolecular interaction might be correlated with a double-layered filament within one fibril as observed by atomic force microscopy (Anderson et al. 2006). When the α-helical structure is mostly lost and the intermolecular interaction is largely weakened, the amyloid formation can not take place due to failure of nucleation as illustrated in Figure 13. After nuclei are formed as fibril seeds, the elongation requires stable interactions between nuclei and proteins. As amyloid fibrils have been proposed to have hydrophobic interior (Buchete & Hummer 2007; Carroll et al. 2006), the area of the hydrophobic surface is important in fibril elongation. The hydrophobicity at the ANS-binding pockets that accept energy from Trp is induced significantly by TMAO, and the high hydrophobicity promotes hydrophobic interactions of nuclei and proteins to form the hydrophobic interior. Notably, in the presence of low concentration of TMAO, the amount of fibrils is significantly increased, but the fibril length is shortened in the middle of growth phase. This phenomenon could be due to adjustment of interaction between nuclei under high hydrophobicity as judged by long growth phase in the presence of TMAO. Taking togther these findings, a certain amount of α-helical conformation seems to be required in the structural conversion of prion proteins in nucleation, and hydrophobic interaction is essential in fibril elongation.

4. Conclusion

In this study, we have investigated the structural effect of osmolytes TMAO on MoPrP proteins and the features of mouse prion fibrils. Low concentration of TMAO alters α-helical structures resulting deceleration of nucleation serving as fibril seeds, but TMAO enhances hydrophobicity promoting fibril growth. High concentration of TMAO inhibits amyloid formation completely by inducing loss of α-helical conformation. This study provides more information in the details of molecular structure and interaction in amyloid formation. These findings are essential in further search for therapeutic therapies for prion disease.

5. Acknowledgment

We are grateful to National Science Council for financial support (Project 100-2321-B-194-001). We also thank Dr. Raymond Chung for editing the manuscript. Usage of PyMol graphics packages and WICF ImageJ software is gratefully acknowledged.

6. References

Abedini, A. and Raleigh, D. P. (2009). A role for helical intermediates in amyloid formation by natively unfolded polypeptides? *Phys Biol*, 6, 1, 15005.

Anderson, M., Bocharova, O. V., Makarava, N., et al. (2006). Polymorphism and ultrastructural organization of prion protein amyloid fibrils: an insight from high resolution atomic force microscopy. *J Mol Biol*, 358, 2, 580-596.

Apetri, A. C., Surewicz, K. and Surewicz, W. K. (2004). The effect of disease-associated mutations on the folding pathway of human prion protein. *J Biol Chem*, 279, 17, 18008-18014.

Arakawa, T. and Timasheff, S. N. (1985). The stabilization of proteins by osmolytes. *Biophys J*, 47, 3, 411-414.

Baskakov, I. and Bolen, D. W. (1998). Forcing thermodynamically unfolded proteins to fold. *J Biol Chem*, 273, 9, 4831-4834.

Baskakov, I., Wang, A. and Bolen, D. W. (1998). Trimethylamine-N-oxide counteracts urea effects on rabbit muscle lactate dehydrogenase function: a test of the counteraction hypothesis. *Biophys J*, 74, 5, 2666-2673.

Bocharova, O. V., Breydo, L., Salnikov, V. V., et al. (2005). Copper(II) inhibits in vitro conversion of prion protein into amyloid fibrils. *Biochemistry*, 44, 18, 6776-6787.

Bocharova, O. V., Breydo, L., Salnikov, V. V., et al. (2005). Synthetic prions generated in vitro are similar to a newly identified subpopulation of PrPSc from sporadic Creutzfeldt-Jakob disease. *Protein Sci*, 14, 5, 1222-1232.

Bolen, D. W. and Baskakov, I. V. (2001). The osmophobic effect: natural selection of a thermodynamic force in protein folding. *J Mol Biol*, 310, 5, 955-963.

Breydo, L., Bocharova, O. V., Makarava, N., et al. (2005). Methionine oxidation interferes with conversion of the prion protein into the fibrillar proteinase K-resistant conformation. *Biochemistry*, 44, 47, 15534-15543.

Brown, D. R., Schmidt, B. and Kretzschmar, H. A. (1998). Effects of copper on survival of prion protein knockout neurons and glia. *J Neurochem*, 70, 4, 1686-1693.

Buchete, N. V. and Hummer, G. (2007). Structure and dynamics of parallel beta-sheets, hydrophobic core, and loops in Alzheimer's A beta fibrils. *Biophys J*, 92, 9, 3032-3039.

Calzolai, L. and Zahn, R. (2003). Influence of pH on NMR structure and stability of the human prion protein globular domain. *J Biol Chem*, 278, 37, 35592-35596.

Carroll, A., Yang, W., Ye, Y., et al. (2006). Amyloid fibril formation by a domain of rat cell adhesion molecule. *Cell Biochem Biophys*, 44, 2, 241-249.

Celinski, S. A. and Scholtz, J. M. (2002). Osmolyte effects on helix formation in peptides and the stability of coiled-coils. *Protein Sci*, 11, 8, 2048-2051.

Chiti, F. and Dobson, C. M. (2009). Amyloid formation by globular proteins under native conditions. *Nat Chem Biol*, 5, 1, 15-22.

Donne, D. G., Viles, J. H., Groth, D., et al. (1997). Structure of the recombinant full-length hamster prion protein PrP(29-231): the N terminus is highly flexible. *Proc Natl Acad Sci U S A*, 94, 25, 13452-13457.

Gossert, A. D., Bonjour, S., Lysek, D. A., et al. (2005). Prion protein NMR structures of elk and of mouse/elk hybrids. *Proc Natl Acad Sci U S A*, 102, 3, 646-650.

Granata, V., Palladino, P., Tizzano, B., et al. (2006). The effect of the osmolyte trimethylamine N-oxide on the stability of the prion protein at low pH. *Biopolymers*, 82, 3, 234-240.

Griffith, J. S. (1967). Self-replication and scrapie. *Nature*, 215, 5105, 1043-1044.

Gursky, O. (1999). Probing the conformation of a human apolipoprotein C-1 by amino acid substitutions and trimethylamine-N-oxide. *Protein Sci*, 8, 10, 2055-2064.

Horwich, A. L. and Weissman, J. S. (1997). Deadly conformations--protein misfolding in prion disease. *Cell*, 89, 4, 499-510.

James, T. L., Liu, H., Ulyanov, N. B., et al. (1997). Solution structure of a 142-residue recombinant prion protein corresponding to the infectious fragment of the scrapie isoform. *Proc Natl Acad Sci U S A*, 94, 19, 10086-10091.

Kuwata, K., Li, H., Yamada, H., et al. (2002). Locally disordered conformer of the hamster prion protein: a crucial intermediate to PrPSc? *Biochemistry*, 41, 41, 12277-12283.

Lee, C. I. and Chang, N. Y. (2010). Characterizing the denatured state of human prion 121-230. *Biophys Chem*, 151, 1-2, 86-90.

Lee, S., Antony, L., Hartmann, R., et al. (2010). Conformational diversity in prion protein variants influences intermolecular beta-sheet formation. *EMBO J*, 29, 1, 251-262.

LeVine, H., 3rd (1999). Quantification of beta-sheet amyloid fibril structures with thioflavin T. *Methods Enzymol*, 309, 274-284.

Lin, T. Y. and Timasheff, S. N. (1994). Why do some organisms use a urea-methylamine mixture as osmolyte? Thermodynamic compensation of urea and trimethylamine N-oxide interactions with protein. *Biochemistry*, 33, 42, 12695-12701.

Makarava, N. and Baskakov, I. V. (2008). The same primary structure of the prion protein yields two distinct self-propagating states. *J Biol Chem*, 283, 23, 15988-15996.

Mouillet-Richard, S., Ermonval, M., Chebassier, C., et al. (2000). Signal transduction through prion protein. *Science*, 289, 5486, 1925-1928.

Nandi, P. K., Bera, A. and Sizaret, P. Y. (2006). Osmolyte trimethylamine N-oxide converts recombinant alpha-helical prion protein to its soluble beta-structured form at high temperature. *J Mol Biol*, 362, 4, 810-820.

Nicholson, E. M., Peterson, R. W. and Scholtz, J. M. (2002). A partially buried site in homologous HPr proteins is not optimized for stability. *J Mol Biol*, 321, 2, 355-362.

Nicoll, A. J., Trevitt, C. R., Tattum, M. H., et al. (2010). Pharmacological chaperone for the structured domain of human prion protein. *Proc Natl Acad Sci U S A*, 107, 41, 17610-17615.

Ostapchenko, V. G., Makarava, N., Savtchenko, R., et al. (2008). The polybasic N-terminal region of the prion protein controls the physical properties of both the cellular and fibrillar forms of PrP. *J Mol Biol*, 383, 5, 1210-1224.

Prusiner, S. B. (1982). Novel proteinaceous infectious particles cause scrapie. *Science*, 216, 4542, 136-144.

Prusiner, S. B. (1997). Prion diseases and the BSE crisis. *Science*, 278, 5336, 245-251.

Prusiner, S. B. (1998). Prions. *Proc Natl Acad Sci U S A*, 95, 23, 13363-13383.

Qu, Y., Bolen, C. L. and Bolen, D. W. (1998). Osmolyte-driven contraction of a random coil protein. *Proc Natl Acad Sci U S A*, 95, 16, 9268-9273.

Riek, R., Hornemann, S., Wider, G., et al. (1996). NMR structure of the mouse prion protein domain PrP(121-321). *Nature*, 382, 6587, 180-182.

Seifert, G., Schilling, K. and Steinhauser, C. (2006). Astrocyte dysfunction in neurological disorders: a molecular perspective. *Nat Rev Neurosci*, 7, 3, 194-206.

Singh, R., Haque, I. and Ahmad, F. (2005). Counteracting osmolyte trimethylamine N-oxide destabilizes proteins at pH below its pKa. Measurements of thermodynamic parameters of proteins in the presence and absence of trimethylamine N-oxide. *J Biol Chem*, 280, 12, 11035-11042.

Tatzelt, J., Prusiner, S. B. and Welch, W. J. (1996). Chemical chaperones interfere with the formation of scrapie prion protein. *EMBO J*, 15, 23, 6363-6373.

Telling, G. C., Scott, M., Mastrianni, J., et al. (1995). Prion propagation in mice expressing human and chimeric PrP transgenes implicates the interaction of cellular PrP with another protein. *Cell*, 83, 1, 79-90.

Tsong, T. Y. and Baldwin, R. L. (1972). A sequential model of nucleation-dependent protein folding: kinetic studies of ribonuclease A. *J Mol Biol*, 63, 3, 453-469.

Uversky, V. N., Li, J. and Fink, A. L. (2001). Trimethylamine-N-oxide-induced folding of alpha-synuclein. *FEBS Lett*, 509, 1, 31-35.

Whittal, R. M., Ball, H. L., Cohen, F. E., et al. (2000). Copper binding to octarepeat peptides of the prion protein monitored by mass spectrometry. *Protein Sci*, 9, 2, 332-343.

Will, R. G., Ironside, J. W., Zeidler, M., et al. (1996). A new variant of Creutzfeldt-Jakob disease in the UK. *Lancet*, 347, 9006, 921-925.

Zahn, R., Liu, A., Luhrs, T., et al. (2000). NMR solution structure of the human prion protein. *Proc Natl Acad Sci U S A*, 97, 1, 145-150.

Part 4

Motor Neuron Diseases

16

Modeling Spinal Muscular Atrophy in Mouse: A Disease of Splicing, Stability, and Timing

Thomas W. Bebee and Dawn S. Chandler
The Center for Childhood Cancer at the Research Institute at Nationwide Children's Hospital, Columbus, Ohio;
The Department of Pediatrics, The Ohio State University, Columbus, Ohio;
United States of America

1. Introduction

Proximal spinal muscular atrophy (SMA) is a progressive neurodegenerative disease associated with the loss of alpha motor neurons in the lumbar spinal cord. The loss of these motor neurons leads to the progressive atrophy of the associated proximal muscles, eventual respiratory distress, and death. SMA occurs in about 1 in 6,000 to 10,000 live births and is a leading genetic cause of infant mortality (Burnett et al. 2009). SMA is subdivided into several groupings based on disease onset, severity, and outcome. The most severe form of SMA is referred to as type 0, or embryonic SMA, wherein patients are born with severe muscle atrophy and have expected lifespans of less than 6 months. The most common type of SMA is type I, which is characterized by disease onset within 6 months and mortality by age 2. Children with SMA type I often fail to sit unaided or walk, have difficulty breathing, and often require respiratory assistance. SMA type II children experience disease onset between 6 to 18 months and will not gain the ability to walk. Two forms of SMA are characterized by disease onset later in life and have unaltered life expectancies: juvenile and adult onset SMA, or type III and IV, respectively. Juvenile onset SMA type III is distinguished by disease onset after the age of 2, but there is variability of onset that can extend to early teen years. Type III children are often able to walk, and the ability to remain ambulatory throughout life can further subdivide this juvenile onset SMA. The least severe form of SMA is adult onset SMA type IV. This form of SMA does not emerge until the adult years and often presents with difficulty in performing previously attainable activities, such as climbing stairs (Zerres et al. 1995; Zerres et al. 1997; Zerres et al. 1997).
In SMA disease progression, the inability to achieve normal motor function is often the primary indication of disease. The level of motor function decline in SMA disease progression can be measured by the loss of functional motor units in SMA patients. In severe forms of SMA, there is a rapid loss of motor neurons innervating proximal muscles. This measure of reduced motor units can be observed by evaluating the Compound Motor Action Potential (CMAP) and Motor Unit Number Estimation (MUNE). The total number of innervated motor units is reduced in SMA disease as measured by these two tests and is correlated with age, severity of disease, and disease progression (Swoboda et al. 2005). The loss of motor neurons early in the onset of disease argues for the significance of motor neurons in disease, although additional components of the disease may provide for the

rapid degeneration of SMA patients in late disease. Respiratory weakness is a common feature of both severe and milder forms of SMA. Children with type I or II SMA will often require respiratory assistance by way of Bi-level Positive Airway Pressure (BiPAP) (Bach et al. 2003), just as less severe forms of SMA also exhibit respiratory weakness that may require assistive breathing and respiratory therapy. While SMA is most directly associated with motor neuron loss, neuronal defects in sensory neurons are also observed in severe SMA patients (Rudnik-Schoneborn et al. 2003). A new emerging component of SMA is cardiac involvement in a subset of severe SMA patients, such as congenital cardiac defects and bradycardia (Bach et al. 2003; Rudnik-Schoneborn et al. 2008).

2. Genetic cause of SMA, reduced levels of SMN protein

The decreased level of the crucial Survival Motor Neuron (SMN) protein is the cause of SMA disease. The low levels of SMN protein are due to the loss of the essential Survival Motor Neuron-1 (*SMN1*) gene located on chromosome 5q13. SMA patients have lost *SMN1* by mutation or deletion, and the functional loss of *SMN1* is the disease locus of SMA (Lefebvre et al. 1995). In mice, the loss of the homologous *Smn* gene results in embryonic lethality (Schrank et al. 1997; Hsieh-Li et al. 2000); however, humans carry a duplication of the *SMN1* gene, *SMN2*, which encodes the same SMN protein. All SMA patients are genetically comprised of *SMN1* gene loss (mutation or deletion) with variable copy numbers of *SMN2* (Lefebvre et al. 1995; Lefebvre et al. 1997; McAndrew et al. 1997). The copy number of *SMN2* inversely correlates with the severity of SMA, where higher copy numbers of *SMN2* increase SMN protein and, therefore, decrease the severity of disease (Lefebvre et al. 1997; McAndrew et al. 1997). SMA patients that have 1-2 copies of *SMN2* are often associated with severe SMA type I, and SMA patients with higher *SMN2* copy number exhibit SMA type II-IV (Lefebvre et al. 1997).

The incomplete compensation for the loss of *SMN1* by *SMN2* is due to the inefficient splicing of the *SMN2* pre-mRNA (Lefebvre et al. 1995; Lorson et al. 1999). The altered splicing is due primarily to a single silent C>T point mutation in exon 7 that reduces recognition of exon 7 by the splicing machinery (Lorson et al. 1999). The functional role of the C>T mutation in exon 7 skipping can be explained by two models. The first model describes the loss of a putative exon splicing enhancer for SF2/ASF (SRSF1), where reduced binding of SF2/ASF (SRSF1) is associated with *SMN2* exon 7 skipping (Lorson et al. 2000; Cartegni et al. 2002; Cartegni et al. 2006). The second model is explained by the generation of an exonic splicing silencer for hnRNP A1 (Kashima et al. 2003; Kashima et al. 2007). Both of these models functionally explain the alteration in the recognition of exon 7 via the C>T point mutation that generates transcripts lacking exon 7 (ΔX7) from *SMN2*. The complex splicing regulation of *SMN* exon 7 beyond the critical C>T mutation has been recently reviewed (Bebee et al. 2010; Singh et al. 2011).

SMA is a disease associated with reduced splicing efficiency of SMN encoding transcripts. Furthermore, the significance of reduced SMN protein in normal cellular maintenance is underscored by the importance of *SMN* in splicing. SMN is crucial for splicing, as the SMN protein is the primary scaffolding protein involved in the maturation of the core splicing factors, or U snRNPs (Fischer et al. 1997; Liu et al. 1997; Pellizzoni et al. 1999; Meister et al. 2001; Pellizzoni et al. 2002). The SMN protein, in complex with several other components, comprises the SMN complex (Paushkin et al. 2002). The SMN complex loads the heptameric Sm ring (Raker et al. 1996) onto the Sm site of U snRNPs, completing the processing of the splicing core components for function in canonical splicing of nascent transcripts (Fischer et al. 1997; Liu et al. 1997). In SMA, the SMN protein levels are reduced due to loss of *SMN1*, and the primary product of *SMN2* is the SMNΔ7 protein produced by the transcripts lacking exon 7 (Lefebvre et al. 1995; Lefebvre et al. 1997). The SMNΔ7 protein is unstable and exhibits reduced protein function (Wang et al. 2001; Cho et al. 2010). However, a portion of *SMN2* transcripts encode full-length SMN protein sufficient for birth, but insufficient for motor neuron maintenance. The ability of *SMN2* to generate full-length transcripts provides for potential therapeutic intervention by increasing transcription or correcting the splicing of *SMN2* to increase the pools of SMN to levels consistent with normal development.

3. Genetic modeling of SMA in mouse

The duplication event of *SMN1* that generated *SMN2* occurred late in evolutionary history, and thus, mice carry only a single *Smn* gene homologous to *SMN1* (Bergin et al. 1997; Rochette et al. 2001). After identification of the gene responsible for SMA disease, efforts to model the human disease in mice began by generating null alleles of the mouse *Smn* gene (Summarized in Table 1). Null alleles of the *Smn* gene were generated by replacing exon 2 or 7 with reporter cassettes, and from these experiments the Smn gene was found to be essential as *Smn* -/- mice were embryonic lethal at the eight cell stage post fertilization (Schrank et al. 1997; Hsieh-Li et al. 2000). The requirement of SMN for survival is congruent with the function of SMN in maturation of the splicing machinery as an essential function for viability in eukaryotes. Mice heterozygous for the *Smn* null alleles have normal lifespans and do not exhibit haploinsufficiency; however, they do develop a mild form of SMA with muscle weakness and motor neuron loss later in life (Jablonka et al. 2000; Monani et al. 2000).

SMA is a disease of reduced SMN protein, and although the loss of Smn represents the loss of *SMN1* seen in SMA patients, this does not fully model the genetics of SMA. To more closely recapitulate the etiology of SMA, bac transgenes that included *SMN2* were introduced into the *Smn* null mice (Hsieh-Li et al. 2000; Monani et al. 2000). The *SMN2* in the bac transgenes exhibit splicing defects similar to *SMN2*, as exon 7 is primarily skipped and low SMN expression is seen. The level of SMN protein generated from the *SMN2* transgenes was sufficient to correct the embryonic lethality in *Smn* null mice. The rescue by *SMN2* in *Smn* null mice is in accordance with the observation that all SMA patients have *SMN2* present. Moreover, increased copy numbers of *SMN2* led to variable severities of SMA that stratify human SMA disease. Mice with 2 copies of *SMN2* ("Line89") exhibited severe SMA with an average lifespan of 4-6 postnatal days, but an increase of the *SMN2* copy number to 8 rescued the Line89 mice from SMA disease (Monani et al. 2000). Mice generated using a second *Smn* null allele (disruption of *Smn* exon 7) in combination with an *SMN2* bac transgene, termed the Taiwanese or Hsieh-Li mice, generated mice that exhibited severe to mild SMA. Hsieh-Li mice with 2 copies of *SMN2* survived 1 week and mice with 4 copies of *SMN2* had normal survival but developed peripheral necrosis (Hsieh-Li et al. 2000). A simplified crossing scheme of these mice now allows for independent generation of both the severe mice that survive 10 days, as well as the mild mice with normal survival (Riessland et al. 2010).

In severe SMA mouse models, reduced SMN protein, loss of anterior horn lumbar motor neurons, and muscle atrophy lead to the observed reduction in survival of 6-10 days (Hsieh-Li et al. 2000; Monani et al. 2000). Interestingly, the lifespan of the severe Line89 mouse was extended to PND13.5 by transgenic over-expression of the SMNΔ7 transcript (Le et al. 2005).

Genotype	Phenotype and Notes	Shorthand	References
Smn-/-	Embryonic lethal at preimplantation (8 cell stage). *Smn* exon 2 knockout.	*Smn* knockout	Schrank 1997
Smn+/-	Grossly normal with normal lifespan in the heterozygous *Smn* exon 2 knockout mice. Motor neuron loss in spinal cord: 40% at 6 months, 54% at 12 months.	Line89 het carrier	Jablonka 2000
Smn-/-; SMN2(2Hung)+/+	Bac transgene (115 kb) including human *SMN2*, *SERF1* and part of *NAIP* genes; rescues embryonic lethality of *Smn-/-* (HPRT knockout of *Smn* exon 7). Variable *SMN2* copy number, with increasing copy number lessening disease severity (Type I-III).	Taiwanese or Hsieh-Li	Hsieh-Li 2000
Smn-/-; SMN2(89Ahmb)+/+	Transgene containing *SMN2* (35.5 kb); rescues *Smn-/-* (exon 2 null allele) embryonic lethality. 2 copies of *SMN2* in the mice have severe SMA and die postnatally with mean survival PND4-6. Motor neuron loss PND5. Eight copies of *SMN2* rescue SMA phenotype.	Line89	Monani 2000
SmnF7/Δ7; NSE-Cre	Cre-mediated *Smn* exon 7 excision in neurons. Mice develop a SMA like pathology with progressive motor neuron loss (cell body number and axon number) in the lumbar spinal cord, muscle atrophy, and have a mean survival of 25 days.	F7 or exon 7 floxed	Frugier 2000, Cifuentes-Diaz 2002
SmnF7/Δ7; HSA-Cre	Cre-mediated *Smn* exon 7 loss in skeletal muscle. Muscle cell death and dystrophy-like pathology, with a mean survival of 33 days.	F7 or exon 7 floxed	Cifuentes-Diaz 2001
Smn-/-; SMN2(89Ahmb)+/+; SMN1(A2G)+/-	Heterozygous expression of *SMN1* A2G patient mutation transgene increase survival of Line89 mice to ~227 days, but is dependent upon *SMN2* (2 copies). Reduced motor neuron number in spinal cord (29%) and facial nucleus (19%) at 3.5 months. ~25% reduction in spinal motor axon by 5 months, muscle atrophy, and axonal sprouting in gastrocnemius and triceps. Homozygous A2G are phenotypically normal.	A2G	Monani 2003

Table 1. Mouse models of SMA. (continues on next page)

Genotype	Phenotype and Notes	Shorthand	References
SmnF7/F7; Alfp-Cre	Cre-mediated *Smn* exon 7 excision in hepatocytes is embryonic lethal at E18.5.	F7 or exon 7 floxed	Vitte 2004
Smn-/-; SMN2(89Ahmb)+/+; SMNΔ7+/+	Expression of the SMNΔ7 transgene in Line89 mice extend survival to ~13.5 days. Motor neuron loss by PND9, weight and motor deficits, and muscle atrophy.	SMNΔ7	Le 2005
Smn-/-; SMN2(89Ahmb)+/+; SMN1(A111G)+/-	Transgene of *SMN1* A111G patient mutation rescues Line89 mice. Survival is normal but requires *SMN2* (2 copies). Gastrocnemius muscle hypertrophy at 10 months and rescued the deficits in snRNP assembly seen in the Line89 mice.	A111G	Workman 2009
Smn2B/-	Mutation of exonic enhancer in *Smn* exon 7 leads to low Smn protein levels and mean survival of 28 days. Muscle weakness and atrophy, and reduced motor neurons at PND21.	2B	Bowerman 2009, Bowerman 2010
Smn-/-; SMN2(N11)+/-; SMN2(N46)+/-	Mice with three copies of *SMN2* from N11(one copy) and N46 (two copies) alleles have a mean survival of 14-16 days. Muscle atrophy and motor neuron loss by PND15. Respiratory deficits and NMJ defects in diaphragm.	3 copy *SMN2*	Michaud 2010
SmnF7/-; SMN2(89Ahmb)+/+; Olig2-Cre	Cre-mediated *Smn* exon 7 excision in motor neuron progenitor cells that also express basal SMN from *SMN2*. 70% survival to 12 months, motor neuron loss in spinal cord, muscle atrophy, and reduced sensory neuron innervation and number in DRG.	Olig2-Cre SMA	Park 2010
SmnC>T	*Smn* gene carrying the *SMN2* exon 7 C>T mutation induces exon 7 skipping and reduces Smn protein. Mild SMA disease onset at 60 days associated with hind limb weakness, reduced activity and rearing, and muscle hypertrophy in gastrocnemius. Normal survival.	*Smn C>T*	Gladman 2010

Table 1. (continued) Mouse models of SMA

The mechanism of life extension in this severe SMA mouse model is not easily understood but begs the question of whether the SMNΔ7 protein has a functional role in normal development and/or neuroprotection. Another transgene that modified the survival of the severe Line89 mice is the *SMN1* A2G mutation. The A2G transgene alone was unable to rescue the *Smn* null mice; however, survival extension through expression of the A2G transgene was contingent upon expression of SMN from the *SMN2* transgene. The transgenic A2G mouse develops mild SMA early in life, though survival is near 1 year and the mice with SMA pathology can appear normal until disease progression late in life. The A2G mice are associated with motor neuron defects such as motor neuron loss, branching, neurofilament accumulation, and failure to respond to repeated stimuli (Monani et al. 2003; Kariya et al. 2008). The milder SMA phenotype may be explained by the partial ability of the A2G mutant SMN protein to bind to normal full-length SMN. This binding is greater than that of the SMNΔ7 protein, arguing the potential for partial rescue of SMN complex formation in the A2G SMA mouse model (Monani et al. 2003).

SMA mouse models that carry the *SMN2* gene can be used to evaluate the expression and splicing of *SMN2* in tissues otherwise inaccessible in SMA patients, such as the central nervous system (CNS). Furthermore, the effect of disease progression and therapies targeting correction of *SMN2* can also be evaluated in mice that have the *SMN2* bac transgenes. The short lifespan of the severe SMA mouse models also allows for rapid evaluation of treatments aimed at increasing SMN, as changes in survival can readily be addressed in the short-lived mice. However, the short lifespan of these SMA models does not allow for therapeutic intervention at later time-points in development and SMA disease. Further attempts to modulate the lifespan of the severe SMA by simply titrating the copy number of *SMN2* in mice have proven difficult. One group generated two *SMN2* transgenic lines that harbor 1 or 2 copies of *SMN2* per allele (lines N11 and N46). When combined to generate a 3 copy *SMN2* mouse, the survival was extended to PND14-16 with some outlier longer lived mice (Michaud et al. 2010). This average survival is similar to the SMNΔ7 mice and is accompanied by severe muscle weakness and atrophy late in disease, motor neuron loss by PND13, abnormal EMG, and NMJ defects. These mice also exhibit respiratory deficiencies associated with reduced volume and frequency. Additional allelic series of mice have been generated harboring alterations in the *Smn* gene and *SMN* hybrid alleles to titrate SMN protein levels in mice (These mice can be found on the Jackson Laboratories web site http://jaxmice.jax.org/list/ra1733.html).

Successful generation of SMA mouse models was achieved through the loss of Smn protein using *Smn* null alleles in combination with transgenic expression of SMN from *SMN2* and other SMN transgenes. However, to simplify the genetics of modeling SMA in mice, it would be desirable to place both the gene loss and modifier expression in the same locus. The cosegregation of these two genetic events would allow for regulation of transcription and splicing in the endogenous genetic locus. The *Smn* C>T allele was engineered by introducing the *SMN2* exon 7 C>T mutation in the murine *Smn* gene. The *Smn* C>T mouse mimics the genetics of SMA patients, and recapitulates the splicing defect of *SMN2*, wherein exon 7 is skipped due to the C>T mutation. These mice exhibit reduced total *Smn* protein and a mild SMA phenotype characterized by hind limb weakness and inactivity consistent with type III SMA (Gladman et al. 2010). A second *Smn* C>T allele has been engineered (*Smn* C-T-Neo); however, this allele harbors the exon 7 C>T mutation with the neo cassette in intron 7 and additional sequences at the 5′ end of exon 8. The splicing pattern of this mouse allele is primarily exon 7 skipped transcripts, and as such, produces very low Smn protein levels leading to embryonic lethality. The *Smn* C-T-Neo mouse has been used as an inducible *Smn* allele as the low Smn protein levels can be increased by the removal of the neo cassette; however, this must be done early in embryonic development (E7.5) or the embryo will be resorbed (Hammond et al. 2010).

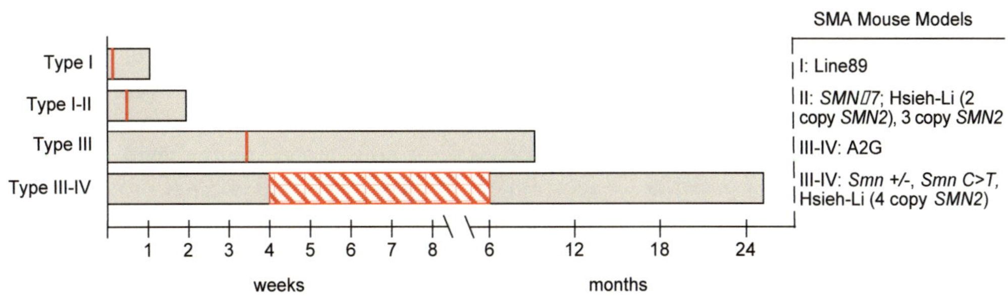

Fig. 1. SMA mouse models: survival and disease onset. Graphical representations of mean survivals of SMA mouse models types I-IV are shown by grey bars. Time scale is in weeks 0-8 and in months 6-24. A red line indicates the disease onset of SMA phenotype. For the mild SMA mouse models, a red-hashed box indicates variable onset in the listed SMA mouse models (i.e.: *Smn* +/- is 6 months, *Smn* C>T is 8 weeks, and Hsieh-Li (4 copy *SMN2*) has tail necrosis starting at 4 weeks)

Mutations in the mouse exon splicing enhancer for Tra2beta (2B) in exon 7 produces high levels of skipped transcripts in the absence of the C>T mutation (DiDonato et al. 2001). The mutation in the Tra2Beta enhancer is not associated with SMA mutations, and though it does induce exon 7 skipping, it does not recapitulate the splicing defect of *SMN2*. A mouse with the Tra2beta mutation in *Smn* (*Smn2B*-Neo) has low Smn protein levels that are associated with reduced size at two weeks, a lifespan of one month, and motor neuron loss late in disease progression (Bowerman et al. 2009; Bowerman et al. 2010). *Smn* alleles that genetically simplify and model SMA disease provide for evaluation of Smn protein reduction in SMA disease progression and can be used in evaluating therapeutic regimes for SMA. In choosing the appropriate mouse model to test therapeutics the survival and disease onset will be crucial considerations (graphically represented in Fig. 1).

4. Addressing the tissue specificity and timing of SMN expression in mouse models of SMA

The requirement for SMN expression in survival and motor neuron maintenance was evident in the genetic modelling of SMA in mice. However, the spatial and temporal requirement for SMN expression in tissues affected by SMA was not initially evaluated. To evaluate the requirement of SMN in specific tissues for SMA disease pathology, the deletion (Table 1) and expression of SMN in specific tissues (Table 2) has been tested in mice. An inducible *Smn* allele in which exon 7 is flanked by loxP sites (F7 allele) can replicate the loss of exon 7 (Frugier et al. 2000). This model has been utilized to knockout *Smn* exon 7 in a variety of tissues such as neurons, muscles, and liver by tissue specific Cre expression. The removal of exon 7 by Cre recombinase is irreversible and is associated with cell death in the target tissue being tested (Frugier et al. 2000; Cifuentes-Diaz et al. 2001; Vitte et al. 2004). The loss of full-length SMN through use of the inducible F7 *Smn* allele in neurons lead to neuronal cell death and mice exhibiting SMA pathology associated with motor neuron loss, whereas loss in muscle leads to a muscular dystrophy-like phenotype in the absence of motor neuron loss (Frugier et al. 2000; Cifuentes-Diaz et al. 2001). In an inverse experiment, increased expression of SMN was isolated to either neurons or muscle by tissue specific promoters in the severe Line89 mice. Rescue of the SMA phenotype was observed in neuronal expression of SMN whereas muscle expression did not rescue the SMA disease (Gavrilina et al. 2008). Together, these studies argue that the expression of SMN is a requirement for basic cellular maintenance and that SMN expression in neurons can rescue the SMA phenotype.

The targeted excision of *Smn* exon 7 (F7) can remove Smn protein rather than reduce the levels, as is seen in SMA patients. To recapitulate the reduced levels of SMN protein, the F7 targeted deletion was used in motor neuron progenitor cells in conjunction with low levels of SMN generated by two copies of the *SMN2* transgene. SMN reduction restricted to motor neuron precursors resulted in a mild SMA pathology, survival rate of 70% at one year, reduced weight and muscle mass, and central and peripheral nerve dysfunction. This study reports a direct effect of reduced SMN protein levels in motor neurons leading to SMA pathology in mice. The reduced severity of SMA may be explained by the presence of normal levels of SMN in other cell types, which would also have reduced SMN protein levels in SMA disease (Park et al. 2010).

The evaluation of SMA mouse models has elucidated changes that occur early and late in disease progression. Thus, the timing of SMN replacement in disease may alter the therapeutic benefit of SMN replacement for disease correction. This consideration has been addressed in severe SMA mouse models in both genetic and therapy based experiments. Most drug treatment regimes require early administration to allow for survival extension and improvement of phenotype in severe mouse models of SMA, including prenatal treatment for Line89 mice (Riessland et al. 2010). Gene therapy using scAAV9 SMN expression argues that early postnatal expression of SMN in motor neurons is required for survival extension, with the greatest success at PND1. However, the rescue observed by systemic delivery of the viral vector required transduction of motor neurons in the CNS (Foust et al. 2010; Valori et al. 2010; Dominguez et al. 2011). Accordingly, the inability to rescue survival at later time-points may be a result of limited access to the CNS by the maturation of the blood brain barrier. The use of RNA molecules that mediate splicing correction can extend survival when administered early postnatally as well (Baughan et al. 2009; Coady et al. 2010; Passini et al. 2010). The ability of each of these therapeutic modalities requires access to the CNS and motor neurons for effective therapeutic benefit in SMA mouse models.

The use of genetic models of induced SMN expression can bypass the limitation of other therapeutic strategies to determine the therapeutic window in SMA mouse models. Genetic induction of *Smn* from embryonic lethal *Smn* hypomorphic alleles can prevent early embryonic lethality when induced early in utero (E7.5) (Hammond et al. 2010). Recently, genetic induction of SMN expression using a high expressing doxycycline inducible SMN transgene showed similar survival extension in the severe SMNΔ7 mice, comparable to that of scAAV9 SMN treatment (Foust et al. 2010; Le et al. 2011). In the doxycycline inducible SMN model, induction in embryos (E13.5) had the greatest survival extension to over 200 days, whereas neonatally treated (PND0-3) SMNΔ7 mice survived 86 days. Interestingly, the removal of doxycycline (i.e.: SMN over-expression ceased) at weaning (28 days) did not lend to rapid decline or death, arguing that lower levels of SMN expression may be sufficient later in life (Le et al. 2011). Together, these data argue for the requirement of early postnatal expression of SMN for therapeutic benefit in severe SMA mouse models, and SMN expression in motor neurons is required for considerable increase in mean lifespan. A still unresolved question is whether the same timing of SMN replacement will be required for treatment in milder SMA mouse models, or if a later therapeutic window exists. Some evidence offers that late treatment in mild SMA may be beneficial as the use of ASOs that correct *SMN2* splicing in the Hsieh-Li (4 copy *SMN2*) mouse can reduce tail necrosis seen in these mice (Hua et al. 2010).

Genotype	Phenotype and Notes	Shorthand	References
Smn-/-; SMN2(89Ahmb)+/+; PrP92-SMN+/+	SMN expression in neurons under the prion promoter (PrP) recues disease in Line89 mice.	Neuronal SMN	Gavrillina 2008
Smn-/-; SMN2(89Ahmb)+/+; HAS63-SMN+/+	SMN expression in muscle under the human skeletal actin (HAS) promoter does not rescue SMA disease in Line89 mice. Leaky expression in neurons can afford moderate rescue in Line89 mice.	Muscle SMN	Gavrillina 2008
Smn-/-; SMN2(89Ahmb)+/+; SMNΔ7+/+; ROSA26rtTA+/+; Luci-TRE-SMN+/+	Induction of SMN expression by doxycycline within 3 days. Embryonic (E13) and PND0 treatment extend survival, mean 100 days but can extend to 200 days, and corrects NMJ defects. Removal of doxycycline at 28 days exhibits continued survival and rescue of NMJ defects.	Doxycycline Inducible SMN	Le 2011
SmnC-T-Neo/C-T-Neo;CreEsr1 and Smn2B-Neo/2B-Neo;CreEsr1	Tamoxifen induced Cre-mediated excision of the neomycin cassette alters the hypomorphic *C-T-Neo* and *2B-Neo* alleles from ~5% SMN to ~30% and 16%, respectively. Early (E7.5) tamoxifen treatment can rescue to embryonic lethality and resorption of the *C-T-Neo* mouse early in embryonic development, though the ability to rescue animals to birth has not been shown.	Inducible *Smn* hypomorphic alleles	Hammond 2011
Smn +/+; Tg SMN2; CreERT2	Inducible SMN expression is under control of tamoxifen inducible Cre (CreERT2). Tamoxifen administration in embryonic (E13.5), neonatal (PND1.5), and weanling (4 week old) mice induces SMN expression. Ability to rescue survival has not yet assessed in SMA mouse models.	Tamoxifen Inducible SMN	Bebee 2011

Table 2. Inducible SMN mouse models

5. SMN snRNP function and splicing in SMA mouse models

The best-characterized function of SMN is the maturation of the core snRNPs required for splicing (Fig. 2). To test the effect of reduced SMN levels on snRNP assembly in SMA, the maturation of both major (U2) and minor (U12) snRNPs were assessed in severe Line 89 mice. In these severe mice, the reduction of SMN protein correlated with reduced maturation of a subset of snRNPs, especially the minor spliceosomal pathway U11 and U12 snRNPs (Gabanella et al. 2007). In the SMNΔ7 mice, reduced U4 snRNP maturation was also reduced in the brain and kidney. The relative levels of snRNAs in the SMNΔ7 mice were altered in disease progression, with the minor spliceosome again showing the greatest reduction at PND11 in the SMA mouse models (Zhang et al. 2008). To genetically evaluate perturbations of snRNP assembly in SMA disease, a transgene of the mild SMA mutation in *SMN1* (A111G) was expressed in Line89 mice. Expression of the A111G transgene extended survival to a normal lifespan with no observable phenotype, though the A111G mice showed signs of muscle hypertrophy in the gastrocnemius at 10 months of age. The survival extension was *SMN2* dependent as A111G failed to rescue the *Smn* -/- mice alone, arguing

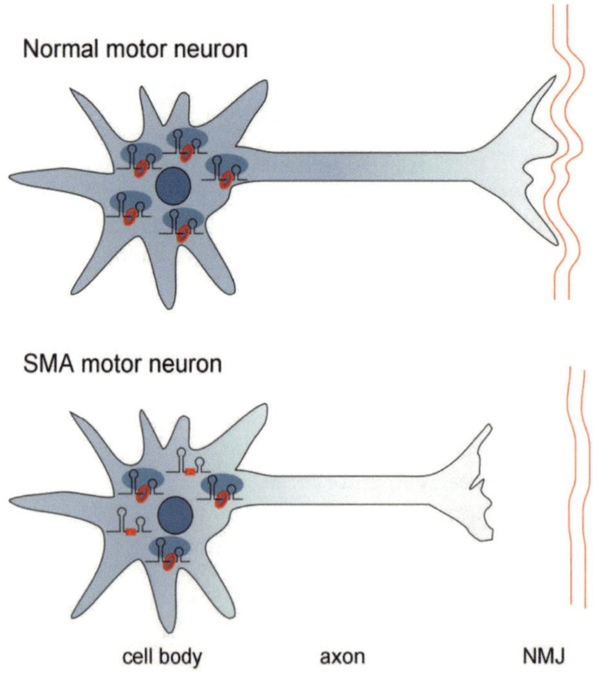

Fig. 2. SMN function in motor neurons. Normal and SMA motor neurons are depicted with blue shading corresponding to SMN protein levels. The SMN complex (blue oval) loads the Sm core (red circle) onto the Sm site (red box) of U snRNAs. In normal motor neurons sufficient SMN is present to form the mature U snRNPs, whereas SMA motor neurons lack sufficient SMN to mature all U snRNAs. Reduced SMN leads to motor neuron loss and dysfunction, which can be seen by immaturity of the NMJ and eventual loss of motor neurons by retraction of the axonal processes and cell death. While U snRNP maturation is the primary function of SMN, other functions of SMN in the axon or at the NMJ may still contribute to SMA pathology

for intragenic complementation between the SMN from *SMN2* and the mutant A111G SMN protein. Analysis of snRNP assembly in the severe Line89 mice also showed reduced U4 and minor spliceosomal snRNP maturation that was subsequently rescued by the expression of the A111G transgene (Workman et al. 2009).

The impact of SMN reduction in mice leads to reduced maturation and relative levels of snRNAs during SMA disease progression. The impact of the alteration in the maturation of the core splicing machinery on splicing in SMA disease was addressed in the severe mouse models of SMA at early and late stage disease. Evaluation of SMNΔ7 mice prior to disease (PND1) and early in disease (PND7) did not show differences in splicing, but later in disease progression (PND11 and 13), global splicing changes were observed using a splicing sensitive microarray (Zhang et al. 2008; Baumer et al. 2009). Major changes in splicing of neuronal and cellular damage genes were observed (Baumer et al. 2009). In the more severe Line89 mice, gene expression analysis in PND1 mice did not show major expression changes in the presymptomatic mice. However, genes involved in extracellular matrix, myelination, and cellular growth factors showed major changes in late disease progression at PND5 (Murray et al. 2010). These observations set SMA as a global splicing disease late in disease progression, which may account either for the effect of cellular stress on global splicing or a global alteration in snRNPs that contribute to disease in mouse models of SMA. While the importance of SMN protein in other non-snRNP associated neuronal functions in still under evaluation, it is clear that the reduction of SMN directly correlates with reduced maturation of snRNPs. As *SMN2* is itself improperly spliced, the potential for reduced exon 7 inclusion when SMN is low was evaluated using in vitro splicing assays. Extracts prepared from cells expressing low levels of SMN reduced inclusion of *SMN* exon 7, implicating a negative feedback loop effect of low SMN protein levels on exon 7 inclusion. This could be associated with the weak definition of exon 7, making the *SMN* transcript more susceptible to low levels of mature snRNPs required for canonical splicing (Jodelka et al. 2010).

6. Neurological manifestations in SMA mouse models

SMA is a disease of motor neurons, and as such mouse models of SMA have been evaluated for both the loss of motor neurons in the development of SMA disease, as well as other neurological manifestations in the SMA mouse models. Neuronal evaluation of the SMA mouse models has uncovered the timing of motor neuron loss and populations of neurons affected in the SMA mice. The neurological manifestations and major findings in the SMA mouse models have been outlined below.

The loss of motor neurons in SMA as observed in SMA patients was the first neuronal cell types evaluated in models of SMA mice. Histological analyses of motor neuron populations in the spinal cord of SMA mouse models have demonstrated that the loss of motor neurons is also seen during the progression of the disease in mice. Surprisingly, the loss of motor neurons in the spinal cord is a late marker of disease, occurring after a motor deficit is already observed and late in disease progression (Hsieh-Li et al. 2000; Jablonka et al. 2000; Monani et al. 2000; Monani et al. 2003; Le et al. 2005; Avila et al. 2007; Kariya et al. 2008; Bowerman et al. 2009; Michaud et al. 2010; Park et al. 2010; Riessland et al. 2010). The development of motor neurons was thus further analysed in the most severe mice (Line 89) during embryonic and neonatal development. In the Line89 mice the neuronal pathfinding and development of motor neurons appears normal in this SMA mouse model, although some abnormal axonal swelling were more pronounced in the SMA mouse model compared to control littermates (McGovern et al. 2008). The presence of motor function deficits in the SMA mouse models prior to motor neuron loss raised the question of whether motor neuron function was compromised. To evaluate the function of the motor neurons, both anatomical and electrophysiological analyses have been performed in severe and mild SMA mouse models. In severe and mild models of SMA, accumulation of neurofilament in the presynaptic termini of motor neurons, disorganization of the postsynaptic NMJ, reduced synaptic vesicle release, and motor neuron sprouting have been reported (Cifuentes-Diaz et al. 2001; Monani et al. 2003; Kariya et al. 2008; McGovern et al. 2008; Murray et al. 2008; Kong et al. 2009; Ling et al. 2010; Michaud et al. 2010; Park et al. 2010; Lee et al. 2011). The changes at the NMJ are also associated with expression of immature isoforms of both the acetylcholine receptor (AChR) and myosin heavy chain (MyHC) (Kariya et al. 2008; Lee et al. 2011). The loss of motor neurons and changes in expression of genes involved in myelination, growth factor signalling, and extracellular matrix are associated with late stage of disease in SMA mouse models (Murray et al. 2010). The susceptibility of motor neurons holds true from mouse to human, in addition the susceptibility can also differ in subpopulations of motor neurons in a single muscle such as the levator auris longus (LAL) muscle (Murray et al. 2008; Murray et al. 2010; Ruiz et al. 2010).

The defects observed in motor neuron function followed by loss of motor neurons late in disease raised the question of whether other neuronal populations were affected in the SMA mouse models. Defects in sensory neurons have been reported in SMA patients (Rudnik-Schoneborn et al. 2003), and the 3 copy *SMN2* mouse also exhibited latency in response to heat (Michaud et al. 2010). The potential for sensory neuron malfunction in SMA was further evaluated in the SMNΔ7 mouse model. A reduction in the input of sensory neurons to the motor neurons of the spinal cord as well as perturbation of the neuronal circuitry was evident as early as PND4 in the SMNΔ7 mice (Ling et al. 2010; Mentis et al. 2011). Furthermore, the reduction of sensory input into lumbar motor neurons was also observed in the Olig2-Cre mouse even when the sensory neurons did not have reduced SMN protein (Park et al. 2010). The reduction of SMN protein also has consequences for neuronal growth and development as evidenced by reduced neuronal numbers in the brain and eye of severe SMA mouse models Line89 and *Smn* 2B (Liu et al. 2010; Wishart et al. 2010). The modelling of SMA in mice have recapitulated the motor neuron loss as is seen in SMA patients, as well as identified neuronal populations affected by reduced SMN levels in the SMA mouse models.

7. Cardiac and pulmonary involvement

Reports of cardiac defects including congenital heart defects, bradycardia, left ventricular cardiomyopathy, and sympathetic-vagal imbalance have recently been reported in severe SMA mouse models (Bevan et al. 2010; Heier et al. 2010; Shababi et al. 2010). Evaluation of 63 severe SMA type I patients reported that 24% presented with severe bradycardia (Bach 2007). In the severe SMNΔ7 mouse model bradycardia was also present due to reduced autonomic innervation, and in turn increased vagal tone. Anatomical analysis of SMNΔ7 mice hearts was positive for dilated cardiomyopathy and reduced contractile function (Bevan et al. 2010; Heier et al. 2010). Therapies aimed at increasing SMN protein by treatment with scAAV9 SMN or TSA were able to improve heart function and survival in the treated SMNΔ7 mice (Bevan et al. 2010; Heier et al. 2010). A third group reported congenital defects present in the severe Line89 mice in the left ventricular septum and wall, but these abnormalities were not observed in the SMNΔ7 mice. However, fibrotic deposition and oxidative stress markers accumulated in the SMNΔ7 heart as disease progressed (Shababi et al. 2010). The collective effect of changes in the heart of SMA models decreases the functional output and implicates additional neuronal targets by way of autonomic neuronal dysfunction in SMA mouse models. As cardiac involvement has not been reported in most severe SMA patients, further analysis of patients to identify cardiac defects will be required to determine if cardiac treatment is a consideration for SMA patients.

Respiratory complications are common during SMA disease progression and are often associated with mortality in severe SMA. Long-term respiratory treatment is often requirement in both severe and mild SMA patients. The 3 copy *SMN2* mice appear normal at PND1 but have reduced numbers of innervated NMJ in the diaphragm at PND9, associated with reduced respiratory capacity starting at PND7 (Michaud et al. 2010). Similar structural defects at the NMJ in the diaphragm of SMA type I patients have also been reported (Kariya et al. 2008). Analysis of the most severe SMA mouse model (Line89) from E10.5 to PND2 for motor neuron developmental defects showed the diaphragm was not affected; however, intercostal muscle denervation was observed (Kariya et al. 2008; McGovern et al. 2008). The defects in motor neurons of the diaphragm and intercostal muscles may account for respiratory deficiency in mouse models of SMA, and may be a point of therapeutic intervention in SMA patients.

8. Therapeutic approaches in SMA treatment

The severity of SMA is directly associated with low SMN protein levels, thus the reintroduction of SMN would predict correction of the disease. The presence of *SMN2* in all SMA patients provides for a direct therapeutic target to increase SMN levels. Therapeutic approaches for increasing transcriptional activity of *SMN2*, splicing correction of *SMN2* exon 7, or stability of SMN protein are major considerations in development of SMA therapies. Additionally, increasing SMN levels by gene therapy or treating the disease pathology in an SMN independent manner are alternative approaches in SMA therapeutic development. Mouse models of SMA have enabled the evaluation of these therapeutic approaches in pre-clinical therapeutic regimes for treatment of SMA.

Small molecules or drugs were the first therapies evaluated for treatment of SMA in mouse models of SMA. Many of the initial drugs are FDA approved drugs and transcriptional activators, histone deacetylase (HDAC) inhibitors. These drugs increased SMN levels by transcriptional activity, splicing of *SMN2* exon 7, and/or SMN protein stability (Chang et al. 2001; Avila et al. 2007; Mattis et al. 2008; Narver et al. 2008; Tsai et al. 2008; Riessland et al. 2010; Mentis et al. 2011). Additional drugs have been used that target increased stability of SMN, read through of *SMN2* transcripts, incorporation of *SMN2* exon 7, as well as second-generation drugs that work via multiple mechanisms (Garbes et al. 2009; Hastings et al. 2009; Butchbach et al. 2010). These drugs improved SMN protein levels and SMA phenotype, and often the extension of survival observed in treatment of severe SMA mouse models was 30%. However, in current clinical trials in SMA patients, these therapies have proven ineffectual (Chen et al. 2010).

Drug correction of *SMN2* splicing underscores the importance of targeting the correction of *SMN2* splicing as a mode for increased SMN expression. The use of RNA based therapies aimed at increasing exon 7 inclusion can be achieved by sequestering a negatively acting sequence in the pre-mRNA and preventing it negative function (Singh et al. 2006; Hua et al. 2007; Williams et al. 2009; Hua et al. 2010; Passini et al. 2010), recruiting positively acting splicing factors to exon 7 (Baughan et al. 2009; Meyer et al. 2009; Voigt et al. 2010), blocking exon 8 inclusion (Dickson et al. 2008), or providing an RNA substrate used in the splicing reaction (trans-splicing) (Coady et al. 2010). These techniques have successfully increased exon 7 inclusion and SMN levels, and have improved survival and phenotype in SMA mouse models.

To reintroduce SMN, viral gene therapies that encode SMN can correct disease if SMN is expressed in the appropriate tissues and cell types. Self-complimentary adeno-associated virus serotype 9 (scAAV9) can transduce motor neurons in mice when administered early postnatally, and the expression of SMN in motor neurons can reduce disease pathology, as well as extend survival in the SMNΔ7 mouse model (Foust et al. 2010; Valori et al. 2010; Dominguez et al. 2011). The requirement for early expression of SMN using scAAV9 argues that SMN is required early postnatally for disease correction. However, the ability of the viral treatment to reach the spinal cord and motor neurons was reduced after PND5. The early therapeutic window outlined by scAAV9 treatment likely represents a limitation of viral gene therapy, and does not necessarily reflect the therapeutic window for SMN replacement.

Most SMA patients present with disease after motor neuron loss and motor function has already occurred. Treatment of the disease pathology may afford therapeutic intervention even in the absence of altering SMN levels. Cell based therapies to replace the lost motor neurons have initially been tested by transplanting normal cells that were programmed to mature into motor neurons. These cells were injected in the spinal cord, engrafted in the spinal cord, and can improve function and survival in the SMNΔ7 mice (Corti et al. 2008). Furthermore, increasing muscle mass by inhibiting myostatin with the antagonist follistatin can reduce muscle loss and improve function and survival, though transgenic overexpression of follistatin in SMNΔ7 mice failed to improve the survival of the mice (Rose et al. 2009; Sumner et al. 2009). As therapeutic development for SMA continues, the use of SMA mouse models will continue to be instrumental in pre-clinical testing of therapies for SMA.

9. Summary and conclusion

The modeling of SMA in mice has successfully recapitulated many components of SMA pathology associated with reduced levels of SMN protein. The use of these SMA mouse models has proven invaluable in further understanding the etiology of SMA disease, uncovering the neurological manifestations of SMA disease, and the importance of when and where SMN expression is required for correction of SMA pathology in mice. The use of mouse models of SMA to determine the pathological manifestations in SMA and testing therapeutic approaches continues as the need for therapies for this devastating disease remains.

10. Acknowledgements

This work was funded by the Association Francaise Contre les Myopathies (AFM) (14278 to D.S.C.) and by student fellowships from the Research Institute at Nationwide Children's Hospital and the Jeffrey J. Seilhamer Cancer Foundation (T.W.B.). We would like to thank Casey Gentis for editorial support in submission of this work.

11. References

Avila, A. M., B. G. Burnett, A. A. Taye, F. Gabanella, M. A. Knight, P. Hartenstein, Z. Cizman, N. A. Di Prospero, L. Pellizzoni, K. H. Fischbeck and C. J. Sumner (2007). "Trichostatin A increases SMN expression and survival in a mouse model of spinal muscular atrophy." *The Journal of clinical investigation* 117(3): 659-671.

Bach, J. R. (2007). "Medical considerations of long-term survival of Werdnig-Hoffmann disease." *American journal of physical medicine & rehabilitation / Association of Academic Physiatrists* 86(5): 349-355.

Bach, J. R., J. Vega, J. Majors and A. Friedman (2003). "Spinal muscular atrophy type 1 quality of life." *American journal of physical medicine & rehabilitation / Association of Academic Physiatrists* 82(2): 137-142.

Baughan, T. D., A. Dickson, E. Y. Osman and C. L. Lorson (2009). "Delivery of bifunctional RNAs that target an intronic repressor and increase SMN levels in an animal model of spinal muscular atrophy." *Human molecular genetics* 18(9): 1600-1611.

Baumer, D., S. Lee, G. Nicholson, J. L. Davies, N. J. Parkinson, L. M. Murray, T. H. Gillingwater, O. Ansorge, K. E. Davies and K. Talbot (2009). "Alternative splicing events are a late feature of pathology in a mouse model of spinal muscular atrophy." *PLoS genetics* 5(12): e1000773.

Bebee, T. W., J. T. Gladman and D. S. Chandler (2010). "Splicing regulation of the survival motor neuron genes and implications for treatment of spinal muscular atrophy." *Front Biosci* 15: 1191-1204.

Bergin, A., G. Kim, D. L. Price, S. S. Sisodia, M. K. Lee and B. A. Rabin (1997). "Identification and characterization of a mouse homologue of the spinal muscular atrophy-determining gene, survival motor neuron." *Gene* 204(1-2): 47-53.

Bevan, A. K., K. R. Hutchinson, K. D. Foust, L. Braun, V. L. McGovern, L. Schmelzer, J. G. Ward, J. C. Petruska, P. A. Lucchesi, A. H. Burghes and B. K. Kaspar (2010). "Early heart failure in the SMNDelta7 model of spinal muscular atrophy and correction by postnatal scAAV9-SMN delivery." *Human molecular genetics* 19(20): 3895-3905.

Bowerman, M., C. L. Anderson, A. Beauvais, P. P. Boyl, W. Witke and R. Kothary (2009). "SMN, profilin IIa and plastin 3: a link between the deregulation of actin dynamics and SMA pathogenesis." *Molecular and cellular neurosciences* 42(1): 66-74.

Bowerman, M., A. Beauvais, C. L. Anderson and R. Kothary (2010). "Rho-kinase inactivation prolongs survival of an intermediate SMA mouse model." *Human molecular genetics* 19(8): 1468-1478.

Burnett, B. G., T. O. Crawford and C. J. Sumner (2009). "Emerging treatment options for spinal muscular atrophy." *Current treatment options in neurology* 11(2): 90-101.

Butchbach, M. E., J. Singh, M. Thorsteinsdottir, L. Saieva, E. Slominski, J. Thurmond, T. Andresson, J. Zhang, J. D. Edwards, L. R. Simard, L. Pellizzoni, J. Jarecki, A. H. Burghes and M. E. Gurney (2010). "Effects of 2,4-diaminoquinazoline derivatives on SMN expression and phenotype in a mouse model for spinal muscular atrophy." *Hum Mol Genet* 19(3): 454-467.

Cartegni, L., M. L. Hastings, J. A. Calarco, E. de Stanchina and A. R. Krainer (2006). "Determinants of exon 7 splicing in the spinal muscular atrophy genes, SMN1 and SMN2." *Am J Hum Genet* 78(1): 63-77.

Cartegni, L. and A. R. Krainer (2002). "Disruption of an SF2/ASF-dependent exonic splicing enhancer in SMN2 causes spinal muscular atrophy in the absence of SMN1." *Nat Genet* 30(4): 377-384.

Chang, J. G., H. M. Hsieh-Li, Y. J. Jong, N. M. Wang, C. H. Tsai and H. Li (2001). "Treatment of spinal muscular atrophy by sodium butyrate." *Proceedings of the National Academy of Sciences of the United States of America* 98(17): 9808-9813.

Chen, T. H., J. G. Chang, Y. H. Yang, H. H. Mai, W. C. Liang, Y. C. Wu, H. Y. Wang, Y. B. Huang, S. M. Wu, Y. C. Chen, S. N. Yang and Y. J. Jong (2010). "Randomized, double-blind, placebo-controlled trial of hydroxyurea in spinal muscular atrophy." *Neurology* 75(24): 2190-2197.

Cho, S. and G. Dreyfuss (2010). "A degron created by SMN2 exon 7 skipping is a principal contributor to spinal muscular atrophy severity." *Genes & development* 24(5): 438-442.

Cifuentes-Diaz, C., T. Frugier, F. D. Tiziano, E. Lacene, N. Roblot, V. Joshi, M. H. Moreau and J. Melki (2001). "Deletion of murine SMN exon 7 directed to skeletal muscle leads to severe muscular dystrophy." *The Journal of cell biology* 152(5): 1107-1114.

Cifuentes-Diaz, C., T. Frugier, F. D. Tiziano, E. Lacene, N. Roblot, V. Joshi, M. H. Moreau and J. Melki (2001). "Deletion of murine SMN exon 7 directed to skeletal muscle leads to severe muscular dystrophy." *J Cell Biol* 152(5): 1107-1114.

Coady, T. H. and C. L. Lorson (2010). "Trans-splicing-mediated improvement in a severe mouse model of spinal muscular atrophy." *J Neurosci* 30(1): 126-130.

Corti, S., M. Nizzardo, M. Nardini, C. Donadoni, S. Salani, D. Ronchi, F. Saladino, A. Bordoni, F. Fortunato, R. Del Bo, D. Papadimitriou, F. Locatelli, G. Menozzi, S. Strazzer, N. Bresolin and G. P. Comi (2008). "Neural stem cell transplantation can ameliorate the phenotype of a mouse model of spinal muscular atrophy." *The Journal of clinical investigation* 118(10): 3316-3330.

Dickson, A., E. Osman and C. L. Lorson (2008). "A negatively acting bifunctional RNA increases survival motor neuron both in vitro and in vivo." *Human gene therapy* 19(11): 1307-1315.

DiDonato, C. J., C. L. Lorson, Y. De Repentigny, L. Simard, C. Chartrand, E. J. Androphy and R. Kothary (2001). "Regulation of murine survival motor neuron (Smn) protein levels by modifying Smn exon 7 splicing." *Human molecular genetics* 10(23): 2727-2736.

Dominguez, E., T. Marais, N. Chatauret, S. Benkhelifa-Ziyyat, S. Duque, P. Ravassard, R. Carcenac, S. Astord, A. Pereira de Moura, T. Voit and M. Barkats (2011). "Intravenous scAAV9 delivery of a codon-optimized SMN1 sequence rescues SMA mice." *Human molecular genetics* 20(4): 681-693.

Fischer, U., Q. Liu and G. Dreyfuss (1997). "The SMN-SIP1 complex has an essential role in spliceosomal snRNP biogenesis." *Cell* 90(6): 1023-1029.

Foust, K. D., X. Wang, V. L. McGovern, L. Braun, A. K. Bevan, A. M. Haidet, T. T. Le, P. R. Morales, M. M. Rich, A. H. Burghes and B. K. Kaspar (2010). "Rescue of the spinal muscular atrophy phenotype in a mouse model by early postnatal delivery of SMN." *Nat Biotechnol* 28(3): 271-274.

Frugier, T., F. D. Tiziano, C. Cifuentes-Diaz, P. Miniou, N. Roblot, A. Dierich, M. Le Meur and J. Melki (2000). "Nuclear targeting defect of SMN lacking the C-terminus in a mouse model of spinal muscular atrophy." *Human molecular genetics* 9(5): 849-858.

Gabanella, F., M. E. Butchbach, L. Saieva, C. Carissimi, A. H. Burghes and L. Pellizzoni (2007). "Ribonucleoprotein Assembly Defects Correlate with Spinal Muscular Atrophy Severity and Preferentially Affect a Subset of Spliceosomal snRNPs." *PLoS ONE* 2(9): e921.

Garbes, L., M. Riessland, I. Holker, R. Heller, J. Hauke, C. Trankle, R. Coras, I. Blumcke, E. Hahnen and B. Wirth (2009). "LBH589 induces up to 10-fold SMN protein levels by several independent mechanisms and is effective even in cells from SMA patients non-responsive to valproate." *Human molecular genetics* 18(19): 3645-3658.

Gavrilina, T. O., V. L. McGovern, E. Workman, T. O. Crawford, R. G. Gogliotti, C. J. DiDonato, U. R. Monani, G. E. Morris and A. H. Burghes (2008). "Neuronal SMN expression corrects spinal muscular atrophy in severe SMA mice while muscle-specific SMN expression has no phenotypic effect." *Hum Mol Genet* 17(8): 1063-1075.

Gladman, J. T., T. W. Bebee, C. Edwards, X. Wang, Z. Sahenk, M. M. Rich and D. S. Chandler (2010). "A humanized Smn gene containing the SMN2 nucleotide alteration in exon 7 mimics SMN2 splicing and the SMA disease phenotype." *Human molecular genetics* 19(21): 4239-4252.

Hammond, S. M., R. G. Gogliotti, V. Rao, A. Beauvais, R. Kothary and C. J. DiDonato (2010). "Mouse survival motor neuron alleles that mimic SMN2 splicing and are inducible rescue embryonic lethality early in development but not late." *PLoS ONE* 5(12): e15887.

Hastings, M. L., J. Berniac, Y. H. Liu, P. Abato, F. M. Jodelka, L. Barthel, S. Kumar, C. Dudley, M. Nelson, K. Larson, J. Edmonds, T. Bowser, M. Draper, P. Higgins and A. R. Krainer (2009). "Tetracyclines that promote SMN2 exon 7 splicing as therapeutics for spinal muscular atrophy." *Sci Transl Med* 1(5): 5ra12.

Heier, C. R., R. Satta, C. Lutz and C. J. DiDonato (2010). "Arrhythmia and cardiac defects are a feature of spinal muscular atrophy model mice." *Human molecular genetics* 19(20): 3906-3918.

Hsieh-Li, H. M., J. G. Chang, Y. J. Jong, M. H. Wu, N. M. Wang, C. H. Tsai and H. Li (2000). "A mouse model for spinal muscular atrophy." *Nat Genet* 24(1): 66-70.

Hua, Y., K. Sahashi, G. Hung, F. Rigo, M. A. Passini, C. F. Bennett and A. R. Krainer (2010). "Antisense correction of SMN2 splicing in the CNS rescues necrosis in a type III SMA mouse model." *Genes Dev* 24(15): 1634-1644.

Hua, Y., K. Sahashi, G. Hung, F. Rigo, M. A. Passini, C. F. Bennett and A. R. Krainer (2010). "Antisense correction of SMN2 splicing in the CNS rescues necrosis in a type III SMA mouse model." *Genes & development* 24(15): 1634-1644.

Hua, Y., T. A. Vickers, B. F. Baker, C. F. Bennett and A. R. Krainer (2007). "Enhancement of SMN2 exon 7 inclusion by antisense oligonucleotides targeting the exon." *PLoS biology* 5(4): e73.

Jablonka, S., B. Schrank, M. Kralewski, W. Rossoll and M. Sendtner (2000). "Reduced survival motor neuron (Smn) gene dose in mice leads to motor neuron degeneration: an animal model for spinal muscular atrophy type III." *Hum Mol Genet* 9(3): 341-346.

Jodelka, F. M., A. D. Ebert, D. M. Duelli and M. L. Hastings (2010). "A feedback loop regulates splicing of the spinal muscular atrophy-modifying gene, SMN2." *Human molecular genetics* 19(24): 4906-4917.

Kariya, S., G. H. Park, Y. Maeno-Hikichi, O. Leykekhman, C. Lutz, M. S. Arkovitz, L. T. Landmesser and U. R. Monani (2008). "Reduced SMN protein impairs maturation of the neuromuscular junctions in mouse models of spinal muscular atrophy." *Human molecular genetics* 17(16): 2552-2569.

Kashima, T. and J. L. Manley (2003). "A negative element in SMN2 exon 7 inhibits splicing in spinal muscular atrophy." *Nat Genet* 34(4): 460-463.

Kashima, T., N. Rao, C. J. David and J. L. Manley (2007). "hnRNP A1 functions with specificity in repression of SMN2 exon 7 splicing." *Human molecular genetics* 16(24): 3149-3159.

Kong, L., X. Wang, D. W. Choe, M. Polley, B. G. Burnett, M. Bosch-Marce, J. W. Griffin, M. M. Rich and C. J. Sumner (2009). "Impaired synaptic vesicle release and immaturity of neuromuscular junctions in spinal muscular atrophy mice." *The Journal of neuroscience : the official journal of the Society for Neuroscience* 29(3): 842-851.

Le, T. T., V. L. McGovern, I. E. Alwine, X. Wang, A. Massoni-Laporte, M. M. Rich and A. H. Burghes (2011). "Temporal requirement for high SMN expression in SMA mice." *Human molecular genetics.*

Le, T. T., L. T. Pham, M. E. Butchbach, H. L. Zhang, U. R. Monani, D. D. Coovert, T. O. Gavrilina, L. Xing, G. J. Bassell and A. H. Burghes (2005). "SMNDelta7, the major product of the centromeric survival motor neuron (SMN2) gene, extends survival in mice with spinal muscular atrophy and associates with full-length SMN." *Hum Mol Genet* 14(6): 845-857.

Lee, Y. I., M. Mikesh, I. Smith, M. Rimer and W. Thompson (2011). "Muscles in a mouse model of spinal muscular atrophy show profound defects in neuromuscular development even in the absence of failure in neuromuscular transmission or loss of motor neurons." *Developmental biology* 356(2): 432-444.

Lefebvre, S., L. Burglen, S. Reboullet, O. Clermont, P. Burlet, L. Viollet, B. Benichou, C. Cruaud, P. Millasseau, M. Zeviani and et al. (1995). "Identification and characterization of a spinal muscular atrophy-determining gene." *Cell* 80(1): 155-165.

Lefebvre, S., P. Burlet, Q. Liu, S. Bertrandy, O. Clermont, A. Munnich, G. Dreyfuss and J. Melki (1997). "Correlation between severity and SMN protein level in spinal muscular atrophy." *Nat Genet* 16(3): 265-269.

Ling, K. K., M. Y. Lin, B. Zingg, Z. Feng and C. P. Ko (2010). "Synaptic defects in the spinal and neuromuscular circuitry in a mouse model of spinal muscular atrophy." *PLoS ONE* 5(11): e15457.

Liu, H., D. Shafey, J. N. Moores and R. Kothary (2010). "Neurodevelopmental consequences of Smn depletion in a mouse model of spinal muscular atrophy." *J Neurosci Res* 88(1): 111-122.

Liu, Q., U. Fischer, F. Wang and G. Dreyfuss (1997). "The spinal muscular atrophy disease gene product, SMN, and its associated protein SIP1 are in a complex with spliceosomal snRNP proteins." *Cell* 90(6): 1013-1021.

Lorson, C. L. and E. J. Androphy (2000). "An exonic enhancer is required for inclusion of an essential exon in the SMA-determining gene SMN." *Human molecular genetics* 9(2): 259-265.

Lorson, C. L., E. Hahnen, E. J. Androphy and B. Wirth (1999). "A single nucleotide in the SMN gene regulates splicing and is responsible for spinal muscular atrophy." *Proceedings of the National Academy of Sciences of the United States of America* 96(11): 6307-6311.

Mattis, V. B., M. E. Butchbach and C. L. Lorson (2008). "Detection of human survival motor neuron (SMN) protein in mice containing the SMN2 transgene: applicability to preclinical therapy development for spinal muscular atrophy." *J Neurosci Methods* 175(1): 36-43.

McAndrew, P. E., D. W. Parsons, L. R. Simard, C. Rochette, P. N. Ray, J. R. Mendell, T. W. Prior and A. H. Burghes (1997). "Identification of proximal spinal muscular atrophy carriers and patients by analysis of SMNT and SMNC gene copy number." *Am J Hum Genet* 60(6): 1411-1422.

McGovern, V. L., T. O. Gavrilina, C. E. Beattie and A. H. Burghes (2008). "Embryonic motor axon development in the severe SMA mouse." *Hum Mol Genet* 17(18): 2900-2909.

Meister, G., D. Buhler, R. Pillai, F. Lottspeich and U. Fischer (2001). "A multiprotein complex mediates the ATP-dependent assembly of spliceosomal U snRNPs." *Nature cell biology* 3(11): 945-949.

Mentis, G. Z., D. Blivis, W. Liu, E. Drobac, M. E. Crowder, L. Kong, F. J. Alvarez, C. J. Sumner and M. J. O'Donovan (2011). "Early functional impairment of sensory-motor connectivity in a mouse model of spinal muscular atrophy." *Neuron* 69(3): 453-467.

Meyer, K., J. Marquis, J. Trub, R. Nlend Nlend, S. Verp, M. D. Ruepp, H. Imboden, I. Barde, D. Trono and D. Schumperli (2009). "Rescue of a severe mouse model for spinal muscular atrophy by U7 snRNA-mediated splicing modulation." *Human molecular genetics* 18(3): 546-555.

Michaud, M., T. Arnoux, S. Bielli, E. Durand, Y. Rotrou, S. Jablonka, F. Robert, M. Giraudon-Paoli, M. Riessland, M. G. Mattei, E. Andriambeloson, B. Wirth, M. Sendtner, J. Gallego, R. M. Pruss and T. Bordet (2010). "Neuromuscular defects and breathing disorders in a new mouse model of spinal muscular atrophy." *Neurobiology of disease* 38(1): 125-135.

Monani, U. R., M. T. Pastore, T. O. Gavrilina, S. Jablonka, T. T. Le, C. Andreassi, J. M. DiCocco, C. Lorson, E. J. Androphy, M. Sendtner, M. Podell and A. H. Burghes (2003). "A transgene carrying an A2G missense mutation in the SMN gene modulates phenotypic severity in mice with severe (type I) spinal muscular atrophy." *J Cell Biol* 160(1): 41-52.

Monani, U. R., M. Sendtner, D. D. Coovert, D. W. Parsons, C. Andreassi, T. T. Le, S. Jablonka, B. Schrank, W. Rossoll, T. W. Prior, G. E. Morris and A. H. Burghes (2000). "The human centromeric survival motor neuron gene (SMN2) rescues embryonic lethality in Smn(-/-) mice and results in a mouse with spinal muscular atrophy." *Hum Mol Genet* 9(3): 333-339.

Murray, L. M., L. H. Comley, D. Thomson, N. Parkinson, K. Talbot and T. H. Gillingwater (2008). "Selective vulnerability of motor neurons and dissociation of pre- and post-synaptic pathology at the neuromuscular junction in mouse models of spinal muscular atrophy." *Human molecular genetics* 17(7): 949-962.

Murray, L. M., S. Lee, D. Baumer, S. H. Parson, K. Talbot and T. H. Gillingwater (2010). "Pre-symptomatic development of lower motor neuron connectivity in a mouse model of severe spinal muscular atrophy." *Human molecular genetics* 19(3): 420-433.

Narver, H. L., L. Kong, B. G. Burnett, D. W. Choe, M. Bosch-Marce, A. A. Taye, M. A. Eckhaus and C. J. Sumner (2008). "Sustained improvement of spinal muscular atrophy mice treated with trichostatin A plus nutrition." *Annals of neurology* 64(4): 465-470.

Park, G. H., Y. Maeno-Hikichi, T. Awano, L. T. Landmesser and U. R. Monani (2010). "Reduced survival of motor neuron (SMN) protein in motor neuronal progenitors functions cell autonomously to cause spinal muscular atrophy in model mice expressing the human centromeric (SMN2) gene." *The Journal of neuroscience : the official journal of the Society for Neuroscience* 30(36): 12005-12019.

Park, G. H., Y. Maeno-Hikichi, T. Awano, L. T. Landmesser and U. R. Monani (2010). "Reduced survival of motor neuron (SMN) protein in motor neuronal progenitors functions cell autonomously to cause spinal muscular atrophy in model mice expressing the human centromeric (SMN2) gene." *J Neurosci* 30(36): 12005-12019.

Passini, M. A., J. Bu, E. M. Roskelley, A. M. Richards, S. P. Sardi, C. R. O'Riordan, K. W. Klinger, L. S. Shihabuddin and S. H. Cheng (2010). "CNS-targeted gene therapy improves survival and motor function in a mouse model of spinal muscular atrophy." *J Clin Invest* 120(4): 1253-1264.

Paushkin, S., A. K. Gubitz, S. Massenet and G. Dreyfuss (2002). "The SMN complex, an assemblyosome of ribonucleoproteins." *Current opinion in cell biology* 14(3): 305-312.

Pellizzoni, L., J. Baccon, J. Rappsilber, M. Mann and G. Dreyfuss (2002). "Purification of native survival of motor neurons complexes and identification of Gemin6 as a novel component." *The Journal of biological chemistry* 277(9): 7540-7545.

Pellizzoni, L., B. Charroux and G. Dreyfuss (1999). "SMN mutants of spinal muscular atrophy patients are defective in binding to snRNP proteins." *Proceedings of the National Academy of Sciences of the United States of America* 96(20): 11167-11172.

Raker, V. A., G. Plessel and R. Luhrmann (1996). "The snRNP core assembly pathway: identification of stable core protein heteromeric complexes and an snRNP subcore particle in vitro." *The EMBO journal* 15(9): 2256-2269.

Riessland, M., B. Ackermann, A. Forster, M. Jakubik, J. Hauke, L. Garbes, I. Fritzsche, Y. Mende, I. Blumcke, E. Hahnen and B. Wirth (2010). "SAHA ameliorates the SMA phenotype in two mouse models for spinal muscular atrophy." *Hum Mol Genet* 19(8): 1492-1506.

Riessland, M., B. Ackermann, A. Forster, M. Jakubik, J. Hauke, L. Garbes, I. Fritzsche, Y. Mende, I. Blumcke, E. Hahnen and B. Wirth (2010). "SAHA ameliorates the SMA phenotype in two mouse models for spinal muscular atrophy." *Human molecular genetics* 19(8): 1492-1506.

Rochette, C. F., N. Gilbert and L. R. Simard (2001). "SMN gene duplication and the emergence of the SMN2 gene occurred in distinct hominids: SMN2 is unique to Homo sapiens." *Human genetics* 108(3): 255-266.

Rose, F. F., Jr., V. B. Mattis, H. Rindt and C. L. Lorson (2009). "Delivery of recombinant follistatin lessens disease severity in a mouse model of spinal muscular atrophy." *Hum Mol Genet* 18(6): 997-1005.

Rudnik-Schoneborn, S., H. H. Goebel, W. Schlote, S. Molaian, H. Omran, U. Ketelsen, R. Korinthenberg, D. Wenzel, H. Lauffer, M. Kreiss-Nachtsheim, B. Wirth and K. Zerres (2003). "Classical infantile spinal muscular atrophy with SMN deficiency causes sensory neuronopathy." *Neurology* 60(6): 983-987.

Rudnik-Schoneborn, S., R. Heller, C. Berg, C. Betzler, T. Grimm, T. Eggermann, K. Eggermann, R. Wirth, B. Wirth and K. Zerres (2008). "Congenital heart disease is a feature of severe infantile spinal muscular atrophy." *Journal of medical genetics* 45(10): 635-638.

Ruiz, R., J. J. Casanas, L. Torres-Benito, R. Cano and L. Tabares (2010). "Altered intracellular Ca2+ homeostasis in nerve terminals of severe spinal muscular atrophy mice." *The Journal of neuroscience : the official journal of the Society for Neuroscience* 30(3): 849-857.

Schrank, B., R. Gotz, J. M. Gunnersen, J. M. Ure, K. V. Toyka, A. G. Smith and M. Sendtner (1997). "Inactivation of the survival motor neuron gene, a candidate gene for human spinal muscular atrophy, leads to massive cell death in early mouse embryos." *Proc Natl Acad Sci U S A* 94(18): 9920-9925.

Shababi, M., J. Habibi, H. T. Yang, S. M. Vale, W. A. Sewell and C. L. Lorson (2010). "Cardiac defects contribute to the pathology of spinal muscular atrophy models." *Human molecular genetics* 19(20): 4059-4071.

Singh, N. K., N. N. Singh, E. J. Androphy and R. N. Singh (2006). "Splicing of a critical exon of human Survival Motor Neuron is regulated by a unique silencer element located in the last intron." *Molecular and cellular biology* 26(4): 1333-1346.

Singh, N. N. and R. N. Singh (2011). "Alternative splicing in spinal muscular atrophy underscores the role of an intron definition model." *RNA biology* 8(4).

Sumner, C. J., C. D. Wee, L. C. Warsing, D. W. Choe, A. S. Ng, C. Lutz and K. R. Wagner (2009). "Inhibition of myostatin does not ameliorate disease features of severe spinal muscular atrophy mice." *Human molecular genetics* 18(17): 3145-3152.

Swoboda, K. J., T. W. Prior, C. B. Scott, T. P. McNaught, M. C. Wride, S. P. Reyna and M. B. Bromberg (2005). "Natural history of denervation in SMA: relation to age, SMN2 copy number, and function." *Annals of neurology* 57(5): 704-712.

Tsai, L. K., M. S. Tsai, C. H. Ting and H. Li (2008). "Multiple therapeutic effects of valproic acid in spinal muscular atrophy model mice." *Journal of molecular medicine* 86(11): 1243-1254.

Valori, C. F., K. Ning, M. Wyles, R. J. Mead, A. J. Grierson, P. J. Shaw and M. Azzouz (2010). "Systemic delivery of scAAV9 expressing SMN prolongs survival in a model of spinal muscular atrophy." *Science translational medicine* 2(35): 35ra42.

Valori, C. F., K. Ning, M. Wyles, R. J. Mead, A. J. Grierson, P. J. Shaw and M. Azzouz (2010). "Systemic delivery of scAAV9 expressing SMN prolongs survival in a model of spinal muscular atrophy." *Sci Transl Med* 2(35): 35ra42.

Vitte, J. M., B. Davoult, N. Roblot, M. Mayer, V. Joshi, S. Courageot, F. Tronche, J. Vadrot, M. H. Moreau, F. Kemeny and J. Melki (2004). "Deletion of murine Smn exon 7 directed to liver leads to severe defect of liver development associated with iron overload." *The American journal of pathology* 165(5): 1731-1741.

Voigt, T., K. Meyer, O. Baum and D. Schumperli (2010). "Ultrastructural changes in diaphragm neuromuscular junctions in a severe mouse model for Spinal Muscular Atrophy and their prevention by bifunctional U7 snRNA correcting SMN2 splicing." *Neuromuscular disorders : NMD* 20(11): 744-752.

Wang, J. and G. Dreyfuss (2001). "Characterization of functional domains of the SMN protein in vivo." *The Journal of biological chemistry* 276(48): 45387-45393.

Williams, J. H., R. C. Schray, C. A. Patterson, S. O. Ayitey, M. K. Tallent and G. J. Lutz (2009). "Oligonucleotide-mediated survival of motor neuron protein expression in CNS improves phenotype in a mouse model of spinal muscular atrophy." *The Journal of neuroscience : the official journal of the Society for Neuroscience* 29(24): 7633-7638.

Wishart, T. M., J. P. Huang, L. M. Murray, D. J. Lamont, C. A. Mutsaers, J. Ross, P. Geldsetzer, O. Ansorge, K. Talbot, S. H. Parson and T. H. Gillingwater (2010). "SMN deficiency disrupts brain development in a mouse model of severe spinal muscular atrophy." *Human molecular genetics* 19(21): 4216-4228.

Workman, E., L. Saieva, T. L. Carrel, T. O. Crawford, D. Liu, C. Lutz, C. E. Beattie, L. Pellizzoni and A. H. Burghes (2009). "A SMN missense mutation complements SMN2 restoring snRNPs and rescuing SMA mice." *Human molecular genetics* 18(12): 2215-2229.

Zerres, K., S. Rudnik-Schoneborn, R. Forkert and B. Wirth (1995). "Genetic basis of adult-onset spinal muscular atrophy." *Lancet* 346(8983): 1162.

Zerres, K., S. Rudnik-Schoneborn, E. Forrest, A. Lusakowska, J. Borkowska and I. Hausmanowa-Petrusewicz (1997). "A collaborative study on the natural history of childhood and juvenile onset proximal spinal muscular atrophy (type II and III SMA): 569 patients." *Journal of the neurological sciences* 146(1): 67-72.

Zerres, K., B. Wirth and S. Rudnik-Schoneborn (1997). "Spinal muscular atrophy--clinical and genetic correlations." *Neuromuscular disorders : NMD* 7(3): 202-207.

Zhang, Z., F. Lotti, K. Dittmar, I. Younis, L. Wan, M. Kasim and G. Dreyfuss (2008). "SMN deficiency causes tissue-specific perturbations in the repertoire of snRNAs and widespread defects in splicing." *Cell* 133(4): 585-600.

17

Wallerian Degeneration in Injury and Diseases: Concepts and Prevention

Bruno S. Mietto[1], Rodrigo M. Costa[1],
Silmara V. de Lima[1], Sérgio T. Ferreira[1,2] and Ana M. B. Martinez[1]
[1]*Program of Basic and Clinical Neuroscience,*
[2]*Institute of Medical Biochemistry, Federal University of Rio de Janeiro,*
Brazil

1. Introduction

The axon is a highly specialized compartment of neurons. Besides their basic function connecting neurons to their targets, axons play key roles in the nervous system. They are involved in the transport of several molecules indispensable to neuronal activity, act as sensors to guidance cues during development and regeneration, and are essential to maintain normal glial cell functions and myelin sheath assembly (Nave & Trap 2008). Recent evidence indicates that mRNA and Schwann cells-delivered ribosomes can be found within the axoplasm, suggesting that axons may be capable of synthesizing specific proteins (Court et al., 2008). However, most axonal structural proteins are synthesized in the neuronal cell body and transported along the length of the axon. Interruption of this supply leads to a degenerative process known as Wallerian degeneration (WD) in the distal portion of the axon (Coleman, 2005). WD is triggered by intrinsic degenerative pathways that are not correlated to cellular apoptosis (Finn et al., 2000). Axon degeneration is a final common pathway observed not only after a traumatic nerve injury, but also in many neurodegenerative disorders (e.g., Parkinson`s and Alzheimer`s diseases) and in demyelinating diseases such as multiple sclerosis (Coleman, 2005; Coleman & Freeman, 2010). Uncovering the mechanisms that trigger and control axon degeneration is extremely relevant, as such knowledge may offer novel tools to treat severed or damaged axons as well as several neurodegenerative disorders in which WD takes place. In this chapter, we will review the basic concepts of WD, with emphasis on the mechanisms that control axon degeneration following trauma. Next, we will address the issue whether or not current anti-degenerative strategies are efficient and can be envisioned to be applied to humans in the near future.

2. Overview of Wallerian degeneration

WD is classically referred to as a series of degenerative processes triggered in the distal portion of axons after a traumatic injury. WD was originally described by Augustus Waller in 1850 based on his observations in transected glossopharyngeal and hypoglossal nerves (Waller, 1850). Waller observed that, upon transection, the distal nerve stump underwent typical morphological alterations which resulted in total nerve fiber fragmentation followed by disintegration. Although Waller`s description of WD was based on studies with transected peripheral nerves, the main features of WD are observed after many types of insults (crush, transection, chemical and/or toxic) both in the central nervous system (CNS) and in the peripheral nervous system (PNS), and are also present in the course of neurodegenerative and demyelinating diseases, suggesting a common triggering mechanism (Coleman & Perry, 2002).

Axons respond rapidly to an injury. Just a few hours after lesion, ultra-structural analysis reveals swollen axons with their axoplasms filled with an amorphous matrix (Figure 1) resulting from the fact that the major cytoskeleton proteins (microtubules and neurofilaments) are being degraded by activation of ubiquitin-proteasome system (UPS) and calcium-dependent proteases, respectively (to review, see Vargas & Barres, 2007). This event is called granular disintegration of the axonal cytoskeleton resulting in complete degradation of axonal organelles and proteins and is the main ultra-structural characteristic of axons undergoing WD in the PNS. In central nerve fibers, axon disruption may present in two distinct patterns of axoplasm degeneration, as based on the ultra-structural aspect of the axoplasm (Figure 1) (Narciso et al., 2001).

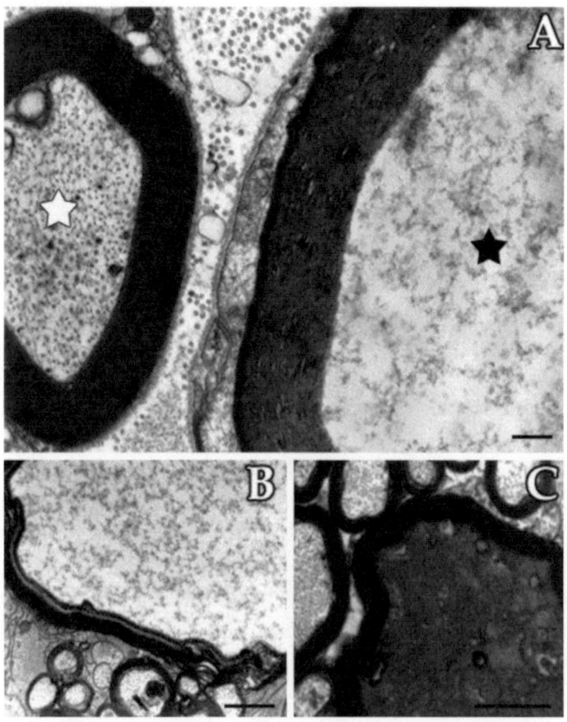

Fig. 1. Ultra-structural images showing different aspects of axon degeneration. Image A represents a sciatic nerve transverse ultra-thin section 48 hours after crush injury in C57BL/6 mice. Note a normal nerve fiber (white star) next to a fiber showing aspects of degeneration with the dissolution of its axoplasmic elements (black star). Images B and C show ultra-thin sections of rat optic nerve, 96 hours after crush injury. Note in B one fiber undergoing watery degeneration, whereas panel C shows a fiber undergoing dark degeneration. Scale bar = 0.3 μm (A) and 1 μm (B and C)

With the onset of WD, the axon will progressively deteriorate and the myelin lamellae will be disrupted into small fragments known as myelin ovoids (Lubińska, 1977) (Figure 2). To date, this criterion is widely used by several groups to study WD in different models (Farah et al., 2011; Narciso et al., 2009).

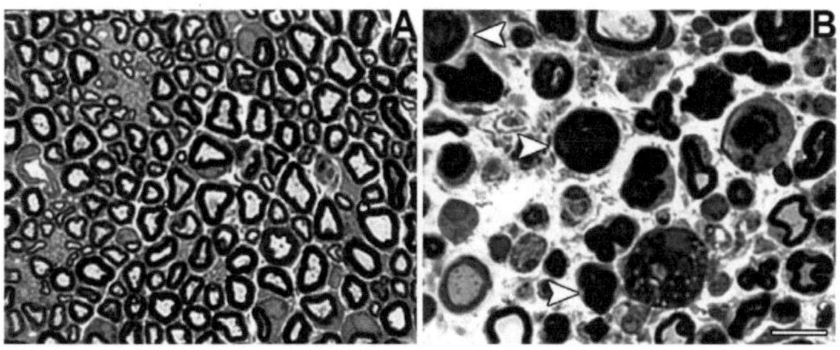

Fig. 2. Wallerian degeneration in C57BL/6 sciatic nerve after crush injury. A. Semi-thin transverse section (toluidine blue staining) from a normal mouse sciatic nerve. B. Semi-thin transverse section from an injured mouse sciatic nerve 96 hours after crush. Note the presence of myelin ovoids (arrowheads). Scale bar = 20 μm

At a later stage of degeneration, myelin and axonal debris will be removed by resident and newly-recruited inflammatory cells (monocytes/macrophages) and microglia (in the CNS) and by Schwann cells (in PNS). The clearance of debris is crucial to create a favorable microenvironment for axon regrowth, since myelin-proteins block axon regeneration by inducing growth-cone collapse (Yiu & He, 2006). During WD, there is an important inflammatory reaction which is highly regulated by immune cells (monocytes/macrophages, T and B lymphocytes, dendritic cells, neutrophils) and by resident non-neuronal cells (microglia and astrocytes in the CNS and Schwann cells in the PNS) (Hawthorne & Popovich, 2011; Sanders & Jones, 2006). Activation of these cells is temporally-orchestrated and triggers the release of several inflammatory molecules that may favor axon degeneration or regeneration. Whether an exacerbated or attenuated inflammatory reaction would be beneficial or harmful to lesioned nerves is still a matter of investigation. Several reports indicate that, in the damaged PNS, inflammation enhances axons regeneration by augmenting macrophages recruitment and myelin debris clearance (Barrete et al., 2008; Narciso et al., 2009). On the other hand, in the damaged CNS, the scenario is not simple: some reports show that recruited macrophages favor axon regeneration (Leon et al., 2000; Yin et al., 2006), while other studies show that it can also be toxic to neurons (Gensel et al., 2009; Popovich & Longbrake, 2008). These conflicting results are currently subject of an intense debate among neuro-immunological researchers and represent an important challenge in the field of neurotrauma (for a review, see Crutcher et al., 2006).

Since Waller`s seminal observations, much has been done in the field of WD. Much of this knowledge was produced with the development of the electron microscope, which allowed researchers to explore in detail the ultra-structural alterations of damaged axons. For a long time, much attention was given to the main mechanisms that control neuronal cell body death; however, to this date, there are several unsolved questions, many of them related to the molecular and cellular pathways that regulate axon destruction, that make this a challenging field for neuroscientists.

3. Molecular and cellular basis of WD

The cascade of events that takes place during axonal degeneration follows a very coordinated sequence determined by the type of nerve fiber affected (motor or sensory neurons, myelinated or unmyelinated fibers), the type and severity of injury, which may vary from a slight crush to complete transection, and by consequences such as deficits in axonal transport (Coleman, 2005) or demyelination (De Vos et al., 2008; Nave & Trapp, 2008). All these factors can affect limb function and recovery in different ways and with different timeframes. But, independently of how severe was the injury, axonal degeneration will occur in a defined fashion. The sequence of steps in axonal degeneration will be discussed in this section. In order to understand the process of axonal degeneration in more detail, however, we first need to cover some basic concepts on axon structure and function.

Each neuron has a highly specialized cylinder-like process that ensures the conduction of information from the cell body to the nerve terminals (Debanne et al., 2011). This process is called "axon" and differs from the other protrusions named "dendrites" in terms of its particular structure and function. The axon emerges from the cell body and varies in length and thickness depending on the function and region of the body it innervates (Wang et al., 2008). Another important feature of axon morphology is the presence or not of a myelin sheath, made by oligodendrocytes in the CNS and by Schwann cells in the PNS. The axonal cylindrical shape is due to the highly organized cytoskeleton components, mainly microtubules and neurofilaments, which are longitudinally aligned along axons. These cytoskeletal components are also responsible for maintenance of axon thickness and are directly implicated in axonal transport of cargoes in association with motor proteins such as dynein and kinesins (De Vos et al., 2008; Perrot et al., 2008).

As previously mentioned, WD is described as the degeneration of axons distal to the point of injury (Waller, 1850). Axonal degeneration is triggered by a large Ca^{2+} influx (George et al., 1995; Martinez & Ribeiro, 1998; Schlaepfer, 1971, 1974), attributed to reversal of the function of the plasma membrane Na^+/Ca^{2+} exchanger as a consequence of dysfunction of the Na^+-K^+ ATPase (reviewed in LoPachin & Lehning, 1997). This intracellular Ca^{2+} overload is presumed to cause disruption of mitochondrial oxidative phosphorylation, excessive formation of free radicals (Anderson et al., 1995; Young et al., 1982) and activation of calpains, calcium-activated neutral cysteine proteases that are responsible for cytoskeleton breakdown and myelin protein degradation (Martinez & Canavarro, 2000; Stokes et al., 1983) (Figure 1). Cytoskeleton disruption leads to failure of axon structural integrity and of important intracellular mechanisms such as axonal trafficking of cargoes and energy supply (De Vos et al., 2008). Intracellular calcium stores are also involved in important cellular changes that boost secondary degeneration (Staal et al., 2010). Another intra-axonal degradation mechanism is the activation of the UPS, which has been implicated as a common mechanism for selective protein degradation in a variety of biological processes including axonal degradation during WD (Zhai et al., 2003). Axon swelling and myelin sheath degradation are the next steps in WD. At this stage, it is possible to observe a bead-like pattern formation along the degenerating axon, classically known as myelin ovoids; this is followed by disconnection and complete degradation of the distal stump (Vargas & Barres, 2007) (Figure 2).

One of the key events in WD is the clearance of axon and myelin debris. Immediately after axonal fragmentation and degradation, Schwann cells in the PNS enter continuous cell division, degrade their own membrane and phagocyte myelin and axonal debris (Liu et al.,

1995; Murinson et al., 2005). Besides, macrophage recruitment and infiltration is initiated via cytokine and chemokine signalling, enhancing myelin debris clearance and creating an appropriated environment for axonal regeneration in the PNS. A different scenario is observed in the CNS, where oligodendrocytes undergo apoptosis and are not involved in myelin debris phagocytosis and signaling for macrophage help. This results in delayed macrophage recruitment, exposure of myelin inhibitory proteins, formation of an astroglial scar and secretion of inhibitory molecules such as chondroitin-sulphate proteoglycans which result in a hostile microenvironment for axon regeneration (George & Griffin, 1994) and establish irreversible loss of function of the target organs. In contrast, microglia, which are considered the resident macrophages of the CNS, are activated after an injury by pro-inflammatory cytokines, among other signals, and undergo several rounds of cell division and morphological changes in order to help phagocytosis of dead cells and myelin debris (Ferrer et al., 1990; Kreutzberg, 1995).

An important tool to better understand the steps and mechanisms involved in WD was the discovery of the slow Wallerian degeneration mouse (Wld^S) (Lunn et al., 1989). In these mutant mice, the active process of neurodegeneration and synapse breakdown after an experimental injury presents a ten-fold delay (Lunn et al., 1989). The chimeric *Wld*^{S} gene resulted from a spontaneous mutation in the C57BL/6 mouse strain, causing a tandem triplication in the distal region of chromosome 4 (Conforti et al., 2000), and is known to protect axons in both CNS and PNS from degeneration induced by injury, neurotoxins and neurodegenerative diseases (Wang et al., 2001). The mutation on chromosome 4 comprises a stable 85-kb tandem triplication encoding the N-terminal 70 amino acids of the multiubiquitination factor Ube4b fused in frame to the nuclear nicotinamide adenine dinucleotide (NAD) producing enzyme nicotinamide mononucleotide adenylyltransferase (Nmnat1) (Coleman et al., 1998; Mi et al., 2003). Interestingly, some research groups have described a significant therapeutic potential for this mutation. The *Wld*^{S} gene can be used to confer neuroprotection using delivery methods such as gene therapy (Wang et al., 2001), with the advantage of no side or detrimental effects on other non-neuronal cell types (Wishart et al., 2009).

The differences between CNS and PNS, as pointed out here, include important features regarding molecular mechanisms in nervous system degeneration. Therapeutic approaches such as anti-degenerative strategies must thus be designed and tested according to the target region of the nervous system, type of injury and severity.

4. Anti-degenerative strategies

The main goal of an anti-degenerative strategy is to halt the progress of neurodegeneration in order to rescue neural and non-neural cells from death. Delaying degeneration can also represent a useful approach to open a time-window in which to introduce combinations treatments, e.g., administration of trophic factors. To achieve its goal, such approach should down-regulate genes related to cellular degeneration and up-regulate those related to regeneration. However, this scenario is not simple. During WD, innumerous signaling pathways are triggered within the neuron´s cell body, axon, synaptic terminals and also in glial cells. To make things worse, we still do not know with certainty the identities of the main proteins that control WD. Nonetheless, based on results from animal model experiments, promising strategies have been proven to be effective in modulating WD progression, raising hopes that they may, in the near future, be applied to humans.

Importantly, several studies have shown that the mechanisms that activate neuronal cell death pathways and axonal degeneration are different from each other. Blocking neuronal death does not prevent axonal degeneration, and inhibiting axonal degeneration does not necessarily block neuronal death (Beirowsky et al., 2008; Vohra et al., 2010). In an attempt to block or decrease tissue damage after neuronal injury, one should simultaneously take into consideration the need to inhibit neuronal death, prevent axonal degeneration and, finally, stimulate neuronal regeneration.

4.1 Neuronal survival

Following a lesion to peripheral nerves, there are molecular and cellular events that occur within the axons acutely after injury and that are followed by other alterations in non-neuronal and neuronal cells. These changes culminate in the activation of signals responsible for initiating the regeneration program but also activate neuronal death pathways (Chen et al., 2007; Makwana & Raivich, 2005). The interruption of axonal transport is one of the first events that take place after injury and its impact on the flow of trophic factors, specially the retrograde transport of ciliary neurotrophic factor (CNTF), brain-derived neurotrophic factor (BDNF) and nerve growth factor (NGF) from target areas, promotes neuronal death (Koliatsos et al., 1993; Sendtner et al., 1997). On the other hand, activation of the signal transducer and activator of transcription 3 (STAT3) and its retrograde transport activates genes important for axonal regeneration (Cafferty et al., 2004). The main components of the axoplasm, the microtubules and neurofilaments, are degraded through the UPS and calpain, respectively (Ehlers, 2004; Zhai et al., 2003), leading to disconnection of the neuronal cell bodies to their targets (Makwana & Raivich, 2005).

Numerous studies have shown the effects of neutrophic factor and neurotrophins (NT) on neuronal survival after injury (Arenas & Persson, 1994; Koliatsos et al., 1993; Yan et al., 1992). Administration of NGF after sciatic nerve transection completely prevented cell loss of dorsal root ganglia neurons (Otto et al., 1987). CNTF and BDNF also prevent death of motor neurons after axotomy (Koliatsos et al., 1993; Yan et al., 1992). This role in preventing neuronal death is important to preserve a certain amount of neuronal cells that can potentially regenerate, resulting in better functional recovery (Chen et al., 2007). The importance of NT in neuronal survival after injury was first appreciated when researchers found that the levels of some NT and neurotrophic factors, and also their receptors, change after lesion and this could account for the roles of different NT on neuronal survival and regeneration (Funakoshi et al., 1993). Funakoshi and collaborators (1993) demonstrated changes in the profile of NT and their receptors at different times after lesion to the sciatic nerve. They showed that levels of BDNF mRNA in the neuronal cell body did not change after sciatic nerve transection but, in contrast, there was a marked increase in the proximal stump. They also found an increase in BDNF mRNA levels at the target, the gastrocnemius muscle, two weeks after lesion. In the case of NT-3, mRNA levels decreased in the cell body after injury but returned to baseline levels 3 days after, while levels in the sciatic nerve dropped within hours after lesion and came back to baseline levels by 2 weeks after the injury. For NT-4, there was no change in the levels of mRNA in the cell body, but there was a 5 -fold increase in the proximal stump and a strong decrease in the neuronal target; this latter event suggests that expression of NT-4 by target organs depends upon neuronal stimulation. Concomitant with changes in the expression of NT, the levels of their receptors also changed and this occurred specially in the nerve's proximal stump. All these changes are important to support neuronal survival after damage and they imply that these factors are produced by glial cells and targets organs in an attempt to promote neuronal survival, regeneration and re-myelination of the growing axons (Chan et al., 2001; Cosgaya et al., 2002).

Another strategy that has been used to prevent cell death is the use of apoptotic and necrotic blockers with the aim of inhibiting activation of cell death pathways. However, the outcomes from these strategies have only impacted on neuronal survival, and not on axonal neuroprotection and regeneration. For example, overexpression of Bcl-2, a mitochondrial protein that inhibits the intrinsic pathway of caspase activation, enhances retinal ganglion cell (RGC) survival after injury, but its effect is only temporary (for a review, see Isenmann et al., 2003). Moreover, BCL-2 overexpression results only in histological improvement after traumatic brain injury without better behavior outcomes (Tehranian et al., 2006). Calpains are also involved in cell death after injury and are implicated in necrotic and apoptotic pathways (McKernan et al., 2007; Paquet-Durand et al., 2007). *In vitro* studies have shown that by inhibiting calpain activation it is possible to attenuate apoptosis in RGC after injury to the optic nerve (Smith et al., 2011). Although calpain inhibition can affect neuronal survival and provide axonal neuroprotection, there is no evidence that its inhibition can promote axonal neuroprotection and neuronal survival at the same time, which is another indicative that neuronal death and axonal degeneration are triggered and controlled by distinct pathways.

4.2 Axonal neuroprotection

As mentioned above, one of the first events triggered upon injury is the degradation of cytoskeleton proteins by calpains. Several studies have shown positive effects of calpain inhibition in different types of lesion and animal models of CNS and PNS disorders, but the precise relationship between calpain activation and neuronal death is not fully understood (Couto et al., 2004; Kieran & Greensmith, 2004; McKernan et al., 2007). It has been shown that use of calpain inhibitors improves the outcomes of muscle function and cell survival after PNS injury (Kieran & Greensmith, 2004). Application of a calpain inhibitor in the distal target organ improved the rate of cell survival and muscular function 12 weeks after a crush lesion of the sciatic nerve (Harding et al., 1996). To test whether calpain inhibition in neuronal cell bodies would have an impact on neuronal survival and muscle function, Kieran & Greensmith (2004) delivered a calpain inhibitor to the spinal cord after injuring the sciatic nerve. Twelve weeks later they observed an improvement in neuronal survival and muscle function, suggesting that calpain inhibition plays an important role on both neuronal survival and axonal neuroprotection. Couto and collaborators (2004) showed that a calpain inhibitor applied to the site of a crush injury had a neuroprotective effect on optic nerve fibers 4 days after injury (Figure 3), while Silmara de Lima and collaborators (unpublished dada) observed that the delay in axonal degeneration promoted by calpain inhibition had no effect on RGC survival 14 days after optic nerve lesion. These results are important since the delay in the onset of WD can create a time-window to add other strategies and investigate whether different types of combinational treatments can lead to better results.

Sodium or calcium channel blockers have also been used in anti-degenerative strategies to prevent axonal disintegration. Lo and colleagues (2003) demonstrated that neuroprotection to spinal cord axons was achieved using a sodium channel blocker in a model of experimental allergic encephalomyelitis. Those authors reported that, besides preventing axonal degeneration, nerve fibers from animals treated with the sodium channel blocker maintained the ability to conduct action potentials. Calcium channel blockers also proved effective in protecting axons from degeneration and improving neuronal survival in models of spinal cord and optic nerve injury, with loss of myelin basic protein and alterations in spinal cord evoked potentials attenuated in the former case (Winkler et al., 2003), and RGC survival increased in the latter (Karim et al., 2006).

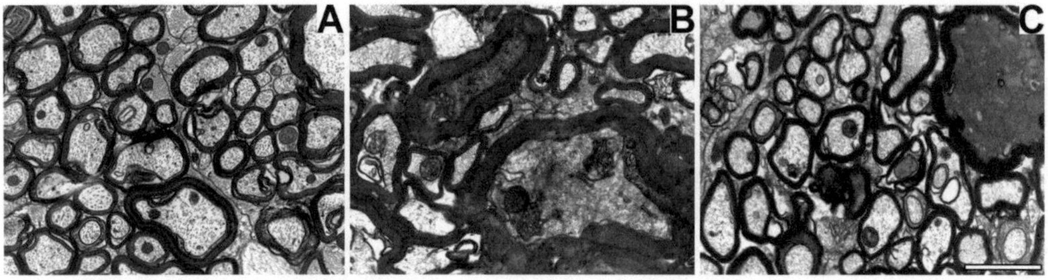

Fig. 3. Transverse ultrathin section from rat optic nerve. A represents a normal optic nerve. B shows a 4 day-injured optic nerve with numerous axons undergoing WD. C shows a 4 day post-injury optic nerve treated with calpain inhibitor prior to the lesion and during the survival time. Note that there are more intact fibers with preserved axoplasm when compared to the image in B. Scale bar = 2 μm

Another important system involved in WD is the UPS, which has been implicated in many biological processes including protein degradation and axonal pathfinding (Campbell & Holt, 2001). The involvement of UPS in the early stages of WD was demonstrated in explanted superior cervical ganglion neurons by Zhai and collaborators (2003), who showed that they could delay axonal degeneration by using a UPS inhibitor. In the same study, they showed that by combining UPS and calpain inhibitors there was also a delay in axonal degeneration. However, better results were obtained when the UPS inhibitor was used prior to the lesion, suggesting that the UPS is involved in the early phase of WD. According to Walker and collaborators (2001), microtubule degradation is sufficient to trigger axonal degeneration, whereas neurofilament disruption *per se* does not affect the distribution of microtubules and other elements of the axon cytoskeleton. For these reasons, maintaining the integrity of axons and improving neuronal survival may be a way to promote a better outcome after nerve fiber injury and to accelerate functional recovery. Therefore, the combined use of calpain and UPS inhibitors may be a promising approach for testing in clinical trials, as inhibitors can be applied peripherally onto neuronal targets.

Another promising strategy is to prevent or slow down axonal degeneration using pharmacological agents. For example, Da Costa et al. (2010) recently showed that intra-peritoneal injections of 2,4-dinitrophenol (DNP) every 24 hours following injury significantly reduced axonal degeneration in a mouse model of sciatic nerve crush injury.

Besides, expression of amyloid precursor protein (APP) and neuregulin-1 (NRG1) were increased in sciatic nerve longitudinal sections after DNP treatment. APP is related to neuronal development, growth and survival (reviewed in Gralle & Ferreira, 2007) and NRG1 plays important roles in development and neurodegeneration (Falls, 2003) and is involved in myelin thickness control (Michailov et al., 2004). DNP is a well-known uncoupler of mitochondrial oxidative phosphorylation (Parascandola, 1974). However, at low concentrations, insufficient to produce mitochondrial uncoupling, DNP has been shown to be a powerful neuroprotective agent against a variety of insults (reviewed in De Felice & Ferreira, 2006; De Felice et al., 2007).

5. Conclusions and perspectives

Since Waller's first experiments and important observations, huge advances have been made in terms of imaging technology, molecular biology tools, genomics and chemical compound synthesis and screening. All this progress has allowed a detailed view of the mechanisms and molecular intimacy of degenerating axons. From accurate freehand drawings to live 3D multiphoton microscopy, researchers have unveiled some of the mysteries behind the dynamics of morphological changes of injured nerves. However, we still face some basic questions regarding axon degeneration: What are the main molecular pathways that trigger axon breakdown after injury? Can we manipulate these key molecules in order to prevent axon degeneration? Furthermore, although it is possible to precisely monitor specific events during degeneration, there are still many open questions about how efficient and which is the best anti-degenerative strategy depending on the type of injury, lesioned region (PNS or CNS) and how far from the cell bodies were the axons damaged. The time between the injury and the beginning of treatment is also a big issue in terms of WD progression and is an important factor regarding limb function recovery. The crosstalk between basic and clinical research is one of the key points in developing new strategies and testing therapeutic hypothesis. Longitudinal screenings on different types of injuries and evaluations of therapies that were applied to each single subject may help to create a blueprint for a personalized nervous system injury treatment.

6. Acknowledgements

Work in the author´s laboratories is funded by grants from the Brazilian agencies Conselho Nacional de Desenvolvimento Científico e Tecnológico, Fundação de Amparo à Pesquisa do Estado do Rio de Janeiro and Instituto de Neurociência Translacional.

7. References

Anderson, D.K.; Means, E.D.; Waters, T.R. & Spears, C. J. (1995). Spinal cord energy metabolism following compression trauma to the feline spinal cord. *J. Neurosurg.* 53:375–380.

Arenas, E. & Persson, H. (1994). Neurotrophin-3 prevents the death of adult central noradrenergic neurons in vivo. *Nature.* 6461:368-71.

Barrete, B.; Hébert, M.A.; Filadi, M.; Lafortune, K.; Vallières, N.; Gowing, G.; Julien, J.P. & Lacroix, S. (2008). Requirement of myeloid cells for axon regeneration. *J. Neurosci.* 38:9363-9376.

Beirowski, B.; Babetto, E.; Coleman, M.P. & Martin, K.R. (2008). The WldS gene delays axonal but not somatic degeneration in a rat glaucoma model. *Eur. J. Neurosci.* 6:1166-79.

Cafferty, W.B.; Gardiner, N.J.; Das P, Q.J.; McMahon, S.B. & Thompson S.W. (2004). Conditioning injury-induced spinal axon regeneration fails in interleukin-6 knock-out mice. *J. Neurosci.* 18:4432-43.

Campbell, D.S. & Holt, C.E. (2001). Chemotropic responses of retinal growth cones mediated by rapid local protein synthesis and degradation. *Neuron.* 6:1013-26.

Chan, J.R.; Cosgava, J.M.; Wu, Y.J. & Shooter, E.M. (2001). Neurotrophins are key mediators of the myelination program in the peripheral nervous system. *Proc. Natl. Acad. Sci.* 25:14661-8. 2001.

Chen, Z.L.; Yu, W.M. & Strickland, S. (2007). Peripheral regeneration. *Annu. Rev. Neurosci.* 30:209-33.

Coleman, M. (2005). Axon degeneration mechanisms: commonality amid diversity. *Nat. Rev. Neurosci.* 6:889–898.

Coleman, M.P. & Freeman, M.R. (2010). Wallerian degeneration, Wlds and Nmnat. *Annu. Rev. Neurosci.* 33:245-267.

Coleman, M. P.; Conforti, L.; Buckmaster, E.A.; Tarlton, A.; Ewing, R.M.; Brown, M.C.; Lyon, M.F. & Perry, V.H. (1998). An 85-kb tandem triplication in the slow Wallerian degeneration (Wlds) mouse. *Proc. Natl. Acad. Sci. USA.* 95:9985-9990

Coleman, M.P. & Perry, V.H. (2002). Axon pathology in neurological diseases: a neglected therapeutic target. *Trends Neurosci.* 25:532-537.

Conforti, L.; Tarlton, A.; Mack, T.G.; Mi, W. & Buckmaster, E. A. (2000). A Ufd2/D4Cole1e chimeric protein and overexpression of Rbp7 in the slow Wallerian degeneration (WldS) mouse. *Proc. Natl. Acad. Sci. USA.* 97: 11377–11382.

Cosgaya, J.M.; Chan, J.R. & Shooter, E.M. (2002). The neurotrophin receptor p75NTR as a positive modulator of myelination. *Science.* 5596:1245-8.

Court, F.A.; Hendriks, W.T.J.; MacGillavry, H.D.; Alvarez, J. & Van Minnen, J. (2008). Schwann cell to axon transfer of ribosomes: toward a novel understanding of the role of glia in the nervous system. *J. Neurosci.* 43:11024-11029.

Couto, L.A.; Narciso, M.S.; Hokoç, J. N. & Blanco Martinez, A. M. (2004). Calpain inhibitor 2 prevents axonal degeneration of opossum optic nerve fibers. *J Neurosci Res.* 77: 410-419.

Crutcher, K.A.; Gendelman, H.E.; Kipnis, J.; Perez-Polo, J.R.; Perry, V.H.; Popovich, P.G. & Weaver, L.C. (2006). Debate: "is increasing neuroinflammation beneficial for neural repair?". *J Neuroimmune Pharmacol.* 1:165-211.

Da Costa, R.M.; Martinez, A.M.B. & Ferreira, S.T. (2010). 2,4-Dinitrophenol blocks neurodegeneration and preserves sciatic nerve function after trauma. *J. Neurotauma.* 5:829-841.

De Felice, F.G. & Ferreira, S.T. (2006). Novel neuroprotective, neuritogenic and anti-amyloidogenic properties of 2,4-dinitrophenol: The gentle face of Janus. *IUBMB Life* 58:185–191.

De Felice, F.G.; Wasilewska-sampaio, A.P.; Gomes, F.A.; Klein, W.L. & Ferreira, S.T. (2007). Cyclic AMP enhances Abeta oligomerization blockers as potential theraqpeutics agents in Alzheimers diseases. *Curr. Alzheimer Res.* 3:263-271.

De Vos, K.J.; Grierson, A.J.; Ackerley, S. & Miller, C.C. (2008). Role of axonal transport in neurodegenerative diseases. *Annu. Rev. Neurosci.* 31:151–73.

Debanne, D.; Campanac, E.; Bialowas, A.; Carlier, E. & Alcaraz, G. (2011). Axon physiology. *Physiol. Rev.* 91(2):555-602.

Ehlers, M.D. (2004). Deconstructing the axon: Wallerian degeneration and the ubiquitin-proteasome system. *Trends. Neurosci.* 1:3-6.

Falls, D.L. (2003). Neuregulins: Functions, forms, and signaling strategies. *Exp. Cell. Res.* 284:14–30.

Farah, M.H.; Pan, B.H.; Hoffman, P.N.; Ferraris, D.; Tsukamoto, T.; Nguyen, T.; Wong, P.C.; Price, D.L.; Slusher, B.S. & Griffin, J.W. (2011). Reduced BACE1 activity enhances clearance of myelin debris and regeneration of axons in the injured peripheral nervous system. *J. Neurosci.* 15:5744-5754.

Ferrer, I.; Bernet, E.; Soriano, E.; Del Rio, T. & Fonseca, M. (1990). Naturally occurring cell death in the cerebral cortex of the rat and removal of dead cells by transitory phagocytes. *Neuroscience.* 39:451–458.

Finn, J.T.; Weil, M.; Archer, F.; Siman, R.; Srinivasan, A. & Raff, M.C. (2000). Evidence that wallerian degeneration and localized axon degeneration induced by local neurotrophin deprivation do not involve caspases. *J. Neurosci.* 20:1333-1341.

Funakoshi, H.; Frisén, J.; Barbany, G.; Timmusk, T.; Zachrisson, O.; Verge, V.M. & Persson, H. (1993). Differential expression of mRNAs for neurotrophins and their receptors after axotomy of the sciatic nerve. *J. Cell. Biol.* 2:455-65.

Gensel, J.C.; Nakamura, S.; Guan, Z.; Rooijen, N.V.; Ankeny, D.P. & Popovich, P.G. (2009). Macrophages promote axon regeneration with concurrent neurotoxicity. *J. Neurosci.* 12:3956-3968.

George, R. & Griffin, J.W. (1994). Delayed macrophage responses and myelin clearance during Wallerian degeneration in the central nervous system: the dorsal radiculotomy model. *Exp. Neurol.* 129:225–36.

George, E.B.; Glass, J.D. & Griffin, J.W. (1995). Axotomy-induced axonal degeneration is mediated by calcium influx through ion-specific channels. *J. Neurosci.* 15:6445–6452.

Gralle, M. & Ferreira, S.T. (2007). Structure and functions of the human amyloid precursor protein: The whole is more than the sum of its parts. *Prog. Neurobiol.* 82:11–32.

Harding, D.I.; Greensmith, L.; Connold, A.L. & Vrbová, G. (1996). Stabilizing neuromuscular contacts increases motoneuron survival after neonatal nerve injury in rats. *Neuroscience.* 3:799-805.

Hawthorne, A.L. & Popovich, P.G. (2011). Emerging concepts in myeloid cell biology after spinal cord injury. *Neurotherapeutics.* 2:252-261.

Isenmann, S.; Kretz, A. & Cellerino, A. (2003). Molecular determinants of retinal ganglion cell development, survival, and regeneration. *Prog. Retin Eye Res.* 4:483-543.

Karim, Z.; Sawada, A.; Kawakami, H.; Yamamoto, T. & Taniguchi, T. (2006). A new calcium channel antagonist, lomerizine, alleviates secondary retinal ganglion cell death after optic nerve injury in the rat. *Curr. Eye Res.* 3:273-283.

Kieran, D. & Greensmith, L. (2004). Inhibition of calpains, by treatment with leupeptin, improves motoneuron survival and muscle function in models of motoneuron degeneration. *Neuroscience.* 2:427-39.

Koliatsos, V.E.; Clatterbuck, R.E.; Winslow, J.W.; Cayouette, M.H. & Price, D.L. (1993). Evidence that brain-derived neurotrophic factor is a trophic factor for motor neurons in vivo. *Neuron.* 3:359-67.

Kreutzberg, G.W. (1995) The First Line of Defense in Brain Pathologies. *Drug Research.* 45: 357–360

Leon, S.; Yin, Y.; Nguyen, J.; Irwin, N. & Benowitz, L.I. (2000). Lens injury stimulates axon regeneration in the mature rat optic nerve. *J. Neurosci.* 12:4615-4626.

Liu, H.M.; Yang, L.H. & Yang, Y.J. (1995). Schwann cell properties: 3. C-fos expression, bFGF production, phagocytosis and proliferation during Wallerian degeneration. *J. Neuropathol. Exp. Neurol.* 54:487–96.

Lo, A.C.; Saab, C.Y.; Black, J.A. & Waxman, S.G. (2003). Phenytoin protects spinal cord axons and preserves axonal conduction and neurological function in a model of neuroinflammation in vivo. *.J Neurophysiol.* 5:3566-71.

LoPachin, R.M. & Lehning, E.J. (1997) Mechanism of calcium entry during axon injury and degeneration. *Toxicol. Appl. Pharmacol.* 143:233–244

Lubińska, L. (1977). Early course of wallerian degeneration in myelinated fibers of the rat phrenic nerve. *Brain Res.* 1:47-63.

Lunn, E.R.; Perry, V.H.; Brown, M.C.; Rosen, H. & Gordon, S. (1989). Absence of Wallerian degeneration does not hinder regeneration in peripheral nerve. *Eur. J. Neurosci.* 1:27–33.

Makwana, M. & Raivich, G. (2005). Molecular mechanisms in successful peripheral regeneration. *FEBS. J.* 11:2628-38.

Martinez, A.M.B. & Canavarro, S. (2000). Early myelin breakdown following sural nerve crush: a freeze-fracture study. *Braz. J. Med. Biol. Res.* 12:1477-1482.

Martinez, A.M.B. & Ribeiro, L.C.V. (1998). Ultrastructural localization of calcium in peripheral nerve fibers undergoing Wallerian degeneration: an oxalate-pyroantimonate and x-ray microanalysis Study. *J. Submicrosc Cytol Pathol.* 3:451-458.

McKernan, D.P.; Guerin, M.B.; O'Brien, C.J. & Cotter, T.G. (2007). A key role for calpains in retinal ganglion cell death. *Invest. Ophthalmol. Vis. Sci.* 12:5420-5430.

Mi, W.; Glass, J. D. & Coleman, M. P. (2003). Stable inheritance of an 85-kb triplication in C57BL/WldS mice. *Mutat. Res.* 526:33-37.

Michailov, G.V.; Sereda, M.W.; Brinkmann, B.G.; Fischer, T.M.; Haug, B.; Birchmeier, C.; Role, L.; Lai, C.; Schwab, M.H. & Nave, K.A. (2004). Axonal neuregulin-1 regulates myelin sheath thickness. *Science* 304:700–703.

Murinson, B.B.; Archer, D.R.; Li, Y. & Griffin, J.W. (2005). Degeneration of efferent myelinated fibers prompts mitosis in Remak Schwann cells of uninjured C-fibers afferents. *J. Neurosci.* 25:1179-1187.

Narciso, M.S.; Hokoç, J.N. & Martinez, A.M.B. (2001). Watery and dark axons in Wallerian degeneration of the opossum`s optic nerve: different patterns of cytoskeletal breakdown?. *An. Acad. Bras. Cienc.* 2:231-243.

Narciso, M.S.; Mietto, B.S.; Marques, S.A.; Soares, C.P.; Mermelstein, C.S.; El-Cheikh, M.C. & Martinez, A.M.B. (2009). Sciatic nerve regeneration is accelerated in galectin-3 knockout mice. *Exp. Neurol.* 217:7-15.

Nave, K.A. & Trapp, B.D. (2008). Axon-glial signaling and the glial support of axon function. *Annu. Rev. Neurosci.* 31: 535–561.

Otto, D.; Unsicker, K. & Grothe, C. (1987). Pharmacological effects of nerve growth factor and fibroblast growth factor applied to the transectioned sciatic nerve on neuron death in adult rat dorsal root ganglia. *Neurosci. Lett.* 1-2:156-60.

Paquet-Durand, F.; Johnson, L. & Ekström, P. (2007). Calpain activity in retinal degeneration. *J. Neurosci. Res.* 4:693-702.

Parascandola, J. (1974). Dinitrophenol and bioenergetics: A historical perspective. *Mol. Cell Biochem.* 5:69–77.

Perrot, R.; Berges, R.; Bocquet, A. & Eyer, J. (2008). Review of the multiple aspects of neurofilament functions, and their possible contribution to neurodegeneration. *Mol. Neurobiol.* 38:27–65.

Popovich, P.G. & Longbrake, E.E. (2008). Can the immune system be harnessed to repair the CNS?. *Nat. Rev. Neurosci.* 6:481-493.

Sanders, V.M. & Jones, K.J. (2006). Role of immunity in recovery from a peripheral nerve. *J. Neuroimmune. Pharmacol.* 1:11-19.

Schlaepfer, W.W. (1971). Experimental alterations of neurofilaments and neurotubules by calcium and other ions. *Exp. Cell Res.* 67:73–80.

Schlaepfer, W.W. (1974). Calcium-induced degeneration of axoplasm in isolated segments of rat peripheral nerve. *Brain Res.* 69:203–215.

Sendtner, M.; Götz, R.; Holtmann, B. & Thoenen, H. (1997). Endogenous ciliary neurotrophic factor is a lesion factor for axotomized motoneurons I adult mice. *J. Neurosci.* 18:6999-7006.

Smith, A.W.; Das, A.; Guyton, M.K.; Ray, S.K.; Rohrer, B. & Banik N.L. (2011). Calpain inhibition attenuates apoptosis of retinal ganglion cells in acute optic neuritis. *Invest. Ophthalmol. Vis. Sci.* 7:4935-41.

Staal, J.A., Dickson, T.C., Gasperini, R., Liu, Y., Foa, L. & Vickers, J.C. (2010) Initial calcium release from intracellular stores followed by calcium dysregulation is linked to secondary axotomy following transient axonal stretch injury. *J. Neurochem.* 112:1147-1155.

Stokes, B.T.; Fox, P. & Hollinden, G. (1983). Extracellular calcium activity in the injured spinal cord. *Exp. Neurol.* 80:561–572.

Tehranian, R.; Rose, M.E.; Vagni, V.; Griffith, R.P.; Wu, S.; Maits, S.; Zhang, X.; Clark, R.S.; Dixon, C.E.; Kochanek, P.M.; Bernard, O. & Graham, S.H. (2006). Transgenic mice that overexpress the anti-apoptotic Bcl-2 protein have improved histological outcome but unchanged behavioral outcome after traumatic brain injury. Brain Res. 1:126-35.

Vargas, M.E. & Barres, B.A. (2007). Why is Wallerian Degeneration in the CNS so slow? *Ann. Rev. Neurosci.* 30:157-179.

Vohra, B.P.; Sasaki, Y.; Miller, B.R.; Chang, J.; DiAntonio, A. & Milbrandt J. (2010). Amyloid precursor protein cleavage-dependent and -independent axonal degeneration programs share a common nicotinamide mononucleotide adenylyltransferase 1-sensitive pathway. *J. Neurosci.* 41:13729-13738.

Walker, K.L.; Yoo, H.K.; Undamatla, J. & Szaro, B.G. (2001). Loss of neurofilaments alters axonal growth dynamics. *J Neurosci.* 24:9655-66

Waller, A. (1850). Experiments on the section of glossopharyngeal and hypoglossal nerves of the frog and observations of the alternatives produced thereby in the structure of their primitive fibers. *Philos. Trans. R. Soc. Lond. B Biol. Sci.* 140:423–29.

Wang, M.S.; Fang, G.; Culver, D.G.; Davis, A.A.; Rich, M.M. & Glass, J.D. (2001). The WldS protein protects against axonal degeneration: a model of gene therapy for peripheral neuropathy. *Ann. Neurol.* 50:773-9.

Wang, S.S.; Shultz, J.R.; Burish, M.J.; Harrison, K.H.; Hof, P.R.; Towns, L.C.; Wagers, M.W. & Wyatt, K.D. (2008). Functional trade-offs in white matter axonal scaling. *J. Neurosci.* 28:4047–4056.

Winkler, T.; Sharma, H.S.; Stålberg, E.; Badgaiyan, R.D.; Gordh, T. & Westman, J. (2003). An L-type calcium channel blocker, nimodipine influences trauma induced spinal cord conduction and axonal injury in the rat. *Acta Neurochir. Suppl.* 86:425-32.

Wishart, T.M.; Brownstein, D.G.; Thomson, D.; Tabakova, A.M.; Boothe, K.M.; Tsao, J.W. & Gillingwater, T.H. (2009) Expression of the neuroprotective slow Wallerian degeneration (WldS) gene in non-neuronal tissues. *BMC Neurosci.* 10:148.

Yan, Q.; Elliott, J. & Snider, W.D. (1992). Brain-derived neurotrophic factor rescues spinal motor neurons from axotomy-induced cell death. *Nature.* 6406:753-755.

Yin, Y.; Henzl, M.T.; Lorber, B.; Nakazawa, T.; Thomas, T.T.; Jiang, F.; Langer, R.; Benowitz, L.I. (2006). Oncomodulin is a macrophage-derived signal for axon regeneration in retinal ganglion cells. *Nat. Neurosci.* 6:843-852.

Yiu, G. & He, Z. (2006). Glial inhibition of CNS axon regeneration. *Nat Rev Neurosci*. 8:617-627.

Young, W.; Yen, V. & Blight, A. (1982) Extracellular calcium ionic activity in experimental spinal cord contusion. *Brain Res*. 253:105–113.

Zhai, Q.; Wang, J.; Kim, A.; Liu, Q.; Watts, R.; Hoopfer, E.; Mitchison, T.; Luo, L. & He, Z. (2003). Involvement of the ubiquitin-proteasome system in the early stages of wallerian degeneration. *Neuron*. 2:217-25.

18

Mesenchymal Stem Cell Therapy for Apoptosis After Spinal Cord Injury

Venkata Ramesh Dasari[1], Krishna Kumar Veeravalli[1], Jasti S. Rao[1,2], Dan Fassett[2,3] and Dzung H. Dinh[2,3]
[1]*Departments of Cancer Biology and Pharmacology,*
[2]*Neurosurgery*
[3]*Illinois Neurological Institute*
University of Illinois College of Medicine at Peoria, Peoria, Illinois, USA

1. Introduction

Spinal cord injury (SCI) is a devastating clinical problem that has irreversible consequences, results in permanent functional loss, and life time disability (Sekhon and Fehlings, 2001). This debilitating condition often affects young and healthy individuals at the prime of their life, creates enormous physical and emotional cost, and places a significant financial burden to society at large (Ackery et al., 2004). Even though years of research have led to a better understanding in the pathophysiology of permanent neural injuries at the cellular level, much of the mechanism and processes of secondary injury at the molecular level remain to be elucidated. With modern molecular strategies and techniques, breakthroughs in the understanding of neuronal injury and neural regeneration provide new promises for reversal of spinal cord injury that once was thought to be permanent and irreversible (Carlson and Gorden, 2002).

Spinal cord injury involves an initial mechanical or primary injury followed by a series of cellular and molecular secondary events that amplify the extent of the initial damage and results in the progressive destruction of spinal cord tissue. After acute contusion, the spinal cord undergoes a sequential progression of pathologic changes, including micro hemorrhage, cytotoxic edema, neuronal necrosis, axonal fragmentation, demyelination, further secondary cellular destruction and eventually cyst formation (Balentine, 1978; Balentine and Greene, 1984; Coutts and Keirstead, 2008). Damage to the spinal cord results in extensive proliferation of microglia and macrophages in and around the injury epicenter. This acute inflammatory response at the injury site is at least partly responsible for secondary spinal cord injury (Popovich et al., 1997; Carlson et al., 1998; Taoka et al., 1998). The inflammatory cells (particularly macrophages/microglia) mediate tissue damage by producing a variety of cytotoxic factors including interleukins (Rice et al., 2007) and tumor necrosis factor-alpha (TNF-α) (Beattie et al., 2002). White matter breakdown begins at the grey-white matter junction with progressive edema (Dohrmann et al., 1972). Axoplasmic stasis and axonal swelling that contains multiple organelles, mitochondria, neurofilament, and smooth endoplasmic reticulum eventually undergo glandular dissolution and myelin disruption (Bresnahan et al., 1976; Balentine, 1978; Bresnahan, 1978; Balentine and Greene, 1984). Within 4h of injury, neuronal and oligodendroglial cell loss is apparent in the lesion epicenter, and extends rostrally and caudally (Grossman et al., 2001). Within days after the injury polymorphonuclear cells and macrophages begin to infiltrate the injured region (Blight, 1985; Means and Anderson, 1983). And within one week, the central necrotic region begins to show cystic changes. By four weeks, chronic changes have occurred, and a cystic cavity remains with astrocytic gliosis and demyelination of the remaining axons (Wagner et al., 1971). Even years after initial trauma, neuronal and oligodendroglial apoptotic cell death processes continues to contribute to demyelination and Wallerian degeneration (Hagg and Oudega, 2006; Taoka and Okajima, 1998). The wave of post-traumatic tissue destruction, as initiated by secondary injury mechanisms, include disruption of spinal cord vasculature and ischemia, glutamatergic excitotoxicity, oxidative cell stress, lipid peroxidation and inflammation (Nashmi and Fehlings, 2001; Tator and Fehlings, 1991)—all of which alone or in concert can trigger apoptosis, contribute to the permanency of functional motor and sensory deficits (Hagg and Oudega, 2006; Taoka and Okajima, 1998).

Apoptotic cell death has been observed to occur for weeks after injury at distance remote from the point of mechanical impact (Crowe et al., 1997; Emery et al., 1998; Springer et al., 1999). Neurons and oligodendrocytes are especially vulnerable to the toxicity of the acute lesion microenvironment after SCI for several reasons (Choi, 1988). Neurons have a high rate of oxidative metabolism that makes them susceptible to injury by reactive oxygen species (ROS) following ischemia (Juurlink and Paterson, 1998). Compared to their supporting astroglial cells, neurons have lower levels of antioxidant levels (e.g., glutathione) and respond differently to molecular mechanisms involving the activation of Phase II enzymes, which are responsible for neutralization of damaging free radicals (Eftekharpour et al., 2000). Oligodendrocytes are also very susceptible to ROS due to their higher iron content and lower levels of glutathione and its related antioxidant enzymes, (Juurlink and Paterson, 1998). The oxidative stress by induction of ROS and pro-inflammatory cytokines initiates a cascade of oxidative events that lead to cell death due to a combination of necrosis and apoptosis (Crowe et al., 1997). Loss of oligodendroglia causes demyelination, impairs axonal function and survival. In the days to weeks after injury, disrupted neuronal axons and extracellular elements of the necrotic core at the site of injury are removed by recruited inflammatory cells and phagocytes (Dusart and Schwab, 1994), leaving in place fluid-filled cystic cavities at the site of injury (Greitz, 2006).

2. Apoptosis after SCI

Apoptosis is a genetically controlled cell death that is characterized by intact membrane integrity, cytoplasmic and nuclear condensation, loss of cellular volume, membrane bleb formation and nuclear disintegration (Yakovlev and Faden, 2001). The cell eventually fragments into apoptotic bodies, which are then engulfed and degraded by neighboring cells. During apoptosis, morphological changes are often accompanied by internucleosomal cleavage of genomic DNA (Wyllie et al., 1980). In the secondary injury process after SCI, apoptosis has been well documented. Emery *et al.*, (1998) analyzed the spinal cords of 15 patients who had died after traumatic SCI and described evidence of apoptotic cells at the edges of the lesion epicenter and in the adjacent white matter. Apoptotic mechanisms of cell death have been implicated in delayed Wallerian degeneration of white matter after spinal cord injury (Crowe et al., 1997). Oligodendrocytes, microglia, and neurons are susceptible to apoptosis. After SCI, some cellular demise was directly related to post-traumatic necrosis, whereas others die due to apoptosis (Crowe et al., 1997; Emery et al., 1998; Shuman et al., 1997; Springer et al., 1999; Keane et al., 2001; Warden et al., 2001; Beattie et al., 2002). Spinal cord trauma activates upregulation of caspases and calpain and the apoptotic machinery, leading to increased expression of death receptors and their ligands (Banik et al., 1997; Casha et al., 2001; Keane et al., 2001; Springer et al., 1999). However, there are conflicting reports as to the role of cell death in SCI— probably a reflection of the known dual capacity of TNF to be both pro- and anti-apoptotic. Fas/CD95, TNFR1 and TNFR2 have been mainly characterized in the immune system and are primarily involved in regulating inflammatory and apoptotic responses. However, these receptors and their ligands are also detectable in CNS tissue (both normal and traumatized), implicating their roles in neuronal maturation as well as in neurological trauma and disease. Apoptotic pathways triggered after SCI are depicted in Figure 1.

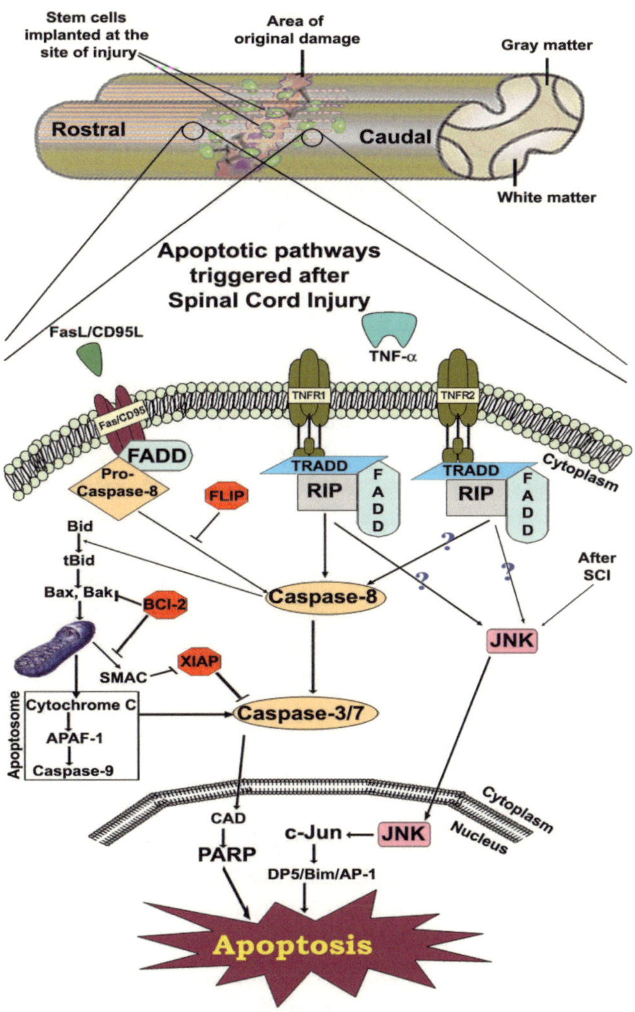

Fig. 1. Apoptotic pathways triggered after SCI

Apoptosis of the cells takes place either rostral or caudal to the area of original damage. These are mainly either Fas-activated or TNF-α or JNK-activated pathways. In Fas-mediated pathway, Fas is activated by Fas ligand, whereby Fas-associated death domain (FADD) and caspase-8 are recruited to Fas to form the death-inducing signaling complex (DISC). Subsequently, caspase-8 can autoactivate and trigger cell death by cleavage of Bid and activation of effector caspases- 3 and -7. The activation and involvement of mitochondria in apoptosis appears to be the main pathway responsible for cell death. In tumor necrosis factor receptor 1 (TNFR1/TNFR2) signaling, early after trauma, increased levels of TNFR1/TNFR2 are activated where they associate with the adaptor protein TRADD, Fas-associated death domain (FADD), TRAF2, TRAF1, and RIP. In later stages after injury, RIP and cIAP-1 appear to dissociate from the TNFR1 complex by an unknown mechanism and this complex signals death by activating caspase-8. In either case, activated caspase-3 translocates to nucleus, and activates CAD resulting in cleavage of PARP leading to apoptotic cell death. In JNK mediated pathway, JNK gets activated after SCI, and translocated to nucleus where it activates c-Jun leading to apoptotic cell death. In mesenchymal stem cell treatment for apoptosis, mesenchymal stem cells are injected at the site of injury or rostral or caudal to the site of injury.

2.1 Apoptosis involving FAS/CD95 and caspases

Fas (CD95 or Apo-1) is a member of the TNFR superfamily and is one of six known death receptors. Fas exists as a 45-kDa, type 1 transmembrane protein with an elongated extracellular domain. This extracellular region contains three cysteine-rich domains (CRDs), which are typical of TNF receptors (Keane et al., 2006). This receptor contains a death domain and plays a central role in the physiological regulation of programmed cell death, and has been implicated in the pathogenesis of various malignancies and diseases of the immune system. The interaction of this receptor with its ligand generates the formation of a death-inducing signaling complex that includes Fas-associated death domain protein (FADD), caspase-8, and caspase-10. The autoproteolytic processing of the caspases in the complex triggers a downstream caspase cascade, and leads to apoptosis. The typical ligand for Fas is FasL (CD95L, Apo-1L, Cd178, TNFSF6), which is a 281–amino acid protein produced as a type 2 transmembrane protein and is highly restricted to immune cells and cells of the CNS. In the nervous system, Fas/CD95 activation can lead to cell death involving neurons and glial cells (D'Souza et al., 1995; Raoul et al., 2002). Activation of Fas/CD95 can also lead to enhanced axonal growth (Desbarats et al., 2003). Fas and FasL are expressed in the normal CNS, and are upregulated in inflamed and degenerated brains (Choi and Benveniste, 2004). Fas and FasL levels have been found to be elevated after SCI (Casha et al., 2001; Dasari et al., 2008; Demjen et al., 2004; Li et al., 2000a). Yoshino *et al.*, (Yoshino et al., 2004) investigated Fas/CD95-mediated apoptosis after SCI using Fas-deficient mutant mice. Mice lacking Fas/FasL showed improved functional recovery, decreased lesion size, and fewer apoptotic cells in the injured cord than control littermates. It appears that Fas-FasL induce apoptosis via both intrinsic and extrinsic pathways. The extrinsic pathway involves Fas-FasL mediated activation of caspase-8, which then directly activates caspase-3 (Salvesen and Dixit, 1999; Stennicke et al., 1998). There was evidence to support the regulation of intrinsic mitochondrial apoptotic pathways by the Bcl-2 family proteins, which consists of both pro-apoptotic (Bid and Bax) and anti-apoptotic (Bcl-2 and Bcl-xL) members (Kim et al., 2000). In addition, the intrinsic pathway can be initiated by the extrinsic pathway, thereby amplifying the apoptotic process. In this scenario, Caspase-8 cleaves Bid into truncated tBid, which translocates from the cytosol into the mitochondria, releasing cytochrome c and activating caspase-3 and -9 (Kuwana et al., 1998; Li et al., 1998; Scaffidi et al., 1998; Stennicke et al., 1998; Verhagen et al., 2000). Also, a mitochondrial apoptotic protein, Apoptosis-inducing factor (AIF), was found capable of inducing neuronal apoptosis when translocated from mitochondria to the nucleus via a caspase-dependent pathway (Tsujimoto, 2003; Tsujimoto and Shimizu, 2000; Yu et al., 2006; Yu et al., 2009).

Strategies to inhibit Fas-FasL cascade may provide effective neuroprotective approaches for mollifying apoptosis after SCI. In one experiment, neutralization of FasL, but not TNF, significantly decreased apoptotic cell death after SCI (Demjen et al., 2004). Mice pretreated with FasL-specific antibodies were capable of initiating active hind-limb movements several weeks after injury with upregulation of growth-associated protein Gap-43 and more abundance in regenerating fibers. Thus, neutralization of FasL appears to diminish apoptotic cell death and promote axonal regeneration and functional improvement in injured adult animals (Demjen et al., 2004). Other experiments have demonstrated that blocking Fas activation using soluble Fas receptors for competitive inhibition or neutralization using anti-FasL antibody diminished brain injury volume and improved outcome in a stroke model of mouse (Gao et al., 2005). The neuroprotective effect of anti-FasL in animal models of SCI, stroke and multiple sclerosis has stimulated considerable interest in elucidation of the role of the Fas/CD95/FasL system in CNS neurons (Demjen et al., 2004; Martin-Villalba et al., 1999; Waldner et al., 1997). However, a true understanding of how FasL antibodies reduce cell death and enhance recovery requires more detailed knowledge. It is not clear if CNS cells exhibit differences in the efficiency of Fas/CD95 signaling and thus can be categorized as type I or type II cells (Keane et al., 2006). The cellular source and target of the ligand in damaged CNS tissue need to be identified, and strategies need to be developed for effective delivering antibodies to the lesion. Recent experimental evidence has provided some knowledge about receptor submembrane localization and the formation of alternative signaling complexes that can alter the fate of cells *in vitro*, but whether these principles hold true *in vivo* remained to be explored. Thus, activation of these signaling pathways might result in promising therapeutic targets for the acute treatment of neurological trauma and disease.

In addition to FasL/CD95 involvement in apoptosis, caspases are also known to be powerful mediators of programmed cell-death in CNS injury and disease processes. All caspases are translated initially as inactive zymogens that are then activated after specific cleavage. They have the following structural features in common: an N-terminal pro-domain of variable length (22 to >200 amino acids), a large subunit (~ 17-20 kDa), a short inter-subunit region (~10 amino acids), and a small subunit (~10 – 12 kDa). The C-terminal portion of the large subunit contains the catalytic cysteine residue. Flanking this are other conserved residues that, together, form the semiconserved pentapeptide sequence QACXG at the active site (Alnemri et al., 1996; Thornberry and Lazebnik, 1998). Pro-caspases are processed by limited proteolysis into their active form, which consists of a large and small subunit dimer. *In vivo*, however, caspases are more conformationally stable as tetramers consisting of two large/small subunit dimers (Eldadah and Faden, 2000). Once activated by specific cleavage to active forms, caspases can activate other procaspases via extrinsic pathway directly or intrinsic pathway by mitochondrial-dependent mechanisms, thereby amplifying the programmed cell death process (Li et al., 1998; Scaffidi et al., 1998; Slee et al., 1999; Yakovlev and Faden, 2001; Yu et al., 2009). Based on their putative functions and sequence homologies, caspases are often categorized into three groups: apoptotic initiators (caspase-2, 8, -9 and -10), apoptotic executioners (caspase- 3, -6, and -7), and inflammatory mediators (caspase -1, -4,-5, -11, -12, and -13) (Alenzi et al., 2010; Thornberry and Lazebnik, 1998). The apoptotic initiators, act at upstream positions within apoptotic pathways; that is, the cell surface and mitochondria. They have in common long N-terminal pro-domains that contain six anti-parallel α-helices with complementary binding capability. Caspases-8 and -10 have two such domains at their N-termini known as death effector domains (DEDs). Caspases-2 and -9 have only one of these domains, which, in the case of these members, are known as caspase recruitment domains (CARDs). These sequences play an important role in localization and activation of specific procaspases. The apoptotic executioners mediate some of the morphological and biochemical manifestations of apoptosis: plasma membrane blebbing, nuclear membrane dissolution, chromatin condensation and margination, and DNA fragmentation. Executioner caspases have short N-terminal pro-domains whose function remains unclear (Eldadah and Faden, 2000). The third group of caspases is inflammatory mediating proteases that are poor substrates for other caspases and their activation pathways are not well understood.

Numerous studies have demonstrated the presence of multiple caspases and apoptosis following SCI (Beattie et al., 2000; Citron et al., 2000; Crowe et al., 1997; Eldadah and Faden, 2000; Keane et al., 2001; Liu et al., 1997; Lou et al., 1998; Springer et al., 1999; Yong et al., 1998). Emery *et al.*, (1998) have reported substantial labeling of active caspase-3 around the injury site in histological study of injured spinal cords from 15 patients who died after traumatic SCI. The involvement of caspase-3 as a major effector in injury-induced neuronal apoptosis was established by using specific caspase inhibitors in various models of ischemic or traumatic injury (Clark et al., 2000; Gillardon et al., 1997; Gottron et al., 1997; Namura et al., 1998; Yakovlev et al., 1997). Caspase-3 can be activated by caspases-8, -9, -11, and -12 (Kang et al., 2000; Wang et al., 1998). Caspases-11 and -12 in turn can be activated by Calpain and Cathepsin B (Nakagawa and Yuan, 2000; Schotte et al., 1998; Yamashima, 2000). Apoptosis therefore plays an important role in the secondary injury processes following traumatic injury to the CNS (Crowe et al., 1997; Keane et al., 2001; Li et al., 1996; Lu et al., 2000). The permanent neurological deficits after spinal cord injury may be due in part to widespread apoptosis in regions distant from and relatively unaffected by the initial injury (Crowe et al., 1997). Caspases were one of the viable therapeutic targets for modulating apoptosis and remain the viable approach to blocking apoptotic cell death (Nicholson, 2000). A number of caspase inhibitors such as z-VAD fmk (N-benzyloxycarbonyl-Val-Ala-Asp-fluoromethylketones) have been developed to avert apoptotic chain events. X-linked inhibitor of apoptosis proteins (XIAP) has been identified as one of the mammalian homologues in the IAP family, and has been demonstrated to inhibit cell death (Ekert et al., 1999). During apoptosis, XIAP is cleaved to generate fragments with distinct specificity for caspases (Deveraux et al., 1999). However, caspase inhibition has yet to be used in clinical setting despite demonstrated efficacy in treatment of various CNS insults of *in vivo* models (Braun et al., 1999; Hara et al., 1997; Li et al., 2000b; Yakovlev et al., 1997). Several SCI experiments using caspase inhibitors have been reported (Li et al., 2000a; Lou et al., 1998; Springer et al., 1999) to mitigate injury-induced programmed cell death.

2.2 Apoptosis involving TNF-α mediated pathway

Tumor necrosis factor (TNF)-α, also known as cachexin or cachectin, is a pro-inflammatory, pro-apoptotic cytokine that elicits diverse biological actions, including the induction of apoptosis (Tracey, 2011). TNF-α is a trimeric protein primarily produced by the brain resident immune cells such as monocytes and macrophages (the microglia cells) in response to various stimuli (Leung and Cahill, 2010). TNF-α is initially synthesized as a 26-kD cell surface-associated molecule (membrane-bound form) which is then cleaved into a soluble 17-kD form by TNF converting enzyme (Grewal, 2009). The known roles of TNF-α have extended from the immune system to neuro-inflammatory domain in the nervous system (Leung and Cahill, 2010). TNF-α induces central sensitization and hyperalgesia by increasing excitatory synaptic transmission (Kawasaki et al., 2008). TNF-α initiates the activation of several cytokines and growth factors, as well as the recruitment of some immune cells. Cytokines exist in 'cascades' and interrupting one cytokine can disrupt the cascade. For example, blocking TNF-α reduces the activity of IL-6 and IL-1b (Fong et al., 1989); whereas blocking IL-1b reduces IL-6 (Goldbach-Mansky et al., 2006); and blocking IL-12 and IL-23 reduces IFN-γ. It is this 'master role' in cytokine function that makes TNF-α an attractive target in SCI and other disorders involving inflammation and apoptosis. TNF-α interacts with two distinct receptors - TNFR-55 (TNFR1, p55, CD120a) and TNFR-75 (TNFR2, p75, CD120b). TNF-α can either bind directly to TNFR1 and TNFR2 through cell-to-cell contact or undergo cleavage and binds in its soluble form (Vandenabeele et al., 1995). All nucleated cells express TNF receptors. TNFR1 is expressed constitutively on most cell types, whereas expression of TNFR2 can be induced by TNF-α, interleukin (IL)-1, and interferon (IFN)-α in rat primary astrocytes (Choi et al., 2005). In addition, TNFR2 expression is restricted to hematopoetic cells and can discriminate between murine and human forms of TNF-α (Tartaglia et al., 1991). The receptors also differ significantly in their binding affinity for homotrimeric TNF-α. Although both receptors can be considered high-affinity, the on–off kinetics of the two differs dramatically. Binding of homotrimeric TNF-α to TNFR1 seems to be essentially irreversible, whereas binding to TNFR2 is associated with rapid on–off kinetics (Choi et al., 2005).

Evidence showed that proinflammatory and proapoptotic cytokines, including TNF-α, IL-1γ, and FasL regulate cellular events and contributes to neuronal damage and functional impairment associated with SCI (Harrington et al., 2005; Lee et al., 2000; Martin-Villalba et al., 1999; Streit et al., 1998). TNF-α levels become elevated in human spinal cord after SCI, reaching a peak within 1h after the initial trauma (Dinomais et al., 2009). The expression of TNF-α is upregulated rapidly at the lesion site after SCI (Hayashi et al., 2000; Streit et al., 1998; Wang et al., 1996; Wang et al., 2002; Yan et al., 2001). TNF-α can induce apoptosis of oligodendrocytes and neuronal cell line *in vitro* (D'Souza et al., 1995; Sipe et al., 1996). Rapid accumulation of TNF-α may act as an external signal initiating apoptosis after SCI in neurons and glial cells (Lee et al., 2000; Shuman et al., 1997). Neutralization of TNF-α reduced the number of apoptotic cells after SCI (Lee et al., 2000). Apoptosis induced by TNF-α after SCI could be mediated in part by nitric oxide via upregulation of inducible nitric oxide synthase (iNOS) (Yune et al., 2003). Although, few studies indicate a neuroprotective role of TNF-α and NOS expression in SCI, several investigators support a neurodestructive role of these agents in spinal cord pathology (Bethea et al., 1999; Bethea and Dietrich, 2002; Dolga et al., 2008; Gonz'alez Deniselle et al., 2001; Sharma et al., 1995; Sharma, 2007; Sharma, 2008; Sharma, 2010; Stalberg et al., 1998).

Apoptosis of oligodendrocytes *in vivo* was shown to be induced by the overexpression of TNFR1 (Akassoglou et al., 1998). Following SCI, TNFR1 and TNFR2 expression is elevated in the injured spinal cord and localized on neurons, astrocytes and oligodendrocytes (Yan et al., 2003). TNFR1 and TNFR2 are elevated as soon as 15 min after traumatic SCI in adult rats, reaches the peak at 4h for TNFR2 and 8h for TNFR1, and declines markedly after 1 day and 3 days (Yan et al., 2003). TNFR1 immunoreactivity was demonstrated on cells and afferent fibers of dorsal root and dorsal root ganglia, dorsal root entry zone and within lamina I and II of dorsal horn, whereas TNFR2 expression was absent in these regions (Holmes et al., 2004). These two receptors might work individually or synergistically to mediate the biological activity of TNF-α. It has been suggested that TNF receptors are involved in anti-apoptotic activities through the TNFR1-nuclear factor kappa B (NFκB) signal transduction pathway, which activates a recently identified endogenous caspase inhibitory system that is mediated by cellular inhibitor of apoptosis protein 2 (c-IAP2) (Kim et al., 2001). After TNF binding to TNFR1, a TNFR1 receptor–associated complex (complex-I) forms and contains TRADD, RIP1, TRAF1, TRAF2, and cIAP-1. Complex-I transduce signals that lead to NF-κB activation through recruitment of the IκB kinase 'signalsome' high-molecular-weight complex (Poyet et al., 2000; Zhang et al., 2000). TNFR1$^{-/-}$ mice had greater numbers of apoptotic cells, larger contusion size, and worse functional recovery after SCI. TNFR2$^{-/-}$ mice had similar, although not as pronounced, consequences as the TNFR1$^{-/-}$ mice. However, when new protein synthesis is inhibited prior to TNF stimulation, TNFR1 can initiate apoptosis by activation of apical caspases (Varfolomeev and Ashkenazi, 2004). TNFR1-mediated apoptosis signaling is induced in which TRADD and RIP1 associate with FADD and caspase-8 to form a cytoplasmic complex (complex-II) that dissociates from TNFR1. When complex-I triggers sufficient NF-κB signaling, anti-apoptotic gene expression is induced and the activation of initiator caspases in complex-II is inhibited. If NFκB signaling is deficient, complex-II transduces an apoptotic signal. Thus, early activation of NFκB by complex-I serves as a checkpoint to regulate whether complex-II induces apoptosis at a later time point after TNF binding.

2.3 Apoptosis involving JNK mediated pathway

The mitogen-activated protein kinases (MAPKs) are a family of evolutionally conserved molecules that play a critical role in cell signaling and gene expression. MAPK family includes three major members: c-Jun N-terminal kinase (JNK), p38 and extracellular signal regulated kinase (ERK), representing three different signaling cascades. The JNK pathway is considered as a key mediator of stress-induced apoptosis (Davis, 2000). Examples include neuronal apoptosis induced by NGF withdrawal (Eilers et al., 1998; Park et al., 1996; Xia et al., 1995), excitotoxic stress (Yang et al., 1997b) and UV radiation (Tournier et al., 2000; Tournier et al., 2001), thymocyte apoptosis induced by anti-CD3 antibody (Rincon et al., 1998; Sabapathy et al., 1999) and endothelial cell apoptosis caused by diabetes-associated hyperglycemia (Ho et al., 2000). JNK pathway activation may also contribute to neuronal death in neurodegenerative diseases including Alzheimer's, Parkinson's, Huntington's Diseases and stroke (Gao et al., 2005; Okuno et al., 2004; Yang et al., 1997b). However, the mechanism by which JNK activation triggers apoptotic processes remains to be fully elucidated. Substrates of JNK, including the Bcl-2 family proteins, regulate cytochrome c release which is an important event in apoptosis secondary to mitochondrial dysfunction. After SCI, JNK3 activity itself is induced by the injury, regulating cytochrome C release by phosphorylating Mcl-1, and thereby facilitating the degradation of Mcl-1, which is necessary for induction of apoptosis of oligodendrocytes (Li et al., 2007). Although JNK3 is also activated in neurons after SCI, it did not induce neuronal apoptosis. A potential role for

JNK3 in neurons is regulation of autophagic death instead of apoptotic death as observed in oligodendrocytes (Li et al., 2007). Several studies demonstrated that the anti-apoptotic proteins Bcl-2, Bcl-xL and Mcl-1 are phosphorylated by JNK *in vitro* and *in vivo* (Inoshita et al., 2002; Maundrell et al., 1997; Yamamoto et al., 1999), there by suppressing the anti-apoptotic activity of these proteins. Another possibility is that JNK phosphorylates the transcription factor c-Jun which might in turn mediate the induction of proteins regulating cytochrome c release in apoptosis (Behrens et al., 1999). Indeed, JNK has been found to regulate some pro-apoptotic BH3-only proteins via transcription-dependent mechanisms (Tournier et al., 2000). Two genes in this subfamily, DP5 and Bim, have AP-1 binding sites on their promoters, and transcription appears to be regulated by JNK activity (Davis, 2000; Harris and Johnson, Jr., 2001; Putcha et al., 2001; Putcha et al., 2003; Whitfield et al., 2001; Yang et al., 1997a; Yin et al., 2005).

Substantial increases in p-JNK expression were noticed after SCI (Esposito et al., 2009; Yin et al., 2005). Activated form of JNK was expressed in the apoptotic cells that were stained by oligodendrocyte antibodies 1–3 days after SCI (Nakahara et al., 1999) and both p-JNK and DP5 colocalization were found in neurons and oligodendrocytes undergoing apoptosis after SCI (Yin et al., 2005). Similarly, the transcription factor, c-Jun (which is an exclusive substrate of JNK), was also phosphorylated shortly after traumatic injury. Furthermore, DP5 is also induced after SCI in a JNK-dependent manner. Suppression of JNK activity by SP600125, a JNK inhibitor, or jnk1 knockdown by an antisense oligodeoxynucleotide (ODN) attenuated SCI-induced DP5 upregulation and caspase-3 activation. Following traumatic SCI, JNK activation contributes to activation of caspase 3, and apoptosis of glia and neurons (Yin et al., 2005). Based on these discoveries, it appears that JNK/c-Jun/DP5/Caspase 3 signaling pathway could represent a potential target for therapeutic interventions in SCI.

3. Stem cell therapy for apoptosis after SCI

During the first few days after injury, there are many microenvironmental features that are detrimental to the survival and integration of transplanted stem cells (Hausmann, 2003). The pathophysiologic processes initiated after acute spinal cord injury are extremely complex, and our limited understanding is reflected in the utilization of i.v. steroid trauma protocol as the only currently available neuroprotective strategy. The limited success of pharmacologic treatment has shifted the focus of medical research away from these traditional treatments to other more promising areas such as cell-based therapy, particularly, the application of stem cell biology (Hipp and Atala, 2004; Stanworth and Newland, 2001). Thus, various cellular transplantation strategies have been utilized in different models of SCI (Eftekharpour et al., 2008). The adult spinal cord harbors endogenous stem/progenitor cells, collectively referred to as NPCs, which might be responsible for normal cell turnover. However, the proliferative activity of endogenous NPCs is too limited to support significant self repair after injury. As such, stem cell transplantation has become a very attractive and viable treatment option for not only CNS injury but also other neurodegenerative disease processes such as Parkinson disease, MS, stroke and ALS (Malgieri et al., 2010). The rationale for cell replacement approach for the treatment of SCI are (1) regeneration, which seeks to replace lost or damaged neurons and induce axonal regeneration or modulate plasticity; and (2) repair, which seeks to replace supportive cells such as oligodendrocytes in order to prevent progressive myelin loss and induce remyelination (Totoiu and Keirstead, 2005). Additionally, stem cell transplantation may promote protection of endogenous cells from further cell loss by attenuation of secondary injury process. Non-embryonic sources of adult stem cells, free from many of the ethical and legal concerns associated with embryonic stem cell research, may offer great promise for the advancement of medicine (Moore et al., 2006). At present, the only non-embryonic stem cells easily available in large numbers are found in the bone marrow, adipose tissue and human umbilical cord blood. These multipotent adult stem cells are ideal vehicles for gene therapy, and genetic engineering for therapeutic treatment of various genetic disorders (Pessina and Gribaldo, 2006). Recent studies have shown that transplanted adult stem cells, including mesenchymal stem cells, human umbilical cord blood stem cells into injured spinal cord promote endogenous myelin repair and modulate immune response, stirring the hope of applying their efficacy to other demyelinating diseases such as MS and stroke.

3.1 Mesenchymal stem cells

Mesenchymal stem cells (MSC) are stromal cells from the bone marrow (BM) and appear as spindle-shaped cells in culture (Friedenstein et al., 1974). Human mesenchymal stem cells are multipotent cells that are present in adult marrow, can replicate as undifferentiated cells and have the potential to differentiate to lineages of mesenchymal tissues, including bone, cartilage, fat, tendon, muscle, and marrow stroma (Pittenger et al., 1999). Even though not immortal, they have the ability to expand many folds in culture while retaining their growth and multilineage potential. MSC are identified by the expression of surface markers including CD105 (SH2) and CD73, and are negative for hematopoietic markers such as CD34, CD45 and CD14. MSC attracted interest for their ability to migrate to the injured site and differentiate into multiple cellular phenotypes *in vivo* (Uccelli et al., 2011). The heterogenity of MSC, and their expression of a large number of regulatory proteins, may explain their wide therapeutic features and capacity to respond differently to injuries depending on the microenvironment, despite their low engraftment *in vivo* (Phinney and Prockop, 2007). MSC produce cytokines and a variety of soluble factors regulating several biological activities as demonstrated by their transcriptome analysis (Phinney et al., 2006). They play a major role in the maintenance of local homeostasis via their supporting activity in the survival of non-proliferating hematopoietic stem cells (HSC) niche in the bone marrow (Mendez-Ferrer et al., 2010). These mesenchymal stem cells are derived from the embryonic mesodermal layer and retain the cardinal abilities of stemcellness for self-renewal and multipotentiality to differentiate into various tissue cell types.

MSCs are attractive candidates for cellular therapies because they are easy to isolate, have a broad differentiation potential, and proliferate *in vitro* (Barry, 2003). Bone Marrow and umbilical cord blood are rich sources of these cells, but MSC have also been isolated from fat (Gronthos et al., 2001), skeletal muscle (Jankowski et al., 2002), human deciduous teeth (Miura et al., 2003), and trabecular bone (Noth et al., 2002). In addition, recent data demonstrated that MSC can give rise to cells of non-mesodermal origin such as hepatocytes, epithelial and neural cells (Chagraoui et al., 2003; Ma et al., 2006; Spees et al., 2003; Woodbury et al., 2000). The choice of the tissue source is governed by availability, as well as by the degree of characterization of the cells and the consistency of the preparations. MSCs from bone marrow and umbilical cord blood have been reasonably well defined in terms of surface markers and differentiation pathways. These donor sites provide a readily available autologous source for cell transplantation, alleviating the need for long-term immunosuppression. Mesenchymal stem cells have been used in experimental models of

SCI and in preliminary clinical trials for SCI (Himes et al., 2006; Sykova et al., 2006) with apparent improvement of behavioral outcome. Stem cells are likely to be therapeutically valuable both in providing permissive substrates for axonal regeneration and as 'cellular minipumps' delivering trophic factors that could enhance white matter sparing and/or axonal regeneration (Enzmann *et al.*, 2006). The functional benefits of MSC transplantation in CNS injuries can be explained by their ability to provide the host tissue with growth factors or modulate the host immune system (Garbuzova-Davis et al., 2006). One of the major goals for the therapeutic use of stem cells is to prevent apoptosis or to replace lost cells, particularly oligodendrocytes, in order to facilitate the remyelination of spared axons. Details showing application of unengineered mesenchymal stem cells from various sources and their applications after SCI are provided in Table 1.

3.1.1 Bone marrow derived mesenchymal stem cells

Human MSCs are isolated from a bone marrow (BM) aspirate, which is often harvested from the superior iliac crest of the pelvis. They represent a very minor fraction of the total nucleated cell population in marrow, but can be plated and enriched using standard cell culture techniques. Frequently, the marrow sample is subjected to fractionation on a density gradient solution, such as Percoll, after which the cells are plated. Primary cultures are usually maintained for 12–16 days, and are then detached by trypsinization and subcultured. Morphologically, the cells resemble adherent fibroblasts (Barry, 2003). Under physiological settings bone marrow derived MSC (BMSC) main function is to regulate hematopoiesis. However, when these cells are grown away from their natural environment, they can be readily and effectively propagated and manipulated genetically into cells of the mesodermal lineage but also, under certain experimental circumstances, into cells of the neuronal and glial lineage (Clark and Keating, 1995). The advantages of using bone marrow as a source for stem cells are numerous: they are relatively easy to isolate, the cells grow and expand well in tissue culture. BMSC may be used in autologous transplantation protocols, and these have already received FDA approval for treatment of hematopoietic diseases (Sykova et al., 2006). BMSC therapeutic value relies on their significant anti-proliferative, anti-inflammatory and anti-apoptotic features. These properties have been demonstrated in the treatment of experimental autoimmune encephalomyelitis (EAE), an animal model of multiple sclerosis where inhibition of the autoimmune response resulted in a significant neuroprotection.

BMSC transplantation results in neuroprotection and increased endogenous neuronal survival in experimental brain ischemia, traumatic brain and spinal cord injury models (Uccelli et al., 2011). There is increasing evidence that MSCs possess immunosuppressive features (Bartholomew et al., 2002; Corcione et al., 2006; Di Nicola et al., 2002; Jiang et al., 2005). These immunosuppressive properties in combination with their restorative functions reduce the acute inflammatory response to SCI, minimize cavity formation, as well as diminish astrocyte and microglia/macrophage reactivity (Abrams et al., 2009; Himes et al., 2006; Neuhuber et al., 2005). BMSC administered 1- week post-SCI had better rates of survival since the microenvironment has become less hostile by then. MSC transplantation in an experimental SCI model has been shown to enhance tissue protection and cellular preservation via reduction in injury-induced sensitivity to mechanical trauma (Abrams et al., 2009). These studies indicated that transplanted MSC attenuates acute inflammation and promote functional recovery following SCI (Hofstetter et al., 2002). Clinically, Park *et al.* (2005)

References	Source of Mesenchymal stem cells	Experimental Animals	Route/site of administration	Treatment timing	Treatment outcome
Cízková *et al.*, 2006	Human bone marrow	Rats	Into right femoral vein	7 days after thoracic SCI	Remyelination of spared white matter tracts, enhancing axonal growth and functional recovery
Dasari *et al.*, 2007a	Rat bone marrow	Rats	Injury epicenter	7 days after thoracic SCI	Downregulation of caspase mediated apoptosis, functional recovery of rats
Dasari *et al.*, 2008	Human umbilical cord blood	Rats	Injury epicenter	7 days after thoracic SCI	Downregulation of Fas mediated apoptosis, functional recovery of rats
Dasari *et al.*, 2009	Human umbilical cord blood	Rats	Injury epicenter	7 days after thoracic SCI	Downregulation of TNF-α mediated neuronal apoptosis
Deng *et al.*, 2006	Rhesus monkey bone marrow	Rhesus monkey	Injury epicenter	7 days after thoracic SCI	*de novo* neurogenesis and functional recovery
Gu *et al.*, 2010	Rat bone marrow	Rats	1mm rostral and caudal from injury epicenter	7 days after thoracic SCI	Reduction in lesion volume; axonal regrowth of injured spinal cord.
Hu *et al.*, 2010	Human umbilical cord blood	Rats	2mm rostral and caudal from injury epicenter	24h after thoracic SCI	Increased length of neurofilament positive fibers and increased numbers of growth cone-like structures around the lesion site, functional recovery
Lee *et al.*, 2007	Human bone marrow	Rats	Injury epicenter	7 days after thoracic SCI	Functional recovery
Lim *et al.*, 2007	Umbilical cord blood of canine fetuses	Dogs	Injury epicenter	7 days after balloon compression at the first lumbar vertebra.	Significant improvement in the nerve conduction velocity based on the somatosensory evoked potentials. Functional recovery.
Osaka *et al.*, 2010	Rat bone marrow	Rats	Intravenous (through the femoral vein)	6h, 1d, 3d, 10d, 14d, 21d, 28d after thoracic SCI	Cavitation in the contused spinal cords was less; functional recovery
Parr *et al.*, 2008	Rat bone marrow	Rats	Injury epicenter	9 days after clip compression injury at the thoracic region	Potential axonal guidance through guiding strands of matrix generated by the bone marrow stromal cells
Satake *et al.*, 2004	Rat bone marrow	Rats	Stem cells injected into the subarachnoid space	3, 5, 7 days after thoracic SCI	MSCs differentiated into Nestin-positive, immature neurons or glial cells
Yang *et al.*, 2008	Wharton's jelly of the human umbilical cord	Rats	2mm rostral and caudal to injury epicenter	After complete transection at the thoracic region.	Functional recovery, regenerated axons in the corticospinal tract and neurofilament-positive fibers around the lesion site.
Zeng *et al.*, 2011	Rat bone marrow derived mesenchymal stem cells grown on 3D gelatin sponge (GS) scaffolds	Rats	Injury epicenter	7 days after thoracic SCI	Attenuating inflammation, promoting angiogenesis and reducing cavity formation.

Table 1. Table showing different authors using mesenchymal stem cells for treatment after SCI

evaluated the therapeutic efficacy of combining autologous BMSC transplantation, administered directly into the spinal cord lesion site, with granulocyte macrophage- colony stimulating factor (GM-CSF), given subcutaneously, in six patients with complete SCI. At the 6-month and 18-month follow-up periods, four of the six patients showed neurological improvements by two ASIA grade (from ASIA A to ASIA C), while another improved from ASIA A to ASIA B. Moreover, BMSC transplantation together with GM-CSF was not associated with increased morbidity or mortality. In another clinical trial, safety of autologous bone marrow cell implantation was tested in 20 patients (Sykova et al., 2006). Motor evoked potential, somatosensory evoked potential, magnetic resonance imaging, and ASIA scores were measured in patient follow-up. This study demonstrated that BMSC transplantation is a relatively safe procedure and BMSC-mediated repair can lead to modest improvements in some injured patients. Thus, it is anticipated that a Phase II clinical trial designed to test the efficacy will be initiated in the near future. In another study using human mesenchymal stem cells (hMSCs) derived from adult bone marrow, the transplanted cells were found to infiltrate mainly into the ventrolateral white matter tracts, spreading to adjacent segments rostro-caudal to the injury epicenter, and facilitate recovery from SCI by remyelinating spared white matter tracts and/or by enhancing axonal growth (Cizkova et al., 2006). In our laboratory, we used mesenchymal stem cells from rat bone marrow to evaluate the therapeutic potential after SCI (Dasari et al., 2007a). Immunohistochemistry confirmed a large number of apoptotic neurons and oligodendrocytes in caudal segments 2 mm away from the lesion site. Expression of caspase-3 on both neurons and oligodendrocytes after SCI was significantly downregulated by BMSC. Treatment with BMSC had a positive effect on behavioral outcome and better structural integrity preservation as seen on histopathological analysis. BMSC secrete protective factors that prevent neuronal apoptosis through stimulation of endogenous survival signaling pathways, namely the PI3-K/Akt and the MAPK/Erk1, 2-cascade (Isele et al., 2007). The potential of bone marrow cell transplantation as a method of repair in the injured CNS may serve a number of different purposes that span various therapeutic targets. Animal studies have demonstrated that transplanted MSCs mollify the inflammatory response in the acute setting and reduce the inhibitory effects of scar tissue in the subacute/chronic setting to provide a permissive environment for axonal extension. In addition, grafted cells may provide a source of growth factors to enhance axonal elongation across spinal cord lesions (Wright et al., 2011). Moreover, SCI initiates an innate immune response that participates not only in secondary pathogenesis but also in wound healing (Trivedi et al., 2006). Even though the present data are promising, further research is needed to establish whether bone marrow cell treatments can serve as a safe and efficacious autologous source for the treatment of the injured SCI (Wright et al., 2011). Downregulation of TNF-α expression in macrophages/microglia was observed at an early stage after SCI in rats transplanted with a gelatin sponge scaffold impregnated with rat bone marrow-derived mesenchymal stem cells at the site of injury (Zeng et al., 2011).

3.1.2 Human umbilical cord blood derived mesenchymal stem cells

Human umbilical cord blood collected from umbilical vein following birth is a valuable source of mesenchymal stem cells (hUCB or hUCBSC) and has been used as an alternative source of allogenic donor cells to treat a variety of hematologic, immunologic and oncologic disorders (Broxmeyer et al., 1989; Gluckman et al., 1997; Han et al., 2003; Kim et al., 2002).

Human umbilical cord blood contains a heterogeneous population of cells enriched in hematopoietic stem cells and display a high proliferative capacity (Mayani and Lansdorp, 1998). These mesenchymal multipotent progenitor cells possess the capability of differentiating into diverse functional progenitors, including hematopoietic cell lineages, dendritic cells, cardiomyocytes, mesenchymal stem cell (MSC) progenitors, neural stem cell (NSC) progenitors, keratinocytes, hepatocytes, pancreatic β-cells, and endothelial cells in specific culture conditions *in vitro* and *in vivo* (Brunstein et al., 2007; Hemmoranta et al., 2006; Mimeault and Batra, 2006; Weiss and Troyer, 2006). Complex interactions between adult stem cells, host cells and the specialized microenvironment may influence their behavior (Arai and Suda, 2007; Barrilleaux et al., 2006; Bryder et al., 2006; Moore et al., 2006; Wilson and Stice, 2006). More specifically, the reciprocal interactions of adult stem cells with neighboring cells *via* the formation of adherens junctions and the secretion of diverse soluble factors might contribute to their restricted mobility and the adoption of a quiescent or activated state within niches (Mimeault and Batra, 2006). There are many advantages of human umbilical cord blood as a source of MSC as compared to bone marrow or adipose tissue. First, the collection of cord blood is easy and painless. The cord blood can be stored for later use. Second, hUCBSC are more primitive than MSCs isolated from other tissue sources (Can and Karahuseyinoglu, 2007; Lu et al., 2006; Sarugaser et al., 2005; Wu et al., 2007). Third, hUCBSC have a higher proliferative capacity and a faster population doubling time that remains unaltered after 30 passages. In contrast, BMSC showed significantly slower doubling time which became even longer after 6 passages (Malgieri et al., 2010). Finally, hUCBSC has lower immunogenicity and graft-versus-host reactivity when compared to BMSC (Malgieri et al., 2010). There are four different methods for isolation and purification of hUCBSC: density gradient centrifugation, flow cytometry isolation, attachment screening and two-step enzymatic digestion (Zhang et al., 2006). In our laboratory, the cord blood is subjected to fractionation on a density gradient solution, such as Ficoll, after which the cells are plated. Primary cultures are usually maintained for 12–16 days, and are then detached by trypsinization and subcultured. As such, umbilical cord blood bank represents a rich source of multipotent stem cells that are readily available for transplantation or for generating diverse tissue-specific adult stem/progenitor cells and their further differentiated progeny for cellular therapies of various disorders in humans (Barrilleaux et al., 2006; Brunstein et al., 2007; Mimeault and Batra, 2006).

Human umbilical cord blood stem cells offer great potential for novel therapeutic approaches targeted against many CNS diseases. The therapeutic potential of hUCBSC may either be attributed to the inherent ability of stem cell populations to replace damaged tissues outright, or alternatively, to their ability to repair damaged tissues through neural protection and secretion of neurotrophic factors by various cell types within the graft (Park et al., 2011; Sanberg et al., 2005). Previous studies have reported that hUCBSC are beneficial in reversing the deleterious behavioral effects of spinal cord injury, even when infused 5 days after injury (Saporta et al., 2003). Transplanted hUCBSC differentiate into various neural cells and induce motor function improvement in SCI rat models (Kuh et al., 2005). However, to date, very few reports have utilized hUCBSC in SCI. More thorough experiments are needed to evaluate how hUCBSC modulates improvement after SCI and whether it possesses the potential of tissue plasticity (Enzmann et al., 2006). In our laboratory, using SCI injury model in rats, we transplanted hUCBSC one week after SCI to evaluate neural cell differentiation and functional improvement. We have shown that hUCBSC transdifferentiated into neurons and oligodendrocytes, and downregulated Fas-mediated apoptosis (Dasari et al., 2007b; Dasari et al., 2008). The hUCBSC-transdifferentiated oligodendrocytes facilitate the secretion of neurotrophic hormones NT3 and BDNF and synthesize MBP and PLP, promoting the remyelination of demyelinated axons in the injured spinal cord (Dasari et al., 2007b). Furthermore, apoptotic pathways mediated by both Fas and TNF-α were downregulated by hUCBSC (Dasari et al., 2008). Our findings confirmed that mesenchymal stem cells were able to downregulate apoptotic pathways mediated by Fas and Caspase-3 (Figure 2) (Dasari et al., 2007b; Dasari et al., 2008). In hUCBSC-treated rats, the PI3K/Akt pathway was also involved in anti-apoptotic actions. Further, the structural integrity of the cytoskeletal proteins α-tubulin, MAP-2A and -2B and NF-200 has been maintained with hUCBSC treatments. The locomotor scale scores in hUCBSC-treated rats were significantly improved compared to those of the injured group. Taken together, hUCBSC-mediated down-regulation of Fas and caspases may lead to functional recovery of the hind limbs of rats after SCI. With extension of this study, using RT-PCR microarray and analyzing 84 apoptotic genes, we identified the genes that render the injured spinal cord harmful and the hUCBSC-treated spinal cord conducive to regeneration and repair at 3 weeks (Dasari et al., 2009). We observed that the genes involved in inflammation and apoptosis were up-regulated (phospho-p53 and Bax) in the injured spinal cords of rats (Kotipatruni et al., 2011), whereas the genes involved in neuroprotection were up-regulated in the hUCBSC-treated rats (Dasari et al., 2008). Changes in the expressions of TNF-α, TNFR1 and TNFR2 were detected over 3 weeks after SCI and after transplantation with hUCBSC cells. The expression of P50 and P65 on neurons after SCI was efficiently inhibited by application of hUCBSC. Both the *in vivo* and *in vitro* studies support our hypothesis that the therapeutic mechanism of hUCBSC is inhibition of the neuronal apoptosis during the repair of injured spinal cord. Veeravalli *et al.* (2009a) reported the involvement of tissue plasminogen activator (tPA) after SCI in rats and the role of hUCB stem cells. The tPA expression and activity were studied *in vivo* after SCI in rats and *in vitro* in rat embryonic spinal neurons in response to injury with staurosporine, hydrogen peroxide and glutamate. The expression of tPA increased after SCI and reached peak levels at 3 weeks post-SCI. The MBP expression was minimal at the time of the peak tPA activity and *vice versa*. By contrast, infusion of hUCBSC stem cells down-regulated the elevated tPA activity *in vivo* in rats as well as *in vitro* in the spinal neurons. Further, MMP-2 is upregulated after hUCBSC treatment in spinal cord injured rats and in spinal neurons injured either with staurosporine or hydrogen peroxide. Also, hUCBSC-induced upregulation of MMP-2 diminished formation of the glial scar at the site of injury along with reduced immunoreactivity to chondroitin sulfate proteoglycans. This upregulation of MMP-2 levels and reduction of glial scar formation by hUCBSC treatment after SCI created an environment more favorable for endogenous repair mechanisms (Veeravalli et al., 2009b). There have been an increasing number of studies suggesting that these hUCB derived-$CD34^+$ cells can induce angiogenesis and endo/exogenous neurogenesis in stroke (Taguchi et al., 2004) and SCI (Kao et al., 2008). In addition, Chen *et al.* (2008) recently showed that hUCB cells have the ability to secrete multiple neurotrophic factors. Their study demonstrated elevation of neuroprotective cytokine serum IL-10 levels and depression of TNF-α levels after hUCB cell infusion. Moreover, both GDNF and VEGF could be detected in the injured spinal cord after the transplantation of hUCB cells, promoting angiogenesis and neuronal regeneration.

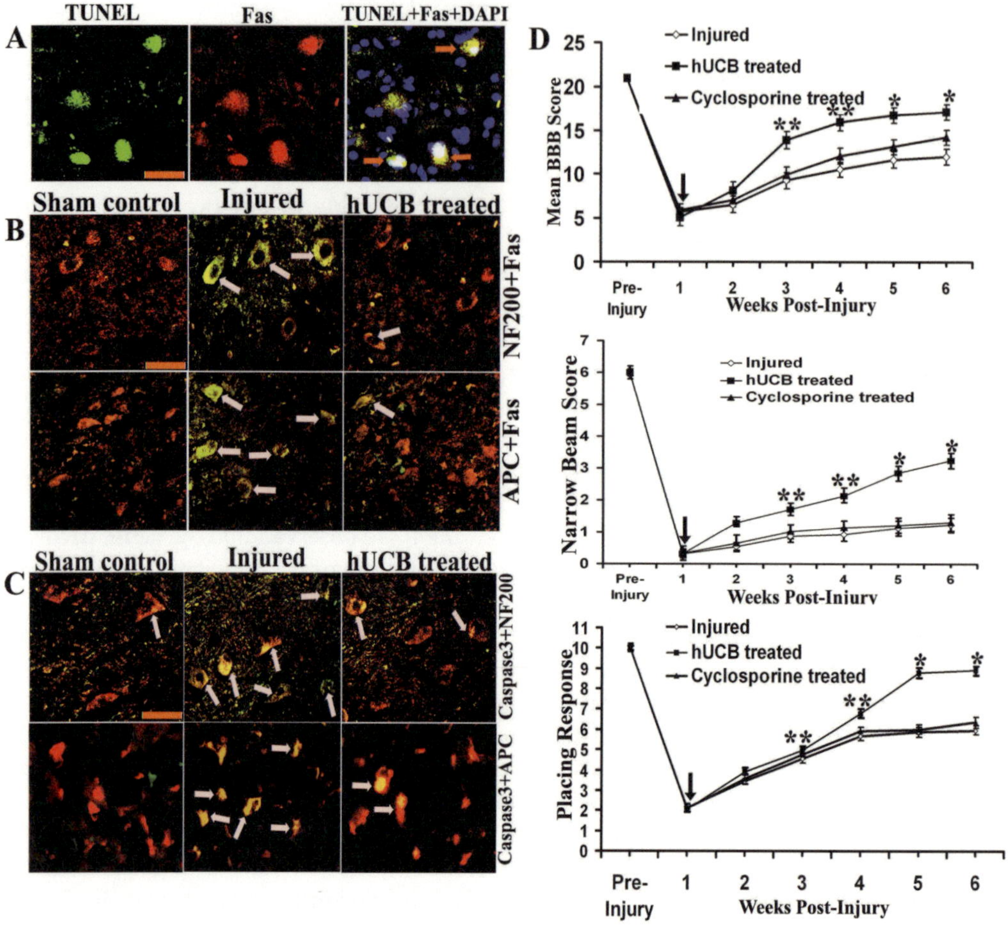

Fig. 2. Fas expression after SCI and treatment with hUCBSC: (A) Fas immunoreactivity on TUNEL positive cells. Expression of Fas (Texas-red conjugated) on TUNEL positive cells (green) from injured sections. (B) Cryo-sections showing co-localization of Fas and NF-200 (specific for neurons) and Fas and APC (mature marker for oligodendrocytes) showing expression of Fas on neurons and oligodendrocytes (↑) undergoing apoptosis. Fas is FITC-conjugated and NF-200 and APC are Texas-red conjugated. Results are from 3 sections between 1 and 2mm caudal to the injury epicenter after 3 weeks SCI (n≥3). (C) Confocal images of cryo-sections illustrate co-localization (yellow) of activated caspase-3 (FITC-conjugated) with NF-200 (Texas-red conjugated) and APC (Texas-red conjugated) within the dorsal region(↑), following spinal cord contusion. For panels A, B and C Bar = 100μm. (D) Top panel shows BBB scores of rats with SCI before and after hUCB transplantation. Repeated-measures of ANOVA followed by Bonferroni's post hoc tests showed that BBB scores in hUCB-grafted animals were significantly higher than those in injured-untreated animals. Each point represents the highest locomotor score achieved each day. Middle panel shows Narrow beam scores of injured and treated rats over a period of 6 weeks and bottom panel shows number of placing responses of injured and treated animals. Arrow (↓) indicates hUCB transplantation point. Error bars indicate ±SEM (n≥5/group) (*p<0.01 and **p<0.05)

4. Conclusions

Transplantation of mesenchymal stem cells into the injured spinal cord and therapeutic applications of mesenchymal stem cells represent exciting new approaches to managing spinal cord injury. Improvements in molecular techniques and strategies along with the availability of modified stem cell lines have fostered our understanding in the mechanism of SCI and advanced the application of stem cell transplantation for treatment of other neurological disorders beyond traumatic brain and spinal cord injury. However, cell-based therapy for SCI is still at an early stage and faces numerous challenges: among them safety problem, patient's genetic diversity and variability, differences in the extent of injury, translational clinical issues, regulatory and ethical concerns. There are numerous ongoing clinical trials utilizing MSC transplantation for treatment of various genetic and neurological disorders. However, the ultimate value of cell-based therapy will need continued expansion of basic scientific knowledge of disease processes and proven therapeutic efficacy via rigorous controlled, randomized, double blind clinical trials.

5. Acknowledgements

This research was supported by a grant from Illinois Neurological Institute to DHD. We also thank Shellee Abraham for manuscript preparation and Diana Meister and Sushma Jasti for manuscript review.

6. References

Abrams M.B., Dominguez C., Pernold K., Reger R., Wiesenfeld-Hallin Z., Olson L. et al. (2009). Multipotent mesenchymal stromal cells attenuate chronic inflammation and injury-induced sensitivity to mechanical stimuli in experimental spinal cord injury. *Restor Neurol Neurosci* 27: 307-321.

Ackery A., Tator C., & Krassioukov A. (2004). A global perspective on spinal cord injury epidemiology. *J Neurotrauma* 21: 1355-1370.

Akassoglou K., Bauer J., Kassiotis G., Pasparakis M., Lassmann H., Kollias G. et al. (1998). Oligodendrocyte apoptosis and primary demyelination induced by local TNF/p55TNF receptor signaling in the central nervous system of transgenic mice: models for multiple sclerosis with primary oligodendrogliopathy. *Am J Pathol* 153: 801-813.

Alenzi F.Q., Lotfy M., & Wyse R. (2010). Swords of cell death: caspase activation and regulation. *Asian Pac J Cancer Prev* 11: 271-280.

Alnemri E.S., Livingston D.J., Nicholson D.W., Salvesen G., Thornberry N.A., Wong W.W. et al. (1996). Human ICE/CED-3 protease nomenclature. *Cell* 87: 171.

Arai F. & Suda T. (2007). Regulation of hematopoietic stem cells in the osteoblastic niche. *Adv Exp Med Biol* 602: 61-67.

Balentine J.D. (1978). Pathology of experimental spinal cord trauma. II. Ultrastructure of axons and myelin. *Lab Invest* 39: 254-266.

Balentine J.D. & Greene W.B. (1984). Ultrastructural pathology of nerve fibers in calcium-induced myelopathy. *J Neuropathol Exp Neurol* 43: 500-510.

Banik N.L., Matzelle D., Gantt-Wilford G., & Hogan E.L. (1997). Role of calpain and its inhibitors in tissue degeneration and neuroprotection in spinal cord injury. *Ann NY Acad Sci* 825: 120-127.

Barrilleaux B., Phinney D.G., Prockop D.J., & O'Connor K.C. (2006). Review: ex vivo engineering of living tissues with adult stem cells. *Tissue Eng* 12: 3007-3019.

Barry F.P. (2003). Biology and clinical applications of mesenchymal stem cells. *Birth Defects Res C Embryo Today* 69: 250-256.

Bartholomew A., Sturgeon C., Siatskas M., Ferrer K., McIntosh K., Patil S. et al. (2002). Mesenchymal stem cells suppress lymphocyte proliferation *in vitro* and prolong skin graft survival *in vivo*. *Exp Hematol* 30: 42-48.

Beattie M.S., Hermann G.E., Rogers R.C., & Bresnahan J.C. (2002). Cell death in models of spinal cord injury. *Prog Brain Res* 137: 37-47.

Beattie M.S., Li Q., & Bresnahan J.C. (2000). Cell death and plasticity after experimental spinal cord injury. *Prog Brain Res* 128: 9-21.

Behrens A., Sibilia M., & Wagner E.F. (1999). Amino-terminal phosphorylation of c-Jun regulates stress-induced apoptosis and cellular proliferation. *Nat Genet* 21: 326-329.

Bethea J.R. & Dietrich W.D. (2002). Targeting the host inflammatory response in traumatic spinal cord injury. *Curr Opin Neurol* 15: 355-360.

Bethea J.R., Nagashima H., Acosta M.C., Briceno C., Gomez F., Marcillo A.E. et al. (1999). Systemically administered interleukin-10 reduces tumor necrosis factor-alpha production and significantly improves functional recovery following traumatic spinal cord injury in rats. *J Neurotrauma* 16: 851-863.

Blight A.R. (1985). Delayed demyelination and macrophage invasion: a candidate for secondary cell damage in spinal cord injury. *Cent Nerv Syst Trauma* 2: 299-315.

Braun J.S., Novak R., Herzog K.H., Bodner S.M., Cleveland J.L., & Tuomanen E.I. (1999). Neuroprotection by a caspase inhibitor in acute bacterial meningitis. *Nat Med* 5: 298-302.

Bresnahan J.C. (1978). An electron-microscopic analysis of axonal alterations following blunt contusion of the spinal cord of the rhesus monkey (*Macaca mulatta*). *J Neurol Sci* 37: 59-82.

Bresnahan J.C., King J.S., Martin G.F., & Yashon D. (1976). A neuroanatomical analysis of spinal cord injury in the rhesus monkey (*Macaca mulatta*). *J Neurol Sci* 28: 521-542.

Broxmeyer H.E., Douglas G.W., Hangoc G., Cooper S., Bard J., English D. et al. (1989). Human umbilical cord blood as a potential source of transplantable hematopoietic stem/progenitor cells. *Proc Natl Acad Sci USA* 86: 3828-3832.

Brunstein C.G., Setubal D.C., & Wagner J.E. (2007). Expanding the role of umbilical cord blood transplantation. *Br J Haematol* 137: 20-35.

Bryder D., Rossi D.J., & Weissman I.L. (2006). Hematopoietic stem cells: the paradigmatic tissue-specific stem cell. *Am J Pathol* 169: 338-346.

Can A. & Karahuseyinoglu S. (2007). Concise review: human umbilical cord stroma with regard to the source of fetus-derived stem cells. *Stem Cells* 25: 2886-2895.

Carlson G.D. & Gorden C. (2002). Current developments in spinal cord injury research. *Spine J* 2: 116-128.

Carlson S.L., Parrish M.E., Springer J.E., Doty K., & Dossett L. (1998). Acute inflammatory response in spinal cord following impact injury. *Exp Neurol* 151: 77-88.

Casha S., Yu W.R., & Fehlings M.G. (2001). Oligodendroglial apoptosis occurs along degenerating axons and is associated with FAS and p75 expression following spinal cord injury in the rat. *Neuroscience* 103: 203-218.

Chagraoui J., Lepage-Noll A., Anjo A., Uzan G., & Charbord P. (2003). Fetal liver stroma consists of cells in epithelial-to-mesenchymal transition. *Blood* 101: 2973-2982.

Chen C.T., Foo N.H., Liu W.S., & Chen S.H. (2008). Infusion of human umbilical cord blood cells ameliorates hind limb dysfunction in experimental spinal cord injury through anti-inflammatory, vasculogenic and neurotrophic mechanisms. *Pediatr Neonatol* 49: 77-83.

Choi C. & Benveniste E.N. (2004). Fas ligand/Fas system in the brain: regulator of immune and apoptotic responses. *Brain Res Brain Res Rev* 44: 65-81.

Choi D.W. (1988). Glutamate neurotoxicity and diseases of the nervous system. *Neuron* 1: 623-634.

Choi S.J., Lee K.H., Park H.S., Kim S.K., Koh C.M., & Park J.Y. (2005). Differential expression, shedding, cytokine regulation and function of TNFR1 and TNFR2 in human fetal astrocytes. *Yonsei Med J* 46: 818-826.

Citron B.A., Arnold P.M., Sebastian C., Qin F., Malladi S., Ameenuddin S. et al. (2000). Rapid upregulation of caspase-3 in rat spinal cord after injury: mRNA, protein, and cellular localization correlates with apoptotic cell death. *Exp Neurol* 166: 213-226.

Cizkova D., Rosocha J., Vanicky I., Jergova S., & Cizek M. (2006). Transplants of human mesenchymal stem cells improve functional recovery after spinal cord injury in the rat. *Cell Mol Neurobiol* 26: 1167-1180.

Clark B.R. & Keating A. (1995). Biology of bone marrow stroma. *Ann N Y Acad Sci* 770: 70-78.

Clark R.S., Kochanek P.M., Watkins S.C., Chen M., Dixon C.E., Seidberg N.A. et al. (2000). Caspase-3 mediated neuronal death after traumatic brain injury in rats. *J Neurochem* 74: 740-753.

Corcione A., Benvenuto F., Ferretti E., Giunti D., Cappiello V., Cazzanti F. et al. (2006). Human mesenchymal stem cells modulate B-cell functions. *Blood* 107: 367-372.

Coutts M. & Keirstead H.S. (2008). Stem cells for the treatment of spinal cord injury. *Exp Neurol* 209: 368-377.

Crowe M.J., Bresnahan J.C., Shuman S.L., Masters J.N., & Beattie M.S. (1997). Apoptosis and delayed degeneration after spinal cord injury in rats and monkeys. *Nat Med* 3: 73-76.

D'Souza S., Alinauskas K., McCrea E., Goodyer C., & Antel J.P. (1995). Differential susceptibility of human CNS-derived cell populations to TNF-dependent and independent immune-mediated injury. *J Neurosci* 15: 7293-7300.

Dasari V.R., Spomar D.G., Cady C., Gujrati M., Rao J.S., & Dinh D.H. (2007a). Mesenchymal stem cells from rat bone marrow downregulate caspase-3-mediated apoptotic pathway after spinal cord injury in rats. *Neurochem Res* 32: 2080-2093.

Dasari V.R., Spomar D.G., Gondi C.S., Sloffer C.A., Saving K.L., Gujrati M. et al. (2007b). Axonal remyelination by cord blood stem cells after spinal cord injury. *J Neurotrauma* 24: 391-410.

Dasari V.R., Spomar D.G., Li L., Gujrati M., Rao J.S., & Dinh D.H. (2008). Umbilical cord blood stem cell mediated downregulation of Fas improves functional recovery of rats after spinal cord injury. *Neurochem Res* 33: 134-149.

Dasari V.R., Veeravalli K.K., Tsung A.J., Gondi C.S., Gujrati M., Dinh D.H. et al. (2009). Neuronal apoptosis is inhibited by cord blood stem cells after spinal cord injury. *J Neurotrauma* 26: 2057-2069.

Davis R.J. (2000). Signal transduction by the JNK group of MAP kinases. *Cell* 103: 239-252.

Demjen D., Klussmann S., Kleber S., Zuliani C., Stieltjes B., Metzger C. et al. (2004). Neutralization of CD95 ligand promotes regeneration and functional recovery after spinal cord injury. *Nat Med* 10: 389-395.

Deng Y.B., Liu X.G., Liu Z.G., Liu X.L., Liu Y., Zhou G.Q. (2006). Implantation of BM mesenchymal stem cells into injured spinal cord elicits de novo neurogenesis and functional recovery: evidence from a study in rhesus monkeys. *Cytotherapy* 8:210-214.

Desbarats J., Birge R.B., Mimouni-Rongy M., Weinstein D.E., Palerme J.S., & Newell M.K. (2003). Fas engagement induces neurite growth through ERK activation and p35 upregulation. *Nat Cell Biol* 5: 118-125.

Deveraux Q.L., Leo E., Stennicke H.R., Welsh K., Salvesen G.S., & Reed J.C. (1999). Cleavage of human inhibitor of apoptosis protein XIAP results in fragments with distinct specificities for caspases. *EMBO J* 18: 5242-5251.

Di Nicola M., Carlo-Stella C., Magni M., Milanesi M., Longoni P.D., Matteucci P. et al. (2002). Human bone marrow stromal cells suppress T-lymphocyte proliferation induced by cellular or nonspecific mitogenic stimuli. *Blood* 99: 3838-3843.

Dinomais M., Stana L., Egon G., Richard I., & Menei P. (2009). Significant recovery of motor function in a patient with complete T7 paraplegia receiving etanercept. *J Rehabil Med* 41: 286-288.

Dohrmann G.J., Wagner F.C., Jr., & Bucy P.C. (1972). Transitory traumatic paraplegia: electron microscopy of early alterations in myelinated nerve fibers. *J Neurosurg* 36: 407-415.

Dolga A.M., Granic I., Blank T., Knaus H.G., Spiess J., Luiten P.G. et al. (2008). TNF-alpha-mediates neuroprotection against glutamate-induced excitotoxicity via NF-kappaB-dependent up-regulation of K2.2 channels. *J Neurochem* 107: 1158-1167.

Dusart I. & Schwab M.E. (1994). Secondary cell death and the inflammatory reaction after dorsal hemisection of the rat spinal cord. *Eur J Neurosci* 6: 712-724.

Eftekharpour E., Holmgren A., & Juurlink B.H. (2000). Thioredoxin reductase and glutathione synthesis is upregulated by t-butylhydroquinone in cortical astrocytes but not in cortical neurons. *Glia* 31: 241-248.

Eftekharpour E., Karimi-Abdolrezaee S., & Fehlings M.G. (2008). Current status of experimental cell replacement approaches to spinal cord injury. *Neurosurg Focus* 24: E19.

Eilers A., Whitfield J., Babij C., Rubin L.L., & Ham J. (1998). Role of the Jun kinase pathway in the regulation of c-Jun expression and apoptosis in sympathetic neurons. *J Neurosci* 18: 1713-1724.

Ekert P.G., Silke J., & Vaux D.L. (1999). Caspase inhibitors. *Cell Death Differ* 6: 1081-1086.

Eldadah B.A. & Faden A.I. (2000). Caspase pathways, neuronal apoptosis, and CNS injury. *J Neurotrauma* 17: 811-829.

Emery E., Aldana P., Bunge M.B., Puckett W., Srinivasan A., Keane R.W. et al. (1998). Apoptosis after traumatic human spinal cord injury. *J Neurosurg* 89: 911-920.

Enzmann G.U., Benton R.L., Talbott J.F., Cao Q., & Whittemore S.R. (2006). Functional considerations of stem cell transplantation therapy for spinal cord repair. *J Neurotrauma* 23: 479-495.

Esposito E., Genovese T., Caminiti R., Bramanti P., Meli R., & Cuzzocrea S. (2009). Melatonin reduces stress-activated/mitogen-activated protein kinases in spinal cord injury. *J Pineal Res* 46: 79-86.

Fong Y., Moldawer L.L., Marano M., Wei H., Barber A., Manogue K. et al. (1989). Cachectin/TNF or IL-1 alpha induces cachexia with redistribution of body proteins. *Am J Physiol* 256: R659-R665.

Friedenstein A.J., Chailakhyan R.K., Latsinik N.V., Panasyuk A.F., & Keiliss-Borok I.V. (1974). Stromal cells responsible for transferring the microenvironment of the hemopoietic tissues. Cloning *in vitro* and retransplantation *in vivo*. *Transplantation* 17: 331-340.

Gao Y., Signore A.P., Yin W., Cao G., Yin X.M., Sun F. et al. (2005). Neuroprotection against focal ischemic brain injury by inhibition of c-Jun N-terminal kinase and attenuation of the mitochondrial apoptosis-signaling pathway. *J Cereb Blood Flow Metab* 25: 694-712.

Garbuzova-Davis S., Willing A.E., Saporta S., Bickford P.C., Gemma C., Chen N. et al. (2006). Novel cell therapy approaches for brain repair. *Prog Brain Res* 157: 207-222.

Gillardon F., Bottiger B., Schmitz B., Zimmermann M., & Hossmann K.A. (1997). Activation of CPP-32 protease in hippocampal neurons following ischemia and epilepsy. *Brain Res Mol Brain Res* 50: 16-22.

Gluckman E., Rocha V., Boyer-Chammard A., Locatelli F., Arcese W., Pasquini R. et al. (1997). Outcome of cord-blood transplantation from related and unrelated donors. Eurocord Transplant Group and the European Blood and Marrow Transplantation Group. *N Engl J Med* 337: 373-381.

Goldbach-Mansky R., Dailey N.J., Canna S.W., Gelabert A., Jones J., Rubin B.I. et al. (2006). Neonatal-onset multisystem inflammatory disease responsive to interleukin-1beta inhibition. *N Engl J Med* 355: 581-592.

Gonz'alez Deniselle M.C., Gonz'alez S.L., & De Nicola A.F. (2001). Cellular basis of steroid neuroprotection in the wobbler mouse, a genetic model of motoneuron disease. *Cell Mol Neurobiol* 21: 237-254.

Gottron F.J., Ying H.S., & Choi D.W. (1997). Caspase inhibition selectively reduces the apoptotic component of oxygen-glucose deprivation-induced cortical neuronal cell death. *Mol Cell Neurosci* 9: 159-169.

Greitz D. (2006). Unraveling the riddle of syringomyelia. *Neurosurg Rev* 29: 251-263.

Grewal I.S. (2009). Overview of TNF superfamily: a chest full of potential therapeutic targets. *Adv Exp Med Biol* 647: 1-7.

Gronthos S., Franklin D.M., Leddy H.A., Robey P.G., Storms R.W., & Gimble J.M. (2001). Surface protein characterization of human adipose tissue-derived stromal cells. *J Cell Physiol* 189: 54-63.

Grossman S.D., Rosenberg L.J., & Wrathall J.R. (2001). Temporal-spatial pattern of acute neuronal and glial loss after spinal cord contusion. *Exp Neurol* 168: 273-282.

Gu W, Zhang F, Xue Q, Ma Z, Lu P, Yu B. (2010). Transplantation of bone marrow mesenchymal stem cells reduces lesion volume and induces axonal regrowth of injured spinal cord. *Neuropathology* 30:205-217.

Hagg T. & Oudega M. (2006). Degenerative and spontaneous regenerative processes after spinal cord injury. *J Neurotrauma* 23: 264-280.

Han I.S., Ra J.S., Kim M.W., Lee E.A., Jun H.Y., Park S.K. et al. (2003). Differentiation of CD34+ cells from human cord blood and murine bone marrow is suppressed by C6 beta-chemokines. *Mol Cells* 15: 176-180.

Hara H., Friedlander R.M., Gagliardini V., Ayata C., Fink K., Huang Z. et al. (1997). Inhibition of interleukin 1beta converting enzyme family proteases reduces ischemic and excitotoxic neuronal damage. *Proc Natl Acad Sci USA* 94: 2007-2012.

Harrington J.F., Messier A.A., Levine A., Szmydynger-Chodobska J., & Chodobski A. (2005). Shedding of tumor necrosis factor type 1 receptor after experimental spinal cord injury. *J Neurotrauma* 22: 919-928.

Harris C.A. & Johnson E.M., Jr. (2001). BH3-only Bcl-2 family members are coordinately regulated by the JNK pathway and require Bax to induce apoptosis in neurons. *J Biol Chem* 276: 37754-37760.

Hausmann O.N. (2003). Post-traumatic inflammation following spinal cord injury. *Spinal Cord* 41: 369-378.

Hayashi M., Ueyama T., Nemoto K., Tamaki T., & Senba E. (2000). Sequential mRNA expression for immediate early genes, cytokines, and neurotrophins in spinal cord injury. *J Neurotrauma* 17: 203-218.

Hemmoranta H., Hautaniemi S., Niemi J., Nicorici D., Laine J., Yli-Harja O. et al. (2006). Transcriptional profiling reflects shared and unique characters for CD34+ and CD133+ cells. *Stem Cells Dev* 15: 839-851.

Himes B.T., Neuhuber B., Coleman C., Kushner R., Swanger S.A., Kopen G.C. et al. (2006). Recovery of function following grafting of human bone marrow-derived stromal cells into the injured spinal cord. *Neurorehabil Neural Repair* 20: 278-296.

Hipp J. & Atala A. (2004). Tissue engineering, stem cells, cloning, and parthenogenesis: new paradigms for therapy. *J Exp Clin Assist Reprod* 1: 3.

Ho F.M., Liu S.H., Liau C.S., Huang P.J., & Lin-Shiau S.Y. (2000). High glucose-induced apoptosis in human endothelial cells is mediated by sequential activations of c-Jun NH(2)-terminal kinase and caspase-3. *Circulation* 101: 2618-2624.

Hofstetter C.P., Schwarz E.J., Hess D., Widenfalk J., El M.A., Prockop D.J. et al. (2002). Marrow stromal cells form guiding strands in the injured spinal cord and promote recovery. *Proc Natl Acad Sci USA* 99: 2199-2204.

Holmes G.M., Hebert S.L., Rogers R.C., & Hermann G.E. (2004). Immunocytochemical localization of TNF type 1 and type 2 receptors in the rat spinal cord. *Brain Res* 1025: 210-219.

Hu S.L., Luo H.S., Li J.T., Xia Y.Z., Li L., Zhang L.J., Meng H., Cui G.Y., Chen Z., Wu N., Lin J.K., Zhu G., Feng H. (2010) Functional recovery in acute traumatic spinal cord injury after transplantation of human umbilical cord mesenchymal stem cells. *Crit Care Med.* 38:2181-2189.

Inoshita S., Takeda K., Hatai T., Terada Y., Sano M., Hata J. et al. (2002). Phosphorylation and inactivation of myeloid cell leukemia 1 by JNK in response to oxidative stress. *J Biol Chem* 277: 43730-43734.

Isele N.B., Lee H.S., Landshamer S., Straube A., Padovan C.S., Plesnila N. et al. (2007). Bone marrow stromal cells mediate protection through stimulation of PI3-K/Akt and MAPK signaling in neurons. *Neurochem Int* 50: 243-250.

Jankowski R.J., Deasy B.M., & Huard J. (2002). Muscle-derived stem cells. *Gene Ther* 9: 642-647.

Jiang X.X., Zhang Y., Liu B., Zhang S.X., Wu Y., Yu X.D. et al. (2005). Human mesenchymal stem cells inhibit differentiation and function of monocyte-derived dendritic cells. *Blood* 105: 4120-4126.

Juurlink B.H. & Paterson P.G. (1998). Review of oxidative stress in brain and spinal cord injury: suggestions for pharmacological and nutritional management strategies. *J Spinal Cord Med* 21: 309-334.

Kang S.J., Wang S., Hara H., Peterson E.P., Namura S., min-Hanjani S. et al. (2000). Dual role of caspase-11 in mediating activation of caspase-1 and caspase-3 under pathological conditions. *J Cell Biol* 149: 613-622.

Kao C.H., Chen S.H., Chio C.C., & Lin M.T. (2008). Human umbilical cord blood-derived CD34+ cells may attenuate spinal cord injury by stimulating vascular endothelial and neurotrophic factors. *Shock* 29: 49-55.

Kawasaki Y., Zhang L., Cheng J.K., & Ji R.R. (2008). Cytokine mechanisms of central sensitization: distinct and overlapping role of interleukin-1beta, interleukin-6, and tumor necrosis factor-alpha in regulating synaptic and neuronal activity in the superficial spinal cord. *J Neurosci* 28: 5189-5194.

Keane R.W., Davis A.R., & Dietrich W.D. (2006). Inflammatory and apoptotic signaling after spinal cord injury. *J Neurotrauma* 23: 335-344.

Keane R.W., Kraydieh S., Lotocki G., Alonso O.F., Aldana P., & Dietrich W.D. (2001). Apoptotic and antiapoptotic mechanisms after traumatic brain injury. *J Cereb Blood Flow Metab* 21: 1189-1198.

Kim G.M., Xu J., Xu J., Song S.K., Yan P., Ku G. et al. (2001). Tumor necrosis factor receptor deletion reduces nuclear factor-kappaB activation, cellular inhibitor of apoptosis protein 2 expression, and functional recovery after traumatic spinal cord injury. *J Neurosci* 21: 6617-6625.

Kim S.K., Koh S.K., Song S.U., Shin S.H., Choi G.S., Kim W.C. et al. (2002). Ex vivo expansion and clonality of CD34+ selected cells from bone marrow and cord blood in a serum-free media. *Mol Cells* 14: 367-373.

Kim T.H., Zhao Y., Barber M.J., Kuharsky D.K., & Yin X.M. (2000). Bid-induced cytochrome c release is mediated by a pathway independent of mitochondrial permeability transition pore and Bax. *J Biol Chem* 275: 39474-39481.

Kotipatruni R.R., Dasari V.R., Veeravalli K.K., Dinh D.H., Fassett D., & Rao J.S. (2011). p53- and Bax-Mediated Apoptosis in Injured Rat Spinal Cord. *Neurochem Res* e-pub ahead of print.

Kuh S.U., Cho Y.E., Yoon D.H., Kim K.N., & Ha Y. (2005). Functional recovery after human umbilical cord blood cells transplantation with brain-derived neutrophic factor into the spinal cord injured rat. *Acta Neurochir (Wien)* 147: 985-992.

Kuwana T., Smith J.J., Muzio M., Dixit V., Newmeyer D.D., & Kornbluth S. (1998). Apoptosis induction by caspase-8 is amplified through the mitochondrial release of cytochrome c. *J Biol Chem* 273: 16589-16594.

Lee K.H., Suh-Kim H., Choi J.S., Jeun S.S., Kim E.J., Kim S.S., Yoon do H., Lee B.H. (2007) Human mesenchymal stem cell transplantation promotes functional recovery following acute spinal cord injury in rats. *Acta Neurobiol Exp (Wars)*. 67:13-22.

Lee Y.B., Yune T.Y., Baik S.Y., Shin Y.H., Du S., Rhim H. et al. (2000). Role of tumor necrosis factor-alpha in neuronal and glial apoptosis after spinal cord injury. *Exp Neurol* 166: 190-195.

Leung L. & Cahill C.M. (2010). TNF-alpha and neuropathic pain--a review. *J Neuroinflammation* 7: 27-38.

Li G.L., Brodin G., Farooque M., Funa K., Holtz A., Wang W.L. et al. (1996). Apoptosis and expression of Bcl-2 after compression trauma to rat spinal cord. *J Neuropathol Exp Neurol* 55: 280-289.

Li H., Zhu H., Xu C.J., & Yuan J. (1998). Cleavage of BID by caspase 8 mediates the mitochondrial damage in the Fas pathway of apoptosis. *Cell* 94: 491-501.

Li M., Ona V.O., Chen M., Kaul M., Tenneti L., Zhang X. et al. (2000a). Functional role and therapeutic implications of neuronal caspase-1 and -3 in a mouse model of traumatic spinal cord injury. *Neuroscience* 99: 333-342.

Li M., Ona V.O., Guegan C., Chen M., Jackson-Lewis V., Andrews L.J. et al. (2000b). Functional role of caspase-1 and caspase-3 in an ALS transgenic mouse model. *Science* 288: 335-339.

Li Q.M., Tep C., Yune T.Y., Zhou X.Z., Uchida T., Lu K.P. et al. (2007). Opposite regulation of oligodendrocyte apoptosis by JNK3 and Pin1 after spinal cord injury. *J Neurosci* 27: 8395-8404.

Lim J.H., Byeon Y.E., Ryu H.H., Jeong Y.H., Lee Y.W., Kim W.H., Kang K. S., Kweon O.K. (2007) Transplantation of canine umbilical cord blood-derived mesenchymal stem cells in experimentally induced spinal cord injured dogs. *J Vet Sci.* 8:275-282.

Liu X.Z., Xu X.M., Hu R., Du C., Zhang S.X., McDonald J.W. et al. (1997). Neuronal and glial apoptosis after traumatic spinal cord injury. *J Neurosci* 17: 5395-5406.

Lou J., Lenke L.G., Ludwig F.J., & O'Brien M.F. (1998). Apoptosis as a mechanism of neuronal cell death following acute experimental spinal cord injury. *Spinal Cord* 36: 683-690.

Lu J., Ashwell K.W., & Waite P. (2000). Advances in secondary spinal cord injury: role of apoptosis. *Spine* 25: 1859-1866.

Lu L.L., Liu Y.J., Yang S.G., Zhao Q.J., Wang X., Gong W. et al. (2006). Isolation and characterization of human umbilical cord mesenchymal stem cells with hematopoiesis-supportive function and other potentials. *Haematologica* 91: 1017-1026.

Ma Y., Xu Y., Xiao Z., Yang W., Zhang C., Song E. et al. (2006). Reconstruction of chemically burned rat corneal surface by bone marrow-derived human mesenchymal stem cells. *Stem Cells* 24: 315-321.

Malgieri A., Kantzari E., Patrizi M.P., & Gambardella S. (2010). Bone marrow and umbilical cord blood human mesenchymal stem cells: state of the art. *Int J Clin Exp Med* 3: 248-269.

Martin-Villalba A., Herr I., Jeremias I., Hahne M., Brandt R., Vogel J. et al. (1999). CD95 ligand (Fas-L/APO-1L) and tumor necrosis factor-related apoptosis-inducing ligand mediate ischemia-induced apoptosis in neurons. *J Neurosci* 19: 3809-3817.

Maundrell K., Antonsson B., Magnenat E., Camps M., Muda M., Chabert C. et al. (1997). Bcl-2 undergoes phosphorylation by c-Jun N-terminal kinase/stress-activated protein kinases in the presence of the constitutively active GTP-binding protein Rac1. *J Biol Chem* 272: 25238-25242.

Mayani H. & Lansdorp P.M. (1998). Biology of human umbilical cord blood-derived hematopoietic stem/progenitor cells. *Stem Cells* 16: 153-165.

Means E.D. & Anderson D.K. (1983). Neuronophagia by leukocytes in experimental spinal cord injury. *J Neuropathol Exp Neurol* 42: 707-719.

Mendez-Ferrer S., Michurina T.V., Ferraro F., Mazloom A.R., Macarthur B.D., Lira S.A. et al. (2010). Mesenchymal and haematopoietic stem cells form a unique bone marrow niche. *Nature* 466: 829-834.

Mimeault M. & Batra S.K. (2006). Concise review: recent advances on the significance of stem cells in tissue regeneration and cancer therapies. *Stem Cells* 24: 2319-2345.

Miura M., Gronthos S., Zhao M., Lu B., Fisher L.W., Robey P.G. et al. (2003). SHED: stem cells from human exfoliated deciduous teeth. *Proc Natl Acad Sci U S A* 100: 5807-5812.

Moore K.E., Mills J.F., & Thornton M.M. (2006). Alternative sources of adult stem cells: a possible solution to the embryonic stem cell debate. *Gend Med* 3: 161-168.

Nakagawa T. & Yuan J. (2000). Cross-talk between two cysteine protease families. Activation of caspase-12 by calpain in apoptosis. *J Cell Biol* 150: 887-894.

Nakahara S., Yone K., Sakou T., Wada S., Nagamine T., Niiyama T. et al. (1999). Induction of apoptosis signal regulating kinase 1 (ASK1) after spinal cord injury in rats: possible involvement of ASK1-JNK and -p38 pathways in neuronal apoptosis. *J Neuropathol Exp Neurol* 58: 442-450.

Namura S., Zhu J., Fink K., Endres M., Srinivasan A., Tomaselli K.J. et al. (1998). Activation and cleavage of caspase-3 in apoptosis induced by experimental cerebral ischemia. *J Neurosci* 18: 3659-3668.

Nashmi R. & Fehlings M.G. (2001). Mechanisms of axonal dysfunction after spinal cord injury: with an emphasis on the role of voltage-gated potassium channels. *Brain Res Brain Res Rev* 38: 165-191.

Neuhuber B., Timothy H.B., Shumsky J.S., Gallo G., & Fischer I. (2005). Axon growth and recovery of function supported by human bone marrow stromal cells in the injured spinal cord exhibit donor variations. *Brain Res* 1035: 73-85.

Nicholson D.W. (2000). From bench to clinic with apoptosis-based therapeutic agents. *Nature* 407: 810-816.

Noth U., Osyczka A.M., Tuli R., Hickok N.J., Danielson K.G., & Tuan R.S. (2002). Multilineage mesenchymal differentiation potential of human trabecular bone-derived cells. *J Orthop Res* 20: 1060-1069.

Okuno S., Saito A., Hayashi T., & Chan P.H. (2004). The c-Jun N-terminal protein kinase signaling pathway mediates Bax activation and subsequent neuronal apoptosis through interaction with Bim after transient focal cerebral ischemia. *J Neurosci* 24: 7879-7887.

Osaka M., Honmou O., Murakami T., Nonaka T., Houkin K., Hamada H., Kocsis J. D. (2010) Intravenous administration of mesenchymal stem cells derived from bone marrow after contusive spinal cord injury improves functional outcome. *Brain Res.* 1343:226-235.

Park D.H., Lee J.H., Borlongan C.V., Sanberg P.R., Chung Y.G., & Cho T.H. (2011). Transplantation of umbilical cord blood stem cells for treating spinal cord injury. *Stem Cell Rev* 7: 181-194.

Park D.S., Stefanis L., Yan C.Y., Farinelli S.E., & Greene L.A. (1996). Ordering the cell death pathway. Differential effects of BCL2, an interleukin-1-converting enzyme family protease inhibitor, and other survival agents on JNK activation in serum/nerve growth factor-deprived PC12 cells. *J Biol Chem* 271: 21898-21905.

Park H.C., Shim Y.S., Ha Y., Yoon S.H., Park S.R., Choi B.H. et al. (2005). Treatment of complete spinal cord injury patients by autologous bone marrow cell transplantation and administration of granulocyte-macrophage colony stimulating factor. *Tissue Eng* 11: 913-922.

Parr A.M., Kulbatski I., Wang X.H., Keating A., Tator C.H. (2008) Fate of transplanted adult neural stem/progenitor cells and bone marrow-derived mesenchymal stromal cells in the injured adult rat spinal cord and impact on functional recovery. *Surg Neurol.* 70:600-607; discussion 607.

Pessina A. & Gribaldo L. (2006). The key role of adult stem cells: therapeutic perspectives. *Curr Med Res Opin* 22: 2287-2300.

Phinney D.G., Baddoo M., Dutreil M., Gaupp D., Lai W.T., & Isakova I.A. (2006). Murine mesenchymal stem cells transplanted to the central nervous system of neonatal versus adult mice exhibit distinct engraftment kinetics and express receptors that guide neuronal cell migration. *Stem Cells Dev* 15: 437-447.

Phinney D.G. & Prockop D.J. (2007). Concise review: mesenchymal stem/multipotent stromal cells: the state of transdifferentiation and modes of tissue repair--current views. *Stem Cells* 25: 2896-2902.

Pittenger M.F., Mackay A.M., Beck S.C., Jaiswal R.K., Douglas R., Mosca J.D. et al. (1999). Multilineage potential of adult human mesenchymal stem cells. *Science* 284: 143-147.

Popovich P.G., Wei P., & Stokes B.T. (1997). Cellular inflammatory response after spinal cord injury in Sprague-Dawley and Lewis rats. *J Comp Neurol* 377: 443-464.

Poyet J.L., Srinivasula S.M., Lin J.H., Fernandes-Alnemri T., Yamaoka S., Tsichlis P.N. et al. (2000). Activation of the Ikappa B kinases by RIP via IKKgamma /NEMO-mediated oligomerization. *J Biol Chem* 275: 37966-37977.

Putcha G.V., Le S., Frank S., Besirli C.G., Clark K., Chu B. et al. (2003). JNK-mediated BIM phosphorylation potentiates BAX-dependent apoptosis. *Neuron* 38:899-914.

Putcha G.V., Moulder K.L., Golden J.P., Bouillet P., Adams J.A., Strasser A. et al. (2001). Induction of BIM, a proapoptotic BH3-only BCL-2 family member, is critical for neuronal apoptosis. *Neuron* 29: 615-628.

Raoul C., Estevez A.G., Nishimune H., Cleveland D.W., deLapeyriere O., Henderson C.E. et al. (2002). Motoneuron death triggered by a specific pathway downstream of Fas. potentiation by ALS-linked SOD1 mutations. *Neuron* 35: 1067-1083.

Rice T., Larsen J., Rivest S., & Yong V.W. (2007). Characterization of the early neuroinflammation after spinal cord injury in mice. *J Neuropathol Exp Neurol* 66: 184-195.

Rincon M., Whitmarsh A., Yang D.D., Weiss L., Derijard B., Jayaraj P. et al. (1998). The JNK pathway regulates the In vivo deletion of immature CD4(+)CD8(+) thymocytes. *J Exp Med* 188: 1817-1830.

Sabapathy K., Hu Y., Kallunki T., Schreiber M., David J.P., Jochum W. et al. (1999). JNK2 is required for efficient T-cell activation and apoptosis but not for normal lymphocyte development. *Curr Biol* 9: 116-125.

Salvesen G.S. & Dixit V.M. (1999). Caspase activation: the induced-proximity model. *Proc Natl Acad Sci USA* 96: 10964-10967.

Sanberg P.R., Willing A.E., Garbuzova-Davis S., Saporta S., Liu G., Sanberg C.D. et al. (2005). Umbilical cord blood-derived stem cells and brain repair. *Ann NY Acad Sci* 1049: 67-83.

Saporta S., Kim J.J., Willing A.E., Fu E.S., Davis C.D., & Sanberg P.R. (2003). Human umbilical cord blood stem cells infusion in spinal cord injury: engraftment and beneficial influence on behavior. *J Hematother Stem Cell Res* 12: 271-278.

Sarugaser R., Lickorish D., Baksh D., Hosseini M.M., & Davies J.E. (2005). Human umbilical cord perivascular (HUCPV) cells: a source of mesenchymal progenitors. *Stem Cells* 23: 220-229.

Satake K., Lou J., Lenke L.G. (2004) Migration of mesenchymal stem cells through cerebrospinal fluid into injured spinal cord tissue. *Spine (Phila Pa 1976).* 29:1971-1979.

Scaffidi C., Fulda S., Srinivasan A., Friesen C., Li F., Tomaselli K.J. et al. (1998). Two CD95 (APO-1/Fas) signaling pathways. *EMBO J* 17: 1675-1687.

Schotte P., Van C.W., Van de C.M., Van L.G., Desmedt M., Grooten J. et al. (1998). Cathepsin B-mediated activation of the proinflammatory caspase-11. *Biochem Biophys Res Commun* 251: 379-387.

Sekhon L.H. & Fehlings M.G. (2001). Epidemiology, demographics, and pathophysiology of acute spinal cord injury. *Spine (Phila Pa)* 26: S2-12.

Sharma H.S. (2007). A select combination of neurotrophins enhances neuroprotection and functional recovery following spinal cord injury. *Ann N Y Acad Sci* 1122: 95-111.

Sharma H.S. (2008). New perspectives for the treatment options in spinal cord injury. *Expert Opin Pharmacother* 9: 2773-2800.

Sharma H.S. (2010). A combination of tumor necrosis factor-alpha and neuronal nitric oxide synthase antibodies applied topically over the traumatized spinal cord enhances neuroprotection and functional recovery in the rat. *Ann N Y Acad Sci* 1199: 175-185.

Sharma H.S., Olsson Y., & Nyberg F. (1995). Influence of dynorphin A antibodies on the formation of edema and cell changes in spinal cord trauma. *Prog Brain Res* 104: 401-416.

Shuman S.L., Bresnahan J.C., & Beattie M.S. (1997). Apoptosis of microglia and oligodendrocytes after spinal cord contusion in rats. *J Neurosci Res* 50: 798-808.

Sipe K.J., Srisawasdi D., Dantzer R., Kelley K.W., & Weyhenmeyer J.A. (1996). An endogenous 55 kDa TNF receptor mediates cell death in a neural cell line. *Brain Res Mol Brain Res* 38: 222-232.

Slee E.A., Harte M.T., Kluck R.M., Wolf B.B., Casiano C.A., Newmeyer D.D. et al. (1999). Ordering the cytochrome c-initiated caspase cascade: hierarchical activation of caspases-2, -3, -6, -7, -8, and -10 in a caspase-9-dependent manner. *J Cell Biol* 144: 281-292.

Spees J.L., Olson S.D., Ylostalo J., Lynch P.J., Smith J., Perry A. et al. (2003). Differentiation, cell fusion, and nuclear fusion during *ex vivo* repair of epithelium by human adult stem cells from bone marrow stroma. *Proc Natl Acad Sci U S A* 100: 2397-2402.

Springer J.E., Azbill R.D., & Knapp P.E. (1999). Activation of the caspase-3 apoptotic cascade in traumatic spinal cord injury. *Nat Med* 5: 943-946.

Stalberg E., Sharma H.S., & Olsson Y. (1998). *Spinal Cord Monitoring. Basic principles, regeneration, pathophysiology and clinical aspects.*, Springer, Wien., New York.

Stanworth S.J. & Newland A.C. (2001). Stem cells: progress in research and edging towards the clinical setting. *Clin Med* 1: 378-382.

Stennicke H.R., Jurgensmeier J.M., Shin H., Deveraux Q., Wolf B.B., Yang X. et al. (1998). Pro-caspase-3 is a major physiologic target of caspase-8. *J Biol Chem* 273: 27084-27090.

Streit W.J., Semple-Rowland S.L., Hurley S.D., Miller R.C., Popovich P.G., & Stokes B.T. (1998). Cytokine mRNA profiles in contused spinal cord and axotomized facial nucleus suggest a beneficial role for inflammation and gliosis. *Exp Neurol* 152: 74-87.

Sykova E., Jendelova P., Urdzikova L., Lesny P., & Hejcl A. (2006). Bone marrow stem cells and polymer hydrogels--two strategies for spinal cord injury repair. *Cell Mol Neurobiol* 26: 1113-1129.

Taguchi A., Soma T., Tanaka H., Kanda T., Nishimura H., Yoshikawa H. et al. (2004). Administration of CD34+ cells after stroke enhances neurogenesis via angiogenesis in a mouse model. *J Clin Invest* 114: 330-338.

Taoka Y. & Okajima K. (1998). Spinal cord injury in the rat. *Prog Neurobiol* 56: 341-358.

Taoka Y., Okajima K., Murakami K., Johno M., & Naruo M. (1998). Role of neutrophil elastase in compression-induced spinal cord injury in rats. *Brain Res* 799: 264-269.

Tartaglia L.A., Weber R.F., Figari I.S., Reynolds C., Palladino M.A., Jr., & Goeddel D.V. (1991). The two different receptors for tumor necrosis factor mediate distinct cellular responses. *Proc Natl Acad Sci USA* 88: 9292-9296.

Tator C.H. & Fehlings M.G. (1991). Review of the secondary injury theory of acute spinal cord trauma with emphasis on vascular mechanisms. *J Neurosurg* 75: 15-26.

Thornberry N.A. & Lazebnik Y. (1998). Caspases: enemies within. *Science* 281: 1312-1316.

Totoiu M.O. & Keirstead H.S. (2005). Spinal cord injury is accompanied by chronic progressive demyelination. *J Comp Neurol* 486: 373-383.

Tournier C., Dong C., Turner T.K., Jones S.N., Flavell R.A., & Davis R.J. (2001). MKK7 is an essential component of the JNK signal transduction pathway activated by proinflammatory cytokines. *Genes Dev* 15: 1419-1426.

Tournier C., Hess P., Yang D.D., Xu J., Turner T.K., Nimnual A. et al. (2000). Requirement of JNK for stress-induced activation of the cytochrome c-mediated death pathway. *Science* 288: 870-874.

Tracey K.J. (2011). Tumor necrosis factor. In: *The Cytokine Handbook*. Thompson A.W. (ed)., pp. 289-304, Academic Press: New York.

Trivedi A., Olivas A.D., & Noble-Haeusslein L.J. (2006). Inflammation and Spinal Cord Injury: Infiltrating Leukocytes as Determinants of Injury and Repair Processes. *Clin Neurosci Res* 6: 283-292.

Tsujimoto Y. (2003). Cell death regulation by the Bcl-2 protein family in the mitochondria. *J Cell Physiol* 195: 158-167.

Tsujimoto Y. & Shimizu S. (2000). Bcl-2 family: life-or-death switch. *FEBS Lett* 466: 6-10.

Uccelli A., Benvenuto F., Laroni A., & Giunti D. (2011). Neuroprotective features of mesenchymal stem cells. *Best Pract Res Clin Haematol* 24: 59-64.

Vandenabeele P., Declercq W., Beyaert R., & Fiers W. (1995). Two tumour necrosis factor receptors: structure and function. *Trends Cell Biol* 5: 392-399.

Varfolomeev E.E. & Ashkenazi A. (2004). Tumor necrosis factor: an apoptosis JuNKie? *Cell* 116: 491-497.

Veeravalli K.K., Dasari V.R., Tsung A.J., Dinh D.H., Gujrati M., Fassett D. et al. (2009a). Human umbilical cord blood stem cells upregulate matrix metalloproteinase-2 in rats after spinal cord injury. *Neurobiol Dis* 36: 200-212.

Veeravalli K.K., Dasari V.R., Tsung A.J., Dinh D.H., Gujrati M., Fassett D. et al. (2009b). Stem Cells Downregulate the Elevated Levels of Tissue Plasminogen Activator in Rats After Spinal Cord Injury. *Neurochem Res* 34: 1183-1194.

Verhagen A.M., Ekert P.G., Pakusch M., Silke J., Connolly L.M., Reid G.E. et al. (2000). Identification of DIABLO, a mammalian protein that promotes apoptosis by binding to and antagonizing IAP proteins. *Cell* 102: 43-53.

Wagner F., Dhormann G., & Bucy P. (1971). Histopathology of transitory traumatic paraplegia in the monkey. *J Neurosurg* 35: 272-276.

Waldner H., Sobel R.A., Howard E., & Kuchroo V.K. (1997). Fas- and FasL-deficient mice are resistant to induction of autoimmune encephalomyelitis. *J Immunol* 159: 3100-3103.

Wang C.X., Nuttin B., Heremans H., Dom R., & Gybels J. (1996). Production of tumor necrosis factor in spinal cord following traumatic injury in rats. *J Neuroimmunol* 69: 151-156.

Wang C.X., Reece C., Wrathall J.R., Shuaib A., Olschowka J.A., & Hao C. (2002). Expression of tumor necrosis factor alpha and its mRNA in the spinal cord following a weight-drop injury. *Neuroreport* 13: 1391-1393.

Wang S., Miura M., Jung Y.K., Zhu H., Li E., & Yuan J. (1998). Murine caspase-11, an ICE-interacting protease, is essential for the activation of ICE. *Cell* 92: 501-509.

Warden P., Bamber N.I., Li H., Esposito A., Ahmad K.A., Hsu C.Y. et al. (2001). Delayed glial cell death following wallerian degeneration in white matter tracts after spinal cord dorsal column cordotomy in adult rats. *Exp Neurol* 168: 213-224.

Weiss M.L. & Troyer D.L. (2006). Stem cells in the umbilical cord. *Stem Cell Rev* 2: 155-162.

Whitfield J., Neame S.J., Paquet L., Bernard O., & Ham J. (2001). Dominant-negative c-Jun promotes neuronal survival by reducing BIM expression and inhibiting mitochondrial cytochrome c release. *Neuron* 29: 629-643.

Wilson P.G. & Stice S.S. (2006). Development and differentiation of neural rosettes derived from human embryonic stem cells. *Stem Cell Rev* 2: 67-77.

Woodbury D., Schwarz E.J., Prockop D.J., & Black I.B. (2000). Adult rat and human bone marrow stromal cells differentiate into neurons. *J Neurosci Res* 61: 364-370.

Wright K.T., Masri W.E., Osman A., Chowdhury J., & Johnson W.E. (2011). Concise review: bone marrow for the treatment of spinal cord injury: mechanisms and clinical applications. *Stem Cells* 29: 169-178.

Wu K.H., Zhou B., Lu S.H., Feng B., Yang S.G., Du W.T. et al. (2007). *In vitro* and *in vivo* differentiation of human umbilical cord derived stem cells into endothelial cells. *J Cell Biochem* 100: 608-616.

Wyllie A.H., Kerr J.F., & Currie A.R. (1980). Cell death: the significance of apoptosis. *Int Rev Cytol* 68: 251-306.

Xia Z., Dickens M., Raingeaud J., Davis R.J., & Greenberg M.E. (1995). Opposing effects of ERK and JNK-p38 MAP kinases on apoptosis. *Science* 270: 1326-1331.

Yakovlev A.G. & Faden A.I. (2001). Caspase-dependent apoptotic pathways in CNS injury. *Mol Neurobiol* 24: 131-144.

Yakovlev A.G., Knoblach S.M., Fan L., Fox G.B., Goodnight R., & Faden A.I. (1997). Activation of CPP32-like caspases contributes to neuronal apoptosis and neurological dysfunction after traumatic brain injury. *J Neurosci* 17: 7415-7424.

Yamamoto K., Ichijo H., & Korsmeyer S.J. (1999). BCL-2 is phosphorylated and inactivated by an ASK1/Jun N-terminal protein kinase pathway normally activated at G(2)/M. *Mol Cell Biol* 19: 8469-8478.

Yamashima T. (2000). Implication of cysteine proteases calpain, cathepsin and caspase in ischemic neuronal death of primates. *Prog Neurobiol* 62: 273-295.

Yan P., Li Q., Kim G.M., Xu J., Hsu C.Y., & Xu X.M. (2001). Cellular localization of tumor necrosis factor-alpha following acute spinal cord injury in adult rats. *J Neurotrauma* 18: 563-568.

Yan P., Liu N., Kim G.M., Xu J., Xu J., Li Q. et al. (2003). Expression of the type 1 and type 2 receptors for tumor necrosis factor after traumatic spinal cord injury in adult rats. *Exp Neurol* 183: 286-297.

Yang C.C., Shih Y.H., Ko M.H., Hsu S.Y., Cheng H, Fu Y.S. (2008) Transplantation of human umbilical mesenchymal stem cells from Wharton's jelly after complete transection of the rat spinal cord. *PLoS One*. 3(10):e3336.

Yang D., Tournier C., Wysk M., Lu H.T., Xu J., Davis R.J. et al. (1997a). Targeted disruption of the MKK4 gene causes embryonic death, inhibition of c-Jun NH2-terminal kinase activation, and defects in AP-1 transcriptional activity. *Proc Natl Acad Sci USA* 94: 3004-3009.

Yang D.D., Kuan C.Y., Whitmarsh A.J., Rincon M., Zheng T.S., Davis R.J. et al. (1997b). Absence of excitotoxicity-induced apoptosis in the hippocampus of mice lacking the Jnk3 gene. *Nature* 389: 865-870.

Yin K.J., Kim G.M., Lee J.M., He Y.Y., Xu J., & Hsu C.Y. (2005). JNK activation contributes to DP5 induction and apoptosis following traumatic spinal cord injury. *Neurobiol Dis* 20: 881-889.

Yong C., Arnold P.M., Zoubine M.N., Citron B.A., Watanabe I., Berman N.E. et al. (1998). Apoptosis in cellular compartments of rat spinal cord after severe contusion injury. *J Neurotrauma* 15: 459-472.

Yoshino O., Matsuno H., Nakamura H., Yudoh K., Abe Y., Sawai T. et al. (2004). The role of Fas-mediated apoptosis after traumatic spinal cord injury. *Spine* 29: 1394-1404.

Yu S.W., Andrabi S.A., Wang H., Kim N.S., Poirier G.G., Dawson T.M. et al. (2006). Apoptosis-inducing factor mediates poly(ADP-ribose) (PAR) polymer-induced cell death. *Proc Natl Acad Sci USA* 103: 18314-18319.

Yu W.R., Liu T., Fehlings T.K., & Fehlings M.G. (2009). Involvement of mitochondrial signaling pathways in the mechanism of Fas-mediated apoptosis after spinal cord injury. *Eur J Neurosci* 29: 114-131.

Yune T.Y., Chang M.J., Kim S.J., Lee Y.B., Shin S.W., Rhim H. et al. (2003). Increased production of tumor necrosis factor-alpha induces apoptosis after traumatic spinal cord injury in rats. *J Neurotrauma* 20: 207-219.

Zeng X., Zeng Y.S., Ma Y.H., Lu L.Y., Du B.L., Zhang W. et al. (2011). Bone Marrow Mesenchymal Stem Cells in a Three Dimensional Gelatin Sponge Scaffold Attenuate Inflammation, Promote Angiogenesis and Reduce Cavity Formation in Experimental Spinal Cord Injury. *Cell Transplant.*

Zhang L., Liu Y., Lu L., Wang A., Xu Z., & Zhu X. (2006). Mesenchymal stem cells derived from human umbilical cord inhibit activation and proliferation of allogenic umbilical cord blood. *Chin J Cancer Biother* 13: 191-195.

Zhang S.Q., Kovalenko A., Cantarella G., & Wallach D. (2000). Recruitment of the IKK signalosome to the p55 TNF receptor: RIP and A20 bind to NEMO (IKKgamma) upon receptor stimulation. *Immunity* 12: 301-311.

19

Modelling Multiple Sclerosis *In Vitro* and the Influence of Activated Macrophages

E.J.F. Vereyken, C.D. Dijkstra and C.E. Teunissen
VU University Medical Center
Amsterdam,
The Netherlands

1. Introduction

Multiple sclerosis (MS) is a chronic inflammatory disease of the central nervous system (CNS). The prevalence of MS is approximately 2 million people worldwide, with an incidence of about 1:1000 in Europe and Northern America, and women are affected more often compared to men, at a ratio of approximately 2:1. It is the most common cause of neurological disability among young adults with an onset generally between 20 and 40 years of age [Pugliatti et al., 2002]. The major neuropathological hallmarks of MS are demyelinating lesions associated with perivascular infiltrates, consisting of macrophages/microglia and lymphocytes. The lesions are characterized by destruction of myelin sheaths, oligodendrocyte death, axonal damage and glial scar formation, called astrogliosis. Demyelination is a central event in MS pathology. Although some remyelination occurs, it ultimately fails [Franklin, 2002]. The cause of the remyelination failure is not clear, although several processes have been suggested to play a role [Franklin and Ffrench-Constant, 2008; Wolswijk, 2002; John et al., 2002]. Not only processes behind remyelination failure remain elusive, also the cellular mechanisms behind the demyelination and axonal damage are largely unknown. Modelling MS both in animals and *in vitro* could help with understanding this.
This chapter will focus on MS pathology and the models that exist for investigating this disease, especially zooming in on *in vitro* models.

2. Multiple sclerosis

2.1 Clinical symptoms and diagnosis

MS is characterized by multiple sclerotic lesions affecting areas such as the cerebellum, cerebrum (periventricular white matter), optic nerve, brainstem and spinal cord [Compston and Coles, 2008]. The clinical symptoms of MS are very heterogeneous depending on the location, size and number of lesions. Symptoms include motor function disturbances, such as muscle weakness, tremor and paralysis, and progressive sensory malfunction, for instance impaired vision. The main criterion for diagnosis of MS is the occurrence of two (or more) independent episodes of clinical symptoms consistent with focal demyelination separated in space (part of the CNS) and time (more than one occasion) [Polman et al., 2011; McDonald et al., 2001]. Magnetic resonance imaging (MRI) techniques have become very important for verification of diagnosis [Barkhof et al., 1997; Nielsen et al., 2005; Polman et al., 2005], for detection of the number and size of the lesions and to differentiate between ongoing inflammation and blood-brain-barrier leakage [Bruck et al., 1997; Miller et al., 1998; Nesbit et al., 1991; Katz et al., 1993]. The presence of oligoclonal bands in cerebrospinal fluid (CSF) of MS patients and elevated immunoglobulin G (IgG) levels are supportive of MS diagnosis [Polman et al., 2011]. Furthermore, they corroborate the inflammatory demyelinating nature of the underlying condition, are used to evaluate alternative diagnoses and to predict clinical definite MS [Correale and de los Milagros Bassani Molinas, 2002]. In approximately 90% of MS patients oligoclonal immunoglobulin bands are detected [Bourahoui et al., 2004]. These oligoclonal bands are also detected in other neurological diseases, although not as consistently and persistently as in MS. In patients with clinically isolated syndrome the presence of oligoclonal bands is predictive for the progression to clinically definite MS [Paolino et al., 1996]. In MS patients the absence of oligoclonal bands is associated with a benign disease course, while high levels of oligoclonal bands are correlated with a severe disease, suggesting that oligoclonal bands may be clinically relevant [Correale and de los Milagros Bassani Molinas, 2002]. The identification of biomarkers for diagnosis and prognosis of MS is the subject of intense ongoing research [Teunissen et al., 2011; Ziemann et al., 2011; Junker et al., 2011; Teunissen et al., 2009]. One example is neurofilament light, which was found to be increased in clinically isolated syndrome patients, especially in those that converted to MS, and was observed to correlate with relapses and the number of gadolinium enhancing lesions [Teunissen et al., 2009].

Four major subtypes of MS with different progression and relapse characteristics have been recognized: the relapsing-remitting (RR-MS), the secondary-progressive (SP-MS), primary progressive (PP-MS) and progressive-relapsing (PR-MS) subtype [Lublin and Reingold, 1996]. Approximately 70% of the cases start with the RR subtype, which is characterized by clinical attacks that are followed by a clinically silent period with almost complete recovery. After a period of 15 to 20 years most cases of the RR-MS subtype develop progressive neurological deterioration without apparent remission, the SP-MS subtype. About 15-20% of MS patients show a progressive disease course without relapses and remissions from the beginning, the PP-MS subtype. Finally, less than 5% suffer from PR-MS, characterized by progressive neurological impairment with occasional relapses.

2.2 Pathology

The major neuropathological hallmarks of MS are multiple focal inflammatory demyelinating lesions spread throughout the CNS. These lesions are associated with perivascular infiltrates containing macrophages and lymphocytes. Other features of MS plaques are axonal damage and loss, oligodendrocyte death and astrogliosis [Charcot, 1868], which is hypertrophy and an abnormal increase in the number of astrocytes. Lesions are classified based on the degree of myelin loss, the presence of inflammatory cells and HLA-DR expression on leukocytes and microglial cells. Four different stages in MS lesions have been identified: (p)reactive, active, chronic active and chronic inactive lesions [van der Valk and De Groot, 2000; de Groot et al., 2001].

In (p)reactive lesions no demyelination is apparent. Clusters of activated microglia can be observed with increased expression of HLA-DR expression and occasionally perivascular leukocyte infiltrations can be seen.

Active lesions are characterized by areas of demyelination containing macrophages, activated microglia and activated hypertrophic astrocytes. Activated astrocytes fill up the lesion area and form a gliotic scar. T-cells and some B-cells can be found, mostly in the perivascular space. The macrophages and microglia in the lesions contain myelin degradation products, such as myelin proteins and lipids, giving them a foamy appearance. The presence of myelin proteins in these macrophages reflect ongoing demyelination, since these myelin proteins are degraded in a known time frame [Bruck et al., 1995; van der Goes A. et al., 2005]. Oligodendrocyte death occurs in these lesions, often via apoptotic mechanisms [Wolswijk, 2000; Rodriguez and Lucchinetti, 1999]. This apoptosis of oligodendrocytes may be a disease initiating event, since it precedes leukocyte infiltration [Barnett and Prineas, 2004; Henderson et al., 2009].

Chronic active lesions are defined by a hypocellular demyelinated centre surrounded by a hypercellular rim with high numbers of foamy macrophages and reactive astrocytes. In these lesions oligodendrocyte numbers are reduced and lymphocytes are present in perivascular spaces.

In chronic inactive lesions almost no cellular infiltrates are present. They are hypocellular, demyelinated and contain widened extracellular spaces and gliotic scar tissue. In the CNS parenchyma and perivascular spaces relatively small numbers of macrophages and lymphocytes still remain. No myelin proteins can be detected in the macrophages.

Next to demyelination, remyelination also occurs [Franklin, 2002]. Remyelination can be restricted to the lesion edge, but can also extend throughout the lesions which are then called shadow-plaques [Bruck et al., 2003; Prineas et al., 1993; Prineas and Connell, 1979; Raine and Wu, 1993; Lassmann et al., 1997]. Oligodendrocyte precursor cells, after maturation into mature oligodendrocytes, generate thin myelin sheaths and could therefore contribute to recovery in MS patients. Remyelination in MS is limited. The cause of remyelination failure in MS is unknown, but several mechanisms have been proposed, such as restricted oligodendrocyte precursor cell migration, maturation and a growth inhibitory environment [Franklin, 2002; Wolswijk, 2002; John et al., 2002; Charles et al., 2002]. Macrophages could play an important role in remyelination as well [Doring and Yong, 2011].

It is clear from the above that macrophages are an important characteristic defining lesion stage. They likely play a central role in lesion formation in MS. In the next sections, we will describe the role of these immune cells in disease and particularly in MS in more detail.

3. Macrophages in MS

3.1 Macrophages and innate immunity

Macrophages (meaning "big eaters") are phagocytic cells that play a vital role in innate immunity, the first line of defense against pathogens. Cells of the innate immune system such as macrophages are able, to some extent, to discriminate between "self" and "non-self" antigens (reviewed by Janeway [Janeway, Jr. and Medzhitov, 2002]). Via a limited number of germline-encoded pattern recognition receptors, macrophages recognize highly conserved structures from bacteria, viruses and fungi. Several different families of pattern recognition receptors have been identified, for example macrophage scavenger receptors and the family of Toll-like receptors [Takeda and Akira, 2005; Akira et al., 2006]. After recognition, the binding of the receptor with its ligand on the pathogen, macrophages usually engulf the pathogen, a process called phagocytosis. This process results in the containment of microbes in the phagosome, which fuses with lysosomal vesicles containing a multitude of microbicidal products. Both oxygen-dependent, called the respiratory burst, and oxygen-independent microbicidal mechanisms exist. The respiratory burst uses an enzymatic complex called nicotinamide adenine dinucleotide phosphate reduced (NADPH) oxidase. Upon stimulation active NADPH oxidase forms. This active complex transfers two electrons from NADPH to two molecules of oxygen to form superoxide anion [DeLeo et al., 1999; Babior, 1999]. From this superoxide anion other ROS, such as hydrogen peroxide, are formed [Babior, 1999]. Oxygen-independent microbicidal mechanisms include acidification of the phagolysosome, nutrient depletion and antimicrobial proteins or peptides.

Macrophages differentiate from circulating monocytes. Once a monocyte migrates into a specific tissue, during steady-state or inflammation, it develops into a macrophage. Macrophages are present in virtually all tissues and usually specialize according to the tissue they are in, for instance osteoclasts (in bone), Kupffer cells (in liver) and microglia (in the CNS) [Gordon and Taylor, 2005].

Next to their role in innate immunity they have an important function in tissue homeostasis, since they are crucial for the clearance of apoptotic cells and the remodeling and repair of tissues after inflammation [Gordon, 1986; Gordon, 1998]. Phagocytosis of apoptotic cells does not induce the expression of inflammatory mediators in unstimulated macrophages [Kono and Rock, 2008].

During an infection macrophages also clear cellular debris of necrotic cells that contain endogenous danger signals, such as heat-shock proteins and nuclear proteins [Zhang and Mosser, 2008]. The detection of these danger signals alters the physiology of the macrophages, including expression of cell surface proteins, cytokines and pro-inflammatory mediators, increasing immune function of macrophages. However, macrophages can respond to many signals in the microenvironment of tissues and not all increase immune function.

3.2 Macrophage activation results in different subtypes

Macrophages are highly plastic cells and are able to respond to a variety of environmental cues changing their phenotype and physiology, resulting in different subtypes of macrophages. These different subtypes of macrophages have different functions in immune response, homeostasis and tissue repair [Gordon, 2003; Mosser, 2003; Mosser and Edwards, 2008].

Based on activation pathways several subtypes of macrophages have been described [Edwards et al., 2006b; Martinez et al., 2008]. The two most studied subtypes are: 1) the classically activated macrophages (CA, also called M1), induced by interferon-gamma (IFN-γ) and lipopolysaccharide (LPS); 2) the alternatively activated macrophages (AA, also called M2), stimulated by IL-4/13 and/or glucocorticoids. In 1992 Stein et al. introduced the concept of alternatively activated macrophages [Stein et al., 1992]. In contrast to the classically activated macrophages, macrophages stimulated with interleukin-4 (IL-4) increased the expression of mannose receptor (MR). Another study showed that Th1 cytokines (e.g. IFN-γ) and Th2 cytokines (e.g. IL-4) induced two distinct functional states in macrophages. Exposure of macrophages to Th2 cytokines led to an upregulation of certain phagocytic receptors and arginase, which reduced ability to kill intracellular pathogens, while Th1 cytokines led to induction of inducible nitric oxide synthase (iNOS) in macrophages [Modolell et al., 1995].

CA macrophages are cytotoxic and secrete high amounts of oxygen and nitrogen radicals in order to kill pathogens [Nathan and Shiloh, 2000]. CA macrophages also produce pro-inflammatory cytokines [O'Shea and Murray, 2008]. In mice, CA macrophages are

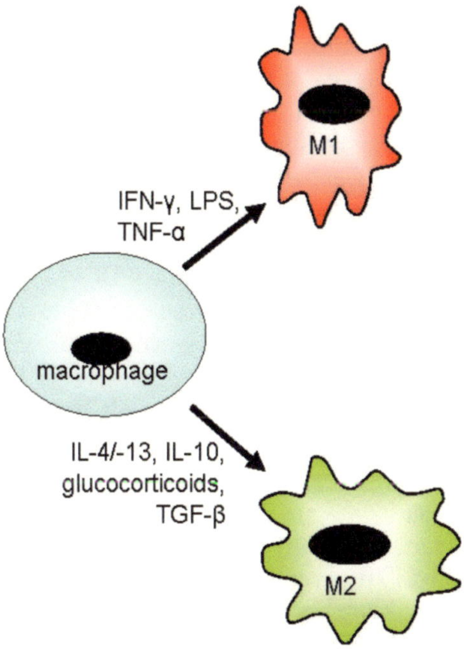

	M1 macrophage
Function	Th1 response, microbicidal, cytotoxic, tumour resistance
Surface markers	MHCII, CD86, CD80, CD40, CD1 1b, FCγRI, FCγRII, CCR7
Cytokines and chemokines	IL-1β, IL-6, IL-8, IL-12, IL-23, TNF-α CCL2, CCL5, CXCL9, CXCL10
Extracellular mediators	Release of superoxide and NO

	M2 macrophage
Function	Th2 response, allergy, parasite response, tissue repair, immunomodulatory
Surface markers	MR (CD206), CD163, CD23, CD36, MSR1, Dectin1, DCIR, MARCO, CCR2, E-cadherin
Cytokines and chemokines	IL-1Ra, IL-10 CCL13, CCL14, CCL16, CCL17, CCL22
Extracellular mediators	Fibronectin 1, IGF, PDGF-C, TGF-β, FXIIIa, collagen IV

Fig. 1. Functions and characteristic markers of macrophage activation types. Macrophages can change their phenotype and function in response to signals from the environment. The most studied phenotypes are M1 and M2 macrophages. M1 macrophages are induced in vitro by IFN-γ, LPS and/or TNF-α, while the induction of the M2 phenotype requires IL-4/13, IL-10, glucocorticoids or TGF-β

characterized by their production of nitric oxide (NO) [Edwards et al., 2006b; MacMicking et al., 1997; Hibbs, Jr., 2002]. Human macrophages derived from circulating monocytes do not generally produce NO [Mosser, 2003], therefore other markers should be used to discriminate between CA and AA macrophages, such as MR, E-cadherin [Van den Bossche J. et al., 2009], CD40 [Zeyda et al., 2007] and Fc-gamma receptor I (FcγRI). CA macrophages are essential for host defence [Gordon and Taylor, 2005; Nathan, 2008] and tumor killing. The pro-inflammatory mediators produced by CA macrophages can cause extensive damage to the host.

AA macrophages seem to play a role in immune suppression and tissue repair, due to production of anti-inflammatory cytokines and extracellular matrix components and lack of production of NO [Edwards et al., 2006b]. The most commonly used distinctive marker for AA macrophages, in mice, is the high expression and activity of arginase [Edwards et al., 2006b]. Due to the activation of arginase, arginine is converted to ornithine, a precursor for polyamines and collagen, which contributes to the production of extracellular matrix [Kreider et al., 2007; Albina et al., 1990; Gratchev et al., 2001; Hesse et al., 2001]. Furtermore, the polyamines produced can influence production of cytokines and suppress clonal expansion of lymphocytes, thereby regulating the immune response [Cordeiro-da-Silva et al., 2004].

Functional differences can be observed between CA and AA macrophages. As mentioned above, due to the production of ROS, CA macrophages are efficient in the killing of bacteria, while AA macrophages do not produce ROS and are therefore less efficient in killing bacteria [Gordon and Taylor, 2005]. Furthermore, CA macrophages are efficient antigen presenting cells, while AA macrophages are not [Edwards et al., 2006b]. CA macrophages are also more efficient in activating T-cell proliferation compared to AA macrophages [Edwards et al., 2006b]. AA macrophages are involved in scar formation, since they enhance fibrogenesis, while CA macrophages do not. AA macrophages stimulate proliferation and activation of fibroblasts, by expression and release of potent fibrogenic growth factors, like transforming growth factor-beta (TGF-β) and platelet derived growth factor (PDGF) [Song et al., 2000]. The angiogenic potential of AA macrophages is higher compared to CA macrophages [Kodelja et al., 1997]. Due to the production of growth factors and stimulation of angiogenesis, AA macrophages are considered tumor promoting. *In vitro* CA macrophages were shown to be cytotoxic to tumor cells but not to normal cells [Romieu-Mourez et al., 2006].

3.3 Macrophages in MS lesion formation and repair

It is widely accepted that macrophages play an important role in MS pathology. Macrophages are implicated in mechanisms that lead to demyelination and axonal damage [Bitsch et al., 2000; Kuhlmann et al., 2002; Trapp et al., 1998; Koning et al., 2007; Huitinga et al., 1990; Heppner et al., 2005; Hendriks et al., 2005; Newman et al., 2001]. Inflammatory infiltrates in MS lesions contain large amounts of macrophages. In experimental autoimmune encephalomyelitis (EAE), an animal model for MS, it has been shown that elimination of infiltrating macrophages reduced both clinical signs and axonal damage [Heppner et al., 2005]. Furthermore, during spinal cord injury (SCI), elimination of infiltrating macrophages increased axonal repair and functional outcome [Popovich et al., 1999; Stirling et al., 2004]. Clinical signs of EAE were significantly enhanced when the macrophage inhibitory signal of CD200/CD200R between neurons and macrophages was blocked [Koning et al., 2007]. This suggests a direct link between increased macrophage activity and aggravated disease course in EAE. Finally, macrophages are able to secrete a plethora of neurotoxic substances, such as matrix metalloproteinases [Newman et al., 2001], reactive oxygen species (ROS) [Nathan and Shiloh, 2000] and nitric oxide (NO) [Smith et al., 2001]. These studies all indicate that macrophages are detrimental.

However the role of macrophages is more complex. Several studies have shown that activated macrophages can actually be beneficial during CNS repair. During SCI macrophages can create a growth-permissive environment in which axonal regeneration can take place [Rapalino et al., 1998; Barrette et al., 2008]. In MS lesions, activated macrophages can be observed in areas with increased growth-associated protein-43 (GAP-43) expression [Teunissen et al., 2006]. *In vitro* AA macrophage conditioned medium has been found to promote axonal outgrowth [Kigerl et al., 2009]. Furthermore, macrophages are beneficial because they remove myelin debris, which is growth inhibiting for axons [Baer et al., 2009; Kotter et al., 2006], they release growth factors [Song et al., 2000; Kodelja et al., 1997] and they support axonal repair [Shechter et al., 2009; Bouhy et al., 2006; Batchelor et al., 2002]. These different roles ascribed to macrophages could be due to polarization in macrophage activation [Edwards et al., 2006a; Mosser and Edwards, 2008; Mantovani et al., 2004a] (Figure 1).

4. Models for MS

4.1 In vivo models

Research on the mechanisms of demyelinating diseases is highly dependent on experimental animal models, due to the inaccessibility of the human brain for experimental research. Most frequently allergic autoimmune encephalitis (EAE) models are used as a model for MS. In EAE, an autoimmune reaction is induced by injection of myelin proteins or myelin-specific inflammatory T-cells into rats or mice. Disability starts with loss of tail tonus, leading to complete paralysis, which can be recovered. Demyelination occurs after a chronic induction paradigm. The model poses very serious discomfort to the many animals involved. Other animal models use viruses or chemical agents such as cuprizone or lysophosphatidylcholine (LPC) to induce demyelination [Ercolini and Miller, 2006; Matsushima and Morell, 2001; Woodruff and Franklin, 1999]. Another model that is currently increasingly used is the mutant shiverer mouse that carries a deletion in the myelin basic protein (MBP) gene [Nave, 1994]. Several drawbacks of using animal models are: i) per animal only one condition can be tested, making the use of many animals unavoidable, ii) investigating the mechanism behind demyelination at a cellular level is difficult, due to the complex interactions of the CNS with the immune system, iii) *in vivo* it is very difficult to control all experimental conditions.

4.2 *In vitro* models

Only few alternative *in-vitro* models for de- and remyelination are available. This is due to the complex interactions between axons, oligodendrocytes and astrocytes needed for the development of multilayered myelin around axons, which cannot be accomplished by cell lines or monolayer cultures. A demyelination model in slice cultures has been described using LPC [Birgbauer et al., 2004; Miron et al., 2010]. Slice cultures contain intact myelin of specific brain areas, and are therefore very suitable for experiments. A drawback, but also advantage, of the use of slice cultures is the fact that the cellular composition of the slice can not be altered. Furthermore, the top and bottom layer of the slice consists of damaged cells, which might influence the behavior of the layers underneath.

Another good and flexible *in vitro* model for the CNS is the culture of 3-dimensional brain spheroids. Spheroids are formed by continuous rotation of a single cell suspension of primary brain cells. These cells aggregate within 24 hours and start to differentiate. The result after 4 weeks of maturation is a spheroid containing all different brain cell types that make 3-dimensional contacts [Figure 2: 3-dimensional aspect of spheroid cultures]. The high level of differentiation is exemplified by the presence of myelinated axons and spontaneous synaptic activity. The model has been used for studying brain development, neurotoxicity, and neurodegenerative diseases [Berglund et al., 2004; Diemel et al., 2004; Honegger and Richelson, 1976].

In previous studies, immune-mediated demyelination has been induced in this model, using anti-myelin antibodies and complement [Diemel et al., 2004; Loughlin et al., 1994]. The major drawback of that model is that only modest and variable effects of antibodies were observed (personal observations C. Teunissen). We were able to induce non-inflammatory demyelination using LPC as well as subsequent recovery after LPC-withdrawal, in rodent brain spheroids. The effect of LPC was specific for myelin, since other CNS cell types present in the cultures were only slightly or not affected [Vereyken et al., 2009]. After cessation of LPC treatment, remyelination was observed in these culture (Figure 3) . These data demonstrate the potential of this model to study several fundamental aspects of de- and remyelination.

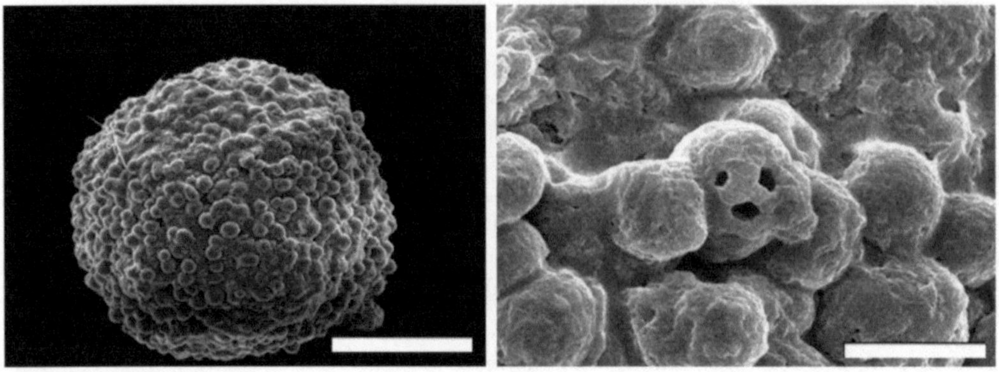

(A) (B)

Fig. 2. Scanning electron microscopy photograph of a cultured spheroid. (A) Example of 3-week-old whole brain spheroids showing a typical three-dimensional appearance. Bar represents 50 mm. (B) Higher magnification than (A), bar represents 5 mm. Teunissen et al 2000 [Teunissen et al., 2000]

5. Macrophage-CNS interaction in an in vitro model for MS

Microglia are present in spheroids, and these can be activated to study the effects of macrophages on myelin formation and demyelination. Alternatively, activated macrophages can be supplemented to the cultures. We set out to study whether the spheroid culture model is suitable for studying effects of supplemented macrophages. An important first question was whether macrophages are able to migrate into the spheroids, which would be a benefit of this model over *in vivo* models as there is no blood brain barrier (BBB) and the influence of BBB interruption can be circumvented. Next, we were especially interested to determine the effects of macrophages on CNS cell types inside the spheroids. Our hypothesis was that CA macrophages would have toxic effects and AA macrophages positive effects on myelin, glia and axonal integrity. No studies so far have addressed the question if these differential macrophage phenotypes have differential effects on intact CNS tissue. Therefore, we also set out to compare the effects of CA and AA macrophages on cellular structures within whole brain spheroid cultures.

5.1 Number of macrophages in spheroids

First, we established whether macrophages could migrate into the spheroids, and whether the numbers were similar for the CA and AA macrophage phenotypes. For this, we cultured rat whole brain spheroids during 4 weeks, to reach optimal myelin development, and exposed them to differently activated macrophages, that were fluorescently labeled, [method of macrophage activation: Vereyken et al., 2011] during maximal 1 week. At several time points, cryostat sections were cut of the spheroids and the number of spheroids containing macrophages were counted.

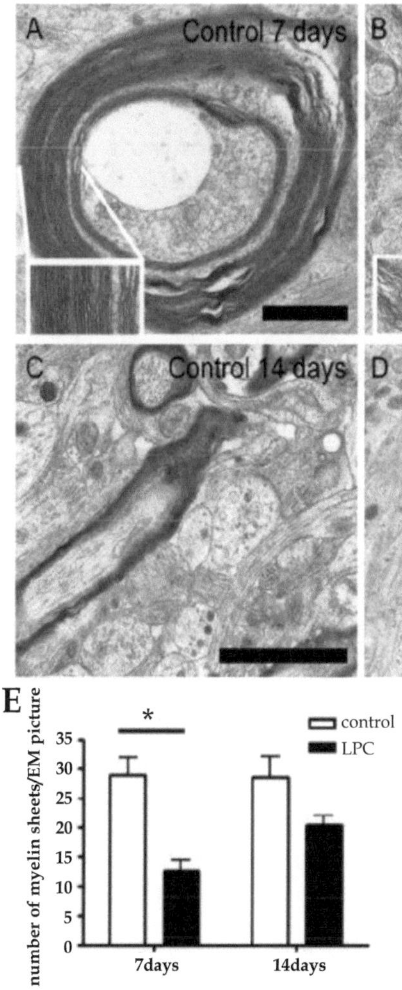

Fig. 3. EM picture of demyelinated rat whole brain spheroid cultures. A: After 4 weeks of culturing the experiment was started at day 0. After 7 days (5 weeks of culturing) multilayered compact myelin was present. See insert for more detail. B: After a week of exposure to LPC (three times addition of 0.12 mM LPC), at day 7 (= week 5 of culturing), the myelin layers were loosely packed. See insert for more detail. C: Control cultures at day 14 (6 week old cultures), show compact myelin. D: At day 14, after 1 week of exposure to LPC and 1 week of recovery, LPC-exposed cultures show compact myelin. Bar is 500 nm. E: Quantification of the number of myelin sheets present in EM pictures from two separate experiments (four pictures from three spheroids). After LPC treatment at 7 days 12.5 myelin sheets per picture were counted. When compared with control spheroids, 29 myelin sheets per picture, a significant decrease of 56% was, therefore, visible. At 14 days, the number of myelin sheets was not significantly different between control, 28 myelin sheets per picture, and LPC treated, 20 myelin sheets per picture, cultures. Results are presented as mean ± SEM. Open bars: control; closed bars: LPC treated; asterisks indicate $P < 0.05$. [Vereyken et al.. 2009]

We observed a temporal pattern. After 1 day no macrophages were visible in the spheroids (data not shown). At 2 days after macrophage addition, low numbers of macrophages were present in spheroids exposed to AA and unstimulated (US) macrophages (data not shown). At 3 days macrophages were observed in 40-70% of the spheroid sections (Figure 4A and D). After 8 days the macrophage numbers were decreased compared to day 3 (data not shown). Most macrophages were associated with spheroids on the outside rim of the spheroid, but several also migrated into the center of the spheroids (Figure 4A, B, C). A larger number of spheroids contained one or more macrophages when exposed to either AA or US macrophages compared to CA macrophages (Figure 4D). These results were in agreement with our previous observations showing that AA macrophages have a higher intrinsic motility compared to CA macrophages [Vereyken et al., 2011]. Furthermore, CA macrophages had been observed to express higher levels of adhesion receptors compared to both AA and US macrophages [Vereyken et al., 2011]. Thus, the lower motility and higher adhesion could contribute to the lower migration of CA macrophages into spheroids.

After induction of demyelination, a similar pattern was observed for the differentially activated macrophages, i.e. a higher percentage of spheroids contained AA and US macrophages (Figure 4E). Taken together, all different macrophage phenotypes could migrate into the spheroids, while the extend of migration differed between phenotypes.

5.2 Effect of differentially activated macrophages on CNS cells in spheroid cultures

Next, we tested whether CA and AA macrophages had and effect on CNS cells in the spheroids and whether the effects were dependent on the macrophage phenotype. We quantified the total immunoreactivity per spheroid section using image analysis software [Vereyken et al., 2009]. Figure 5A-D. show the results of the quantification of the immunereactivity (IR). MBP immunereactivity was 50% increased in spheroid cultures exposed to CA and AA macrophages, compared to control spheroid cultures (spheroids exposed to unstimulated macrophages and spheroid cultures without macrophages). Figure 6A-D shows representative images of MBP staining after exposure of intact spheroids to differently activated macrophages. In control spheroids, MBP IR was present in structures in the center and at the borders (Figure 6A). In the spheroids exposed to unstimulated macrophages a similar picture was observed, although, in some spheroids a higher number of MBP-positive structures near the border was observed (Figure 6B). Note that in this specific section, no intact macrophages are visible, which is likely due to the relatively low numbers of macrophages inside the spheroids in combination with the low thickness of the sections. After exposure to CA macrophages, a higher mean IR was observed at the spheroid border (Figure 6C). The mean IR was also increased in spheroids exposed to AA macrophages (Figure 6D). This increase was mainly observed in the area just below the border.

GFAP IR was not affected by addition of the macrophages. GFAP IR was slightly lower in spheroids exposed to AA macrophages compared to spheroids exposed to CA macrophages (Fig 5B). β-tubulin IR was decreased by 50% in CA macrophage-exposed spheroids compared to control spheroids, not exposed to any macrophages. Tubulin staining was present in center of the control spheroids, as described before [Vereyken et al., 2009]. After exposure of the spheroids to CA macrophages especially the β-tubulin IR in the center of the spheroids was decreased (Figure 5C). A slight increase in GAP-43 IR was observed in spheroids exposed to CA macrophages compared to control spheroids not exposed to macrophages (Figure 5D).

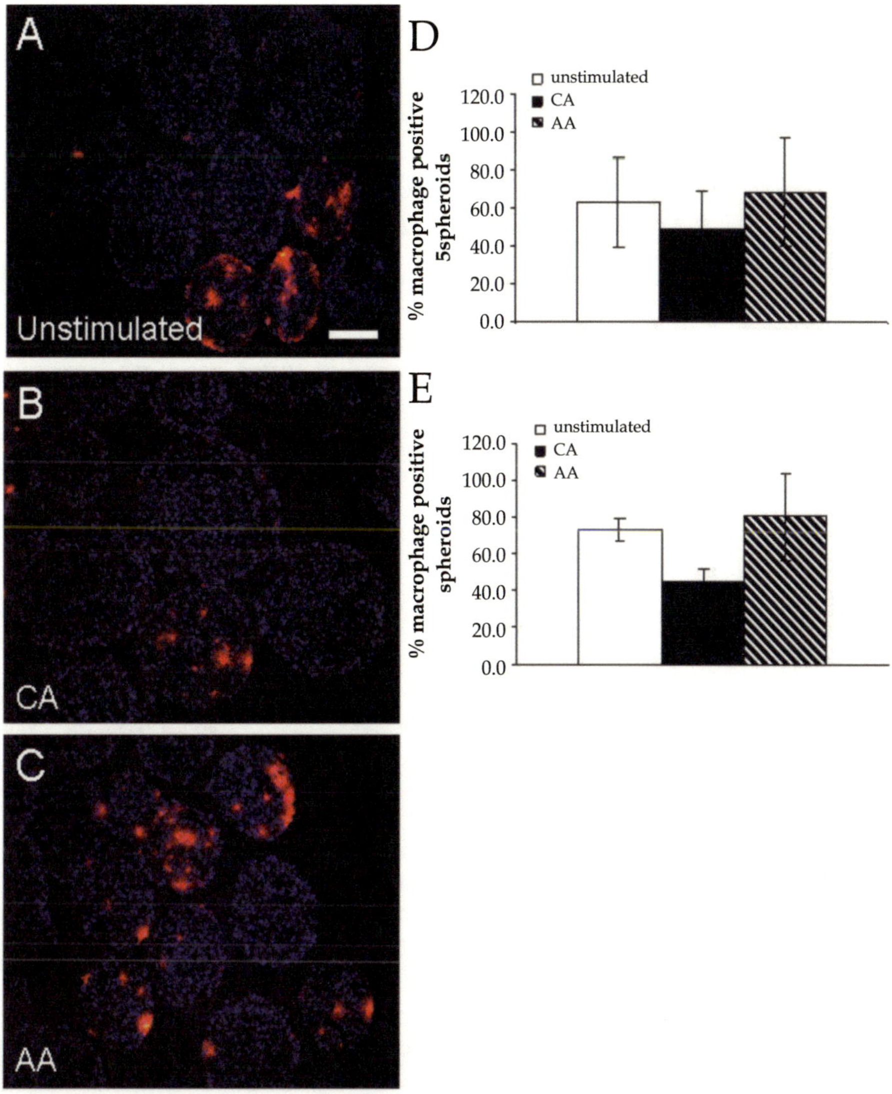

Fig. 4. Migration of macrophages in whole brain spheroid cultures. Mature spheroids were exposed to unstimulated (A); classically activated (CA); of alternatively activated (AA) macrophages during three days. Macrophages were labelled with DiI before addition to the cultures. Sections were prepared and nuclei stained with Hoechst. Bar in A is 200 µm. Figure 4D and E: Quantification of migration of differently activated macrophages in whole brain spheroids. D: The number of positive spheroids was determined as the number of spheroids containing one or more macrophages/total number of control spheroids. A trend could be seen of a lower migration of CA macrophages into spheroids compared to unstimulated and AA macrophages. E: Quantification of migration of macrophages is higher in demyelinated spheroids. Unstimulated macrophages were present in 73% (± 6) of the LPC-demyelineated spheroids. Spheroids exposed to CA macrophages. Only 45% (± 6) of the LPC-demyelineated spheroids were positive for CA macrophages. With AA macrophages the percentage of spheroids positive was 80 % (± 24)

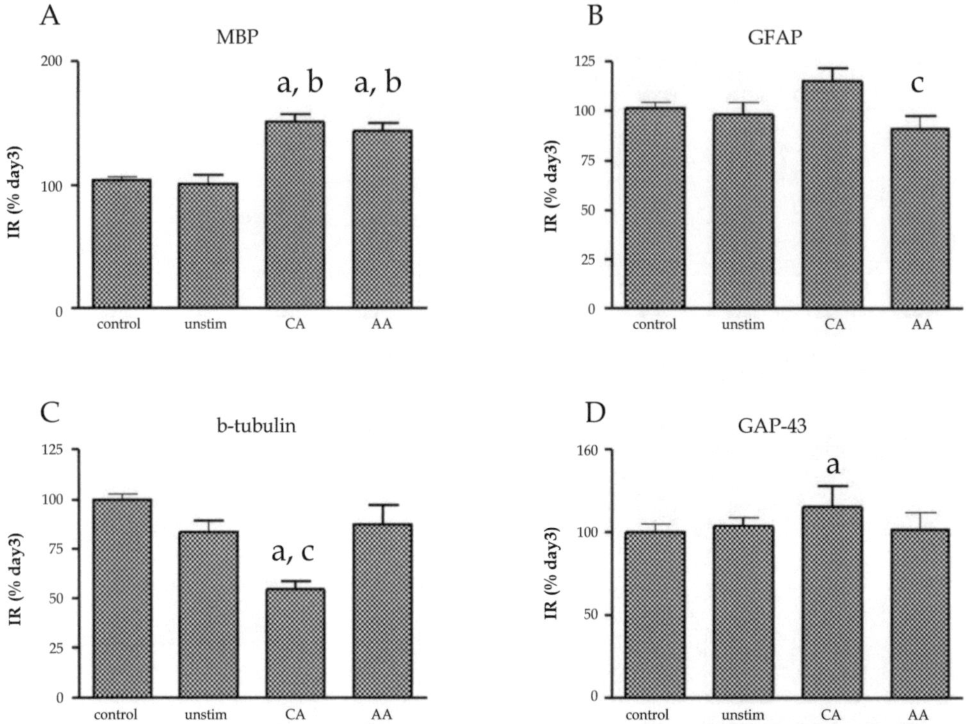

Fig. 5. Quantification of effects of differentially activated macrophages on immunereactivity of specific CNS cell proteins in spheroid cultures. Unstim=unstimulated macrophages; CA: classically activated macrophages; AA: Alternatively activated macrophages. Four-weeks old whole brain spheroid cultures exposed to unstim, CA or AA macrophages during 3 days. a: $P < 0.05$ compared to control; b: $P < 0.05$ compared to unstimulated macrophages; c: $P < 0.05$ for differences between CA and AA macrophages

5.3 Discussion of the experimental results in spheroid cultures

The first aim of the experiments described above was to study whether macrophages can migrate into the spheroid cultures. This was indeed the case. Externally supplemented macrophages can be labeled to trace them within the spheroid and we observed that they can migrate into the center of the spheroid.

The second aim was to study effects of classically and alternatively activated macrophages on cellular structures of whole brain spheroid cultures. Our hypothesis was that CA macrophages would have toxic effects and that AA macrophages have positive effects on myelin and axonal integrity. Our results were in part supportive for this hypothesis: CA macrophages had a slight negative effect on tubulin immune reactivity in intact spheroids, while AA macrophages had no effect on tubulin immune reactivity. This indicates that CA macrophages were toxic to neurons, while AA macrophages were not. These data are in agreement with our observations in monolayers (EJFV Unpublished observation). The GFAP immunereactivity was slightly higher in CA exposed macrophages compared to AA exposed macrophages. However, for many of our read-outs there were no substantial differences between the differently activated macrophages. A similar positive effect of both

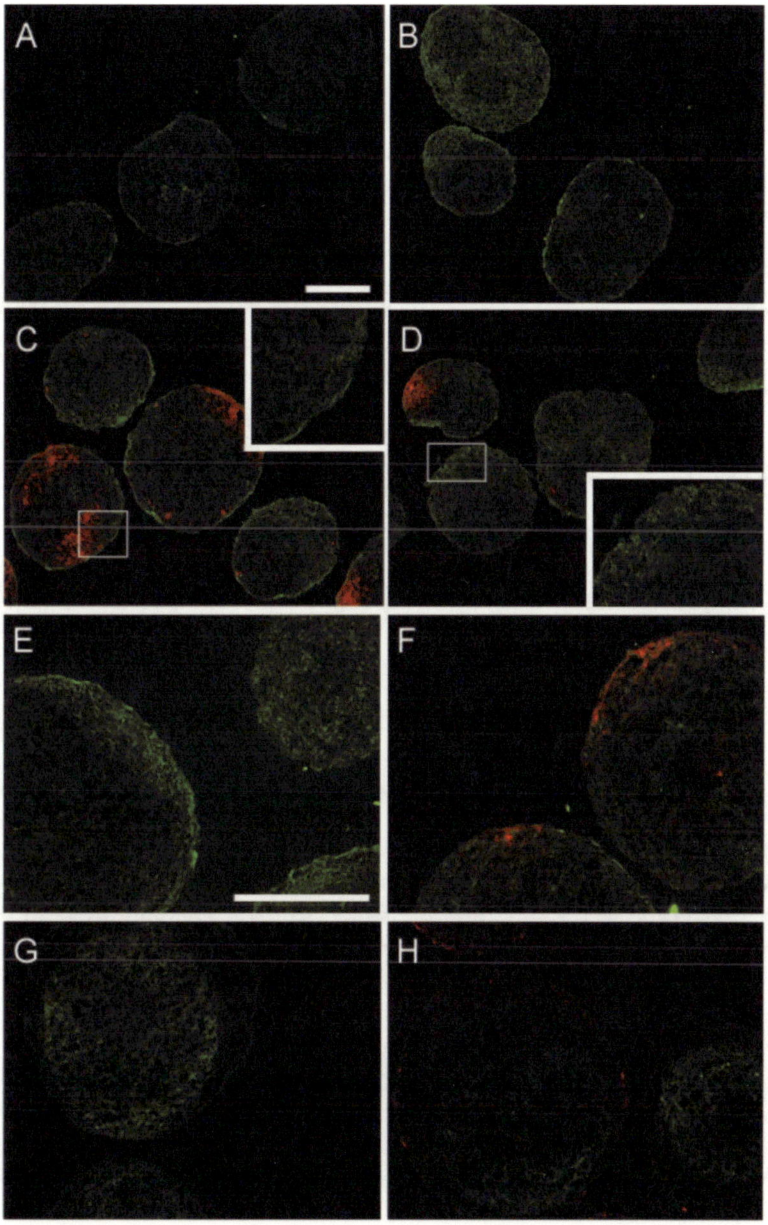

Fig. 6. Effects of differentially activated macrophages on immunereactivity of myelin basic protein (MBP) in spheroid cultures. Four-weeks old whole brain spheroid cultures were exposed to unstim, CA or AA macrophages during 3 days. A: MBP immune reactivity in control spheroids without exposure to macrophages.; B-D: MBP immune reactivity in spheroids exposed to (B) unstimulated macrophages, (C) classically activated (CA) macrophages, and (D) Alternatively activated macrophages (AA). E: GFAP IR in spheroids exposed to CA macrophages; F: GFAP IR in spheroids exposed to AA macrophages. G: β-tubulin IR in control spheroids. H: β-tubulin IR in spheroids exposed to CA macrophages. Bar in A and G= 200 μm

CA and AA macrophages on MBP immunereactivity in spheroids was observed. The lack of large differences between the different macrophage phenotypes could be related to the length of the experiments and the flexibility of the macrophage phenotypes, as a fundamental characteristic of macrophages is their ability to change their phenotype and they could all have a similar phenotype after a few days of contact with the CNS tissue. However, the duration of the experiments was three days, and we observed differences in migration between the phenotypes after 3 days. The different phenotypes do contain similar receptors, and it is possible that MBP expression is influenced by growth factors that may be differently, but at least sufficient on both phenotypes for induction of the observed.
Taken together, our results have shown that CA and AA macrophages can both affect myelin formation in spheroid cultures. Future studies must show whether macrophages can enhance myelin formation after demyelination and the conditions under which they can have regenerative effects.

6. Future perspectives

There are various in vivo and in vitro models for de- and remyelination in MS. The use of each of the models will depend on the research question. In vitro models provide the possibility to study direct effects on CNS cell types, without interference of other processes. Furthermore, access to CNS cell types is not hampered by the blood brain barrier. Furthermore, use of in *in vitro* models leads to a reduction of animal suffering. Nevertheless, we do not expect *in vitro* results to be directly translatable to the human situation and thus an intermediate step *in vivo* will be needed, but this can be on a limited scale when the range of conditions are narrowed by *in vitro* experiments.
In MS lesions, macrophages with the CA phenotype could inhibit repair or propagate lesion formation, since CA macrophages have been shown to be neurotoxic while AA activation abolished the neurotoxic effects. In MS lesions it could therefore be beneficial to reduce the CA phenotype and promote the AA phenotype. Possible mechanisms to skew the macrophage phenotype in the CNS are interesting to investigate, in order to design anti-inflammatory therapies. Here, we discuss these options.

6.1 Skewing of macrophage phenotype

Glucocorticoids are an accepted therapy during MS. Treatment with glucocorticoids might be a means of skewing the activational phenotype, since exposure to glucocorticoids induce a wound healing phenotype in macrophages *in vitro* [Mosser and Edwards, 2008; Gordon, 2003]. A glucocorticoid receptor ligand was found to attenuate experimental autoimmune neuritis, decrease the expression of inflammatory cytokines and iNOS and induce a M2 phenotype *in vitro* [Zhang et al., 2009].
Evidence for the possibility that substances in the periphery can influence CNS cells has been observed previously. In the CNS microglia have been shown to switch cytokine profile, from relatively anti-inflammatory to pro-inflammatory CA phenotype, after induction of Wallerian degeneration followed by systemic injection of LPS [Palin et al., 2008]. The peripheral LPS injection also led to a decrease in neurofilament staining, indicating that neurodegeneration is increased. Similar results were found with a mouse model for prion disease, more inflammation and neuronal apoptosis after systemic LPS injection [Cunningham et al., 2005]. Likewise, glucocorticoids and glatiramer acetate, when applied peripherally, could influence the phenotype of microglia and macrophages inside the CNS.

It would therefore be interesting to determine the effect of glucocorticoid treatment on the macrophage phenotype in the CNS. Furthermore, since in MS lesions the macrophages predominantly express markers of the CA phenotype, it would be useful to study whether AA macrophages that enter a pro-inflammatory environment would be able to keep their phenotype. Could AA macrophages be able to exert positive effects in a pro-inflammatory environment? These questions can be investigated using *in vitro* models, such as the spheroid model, representing the CNS environment.

6.2 Injection of skewed macrophages

Some investigation into direct treatment with AA macrophages has been performed and therapeutic effects have been observed. In a model for murine diabetes a reduction in renal and pancreatic injury was seen after treatment with *in vitro* generated AA macrophages [Zheng et al., 2011]. The injection of AA macrophages reduced disease in a model for colitis [Hunter et al., 2010]. Furthermore, axonal dieback induced by macrophages was reduced after the addition of multipotent adult progenitor cells, which induced the AA phenotype in macrophages *in vitro* [Busch et al., 2011]. During EAE, treatment with substances skewing the macrophage phenotype toward an AA phenotype, such as anti-CCL22 [Dogan et al., 2011] and 2-arachidonoylglycerol [Lourbopoulos et al., 2011], was found to ameliorate the disease course and increase the presence of macrophages with an AA phenotype in the lesions. In a model for relapsing EAE, the injection of AA macrophages, generated in vitro, reduced the development of relapses [Mikita et al., 2011]. Clinical EAE was reversed by the adoptive transfer of AA macrophages, which were induced in vitro with glatiramer acetate [Weber et al., 2007]. Our studies have shown that macrophage migration towards CNS cell types differs upon skewing [Vereyken et al., 2011] and that migration of macrophages in spheroids is limited and varies with skewing of the macrophages (Figure 4E). Microinjection of skewed macrophages into spheroids or co-culture of differently activated macrophages would allow more in depth analysis into the cellular mechanisms behind the effects reported in these studies.

7. Conclusion

Spheroid cultures are a suitable model to test the effects of novel therapeutics on remyelination, e.g. magnitude and speed. Furthermore, this model is very useful to study the mechanism of remyelination and the effects of demyelination, for example on axons. Using spheroid cultures, cells not endogenous to the CNS, like macrophages, can be introduced into the spheroids with relative ease [Loughlin et al., 1994; Loughlin et al., 1997; Pardo and Honegger, 2000] as we demonstrated. Both CA and AA macrophages can have beneficial effects in an MS lesion. The CA macrophages are very efficient in clearing debris, however, they are toxic to neurons. The AA macrophages secrete higher amounts of neurotrophins and are not neurotoxic, however they are less efficient in clearing debris. It would be of great value if an activational status in macrophages could be reached with an increased phagocytic capacity, without the production of neurotoxic substances such as ROS, NO and TNF-α, and with the secretion of growth factors. Future research should therefore focus on the functional activation status of macrophages stimulated with for example glucocorticoids, to enhance the secretion of growth factors and phagocytosis and limit secretion of neurotoxic substances.

8. Acknowledgements

We would like to extend our gratitude towards all who have contributed to the spheroid studies: Marije Bolijn, Priscilla Heijnen, Wia Baron, Sjef Copray, Elga de Vries, Amos Attali and Ilja Boor. Support grant: Dutch MS Research Foundation, grant number: 05-358c. Dutch Research Council (NWO (016.056.024))

9. References

Akira S, Uematsu S, Takeuchi O (2006) Pathogen recognition and innate immunity. *Cell* 124: 783-801

Albina JE, Mills CD, Henry WL, Jr., Caldwell MD (1990) Temporal expression of different pathways of 1-arginine metabolism in healing wounds. *J Immunol* 144: 3877-3880

Babior BM (1999) NADPH oxidase: an update. *Blood* 93: 1464-1476

Baer AS, Syed YA, Kang SU, Mitteregger D, Vig R, Ffrench-Constant C, Franklin RJ, Altmann F, Lubec G, Kotter MR (2009) Myelin-mediated inhibition of oligodendrocyte precursor differentiation can be overcome by pharmacological modulation of Fyn-RhoA and protein kinase C signalling. *Brain* 132: 465-481

Barkhof F, Filippi M, Miller DH, Scheltens P, Campi A, Polman CH, Comi G, Ader HJ, Losseff N, Valk J (1997) Comparison of MRI criteria at first presentation to predict conversion to clinically definite multiple sclerosis. *Brain* 120 (Pt 11): 2059-2069

Barnett MH, Prineas JW (2004) Relapsing and remitting multiple sclerosis: pathology of the newly forming lesion. *Ann Neurol* 55: 458-468

Barrette B, Hebert MA, Filali M, Lafortune K, Vallieres N, Gowing G, Julien JP, Lacroix S (2008) Requirement of myeloid cells for axon regeneration 1. *J Neurosci* 28: 9363-9376

Batchelor PE, Porritt MJ, Martinello P, Parish CL, Liberatore GT, Donnan GA, Howells DW (2002) Macrophages and Microglia Produce Local Trophic Gradients That Stimulate Axonal Sprouting Toward but Not beyond the Wound Edge 1. *Mol Cell Neurosci* 21: 436-453

Berglund CM, Aarum J, Haeberlein SL, Nyengaard JR, Hokfelt T, Sandberg K, Naslund J, Persson MA (2004) Characterization of long-term mouse brain aggregating cultures: evidence for maintenance of neural precursor cells. *J Comp Neurol* 474: 246-260

Birgbauer E, Rao TS, Webb M (2004) Lysolecithin induces demyelination in vitro in a cerebellar slice culture system. *J Neurosci Res* 78: 157-166

Bitsch A, Schuchardt J, Bunkowski S, Kuhlmann T, Bruck W (2000) Acute axonal injury in multiple sclerosis. Correlation with demyelination and inflammation. *Brain* 123 (Pt 6): 1174-1183

Bouhy D, Malgrange B, Multon S, Poirrier AL, Scholtes F, Schoenen J, Franzen R (2006) Delayed GM-CSF treatment stimulates axonal regeneration and functional recovery in paraplegic rats via an increased BDNF expression by endogenous macrophages. *FASEB J* 20: 1239-1241

Bourahoui A, De SJ, Guttierez R, Onraed B, Hennache B, Ferriby D, Stojkovic T, Vermersch P (2004) CSF isoelectrofocusing in a large cohort of MS and other neurological diseases. *Eur J Neurol* 11: 525-529

Bruck W, Bitsch A, Kolenda H, Bruck Y, Stiefel M, Lassmann H (1997) Inflammatory central nervous system demyelination: correlation of magnetic resonance imaging findings with lesion pathology. *Ann Neurol* 42: 783-793

Bruck W, Kuhlmann T, Stadelmann C (2003) Remyelination in multiple sclerosis. *J Neurol Sci* 206: 181-185

Bruck W, Porada P, Poser S, Rieckmann P, Hanefeld F, Kretzschmar HA, Lassmann H (1995) Monocyte/macrophage differentiation in early multiple sclerosis lesions. *Ann Neurol* 38: 788-796

Busch SA, Hamilton JA, Horn KP, Cuascut FX, Cutrone R, Lehman N, Deans RJ, Ting AE, Mays RW, Silver J (2011) Multipotent adult progenitor cells prevent macrophage-mediated axonal dieback and promote regrowth after spinal cord injury. *J Neurosci* 31: 944-953

Charcot M (1868) Histolgie de le sclerose en plaques. *Gaz Hop* 141: 554-558

Charles P, Reynolds R, Seilhean D, Rougon G, Aigrot MS, Niezgoda A, Zalc B, Lubetzki C (2002) Re-expression of PSA-NCAM by demyelinated axons: an inhibitor of remyelination in multiple sclerosis? *Brain* 125: 1972-1979

Compston A, Coles A (2008) Multiple sclerosis. *Lancet* 372: 1502-1517

Cordeiro-da-Silva A, Tavares J, Araujo N, Cerqueira F, Tomas A, Kong Thoo LP, Ouaissi A (2004) Immunological alterations induced by polyamine derivatives on murine splenocytes and human mononuclear cells. *Int Immunopharmacol* 4: 547-556

Correale J, de los Milagros Bassani Molinas (2002) Oligoclonal bands and antibody responses in multiple sclerosis. *J Neurol* 249: 375-389

Cunningham C, Wilcockson DC, Campion S, Lunnon K, Perry VH (2005) Central and systemic endotoxin challenges exacerbate the local inflammatory response and increase neuronal death during chronic neurodegeneration. *J Neurosci* 25: 9275-9284

de Groot CJ, Bergers E, Kamphorst W, Ravid R, Polman CH, Barkhof F, Van der Valk P. (2001) Post-mortem MRI-guided sampling of multiple sclerosis brain lesions: increased yield of active demyelinating and (p)reactive lesions. *Brain* 124: 1635-1645

DeLeo FR, Allen LA, Apicella M, Nauseef WM (1999) NADPH oxidase activation and assembly during phagocytosis. *J Immunol* 163: 6732-6740

Diemel LT, Wolswijk G, Jackson SJ, Cuzner ML (2004) Remyelination of cytokine- or antibody-demyelinated CNS aggregate cultures is inhibited by macrophage supplementation. *Glia* 45: 278-286

Dogan RN, Long N, Forde E, Dennis K, Kohm AP, Miller SD, Karpus WJ (2011) CCL22 regulates experimental autoimmune encephalomyelitis by controlling inflammatory macrophage accumulation and effector function. *J Leukoc Biol* 89: 93-104

Doring A, Yong VW (2011) The good, the bad and the ugly. Macrophages/microglia with a focus on myelin repair. *Front Biosci (Schol Ed)* 3: 846-856

Edwards JP, Zhang X, Frauwirth KA, Mosser DM (2006b) Biochemical and functional characterization of three activated macrophage populations. *J Leukoc Biol* 80: 1298-1307

Edwards JP, Zhang X, Frauwirth KA, Mosser DM (2006a) Biochemical and functional characterization of three activated macrophage populations. *J Leukoc Biol* 80: 1298-1307

Ercolini AM, Miller SD (2006) Mechanisms of immunopathology in murine models of central nervous system demyelinating disease. *J Immunol* 176: 3293-3298

Franklin RJ (2002) Why does remyelination fail in multiple sclerosis? *Nat Rev Neurosci* 3: 705-714

Franklin RJ, Ffrench-Constant C (2008) Remyelination in the CNS: from biology to therapy. *Nat Rev Neurosci* 9: 839-855

Gordon S (1986) Biology of the macrophage. *J Cell Sci Suppl* 4: 267-286

Gordon S (1998) The role of the macrophage in immune regulation. *Res Immunol* 149: 685-688

Gordon S (2003) Alternative activation of macrophages. *Nat Rev Immunol* 3: 23-35

Gordon S, Taylor PR (2005) Monocyte and macrophage heterogeneity. *Nat Rev Immunol* 5: 953-964

Gratchev A, Guillot P, Hakiy N, Politz O, Orfanos CE, Schledzewski K, Goerdt S (2001) Alternatively activated macrophages differentially express fibronectin and its splice variants and the extracellular matrix protein betaIG-H3. *Scand J Immunol* 53: 386-392

Henderson AP, Barnett MH, Parratt JD, Prineas JW (2009) Multiple sclerosis: distribution of inflammatory cells in newly forming lesions. *Ann Neurol* 66: 739-753

Hendriks JJ, Teunissen CE, de Vries HE, Dijkstra CD (2005) Macrophages and neurodegeneration. *Brain Res Brain Res Rev* 48: 185-195

Heppner FL, Greter M, Marino D, Falsig J, Raivich G, Hovelmeyer N, Waisman A, Rulicke T, Prinz M, Priller J, Becher B, Aguzzi A (2005) Experimental autoimmune encephalomyelitis repressed by microglial paralysis. *Nat Med* 11: 146-152

Hesse M, Modolell M, La Flamme AC, Schito M, Fuentes JM, Cheever AW, Pearce EJ, Wynn TA (2001) Differential regulation of nitric oxide synthase-2 and arginase-1 by type 1/type 2 cytokines in vivo: granulomatous pathology is shaped by the pattern of L-arginine metabolism. *J Immunol* 167: 6533-6544

Hibbs JB, Jr. (2002) Infection and nitric oxide. *J Infect Dis* 185 Suppl 1: S9-17

Honegger P, Richelson E (1976) Biochemical differentiation of mechanically dissociated mammalian brain in aggregating cell culture. *Brain Res* 109: 335-354

Huitinga I, Van Rooijen N, De Groot CJ, Uitdehaag BM, Dijkstra CD (1990) Suppression of experimental allergic encephalomyelitis in Lewis rats after elimination of macrophages. *J Exp Med* 172: 1025-1033

Hunter MM, Wang A, Parhar KS, Johnston MJ, van RN, Beck PL, McKay DM (2010) In vitro-derived alternatively activated macrophages reduce colonic inflammation in mice. *Gastroenterology* 138: 1395-1405

Janeway CA, Jr., Medzhitov R (2002) Innate immune recognition. *Annu Rev Immunol* 20: 197-216

John GR, Shankar SL, Shafit-Zagardo B, Massimi A, Lee SC, Raine CS, Brosnan CF (2002) Multiple sclerosis: re-expression of a developmental pathway that restricts oligodendrocyte maturation. *Nat Med* 8: 1115-1121

Junker A, Hohlfeld R, Meinl E (2011) The emerging role of microRNAs in multiple sclerosis. *Nat Rev Neurol* 7: 56-59

Katz D, Taubenberger JK, Cannella B, McFarlin DE, Raine CS, McFarland HF (1993) Correlation between magnetic resonance imaging findings and lesion development in chronic, active multiple sclerosis. *Ann Neurol* 34: 661-669

Kigerl KA, Gensel JC, Ankeny DP, Alexander JK, Donnelly DJ, Popovich PG (2009) Identification of two distinct macrophage subsets with divergent effects causing either neurotoxicity or regeneration in the injured mouse spinal cord. *J Neurosci* 29: 13435-13444

Kodelja V, Muller C, Tenorio S, Schebesch C, Orfanos CE, Goerdt S (1997) Differences in angiogenic potential of classically vs alternatively activated macrophages. *Immunobiology* 197: 478-493

Koning N, Bo L, Hoek RM, Huitinga I (2007) Downregulation of macrophage inhibitory molecules in multiple sclerosis lesions. *Ann Neurol* 62: 504-514

Kono H, Rock KL (2008) How dying cells alert the immune system to danger. *Nat Rev Immunol* 8: 279-289

Kotter MR, Li WW, Zhao C, Franklin RJ (2006) Myelin impairs CNS remyelination by inhibiting oligodendrocyte precursor cell differentiation. *J Neurosci* 26: 328-332

Kreider T, Anthony RM, Urban JF, Jr., Gause WC (2007) Alternatively activated macrophages in helminth infections. *Curr Opin Immunol* 19: 448-453

Kuhlmann T, Lingfeld G, Bitsch A, Schuchardt J, Bruck W (2002) Acute axonal damage in multiple sclerosis is most extensive in early disease stages and decreases over time. *Brain* 125: 2202-2212

Lassmann H, Bruck W, Lucchinetti C, Rodriguez M (1997) Remyelination in multiple sclerosis. *Mult Scler* 3: 133-136

Loughlin AJ, Copelman CA, Hall A, Armer T, Young BC, Landon DN, Cuzner ML (1997) Myelination and remyelination of aggregate rat brain cell cultures enriched with macrophages. *J Neurosci Res* 47: 384-392

Loughlin AJ, Honegger P, Woodroofe MN, Comte V, Matthieu JM, Cuzner ML (1994) Myelin basic protein content of aggregating rat brain cell cultures treated with cytokines and/or demyelinating antibody: effects of macrophage enrichment. *J Neurosci Res* 37: 647-653

Lourbopoulos A, Grigoriadis N, Lagoudaki R, Touloumi O, Polyzoidou E, Mavromatis I, Tascos N, Breuer A, Ovadia H, Karussis D, Shohami E, Mechoulam R, Simeonidou C (2011) Administration of 2-arachidonoylglycerol ameliorates both acute and chronic experimental autoimmune encephalomyelitis. *Brain Res* 1390: 126-141

Lublin FD, Reingold SC (1996) Defining the clinical course of multiple sclerosis: results of an international survey. National Multiple Sclerosis Society (USA) Advisory Committee on Clinical Trials of New Agents in Multiple Sclerosis. *Neurology* 46: 907-911

MacMicking J, Xie QW, Nathan C (1997) Nitric oxide and macrophage function. *Annu Rev Immunol* 15: 323-350

Mantovani A, Sica A, Sozzani S, Allavena P, Vecchi A, Locati M (2004b) The chemokine system in diverse forms of macrophage activation and polarization. *Trends Immunol* 25: 677-686

Mantovani A, Sica A, Sozzani S, Allavena P, Vecchi A, Locati M (2004a) The chemokine system in diverse forms of macrophage activation and polarization. *Trends Immunol* 25: 677-686

Martinez FO, Gordon S, Locati M, Mantovani A (2006) Transcriptional profiling of the human monocyte-to-macrophage differentiation and polarization: new molecules and patterns of gene expression. *J Immunol* 177: 7303-7311

Martinez FO, Sica A, Mantovani A, Locati M (2008) Macrophage activation and polarization. *Front Biosci* 13: 453-461

Matsushima GK, Morell P (2001) The neurotoxicant, cuprizone, as a model to study demyelination and remyelination in the central nervous system. *Brain Pathol* 11: 107-116

McDonald WI, Compston A, Edan G, Goodkin D, Hartung HP, Lublin FD, McFarland HF, Paty DW, Polman CH, Reingold SC, Sandberg-Wollheim M, Sibley W, Thompson A, van den NS, Weinshenker BY, Wolinsky JS (2001) Recommended diagnostic criteria for multiple sclerosis: guidelines from the International Panel on the diagnosis of multiple sclerosis. *Ann Neurol* 50: 121-127

Medzhitov R, Janeway CA, Jr. (2002) Decoding the patterns of self and nonself by the innate immune system. *Science* 296: 298-300

Mikita J, Dubourdieu-Cassagno N, Deloire MS, Vekris A, Biran M, Raffard G, Brochet B, Canron MH, Franconi JM, Boiziau C, Petry KG (2011) Altered M1/M2 activation patterns of monocytes in severe relapsing experimental rat model of multiple sclerosis. Amelioration of clinical status by M2 activated monocyte administration. *Mult Scler* 17: 2-15

Miller DH, Grossman RI, Reingold SC, McFarland HF (1998) The role of magnetic resonance techniques in understanding and managing multiple sclerosis. *Brain* 121 (Pt 1): 3-24

Miron VE, Ludwin SK, Darlington PJ, Jarjour AA, Soliven B, Kennedy TE, Antel JP (2010) Fingolimod (FTY720) enhances remyelination following demyelination of organotypic cerebellar slices. *Am J Pathol* 176: 2682-2694

Modolell M, Corraliza IM, Link F, Soler G, Eichmann K (1995) Reciprocal regulation of the nitric oxide synthase/arginase balance in mouse bone marrow-derived macrophages by TH1 and TH2 cytokines. *Eur J Immunol* 25: 1101-1104

Mosser DM (2003) The many faces of macrophage activation. *J Leukoc Biol* 73: 209-212

Mosser DM, Edwards JP (2008) Exploring the full spectrum of macrophage activation. *Nat Rev Immunol* 8: 958-969

Nathan C (2008) Metchnikoff's Legacy in 2008. *Nat Immunol* 9: 695-698

Nathan C, Shiloh MU (2000) Reactive oxygen and nitrogen intermediates in the relationship between mammalian hosts and microbial pathogens. *Proc Natl Acad Sci U S A* 97: 8841-8848

Nave KA (1994) Neurological mouse mutants and the genes of myelin. *J Neurosci Res* 38: 607-612

Nesbit GM, Forbes GS, Scheithauer BW, Okazaki H, Rodriguez M (1991) Multiple sclerosis: histopathologic and MR and/or CT correlation in 37 cases at biopsy and three cases at autopsy. *Radiology* 180: 467-474

Newman TA, Woolley ST, Hughes PM, Sibson NR, Anthony DC, Perry VH (2001) T-cell- and macrophage-mediated axon damage in the absence of a CNS-specific immune response: involvement of metalloproteinases. *Brain* 124: 2203-2214

Nielsen JM, Korteweg T, Barkhof F, Uitdehaag BM, Polman CH (2005) Overdiagnosis of multiple sclerosis and magnetic resonance imaging criteria. *Ann Neurol* 58: 781-783

O'Shea JJ, Murray PJ (2008) Cytokine signaling modules in inflammatory responses. *Immunity* 28: 477-487

Palin K, Cunningham C, Forse P, Perry VH, Platt N (2008) Systemic inflammation switches the inflammatory cytokine profile in CNS Wallerian degeneration. *Neurobiol Dis* 30: 19-29

Paolino E, Fainardi E, Ruppi P, Tola MR, Govoni V, Casetta I, Monetti VC, Granieri E, Carreras M (1996) A prospective study on the predictive value of CSF oligoclonal bands and MRI in acute isolated neurological syndromes for subsequent progression to multiple sclerosis. *J Neurol Neurosurg Psychiatry* 60: 572-575

Pardo B, Honegger P (2000) Differentiation of rat striatal embryonic stem cells in vitro: monolayer culture vs. three-dimensional coculture with differentiated brain cells. *J Neurosci Res* 59: 504-512

Polman CH, Reingold SC, Banwell B, Clanet M, Cohen JA, Filippi M, Fujihara K, Havrdova E, Hutchinson M, Kappos L, Lublin FD, Montalban X, O'Connor P, Sandberg-Wollheim M, Thompson AJ, Waubant E, Weinshenker B, Wolinsky JS (2011) Diagnostic criteria for multiple sclerosis: 2010 revisions to the McDonald criteria. *Ann Neurol* 69: 292-302

Polman CH, Reingold SC, Edan G, Filippi M, Hartung HP, Kappos L, Lublin FD, Metz LM, McFarland HF, O'Connor PW, Sandberg-Wollheim M, Thompson AJ, Weinshenker BG, Wolinsky JS (2005) Diagnostic criteria for multiple sclerosis: 2005 revisions to the "McDonald Criteria". *Ann Neurol* 58: 840-846

Popovich PG, Guan Z, Wei P, Huitinga I, van RN, Stokes BT (1999) Depletion of hematogenous macrophages promotes partial hindlimb recovery and neuroanatomical repair after experimental spinal cord injury. *Exp Neurol* 158: 351-365

Prineas JW, Barnard RO, Kwon EE, Sharer LR, Cho ES (1993) Multiple sclerosis: remyelination of nascent lesions. *Ann Neurol* 33: 137-151

Prineas JW, Connell F (1979) Remyelination in multiple sclerosis. *Ann Neurol* 5: 22-31

Pugliatti M, Sotgiu S, Rosati G (2002) The worldwide prevalence of multiple sclerosis. *Clin Neurol Neurosurg* 104: 182-191

Raine CS, Wu E (1993) Multiple sclerosis: remyelination in acute lesions. *J Neuropathol Exp Neurol* 52: 199-204

Rapalino O, Lazarov-Spiegler O, Agranov E, Velan GJ, Yoles E, Fraidakis M, Solomon A, Gepstein R, Katz A, Belkin M, Hadani M, Schwartz M (1998) Implantation of stimulated homologous macrophages results in partial recovery of paraplegic rats. *Nat Med* 4: 814-821

Rodriguez M, Lucchinetti CF (1999) Is apoptotic death of the oligodendrocyte a critical event in the pathogenesis of multiple sclerosis?. *Neurology* 53: 1615-1616

Romieu-Mourez R, Solis M, Nardin A, Goubau D, Baron-Bodo V, Lin R, Massie B, Salcedo M, Hiscott J (2006) Distinct roles for IFN regulatory factor (IRF)-3 and IRF-7 in the activation of antitumor properties of human macrophages. *Cancer Res* 66: 10576-10585

Shechter R, London A, Varol C, Raposo C, Cusimano M, Yovel G, Rolls A, Mack M, Pluchino S, Martino G, Jung S, Schwartz M (2009) Infiltrating blood-derived macrophages are vital cells playing an anti-inflammatory role in recovery from spinal cord injury in mice. *PLoS Med* 6: e1000113

Smith KJ, Kapoor R, Hall SM, Davies M (2001) Electrically active axons degenerate when exposed to nitric oxide. *Ann Neurol* 49: 470-476

Song E, Ouyang N, Horbelt M, Antus B, Wang M, Exton MS (2000) Influence of alternatively and classically activated macrophages on fibrogenic activities of human fibroblasts. *Cell Immunol* 204: 19-28

Stein M, Keshav S, Harris N, Gordon S (1992) Interleukin 4 potently enhances murine macrophage mannose receptor activity: a marker of alternative immunologic macrophage activation. *J Exp Med* 176: 287-292

Stirling DP, Khodarahmi K, Liu J, McPhail LT, McBride CB, Steeves JD, Ramer MS, Tetzlaff W (2004) Minocycline treatment reduces delayed oligodendrocyte death, attenuates axonal dieback, and improves functional outcome after spinal cord injury. *J Neurosci* 24: 2182-2190

Takeda K, Akira S (2005) Toll-like receptors in innate immunity. *Int Immunol* 17: 1-14

Teunissen CE, Dijkstra CD, Jasperse B, Barkhof F, Vanderstichele H, Vanmechelen E, Polman CH, Bo L (2006) Growth-associated protein 43 in lesions and cerebrospinal fluid in multiple sclerosis. *Neuropathol Appl Neurobiol* 32: 318-331

Teunissen CE, Iacobaeus E, Khademi M, Brundin L, Norgren N, Koel-Simmelink MJ, Schepens M, Bouwman F, Twaalfhoven HA, Blom HJ, Jakobs C, Dijkstra CD (2009) Combination of CSF N-acetylaspartate and neurofilaments in multiple sclerosis. *Neurology* 72: 1322-1329

Teunissen CE, Koel-Simmelink MJ, Pham TV, Knol JC, Khalil M, Trentini A, Killestein J, Nielsen J, Vrenken H, Popescu V, Dijkstra CD, Jimenez CR (2011) Identification of biomarkers for diagnosis and progression of MS by MALDI-TOF mass spectrometry. *Mult Scler* 17: 838-850

Teunissen CE, Steinbusch HW, Markerink-van Ittersum M., de Bruijn C., Axer H, de Vente J. (2000) Whole brain spheroid cultures as a model to study the development of nitric oxide synthase-guanylate cyclase signal transduction. *Brain Res Dev Brain Res* 125: 99-115

Trapp BD, Peterson J, Ransohoff RM, Rudick R, Mork S, Bo L (1998) Axonal transection in the lesions of multiple sclerosis. *N Engl J Med* 338: 278-285

Van den Bossche J., Bogaert P, Van Hengel J, Guerin CJ, Berx G, Movahedi K, Van den Bergh R., Pereira-Fernandes A, Geuns JM, Pircher H, Dorny P, Grooten J, De Baetselier P., Van Ginderachter JA (2009) Alternatively activated macrophages engage in homotypic and heterotypic interactions through IL-4 and polyamine-induced E-cadherin/catenin complexes. *Blood* 114: 4664-4674

van der Goes A., Boorsma W, Hoekstra K, Montagne L, De Groot CJ, Dijkstra CD (2005) Determination of the sequential degradation of myelin proteins by macrophages. *J Neuroimmunol* 161: 12-20

van der Valk, De Groot CJ (2000) Staging of multiple sclerosis (MS) lesions: pathology of the time frame of MS. *Neuropathol Appl Neurobiol* 26: 2-10

Vereyken EJ, Fluitsma DM, Bolijn MJ, Dijkstra CD, Teunissen CE (2009) An in vitro model for de- and remyelination using lysophosphatidyl choline in rodent whole brain spheroid cultures. *Glia* 57: 1326-1340

Vereyken EJ, Heijnen PD, Baron W, de Vries EH, Dijkstra CD, Teunissen CE (2011) Classically and alternatively activated bone marrow derived macrophages differ in cytoskeletal functions and migration towards specific CNS cell types. *J Neuroinflammation* 8: 58

Weber MS, Prod'homme T, Youssef S, Dunn SE, Rundle CD, Lee L, Patarroyo JC, Stuve O, Sobel RA, Steinman L, Zamvil SS (2007) Type II monocytes modulate T cell-mediated central nervous system autoimmune disease. *Nat Med* 13: 935-943

Wolswijk G (2000) Oligodendrocyte survival, loss and birth in lesions of chronic-stage multiple sclerosis. *Brain* 123 (Pt 1): 105-115

Wolswijk G (2002) Oligodendrocyte precursor cells in the demyelinated multiple sclerosis spinal cord. *Brain* 125: 338-349

Woodruff RH, Franklin RJ (1999) Demyelination and remyelination of the caudal cerebellar peduncle of adult rats following stereotaxic injections of lysolecithin, ethidium bromide, and complement/anti-galactocerebroside: a comparative study. *Glia* 25: 216-228

Zeyda M, Farmer D, Todoric J, Aszmann O, Speiser M, Gyori G, Zlabinger GJ, Stulnig TM (2007) Human adipose tissue macrophages are of an anti-inflammatory phenotype but capable of excessive pro-inflammatory mediator production. *Int J Obes (Lond)* 31: 1420-1428

Zhang X, Mosser DM (2008) Macrophage activation by endogenous danger signals. *J Pathol* 214: 161-178

Zhang Z, Zhang ZY, Schluesener HJ (2009) Compound A, a plant origin ligand of glucocorticoid receptors, increases regulatory T cells and M2 macrophages to attenuate experimental autoimmune neuritis with reduced side effects. *J Immunol* 183: 3081-3091

Zheng D, Wang Y, Cao Q, Lee VW, Zheng G, Sun Y, Tan TK, Wang Y, Alexander SI, Harris DC (2011) Transfused macrophages ameliorate pancreatic and renal injury in murine diabetes mellitus. *Nephron Exp Nephrol* 118: e87-e99

Ziemann U, Wahl M, Hattingen E, Tumani H (2011) Development of biomarkers for multiple sclerosis as a neurodegenerative disorder. *Prog Neurobiol*

20

Amyotrophic Lateral Sclerosis

David S. Shin[1], Ashley J. Pratt[2],
Elizabeth D. Getzoff[2] and J. Jefferson P. Perry[2,3]
[1]Lawrence Berkeley National Laboratory,
[2]The Scripps Research Institute,
[3]Amrita University,
[1,2]USA
[3]India

1. Introduction

Amyotrophic lateral sclerosis (ALS) is a fatal neurodegenerative motor neuron disease for which no successful treatment presently exists. ALS is also termed Charcot's disease (maladie de Charcot), after the French clinician Jean Martin Charcot who first described its features in 1869 (Charcot 1869) or Lou Gehrig's disease in the United States, after the New York Yankees baseball player afflicted with the condition. Within Europe ALS is often referred to as Motor Neuron Disease, describing the cells chiefly affected, although this term may also more generally refer to a wider group of motor neuron diseases.

ALS is characterized by the degeneration of motor cortex, brainstem and/or motor neurons associated with the spinal cord, resulting in muscle weakness and loss of voluntary muscle control. Progressive paralysis ensues, and respiratory failure is the usual cause of death. *Amyotrophic* refers to the lack (*a-*) of muscle (*-myo-*) nourishment (*-trophic*), resulting in wasting of the fibers; *Lateral* refers to the lateral corticospinal tract of affected neurons between the brain and spinal cord; *Sclerosis* is the resultant hardening of the tissue. The incidence of ALS globally ranges from 0.3 to 2.4 cases per 100,000 (Sathasivam 2010). Approximately 95% of ALS cases are random or sporadic (SALS), whereas 5 or more percent are inherited (familial ALS, FALS), with a subset of these arising from known genetic determinants.

Despite the initial description of the disorder about 150 years ago, and significant progress in the understanding of its pathology, ALS remains an ill-defined terminal disease with few medicinal options and an average duration of only a few years. Nonetheless, new developments in ALS research are slowly emerging in diagnostics, in elucidating molecular mechanisms behind the disease, and in generating treatments. Improved technologies and recent research insights, when coupled with meaningful collaborations between scientists and clinicians hold promise for exciting progress. Thus, we discuss here the current understanding of ALS in terms of its clinical presentation, and its molecular and cellular basis. In particular, we highlight new insights into the genetics of the inherited disease, with a focus on the mutant gene products Cu,Zn-superoxide dismutase (Cu,ZnSOD), Fused in Sarcoma/Translated in Lipsarcoma (FUS/TLS) and the Tar-DNA binding protein 43 (TDP-43). The standard care regimen will also be described, along with a focus on novel therapeutic strategies and developments for improving the outlook for patients with this terminal disease.

2. Clinical phenotype

The initial onset of ALS (both FALS and SALS) typically begins with one of several patterns. Seventy five percent of patients have "spinal onset," affecting the limbs (Kiernan et al. 2011). Within this group a "cervical" subset will have muscle weakness in the upper limbs, while symptoms of the "lumbar" subset will arise in the lower limbs. In ALS, affected cells include the upper motor neurons (UMN) in the motor cortex and/or lower motor neurons (LMN) in the brainstem and spinal cord. Presentation of pure UMN symptoms, sometimes referred to as primary lateral sclerosis (PLS), includes decelerated speech, weakness and spasticity, hypereflexia, pseudobulbar affect (inappropriate emotionality including bursts of crying or laughing). Presentation of pure LMN symptoms, known as progressive muscular atrophy (PMA), includes severe weakness and hypereflexia, in addition to loss of muscle tone, muscle atrophy, cramps and twitching (termed fasciculations) (Sathasivam 2010; Lomen-Hoerth 2008). A combination of UMN and LMN symptoms may also occur. Onset is usually asymmetrical, although progressive wasting and spreading will most likely ensue (Swash 1998).

Fewer patients have "bulbar onset" ALS, which targets muscles of the face and neck; this form is more common in women and the elderly (Forbes, Colville, and Swingler 2004; McCombe and Henderson 2010) and has a worse prognosis. Symptoms of the UMN-based bulbar variant (pseudobulbar palsy) include emotional responses (as mentioned above), slurred speech (dysarthria), excessive yawning and jerking of the jaw (Wicks 2007; Kuhnlein et al. 2008). The LMN-based affliction (bulbar palsy) manifests as tongue fasciculation resulting in dysarthria, drooling, difficulties in swallowing (dysphagia) and wasting of the tongue (Kuhnlein et al. 2008). Several rare, additional phenotypes exist, including a respiratory onset form, which shares the poorest prognosis with the bulbar onset form (Chio et al. 2011).

The characteristic clinical course of ALS is a progressive loss of voluntary movement, with symptoms spreading to more distant locations (Haverkamp, Appel, and Appel 1995), and the end result being paralysis and death from respiratory failure. Treatment with a ventilator may assist breathing and improve the quality of life (Radunovic et al. 2009). However, eventually the patient may enter a "locked-in" state, where communication is only possibly with the help of an electronic device, and ultimately, even oculomotor function may be impaired (Sharma et al. 2011). In addition to facial, limb and behavioral impairments, frontotemporal dementia (FTD) occurs in a subset of ALS patients (Murphy, Henry, and Lomen-Hoerth 2007), with negative implications for treatment and survival (Olney et al. 2005). Frontotemporal dementia (FTD) patients can also display ALS-like symptoms, suggesting that some aspects of these two diseases may overlap (Ferrari et al. 2011). Unfortunately, treatment of ALS is mostly palliative; the sole approved drug, riluzole (as discussed in section 4), extends life for only a few months (Miller et al. 2007). Typically, half of diagnosed ALS patients will succumb to the disease within about 3 years, 20-25% within 5 years and a small minority can survive 10 years and beyond (Talbot 2009; Testa et al. 2004; Forsgren et al. 1983). Post-mortem staining of the degenerating tissues in motor neurons of the motor cortex, brainstem and spinal cord with eosin and hematoxylin may reveal Bunina bodies and/or ubiquitin-positive-inclusions of the skein-like or hyaline form (most commonly the Lewy body-like variety), among others (Leigh et al. 1991). Thus, the underlying multi-pathway cellular dyshomeostasis leading to the complicated, heterogeneous clinical phenotypes associated with ALS and its variants so far remains mysterious and is under intense investigation.

The distinction between familial and sporadic cases of ALS is not always clear-cut, due to incomplete genetic penetrance, complicating environmental factors and diagnostic difficulties. FALS has been attributed to approximately 5% of ALS cases (Byrne and Hardiman 2010; Talbot 2010), although higher levels in certain geographical regions have been reported (Haberlandt 1959; Murros and Fogelholm 1983). It has been suggested that even rates for the familial disease as high as 13.5% might be underestimates (Andersen 2006), due to the complicating variable of reduced penetrance in some families, causing miscategorization of some FALS cases as SALS (Williams, Floate, and Leicester 1988). FALS is usually inherited in a Mendelian, autosomal dominant manner (Veltema, Roos, and Bruyn 1990), with autosomal recessive and X-linked modes of inheritance occurring rarely (Donkervoort and Siddique 1993; Andersen et al. 1996). The clinical symptoms of FALS and SALS are generally similar, but may be more homogeneous within individual FALS-afflicted families than between them (Horton, Eldridge, and Brody 1976). The mean age of onset at about 48-52 years for FALS (Mulder et al. 1986; Li, Alberman, and Swash 1988) is earlier than the mean at approximately 56 years for SALS (Li, Alberman, and Swash 1988; Haverkamp, Appel, and Appel 1995) and the survival period is also shorter for FALS than for SALS (Mulder et al. 1986). A small minority of ALS patients exhibit juvenile onset (usually before age 25), which is generally characterized by longer survival (Aggarwal and Shashiraj 2006; Ben Hamida, Hentati, and Ben Hamida 1990). Juvenile-onset ALS can occur in an autosomal dominant form, linked to several known genes (Blair et al. 2000) or in a form that may be recessive or sporadic (Hadano et al. 2001).

The lifetime risk of ALS is about 1 in 400, [in the United Kingdom (Alonso et al. 2009)], yet due to the very short survival rate of about 3 years (Donkervoort and Siddique 1993), the disease prevalence is low, ranging from only 0.8 per 100,000 people (in Mexico) to 8.4 per 100,000 (in Sweden) (Olivares, Esteban, and Alter 1972; Gunnarsson and Palm 1984). The yearly incidence of ALS globally varies only slightly worldwide, from as few as 0.3 diagnoses per 100,000 persons in Hong Kong-China (Fong et al. 1996) to 2.4 cases per 100,000 in Finland (Fong et al. 1996), excepting a few, documented, high-occurrence clusters [e.g. an ALS-Parkinsonism-like disease frequency in Guam of up to 100 times greater than average in the middle of the 20th century (Steele and McGeer 2008)]. More studies of non-Caucasian populations are needed to evaluate ALS rates across all ethnic groups (Cronin, Hardiman, and Traynor 2007). The gender ratio for ALS varies somewhat between studies, and with factors such as age and ethnicity (McCombe and Henderson 2010; Abhinav et al. 2007) but consistently shows an increased risk for males. This variability may be due to regional, environmental or genetic differences among patients or, to a decrease in the skewing of ALS cases toward men over time (Worms 2001). Interestingly, the ratio also tends more toward gender equality in FALS than in SALS (Mulder et al. 1986; Li, Alberman, and Swash 1988).

No diagnostic test for ALS is currently available. The Revised El Escorial criteria (Brooks et al. 2000), developed by the World Federation of Neurology, are a set of findings used in the diagnosis of ALS. They categorize the case as "definite," "probable" or "possible," based on clinical UMN and LMN observations and electrophysiological data. These criteria are commonly used for participation in clinical trials, although they have been suggested to be inappropriate for general clinical practice (Andersen et al. 2005) and not sensitive enough as an early diagnostic tool (Kiernan et al. 2011). Earlier diagnosis is in fact highly associated with a longer survival (Testa et al. 2004; Haverkamp, Appel, and Appel 1995), although the median duration between first symptoms and diagnosis was found to be about a year for many cases (Chio 1999; Spuler et al. 2011). Another measure sometimes used in research or private practice is the revised ALS Functional Rating Scale (ALSFRS-R), a scoring tool to monitor the disease progression of patients (Cedarbaum et al. 1999). These measures and others [e.g. the Awaji criteria, (de Carvalho et al. 2008)] are undoubtedly useful. However, objective laboratory tests (e.g. for ALS-specific blood or cerebrospinal fluid biomarkers) would represent a major stride in diagnosis, and some progress is underway in this area (Turner et al. 2009), though validation is still needed.

Current diagnosis of ALS is typically by process of elimination. The trained clinician will assess the presence of UMN and/or LMN symptoms and any evidence of disease progression, then test to eliminate potentially overlapping syndromes. For FALS, the presence of an affected family member can aid diagnosis, and trigger genetic testing, if appropriate (Andersen 2000). Due to the heterogeneity of presentation (Chio et al. 2011), the exclusion of ALS mimics is a very important part of diagnosis. Conditions with overlapping symptoms may include spinal disease or injury (e.g. compression), enzyme or vitamin deficiency (B-12 etc.), cancers, myopathy, neuropathy, infections such as Lyme or HIV, thyroid problems, myasthenia gravis, Kennedy's disease, Tay-Sachs diseases, lead poisoning and multiple sclerosis, among others (Sathasivam 2010; Lomen-Hoerth 2008; Traynor et al. 2000; Silani et al. 2011). Elimination of these ALS mimics is non-trivial, especially since misdiagnosis is very common (Chio 1999; Traynor et al. 2000). Conversely, false positive diagnosis of ALS (estimated at around 10%) can also have marked impacts on patient prognosis and treatment (Davenport et al. 1996; Ludolph and Knirsch 1999). Magnetic resonance imaging (MRI) is one of the most commonly performed diagnostic tests to image the condition of the brain and neck, to eliminate injury as a cause of symptoms. Electromyography (EMG) and nerve conduction studies are useful for evaluating muscle and nerve status. Blood tests (to determine blood count, erythrocyte sedimentation, specific enzyme abnormalities such as creatine kinase) are also useful (Talbot 2009). Less commonly, CSF tests, psychological tests and muscle biopsies are performed to rule out other conditions. Therefore, diagnosis is made by careful examination of the clinical presentation coupled to evaluation by laboratory tests.

3. Pathophysiology

Despite a multitude of genetic, biochemical, cellular and clinical investigations, current ALS research suggests that there is no definitive single cause for the disease and/or that the cellular pathways involved employ much complexity. Thus, further research is required on all fronts to elucidate the underlying pathophysiological mechanisms. We focus on several key disease-implicated proteins, and discuss advances and controversies in our understanding of how mutations may give rise to the disease. We include our own studies on ALS-linked mutations in Cu,Zn superoxide dismutase (SOD), which account for a very significant proportion of genetically defined FALS cases. We also address other genetic factors and environmental influences that have been implicated in ALS.

3.1 Genetic factors

Many recent significant advances in ALS research result from investigations of genetic lesions and their consequent biological defects leading to the disease. Most of these genetic abnormalities in ALS alter expressed proteins through missense and nonsense mutations, but some genetic linkages are presently not yet connected to a specific underlying protein defect. ALS cases arising from genetic defects have been further divided into subtypes dependent on gene mapping, linkage analysis and phenotype (Table 1). The more characterized subtypes are referred to as ALS1 through ALS14. We have also included in Table 1 several other genes implicated in ALS susceptibility (Al-Chalabi et al. 1999; He and Hays 2004; Munch et al. 2005; Munch et al. 2004). Below, we describe the distribution of >130 distinct mutations in ALS1 (Cu,ZnSOD) within the protein structure, and provide current hypotheses for how this multitude of distinct substitutions affect Cu,ZnSOD structure and function, leading to an ALS phenotype. We also focus on proteins involved in predominately sporadic ALS cases. In particular, we highlight recent results that point to mutation-induced dysfunctions of ALS6 (FUS/TLS) and ALS10 TDP-43 (also involved in certain familial ALS cases), two proteins that are involved in DNA/RNA synthesis and gene regulation, implicating a role for RNA metabolic defects in the disease.

ALS Sub-type	Gene	MIM Gene Number	Locus	Protein	MIM Pheno-type	Age of Onset	Notes
ALS1	*SOD1*	147450	21q22.1 | 21q22.11	Cu,Zn superoxide dismutase	105400	Adult	AD, AR, Sp
ALS2	*ALS2*	606352	2q33.1	Alsin	205100	Juvenile	AR
ALS3	-	-	18q21	-	606640	Adult	AD
ALS4	*SETX*	608465	9q34.13	Senataxin	602433	Juvenile	AD
ALS5	*SPG11*	-	15q15-q21.1	Spatacsin	602099	Any age	AR
ALS6	*FUS*	137070	16p11.2	Fused in sarcoma	608030	Adult	AD, AR, Sp
ALS7	-	-	20p13	-	608031	Adult	AD
ALS8	*VAPB*	605704	20q13.33	VAMP-associated protein B	608627	Adult	AD
ALS9	*ANG*	105850	14q11.1-q11.2	Angiogenin	611895	Adult	AD, Sp
ALS10	*TARDBP*	605078	1p36.22	TDP-43	612069	Adult	AD, Sp
ALS11	*FIG4*	609390	6q21	Phosphoinositide 5-phosphatase	612577	Adult	AD
ALS12	*OPTN*	602432	10p13	Optineurin	613435	Adult	AD, AR, Sp
ALS13	*ATXN2*	601517	12q24.1	Ataxin-2	183090	-	Suscept
ALS14	*VCP*	601023	9p13.3	Valosin-containing protein	613954	Adult	AD
-	*DCTN*	601143	2p13	Dynactin	105400	-	Suscept
-	*NEFH*	162230	22q12.2	Heavy neurofilament subunit	105400	-	Suscept
-	*PRPH*	105400	12q12-q13	Peripherin	105400	-	Suscept
-	*UBQLN2*	-	Xp11.2	Ubiquilin	-	Any age	X-linked

Table 1. ALS subtypes. ALS phenotypes map to many chromosomal loci, and often to specific proteins implicated in the disease. Data for this table were compiled from the Online Mendelian Inheritance in Man® (MIM) website (http://omim.org) and other sources (Pasinelli and Brown 2006; Ticozzi et al. 2011; Boillee, Vande Velde, and Cleveland 2006; Deng et al. 2011) MIM gene and phenotype numbers are included for reference. Abbreviations in Notes column: AD, autosomal dominant; AR, autosomal recessive; Sp, sporadic; Suscept, aids susceptibility to ALS; X-linked, Chromosome X linkage

3.1.1 Cu,Zn superoxide dismutase

Cu,ZnSOD was first isolated from bovine erythrocytes in the late 1930s (Mann and Keilin 1938). The protein was then termed hemocuprein for its copper content, apparent from the blue color of the crystalline protein. In the 1950s, Cu,ZnSOD was purified from brain (Porter and Folch 1957), where it accounts for approximately 1% of neuronal cytosolic protein (Siddique and Deng 1996). McCord and Fridovich biochemically characterized the protein in 1969, and discovered that it catalyzed the dismutation of superoxide radicals to hydrogen peroxide and oxygen (McCord and Fridovich 1969). Reactive oxygen species, such as superoxide, were subsequently linked to aging and to many diseases. This cytosolic protein was discovered to be unusually stable, surviving organic extraction in the original purifications (McCord and Fridovich 1969) and maintaining enzymatic activity under harsh conditions, such as denaturants and heat (Forman and Fridovich 1973; Malinowski and Fridovich 1979; Hallewell et al. 1991). Our labs routinely use heat denaturation of host proteins when purifying Cu,ZnSOD from heterologous expression systems (Shin et al. 2009). This unusual enzymatic stability could be involved ALS etiology.

Members of our groups have analyzed the biochemical, biophysical and structural properties of wild-type and ALS-linked mutant Cu,ZnSOD proteins. The first Cu,ZnSOD X-ray crystal structure (Tainer et al. 1982; Tainer et al. 1983), revealing the fold and structure-based mechanism of catalysis, was from the bovine enzyme and was later followed by our crystal structure of human Cu,ZnSOD (Figure 1) (Parge, Hallewell, and Tainer 1992).

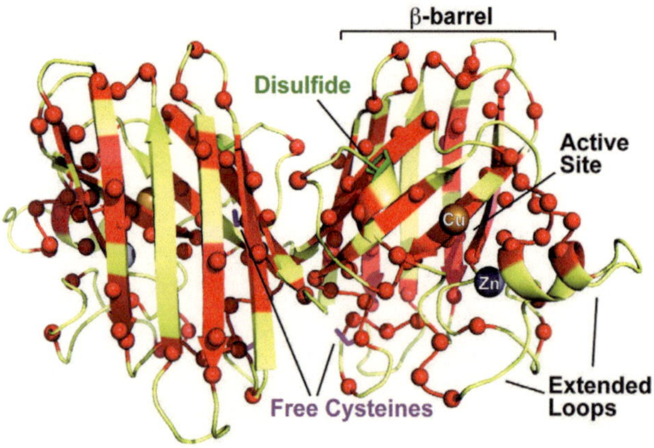

Fig. 1. Human Cu,ZnSOD crystal structure (PDB ID 1PU0) and known ALS mutation sites. Cu,ZnSOD exists as a homodimer and each subunit consists of a single Greek-key motif barrel-like domain, flanked by extended loops that form the active site cleft and house catalytic Cu and Zn ions (large labeled spheres). The smaller red spheres denote Cα ALS mutation site positions mapped onto this cartoon representation of the protein. The conserved disulfide bond (green) in each subunit conveys stability, while free cysteine residues (magenta) are implicated in irreversible unfolding

Our latest published structures of Cu,ZnSOD (Shin et al. 2009) were derived from the eukaryotic thermophile *Alvinella pompejana*, a deep-sea thermal vent worm that we and others discovered contains particularly stable proteins (Burjanadze 2000; Henscheid et al. 2005; Kashiwagi et al. 2010; Piccino et al. 2004). *Alvinella pompejana* Cu,ZnSOD allowed us to obtain both the first sub-angstrom resolution crystal structure of Cu,ZnSOD, and a co-crystal structure with the H_2O_2 product. These structures revealed that the copper ion likely moves within the active site during catalysis (Shin et al. 2009). Structural and computational analyses showed that electrostatic guidance (Getzoff et al. 1992; Getzoff et al. 1983; Perry et al. 2010) aids catalysis, allowing Cu,ZnSOD to be one of the fastest enzymes known.

Our initial structural studies on human Cu,ZnSOD were conducted prior to the discovery that ALS was correlated with mutations in Cu,ZnSOD (Deng et al. 1993; Rosen 1993). Greater than 130 Cu,ZnSOD mutations, occuring at ~70 of the 153 amino acids that comprise a single subunit of human Cu,ZnSOD (Figure 1), are now implicated in causing ALS; the vast majority of these are autosomal dominant in inheritance. These Cu,ZnSOD associated ALS mutations also constitute the majority of ALS cases that have been genetically defined, approximately 20% of FALS cases and ~1-3% of SALS cases. Mapping of the ALS mutations onto the human Cu,ZnSOD structure prompted our suggestion of a 'framework destabilization' hypothesis (Deng et al. 1993). This destabilization hypothesis suggests that ALS SOD mutations promote local unfolding events in Cu,ZnSOD that can drive self-aggregation and potentially aberrant interactions with other proteins, dysregulating the normal cellular functions of this highly abundant protein in neuronal cells.

Alternative hypotheses include a gain of function mechanism, for example a change of SOD chemistry so that the enzyme performs other reactions (such as peroxidation and increased tyrosine nitration), or exhibits an increase or decrease in catalytic activity (Beckman et al. 1993; Brown 1995; Crow et al. 1997; Rosen 1993; Wiedau-Pazos et al. 1996; Wong and Borchelt 1995; Zhang et al. 2002). However, support for these other hypotheses is unclear. Certain mutations are known to make a more active enzyme, while others produce a less active protein, and some have with relatively unchanged chemistry. Some mutations (such as H46R and H48Q) remove copper binding, rendering the protein non-catalytic, thus suggesting that gain of enzymatic function or increased activity is unlikely. Transgenic mice harboring SOD1 mutations present ALS-like symptoms (Gurney et al. 1994), but transgenic SOD1 knockout mice do not (Reaume et al. 1996). This indicates that a loss of normal catalytic activity or a gain of abnormal activity may not be important in propagating ALS. Also, activity-altering mutations would be expected to be focused in and around the active site, rather than occurring across the entire Cu,ZnSOD fold.

Protein aggregates are observed within neural cells from Alzheimer's, Huntington's and Parkinson's individuals (Dobson 2001; Soto 2001; Wanker 2000). Likewise, proteinaceous aggregates were discovered in neurons of ALS patients (Leigh et al. 1991). We observed *in vitro* that purified FALS A4V and H43R mutants form fibrous aggregates, and that two free cysteines within the protein are not required for this aggregation. These two ALS mutants bound Congo Red and Thioflavin T dyes that typically bind amyloid-like β-sheet structures (Figure 2) (DiDonato et al. 2003). Notably, the kinetics of forming aggregates and the binding affinity for dyes were more enhanced for the more clinically aggressive mutant A4V mutant. In cellular inclusions, aggregates were found to be immunoreactive for Cu,ZnSOD, and did not dissociate readily in the presence of detergents or reductants (Bruijn et al. 1998; Durham et al. 1997). Also, the detection of Cu,ZnSOD-containing inclusions often precedes ALS-like symptoms, and the aggregates are similar to Lewy bodies found in Parkinson's disease (Johnston et al. 2000; Kato et al. 2001).

ALS mutant SODs interact and/or co-precipitate with additional proteins to form the inclusions observed in cells from ALS patients; these inclusions resemble those characteristic of other neurodegenerative disease. These associated proteins include 1) proteins involved in stress response pathways, namely Derlin-1 (Nishitoh et al. 2008) and Rac1 (Harraz et al. 2008), 2) chromogramin proteins associated with neurosectretory vesicles (Urushitani et al. 2006), 3) the cytosolic chaperone Hsc70 (Wang et al. 2009), 4) the SOD copper chaperone (Kato et al. 2001), and 5) the dynein complex heavy chain, which is used in neural retrograde transport (Kieran et al. 2005; Zhang et al. 2007). Thus, local destabilizing *SOD1* mutations, leading to interactions and/or co-precipitation of these proteins within aggregates, may impact normal cellular functions. It was also recently discovered that neural membrane fluidity was altered in transgenic ALS mice that harbor a FALS SOD mutation (Miana-Mena et al. 2011). The authors hypothesize that membranes may be altered through lipid peroxidation, yet misfolded SODs may also play a role by interacting with membranes. Other hypotheses for the involvement of mutant SOD in ALS include disruption of the ubiquitin and proteosome system, altering mitochondrial function, playing a role in glutamatergic neurotransmission leading to excitotoxicity, and interference with axonal transport systems (Bastos et al. 2011; Kiernan et al. 2011; Ticozzi et al. 2011). Thus, we suggest that the framework destabilization hypothesis, unlike other suggested hypotheses, provides a unified mechanism for ALS mutant phenotype: This hypothesis encompasses the widespread distribution of ALS mutation sites within the protein, and is further supported by the observed *in vitro* aggregation results and the cellular analyses that are also in keeping with other aggregation-prone neurodegenerative diseases.

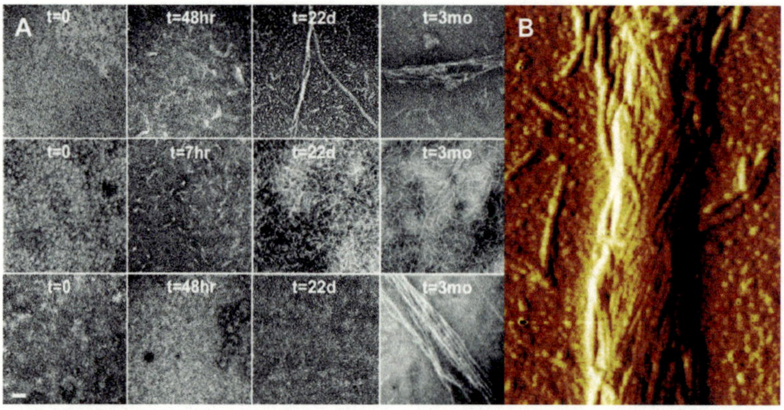

Fig. 2. FALS SOD mutants promote the formation of filamentous aggregates. (A) Electron micrographs of H43R and A4V fibers reveals diameters of 2-15 nm implying a loss of dimer assembly specificity. Samples of H43R (top row), A4V (middle row) and wild-type (bottom row), all in the C6A, C111S SOD background lacking free Cys, were subjected to conditions designed to perturb the SOD fold. The scale bar = 40 nm. (B) Atomic force micrograph (phase mode) of large H43R bundles. Adapted from (DiDonato et al. 2003)

3.1.2 FUS/TLS

The *FUS* gene, representing the ALS6 subtype of amyotrophic lateral sclerosis, encodes the "fused in sarcoma" protein, initially characterized as one of the fusion proteins generated by carcinogenic oncogenes (Crozat et al. 1993; Rabbitts et al. 1993). The alternative name TLS stands for "translocation in liposarcoma", and the gene product is often referred to as FUS/TLS, as we will do for the remainder of this chapter. FUS/TLS is a 526 amino acid protein of the TET family (which stands for **T**ranslocated in liposarcoma/**E**wing's sarcoma/**T**ATA-binding protein-associated factor 15). FUS/TLS binds both DNA and RNA, and like Cu,ZnSOD, is ubiquitously expressed. The protein is divided into distinct motifs and regions, which are responsible for different functions [see Figure 3 and the following reviews (Dormann and Haass 2011; Lagier-Tourenne and Cleveland 2009; Perry, Shin, and Tainer 2010)]. FUS/TLS plays a role in transcription activities within the cell via interactions with a variety of proteins, including transcription factors and hormone receptors (Cassiday and Maher 2002; Lagier-Tourenne and Cleveland 2009) (Cassiday and Maher 2002; Lagier-Tourenne and Cleveland 2009; Law, Cann, and Hicks 2006). FUS/TLS may also function in DNA damage responses by binding to non-coding RNA elements transcribed by the 5' regulatory region of the cell-cycle kinase cyclin D1 gene. This binding event recruits FUS/TLS to interact with and inhibit CREB-binding protein and p300 histone acetelytransferase, further repressing cyclin D1-mediated transcription (Perry, Shin, and Tainer 2010). FUS/TLS has also been implicated in RNA processing, such as splicing, transport and maturation (Lagier-Tourenne and Cleveland 2009). In neurons, FUS/TLS is transported to dendritic spines upon activation of glutamate receptor mGluR5 (Fujii et al. 2005).

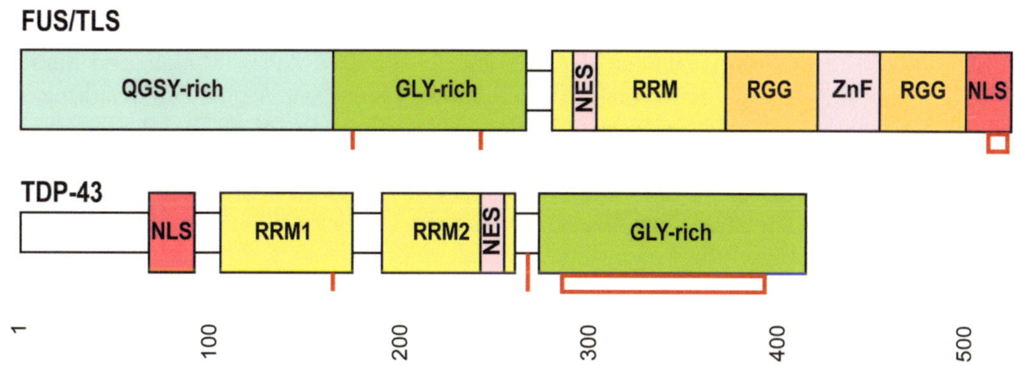

Fig. 3. Schematic diagrams of the FUS/TLS and TDP-43 proteins. Both proteins contain similar motifs, bind DNA and RNA, and are involved in both ALS and FTD. (Top) FUS/TLS contains QGSY- and Gly-rich regions, an RNA recognition motif (RRM) with a nuclear export signal (NES), a pair of RGG-motifs flanking a Zinc-finger (ZnF), and a nuclear localization signal (NLS). (Bottom) The TDP-43 protein has its NLS at the N-terminus, two RRM motifs with the latter containing an NES, and a C-terminal Gly-rich region. Red bars indicate ALS mutation sites, and red boxes indicate ALS hotspots that contain multiple ALS mutation sites. Numbers below indicate amino acid positions

The *FUS* gene was implicated in ALS after the discovery that a locus within chromosome 16 was linked to both autosomal dominant (Ticozzi et al. 2011; Vance et al. 2009) and recessive manifestations of the disease (Kwiatkowski et al. 2009). FUS mutations have since been identified in patients with sporadic ALS, and according to recent reviews [see (Kiernan et al. 2011; Ticozzi et al. 2011)], *FUS* mutants are estimated to account for approximately 4-5% of FALS and 1% of SALS cases. Interestingly, mutations in FUS/TLS are also involved in FTD [see (Mackenzie, Rademakers, and Neumann 2010)]. The disease-promoting mechanisms in mutant *FUS*-mediated ALS are not understood, but aggregate formation has been observed (Deng et al. 2010; Vance et al. 2009; Dormann and Haass 2011). The FUS/TLS mutations tend to cluster mainly at the C-terminal glycine-rich region and NLS (Dormann and Haass 2011; Lagier-Tourenne and Cleveland 2009; Perry, Shin, and Tainer 2010), instead of throughout the entire structure as observed in Cu,ZnSOD. Similar to Cu,ZnSOD mutant pathology is the observation that inclusions containing FUS/TLS are found within the cytosol within diseased neural cells (Dormann et al. 2010). Interestingly, NLS mutations that yield a greater concentration of FUS/TLS within the cytosol correlate with a more rapid onset and aggressiveness of the disease. Also, some of the most severe NLS mutations cause substitutions in amino acids required for an interaction with transportin, a nuclear import receptor (Dormann et al. 2010). Mutant cytosolic FUS/TLS may also be incorporated into stress granules that may serve as an inclusion precursor (Dormann and Haass 2011)).

Additionally, FUS/TLS has been predicted to contain prion-like regions within its amino-acid sequence, which may also contribute to the formation of aggregates (Udan and Baloh 2011).

3.1.3 TDP-43

TDP-43, named for binding to TAR DNA of the human immunodeficiency type 1 virus, is also a DNA and RNA binding protein like FUS/TLS. TDP-43 is encoded by the *TARDBP* gene, and is classified as the ALS10 subtype. TDP-43 is composed of 414 residues, and includes functional motifs shared with FUS/TLS (Figure 3). Functions for TDP-43 include transcriptional regulator (Abhyankar, Urekar, and Reddi 2007; Ayala, Misteli, and Baralle 2008), and TDP-43 was also implicated in binding UG-repeat sequences, resulting in pathogenic consequences that include cystic fibrosis (Mantovani et al. 2007). Like FUS/TLS, TDP-43 has been implicated in both ALS and FTD pathology (Arai et al. 2006; Mackenzie, Rademakers, and Neumann 2010; Dormann and Haass 2011; Perry, Shin, and Tainer 2010). Presently, over 35 mutations in TDP-43 have been implicated in these two diseases, including ~0.5-2% of sporadic ALS cases (Arai et al. 2006) and ~3-5% of autosomal dominant FALS cases (Lagier-Tourenne and Cleveland 2009; Ticozzi et al. 2011). TDP-43 aggregates are also found within diseased neural cells, where the protein is found to be highly ubiquinated and phosphorylated, as well as being truncated (Arai et al. 2006; Neumann et al. 2006). These aggregates are generally localized to the cytoplasm, while nuclear levels of TDP-43 are significantly diminished. Interestingly, analysis of the aggregates suggests that these deposits are not composed of amyloid-like structures (Kwong et al. 2008). Cu,ZnSOD is not found within the TDP-43 or the FUS/TLS aggregates; however, a recent report states that mutant Cu,ZnSOD interacts with TDP-43 (Higashi et al. 2010), and was shown to co-immunoprecipitate with FUS/TLS for a function in stabilizing histone deactylase 6 (HDAC6) mRNA (Kim et al. 2010). ALS mutations in TDP-43 appear to enhance this interaction with FUS/TLS (Ling et al. 2010). Therefore, additional research is required to clearly define these provisional links between TDP-43, FUS/TLS and/or Cu,ZnSOD in ALS pathology.

The majority of mutations found within TDP-43 ALS patients are missense mutations toward the C-terminal end of the protein, beginning at the glycine-rich segment. Recent research has identified the possibility that like FUS/TLS, TDP-43 also contains a prion-like element at its C-terminus. This region contains Gln and Asn residues similar to yeast Q/N prion domains. This represents yet another structural element that may initiate the formation of aggregates within ALS10 type cells. Currently, research on the function of TDP-43 and its roles in various pathologies including ALS and FTD is on the rise. Changes in TDP-43 structure and stability behind its ALS pathology may also influence the expression and activities of various cellular machinery within neural cells [see detailed reviews: (Dormann and Haass 2011; Lagier-Tourenne and Cleveland 2009; Lagier-Tourenne, Polymenidou, and Cleveland 2010; Perry, Shin, and Tainer 2010; Swarup et al. 2011)].

3.1.4 Other ALS subtypes

Research is being initiated on the defective genes for the other, more rare, ALS subtypes [see more detailed reviews (Boillee, Vande Velde, and Cleveland 2006; Kiernan et al. 2011; Pasinelli and Brown 2006; Strong et al. 2007; Ticozzi et al. 2011) for further information on these lesser-characterized ALS subtypes]. Many proteins encoded by these ALS subtype genes share the ability to modulate gene expression and/or RNA metabolism; this includes the *ANG* (ALS9) and *SETX* (ALS4) gene products, along with those of *FUS/TLS*, *TDP-43* and *SOD1* (Strong 2010). Also, the VAPB (ALS8) mutant shares the ability to form aggregates (Suzuki et al. 2009). Notably, the native alsin protein encoded by the *ALS2* gene has been observed to offer protection against Cu,ZnSOD mutational effects in certain cells (Hadano et al. 2007). Many mutations in *ALS2* are nonsense mutations that lead to truncations in the gene product, which can destabilize the protein, resulting in proteasomal degradation (Yamanaka et al. 2003). Another study suggests that alsin loss may cause neurons to be more vulnerable to excitotoxicity, via glutamate receptors (Lai et al. 2006). Co-localization has not yet been observed between Cu,ZnSOD and FUS/TLS or TDP-43. However, optineurin, which is encoded by *OPTN* and represents ALS12, does appear to colocalize with Cu,ZnSOD, FUS/TLS and TDP-43 [see (Ito et al. 2011)], and the interaction of optineruin with at least with the former two, appears to be mutually exclusive. A comprehensive study of a five generation family with ALS lead to the discovery that mutations in UBQLN2, which encodes the ubiquitin-like protein ubiquilin 2, cause dominant X-linked juvenile and adult-onset ALS and ALS/dementia (Deng et al. 2011). Also, excitingly, two very recent research findings have identified the largely uncharacterized locus 9p21 *C9ORF72* gene product to be linked to a significant proportion of dominant cases of ALS/FTD (Renton et al, 2011; DeJesus-Hernandez et al. 2011) Thus, it currently appears that genetic lesions may lead to ALS by different pathways, and continued research will be needed to establish whether there are one, several or many more general mechanistic themes that lead to the ALS phenotypes.

3.2 Other factors

Non-genetic risk factors for ALS, including environmental factors and physical injury, are being actively pursued. Although the effects of these risks of ALS are difficult to deconvolute (e.g. the prevalence of ALS in athletes), the involvement of these factors may enhance underlying, genetic predispositions to the disease, or may indeed have a direct link to ALS.

3.2.1 Diet/Lifestyle

The role of diet in ALS was assessed when considerably higher prevalence levels of ALS were noted in certain Western Pacific populations (50-100-fold). Non-genetic causes for these ALS cases have been suggested to be due to high levels of β-methyl-amino-L-alanine. This non-standard amino acid is highly concentrated in a certain seed that is consumed by animals that provide food for the inhabitants of Guam (Bastos et al. 2011; Ince and Codd 2005). A recent study has highlighted adverse effects from high levels of branched-chain amino acids (BCAAs) on the ion channels of mice. The researchers discovered an increased sodium current within motor neurons, resembling that observed in the transgenic Cu,ZnSOD G93A mouse model for ALS. The increased sodium current promotes hyperexcitability of the cells, which may lead to excitotoxicity, subsequent calcium influx and apoptosis (Carunchio et al. 2010; Manuel and Heckman 2011). BCAAs are commonly used as a supplement by athletes, and therefore might account for the increased incidence of ALS seen in Italian soccer (Chio et al. 2005) and American football (Abel 2007) players.

Smoking was proposed as another potential risk factor for ALS (Kamel et al. 1999), and continues to provoke interest (Armon 2009). Several studies reported no ill effects of smoking on ALS (Schmidt et al. 2010) (Okamoto et al. 2009), others implicated a gender-specific effect (Alonso et al. 2010), and a recent study of 832 ALS patients suggested smoking increased ALS incidence by ~1.4 fold (Wang et al. 2011).

3.2.2 Injury and trauma

Neuronal injury may result in excessive stimulation by α-amino-hydroxy-5-methylisoxasole-4 propionic acid (AMPA), glutamate or kainite, leading to excitotoxcity and downstream apoptosis (Perry, Shin, and Tainer 2010; Beal 1992). Thus, head trauma may be linked to the increased incidence of ALS observed in Italian soccer players, American football players, and military personnel, all of whom more commonly have head injuries (Horner et al. 2008; Miranda et al. 2008). Other forms of trauma, such as electrical shock, have also been correlated to ALS [for a broader list and additional details, see the review by (Bastos et al. 2011)].

3.2.3 Environmental toxins

Exposure to environmental toxins is actively investigated as a potential contributing factor to ALS. Several metals have been implicated in increased risk for ALS after occupational exposure to lead, residency in areas with high levels of selenium, and accidental contact with mercury (Bastos et al. 2011). Inhabitants of Guam who exhibit ALS-like symptoms have been exposed to potentially high levels of aluminum (Wicklund 2005). More complex molecules implicated in increased risk of ALS include formaldehyde, pesticides that are suspected to cause ALS in Italian soccer players, and chemical agents to which military personnel have been subjected. Yet, a causative effect between ALS and such factors is difficult to establish. One reason for this is the relatively small sample size in some of these studies. A second reason is the difficulty in deconvoluting which specific factor or combination of factors contributed to the disease, as in the case for the soccer players. Third, some of the ALS patients within the studies may have had an undetected genetic defect, and the additional environmental factor accelerated the course of the disease.

4. Therapeutic progress

The only approved treatment for ALS is riluzole, which functions to reduce glutamate-induced excitotoxicity in ALS individuals, and is licensed by Sanofi-Aventis with the brand name Rilutek. Riluzole only modestly slows the progression of ALS, with a 9% gain in the probability of surviving one year, and a small beneficial effect for limb function, but not muscle strength (Miller et al. 2007). Several other drugs that gave positive results in animal models failed in human trials. However, additional clinical trials now underway are aimed at producing new ALS therapies by using varied strategic approaches that go beyond the modulation of glutamate levels [reviewed in (Zoccolella, Santamato, and Lamberti 2009)(see http://clinicaltrials.gov)]. Exciting progress in this regard includes the commencement of a phase I clinical trial by Neuralstem that aims to establish the safety and feasibility of using stem cells to treat ALS, by injecting these cells directly into the spinal cord (see http://neurology.emory.edu/ALS/Stem%20Cell.html). This development is based on initial studies showing that human fetal neuronal stem cells could delay the onset and progression in a rat model of ALS (Xu et al. 2006).

The Northeast ALS consortium (NEALS), a non-profit consortium bringing together scientific and clinical investigators from now 97 institutions across in the United States, Puerto Rico, Canada and Ireland, forms a central component of many of the clinical trials (http://www.alsconsortium.org). For example, as part of NEALS, a stage III trial of ceftriaxone, which has been recently observed to modulate glutamate uptake, is being conducted by Massachusetts General Hospital with the National Institute of Neurological

Disorders and Stroke. Ceftriaxone is a semi-synthetic cephalosporin antibiotic, originally approved by the FDA for treating bacterial infections. Combination therapies are also being analyzed, including a phase II a trial by Phoenix Neurological Associates LTD of riluzole in conjunction with tretionin and pioglitazone. Tretinoin, used to treat acute promyelocytic leukemia (Sanz 2006), is a retinoic acid derivative, and as such may have neuroprotective properties (Choi et al. 2009; Lee et al. 2009). The oral anti-diabetic pioglitazone has anti-inflammatory properties that showed positive responses in an ALS mouse model (Schutz et al. 2005). Tamoxifen is currently in stage II clinical trials for treating ALS, based on an observation by clinicians that an ALS patient also receiving tamoxifen for breast cancer had an unusually mild form of the disease (see http://www.alsa.org/research/clinical-trials/trial-tamoxifen.html). Tamoxifen may also help protect cells from glutamate toxicity (Maenpaa et al. 2002) in addition to inhibiting protein kinase C mediated spinal inflammation and prolonging life expectancy in a mouse model of ALS (Traynor et al. 2006; Zoccolella, Santamato, and Lamberti 2009).

Several other compounds with neuroprotective activities are undergoing clinical trials. These include rasagiline, which was reported to have neuroprotective properties in an ALS mouse model (Waibel et al. 2004). Rasagiline is currently used as a therapy for Parkinson's disease, functioning as a selective inhibitor of monoamine oxidase B, and is now under phase II clinical trials for ALS treatment by the University of Kansas. Neuraltus Pharmaceuticals is targeting an anti-inflammatory response through transforming macrophage cells from a neurotoxic to a protective state, with the compound 'NP001' that is now in phase II clinical trials (see http://www.neuraltus.com). Biogen Idec and Knopp Biosciences have an interesting small molecule therapeutic, dexpramipexole, which also has a neuroprotective function, through increasing the efficiency of mitochondria in neurons (Gribkoff and Bozik 2008). Dexpramipexole is the R(+) enantiomer of an already licensed compound, pramipexole, which is used for the treatment of both Parkinson's disease and restless legs syndrome. Pramipexole functions as a non-ergot dopaminergic autoreceptor antagonist, but has dose-limiting side effects that include orthostatic hypotension and hallucination, due its dopaminergic receptor activity. Dempramipexole, on the other hand, has a much lower affinity for dopaminergic receptors, and in phase II trials was well tolerated at levels considerably higher than the maximum daily dose of pramipexole (Bozik et al. 2011). Dexpramipexole also showed positive trends in slowing functional decline and improving survivability in phase II, and is now undergoing a multi-national phase III study.

Approaches specifically targeting Cu,ZnSOD include arimoclomol, a compound developed by CytRx corporation, that activates chaperones to perturb protein aggregation. Arimoclomol was observed to extend life in an ALS mutant Cu,ZnSOD mouse model (indirectly supporting the framework destabilization model for Cu,ZnSOD mutations), and is currently at the Phase II/III stage (Kalmar et al. 2008). Cornell University and the Muscular Dystrophy Association are studying pyrimethamine, an anti-malarial drug shown in one study to substantially reduce Cu,ZnSOD levels in mice (Lange 2008), although a separate study at the University of Massachusetts Medical School did not observe this pyrimethamine effect in either cells or animal models of disease (Wright et al. 2010). Moving away from small molecule based therapies, Isis Pharmaceuticals is taking an siRNA approach to combat FALS mutant Cu,ZnSOD, with Isis-SOD1RX entering into phase I clinical trials. Isis-SOD1RX is antisense oligonucleotide to SOD1 that is infused directly into the cerebral spinal fluid, due to an inability to pass the blood brain barrier. This siRNA was shown to reduce both Cu,ZnSOD protein and mRNA levels throughout the brain and spinal cord in animal models (Smith et al. 2006).

Other recent therapeutic approaches target muscle deficiencies in ALS. Cytokinetics developed 'CK-2107357', an activator of the fast skeletal muscle troponin complex, increasing cellular sensitivity to calcium, which results in an increase in skeletal muscle force and a decrease in the time to muscle fatigue. In phase IIa trials, CK-2107357 showed evidence of clinical effect, as well as being suitably safe and tolerated. Acceleron Pharma is developing ACE-031, a protein therapeutic that builds muscle and increases strength by inhibiting signaling through the activin type IIb cell surface receptor (Cadena et al. 2010). ACE-031 increased skeletal muscle mass and strength in disease models of amyotrophic lateral sclerosis (ALS), muscular dystrophy, glucocorticoid-induced muscle loss and age-related muscle loss (sarcopenia). An extended phase II clinical trial in Canada for Duchenne Muscular Dystrophy was recently terminated, and is pending further analysis of safety data.

5. Future research

Evidently, much work remains on all fronts from uncovering disease mechanisms to developing new therapies for ALS. The very recent publication determining that mutations in ubiquilin 2 are a cause of dominantly inherited X-linked ALS and ALS/dementia has opened up a new area of ALS research (Deng et al. 2011). Ubiquilin 2 functions as part of the protein degradation pathway, revealing pathological roles for this pathway in ALS and suggesting new therapeutic opportunities for treating ALS, since ubiquilin 2 was found in skein-like inclusions of a wide variety of ALS cases (Deng et al. 2011). Another area of important focus is improvement of animal models for ALS, as the utility of these has come into question (Benatar 2007; Bedlack, Traynor, and Cudkowicz 2007). One problem is that treatment in these animal models typical begins before the onset of disease symptoms, whereas this is not possible for ALS individuals, due to a lack of understanding of causative factors and potential differences in pathogenic mechanisms between SALS and FALS. Notably, when guidelines on improving animal study criteria were implemented, therapeutic benefits from a host of compounds that included ceftiaxone and even riluzole were no longer observed (Scott et al. 2008), further highlighting issues with the use and understanding of current models. Improved experimental ALS models will also be of use to further our understanding of the causative factors of SALS, such as potentially toxic effects of smoking on motor neurons. Future therapeutic studies also need to take into consideration overcoming problems within clinical trials, such as the small sample sizes and short durations of study, making assessment of milder effects that are expected with many of the therapeutics more challenging.

Once key advance that is likely to influence the future direction of research is the generation of ALS stem cells from adult skin cells from an individual with ALS (Dimos et al. 2008). Now, stem cells from different patients can be isolated and used to grow different motor neuron cell lines for more detailed analyses, or potentially for high-throughput screening.

6. Conclusions

There has been some exciting progress in our understanding of ALS, including recent developments in the genetics and molecular mechanisms behind this most common form of motor neuron disease. New discoveries include the identification of two ALS-linked proteins, FUS/TLS and TDP-43, which are involved in DNA/RNA metabolism. However, we still have to clearly establish whether aggregation or loss of the wild-type functions of either of these two proteins is the underlying cause of the disease phenotype. Studies behind the pathogenicity of Cu,ZnSOD mutations in ALS are also continuing, with the recent data supporting an initial concept that mutation-induced structural instability of the protein drives aggregation events, which ultimately prove toxic to the neuronal cell. Encouragingly, several distinct therapeutic strategies are in play aiming to at least delay the progression of the disease. These strategies range from small molecule inhibitors, some of which are in later stages of clinical trials, to siRNA and stem cell based approaches. We hope that the rapid pace of research findings and the ongoing clinical trials will shortly produce novel therapies that can help fight against this terrible disease.

7. Acknowledgments

A.J.P. is grateful to the N.S.F. and the Skaggs Institute for Chemical Biology at The Scripps Research Institute for pre-doctoral funding, and E.D.G would like to acknowledge funding from NIH grant GM39345.

8. References

Abel, E. L. 2007. Football increases the risk for Lou Gehrig's disease, amyotrophic lateral sclerosis. *Percept Mot Skills* 104 (3 Pt 2):1251-4.

Abhinav, K., B. Stanton, C. Johnston, J. Hardstaff, R. W. Orrell, R. Howard, J. Clarke, M. Sakel, M. A. Ampong, C. E. Shaw, P. N. Leigh, and A. Al-Chalabi. 2007. Amyotrophic lateral sclerosis in South-East England: a population-based study. The South-East England register for amyotrophic lateral sclerosis (SEALS Registry). *Neuroepidemiology* 29 (1-2):44-8.

Abhyankar, M. M., C. Urekar, and P. P. Reddi. 2007. A novel CpG-free vertebrate insulator silences the testis-specific SP-10 gene in somatic tissues: role for TDP-43 in insulator function. *J Biol Chem* 282 (50):36143-54.

Aggarwal, A., and Shashiraj. 2006. Juvenile amyotrophic lateral sclerosis. *Indian J Pediatr* 73 (3):225-6.

Al-Chalabi, A., P. M. Andersen, P. Nilsson, B. Chioza, J. L. Andersson, C. Russ, C. E. Shaw, J. F. Powell, and P. N. Leigh. 1999. Deletions of the heavy neurofilament subunit tail in amyotrophic lateral sclerosis. *Hum Mol Genet* 8 (2):157-64.

Alonso, A., G. Logroscino, S. S. Jick, and M. A. Hernan. 2009. Incidence and lifetime risk of motor neuron disease in the United Kingdom: a population-based study. *Eur J Neurol* 16 (6):745-51.

Alonso, A., G. Logroscino, S. S. Jick, and M. A. Hernan. 2010. Association of smoking with amyotrophic lateral sclerosis risk and survival in men and women: a prospective study. *BMC Neurol* 10:6.

Andersen, P. M. 2000. Genetic factors in the early diagnosis of ALS. *Amyotroph Lateral Scler Other Motor Neuron Disord* 1 Suppl 1:S31-42.

Andersen, P. M. 2006. Amyotrophic lateral sclerosis associated with mutations in the CuZn superoxide dismutase gene. *Curr Neurol Neurosci Rep* 6 (1):37-46.

Andersen, P. M., G. D. Borasio, R. Dengler, O. Hardiman, K. Kollewe, P. N. Leigh, P. F. Pradat, V. Silani, B. Tomik, and EFNS Task Force Diag Management. 2005. EFNS task force on management of amyotrophic lateral sclerosis: guidelines for diagnosing and clinical care of patients and relatives - An evidence-based review with good practice points. *European Journal of Neurology* 12 (12):921-938.

Andersen, P. M., L. Forsgren, M. Binzer, P. Nilsson, V. Ala-Hurula, M. L. Keranen, L. Bergmark, A. Saarinen, T. Haltia, I. Tarvainen, E. Kinnunen, B. Udd, and S. L. Marklund. 1996. Autosomal recessive adult-onset amyotrophic lateral sclerosis associated with homozygosity for Asp90Ala CuZn-superoxide dismutase mutation. A clinical and genealogical study of 36 patients. *Brain* 119 (Pt 4):1153-72.

Arai, T., M. Hasegawa, H. Akiyama, K. Ikeda, T. Nonaka, H. Mori, D. Mann, K. Tsuchiya, M. Yoshida, Y. Hashizume, and T. Oda. 2006. TDP-43 is a component of ubiquitin-positive tau-negative inclusions in frontotemporal lobar degeneration and amyotrophic lateral sclerosis. *Biochem Biophys Res Commun* 351 (3):602-11.

Armon, C. 2009. Smoking may be considered an established risk factor for sporadic ALS. *Neurology* 73 (20):1693-1698.

Ayala, Y. M., T. Misteli, and F. E. Baralle. 2008. TDP-43 regulates retinoblastoma protein phosphorylation through the repression of cyclin-dependent kinase 6 expression. *Proc Natl Acad Sci U S A* 105 (10):3785-9.

Bastos, A. F., M. Orsini, D. Machado, M. P. Mello, S. Nader, J. G. Silva, A. M. da Silva Catharino, M. R. de Freitas, A. Pereira, L. L. Pessoa, F. R. Sztajnbok, M. A. Leite, O. J. Nascimento, and V. H. Bastos. 2011. Amyotrophic lateral sclerosis: one or multiple causes? *Neurol Int* 3 (1):e4.

Beal, M. F. 1992. Mechanisms of excitotoxicity in neurologic diseases. *FASEB J* 6 (15):3338-44.

Beckman, J. S., M. Carson, C. D. Smith, and W. H. Koppenol. 1993. ALS, SOD and peroxynitrite. *Nature* 364 (6438):584.

Bedlack, R. S., B. J. Traynor, and M. E. Cudkowicz. 2007. Emerging disease-modifying therapies for the treatment of motor neuron disease/amyotropic lateral sclerosis. *Expert Opin Emerg Drugs* 12 (2):229-52.

Ben Hamida, M., F. Hentati, and C. Ben Hamida. 1990. Hereditary motor system diseases (chronic juvenile amyotrophic lateral sclerosis). Conditions combining a bilateral pyramidal syndrome with limb and bulbar amyotrophy. *Brain* 113 (Pt 2):347-63.

Benatar, M. 2007. Lost in translation: treatment trials in the SOD1 mouse and in human ALS. *Neurobiol Dis* 26 (1):1-13.

Blair, I. P., C. L. Bennett, A. Abel, B. A. Rabin, J. W. Griffin, K. H. Fischbeck, D. R. Cornblath, and P. F. Chance. 2000. A gene for autosomal dominant juvenile amyotrophic lateral sclerosis (ALS4) localizes to a 500-kb interval on chromosome 9q34. *Neurogenetics* 3 (1):1-6.

Boillee, S., C. Vande Velde, and D. W. Cleveland. 2006. ALS: a disease of motor neurons and their nonneuronal neighbors. *Neuron* 52 (1):39-59.

Bozik, M. E., J. L. Mather, W. G. Kramer, V. K. Gribkoff, and E. W. Ingersoll. 2011. Safety, Tolerability, and Pharmacokinetics of KNS-760704 (Dexpramipexole) in Healthy Adult Subjects. *J Clin Pharmacol* 51 (8):1177-85.

Brooks, B. R., R. G. Miller, M. Swash, and T. L. Munsat. 2000. El Escorial revisited: revised criteria for the diagnosis of amyotrophic lateral sclerosis. *Amyotroph Lateral Scler Other Motor Neuron Disord* 1 (5):293-9.

Brown, R. H., Jr. 1995. Amyotrophic lateral sclerosis: recent insights from genetics and transgenic mice. *Cell* 80 (5):687-92.

Bruijn, L. I., M. K. Houseweart, S. Kato, K. L. Anderson, S. D. Anderson, E. Ohama, A. G. Reaume, R. W. Scott, and D. W. Cleveland. 1998. Aggregation and motor neuron toxicity of an ALS-linked SOD1 mutant independent from wild-type SOD1. *Science* 281 (5384):1851-4.

Burjanadze, T. V. 2000. New analysis of the phylogenetic change of collagen thermostability. *Biopolymers* 53 (6):523-8.

Byrne, S. C., and O. Hardiman. 2010. Rate of Familial Amyotrophic Lateral Sclerosis - A Systematic Review and Meta-Analysis. *Neurology* 74 (9):A56-A56.

Cadena, S. M., K. N. Tomkinson, T. E. Monnell, M. S. Spaits, R. Kumar, K. W. Underwood, R. S. Pearsall, and J. L. Lachey. 2010. Administration of a soluble activin type IIB receptor promotes skeletal muscle growth independent of fiber type. *J Appl Physiol* 109 (3):635-42.

Carunchio, I., L. Curcio, M. Pieri, F. Pica, S. Caioli, M. T. Viscomi, M. Molinari, N. Canu, G. Bernardi, and C. Zona. 2010. Increased levels of p70S6 phosphorylation in the G93A mouse model of Amyotrophic Lateral Sclerosis and in valine-exposed cortical neurons in culture. *Exp Neurol* 226 (1):218-30.

Cassiday, L. A., and L. J. Maher, 3rd. 2002. Having it both ways: transcription factors that bind DNA and RNA. *Nucleic Acids Res* 30 (19):4118-26.

Cedarbaum, J. M., N. Stambler, E. Malta, C. Fuller, D. Hilt, B. Thurmond, A. Nakanishi, and Bdnf Als Study Grp. 1999. The ALSFRS-R: a revised ALS functional rating scale that incorporates assessments of respiratory function. *Journal of the Neurological Sciences* 169 (1-2):13-21.

Charcot, J.M. 1869. Deux cas d'atrophie musculaire progressive avec lesions de la substance grise et des faisceaux antero-lateraux de la moelle epiniere. *Arch Physiol Neurol Pathol* 2:744-754.

Chio, A. 1999. ISIS Survey: an international study on the diagnostic process and its implications in amyotrophic lateral sclerosis. *J Neurol* 246 Suppl 3:III1-5.

Chio, A., G. Benzi, M. Dossena, R. Mutani, and G. Mora. 2005. Severely increased risk of amyotrophic lateral sclerosis among Italian professional football players. *Brain* 128 (Pt 3):472-6.

Chio, A., A. Calvo, C. Moglia, L. Mazzini, and G. Mora. 2011. Phenotypic heterogeneity of amyotrophic lateral sclerosis: a population based study. *J Neurol Neurosurg Psychiatry* 82 (7):740-6.

Choi, B. K., J. H. Kim, J. S. Jung, Y. S. Lee, M. E. Han, S. Y. Baek, B. S. Kim, J. B. Kim, and S. O. Oh. 2009. Reduction of ischemia-induced cerebral injury by all-trans-retinoic acid. *Exp Brain Res* 193 (4):581-9.

Cronin, S., O. Hardiman, and B. J. Traynor. 2007. Ethnic variation in the incidence of ALS: a systematic review. *Neurology* 68 (13):1002-7.

Crow, J. P., Y. Z. Ye, M. Strong, M. Kirk, S. Barnes, and J. S. Beckman. 1997. Superoxide dismutase catalyzes nitration of tyrosines by peroxynitrite in the rod and head domains of neurofilament-L. *J Neurochem* 69 (5):1945-53.

Crozat, A., P. Aman, N. Mandahl, and D. Ron. 1993. Fusion of CHOP to a novel RNA-binding protein in human myxoid liposarcoma. *Nature* 363 (6430):640-4.

Davenport, R. J., R. J. Swingler, A. M. Chancellor, and C. P. Warlow. 1996. Avoiding false positive diagnoses of motor neuron disease: lessons from the Scottish Motor Neuron Disease Register. *J Neurol Neurosurg Psychiatry* 60 (2):147-51.

de Carvalho, M., R. Dengler, A. Eisen, J. D. England, R. Kaji, J. Kimura, K. Mills, H. Mitsumoto, H. Nodera, J. Shefner, and M. Swash. 2008. Electrodiagnostic criteria for diagnosis of ALS. *Clin Neurophysiol* 119 (3):497-503.

Dejesus-Hernandez M., I.R. Mackenzie, B.F. Boeve, A.L. Boxer, M. Baker, N.J. Rutherford, A.M. Nicholson, N.A. Finch, H. Flynn, J. Adamson, N. Kouri, A. Wojtas, P. Sengdy,

G.Y. Hsuing, A. Karydas A., W.W. Seeley, K.A. Josephs, G. Coppola, D.H. Geshwind, Z.K. Wszolek, H. Feldman, D.S. Knopman, R.C. Petersen, B.L. Miller, D.W. Dickson, K.B. Boylan, N.R. Graff-Radford and R. Rademakers. 2011. Expanded GGGGCC Hexanucleotide Repeat in Noncoding Region of C9ORF72 Causes Chromosome 9p-Linked FTD and ALS. *Neuron* Epub Sept 21.

Deng, H. X., W. Chen, S. T. Hong, K. M. Boycott, G. H. Gorrie, N. Siddique, Y. Yang, F. Fecto, Y. Shi, H. Zhai, H. Jiang, M. Hirano, E. Rampersaud, G. H. Jansen, S. Donkervoort, E. H. Bigio, B. R. Brooks, K. Ajroud, R. L. Sufit, J. L. Haines, E. Mugnaini, M. A. Pericak-Vance, and T. Siddique. 2011. Mutations in UBQLN2 cause dominant X-linked juvenile and adult-onset ALS and ALS/dementia. *Nature.*

Deng, H. X., A. Hentati, J. A. Tainer, Z. Iqbal, A. Cayabyab, W. Y. Hung, E. D. Getzoff, P. Hu, B. Herzfeldt, R. P. Roos, and et al. 1993. Amyotrophic lateral sclerosis and structural defects in Cu,Zn superoxide dismutase. *Science* 261 (5124):1047-51.

Deng, H. X., H. Zhai, E. H. Bigio, J. Yan, F. Fecto, K. Ajroud, M. Mishra, S. Ajroud-Driss, S. Heller, R. Sufit, N. Siddique, E. Mugnaini, and T. Siddique. 2010. FUS-immunoreactive inclusions are a common feature in sporadic and non-SOD1 familial amyotrophic lateral sclerosis. *Ann Neurol* 67 (6):739-48.

DiDonato, M., L. Craig, M. E. Huff, M. M. Thayer, R. M. Cardoso, C. J. Kassmann, T. P. Lo, C. K. Bruns, E. T. Powers, J. W. Kelly, E. D. Getzoff, and J. A. Tainer. 2003. ALS mutants of human superoxide dismutase form fibrous aggregates via framework destabilization. *J Mol Biol* 332 (3):601-15.

Dimos, J. T., K. T. Rodolfa, K. K. Niakan, L. M. Weisenthal, H. Mitsumoto, W. Chung, G. F. Croft, G. Saphier, R. Leibel, R. Goland, H. Wichterle, C. E. Henderson, and K. Eggan. 2008. Induced pluripotent stem cells generated from patients with ALS can be differentiated into motor neurons. *Science* 321 (5893):1218-21.

Dobson, C. M. 2001. Protein folding and its links with human disease. *Biochem Soc Symp* (68):1-26.

Donkervoort, S., and T. Siddique. 1993. Amyotrophic Lateral Sclerosis Overview. *In: Pagon RA, Bird TD, Dolan CR, Stephens K, editors. GeneReviews [Internet]. Seattle (WA): University of Washington, Seattle; 1993-. [updated 2009 Jul 28].*

Dormann, D., and C. Haass. 2011. TDP-43 and FUS: a nuclear affair. *Trends Neurosci.*

Dormann, D., R. Rodde, D. Edbauer, E. Bentmann, I. Fischer, A. Hruscha, M. E. Than, I. R. Mackenzie, A. Capell, B. Schmid, M. Neumann, and C. Haass. 2010. ALS-associated fused in sarcoma (FUS) mutations disrupt Transportin-mediated nuclear import. *EMBO J* 29 (16):2841-57.

Durham, H. D., J. Roy, L. Dong, and D. A. Figlewicz. 1997. Aggregation of mutant Cu/Zn superoxide dismutase proteins in a culture model of ALS. *J Neuropathol Exp Neurol* 56 (5):523-30.

Ferrari, R., D. Kapogiannis, E. D. Huey, and P. Momeni. 2011. FTD and ALS: A Tale of Two Diseases. *Curr Alzheimer Res.*

Fong, K. Y., Y. L. Yu, Y. W. Chan, R. Kay, J. Chan, Z. Yang, M. C. Kwan, K. P. Leung, P. C. Li, T. H. Lam, and R. T. Cheung. 1996. Motor neuron disease in Hong Kong Chinese: epidemiology and clinical picture. *Neuroepidemiology* 15 (5):239-45.

Forbes, R. B., S. Colville, and R. J. Swingler. 2004. The epidemiology of amyotrophic lateral sclerosis (ALS/MND) in people aged 80 or over. *Age Ageing* 33 (2):131-4.

Forman, H. J., and I. Fridovich. 1973. On the stability of bovine superoxide dismutase. The effects of metals. *J Biol Chem* 248 (8):2645-9.

Forsgren, L., B. G. Almay, G. Holmgren, and S. Wall. 1983. Epidemiology of motor neuron disease in northern Sweden. *Acta Neurol Scand* 68 (1):20-9.

Fujii, R., S. Okabe, T. Urushido, K. Inoue, A. Yoshimura, T. Tachibana, T. Nishikawa, G. G. Hicks, and T. Takumi. 2005. The RNA binding protein TLS is translocated to dendritic spines by mGluR5 activation and regulates spine morphology. *Curr Biol* 15 (6):587-93.

Getzoff, E. D., D. E. Cabelli, C. L. Fisher, H. E. Parge, M. S. Viezzoli, L. Banci, and R. A. Hallewell. 1992. Faster superoxide dismutase mutants designed by enhancing electrostatic guidance. *Nature* 358 (6384):347-51.

Getzoff, E. D., J. A. Tainer, P. K. Weiner, P. A. Kollman, J. S. Richardson, and D. C. Richardson. 1983. Electrostatic recognition between superoxide and copper, zinc superoxide dismutase. *Nature* 306 (5940):287-90.

Gribkoff, V. K., and M. E. Bozik. 2008. KNS-760704 [(6R)-4,5,6,7-tetrahydro-N6-propyl-2, 6-benzothiazole-diamine dihydrochloride monohydrate] for the treatment of amyotrophic lateral sclerosis. *CNS Neurosci Ther* 14 (3):215-26.

Gunnarsson, L.-G., and Palm. 1984. Motor Neuron Disease and Heavy Manual Labor: An Epidemiologic Survey of Värmland County, Sweden. *Neuroepidemiology* 3 (4):195-206.

Gurney, M. E., H. F. Pu, A. Y. Chiu, M. C. Dalcanto, C. Y. Polchow, D. D. Alexander, J. Caliendo, A. Hentati, Y. W. Kwon, H. X. Deng, W. J. Chen, P. Zhai, R. L. Sufit, and T. Siddique. 1994. Motor-Neuron Degeneration in Mice That Express a Human Cu,Zn Superoxide-Dismutase Mutation. *Science* 264 (5166):1772-1775.

Haberlandt, W. F. 1959. Genetic aspects of amyotrophic lateral sclerosis and progressive bulbar paralysis. *Acta Genet Med Gemellol (Roma)* 8:369-74.

Hadano, S., C. K. Hand, H. Osuga, Y. Yanagisawa, A. Otomo, R. S. Devon, N. Miyamoto, J. Showguchi-Miyata, Y. Okada, R. Singaraja, D. A. Figlewicz, T. Kwiatkowski, B. A. Hosler, T. Sagie, J. Skaug, J. Nasir, R. H. Brown, S. W. Scherer, G. A. Rouleau, M. R. Hayden, and J. E. Ikeda. 2001. A gene encoding a putative GTPase regulator is mutated in familial amyotrophic lateral sclerosis 2 (vol 29, pg 166, 2001). *Nature Genetics* 29 (3):352-352.

Hadano, S., R. Kunita, A. Otomo, K. Suzuki-Utsunomiya, and J. E. Ikeda. 2007. Molecular and cellular function of ALS2/alsin: implication of membrane dynamics in neuronal development and degeneration. *Neurochem Int* 51 (2-4):74-84.

Hallewell, R. A., K. C. Imlay, P. Lee, N. M. Fong, C. Gallegos, E. D. Getzoff, J. A. Tainer, D. E. Cabelli, P. Tekamp-Olson, G. T. Mullenbach, and et al. 1991. Thermostabilization of recombinant human and bovine CuZn superoxide dismutases by replacement of free cysteines. *Biochem Biophys Res Commun* 181 (1):474-80.

Harraz, M. M., J. J. Marden, W. Zhou, Y. Zhang, A. Williams, V. S. Sharov, K. Nelson, M. Luo, H. Paulson, C. Schoneich, and J. F. Engelhardt. 2008. SOD1 mutations disrupt redox-sensitive Rac regulation of NADPH oxidase in a familial ALS model. *J Clin Invest* 118 (2):659-70.

Haverkamp, L. J., V. Appel, and S. H. Appel. 1995. Natural history of amyotrophic lateral sclerosis in a database population. Validation of a scoring system and a model for survival prediction. *Brain* 118 (Pt 3):707-19.

He, C. Z., and A. P. Hays. 2004. Expression of peripherin in ubiquinated inclusions of amyotrophic lateral sclerosis. *J Neurol Sci* 217 (1):47-54.

Henscheid, K. L., D. S. Shin, S. C. Cary, and J. A. Berglund. 2005. The splicing factor U2AF65 is functionally conserved in the thermotolerant deep-sea worm Alvinella pompejana. *Biochim Biophys Acta* 1727 (3):197-207.

Higashi, S., Y. Tsuchiya, T. Araki, K. Wada, and T. Kabuta. 2010. TDP-43 physically interacts with amyotrophic lateral sclerosis-linked mutant CuZn superoxide dismutase. *Neurochem Int* 57 (8):906-13.

Horner, R. D., S. C. Grambow, C. J. Coffman, J. H. Lindquist, E. Z. Oddone, K. D. Allen, and E. J. Kasarskis. 2008. Amyotrophic lateral sclerosis among 1991 Gulf War veterans: evidence for a time-limited outbreak. *Neuroepidemiology* 31 (1):28-32.

Horton, W. A., R. Eldridge, and J. A. Brody. 1976. Familial motor neuron disease. Evidence for at least three different types. *Neurology* 26 (5):460-5.

Ince, P. G., and G. A. Codd. 2005. Return of the cycad hypothesis - does the amyotrophic lateral sclerosis/parkinsonism dementia complex (ALS/PDC) of Guam have new implications for global health? *Neuropathol Appl Neurobiol* 31 (4):345-53.

Ito, H., K. Fujita, M. Nakamura, R. Wate, S. Kaneko, S. Sasaki, K. Yamane, N. Suzuki, M. Aoki, N. Shibata, S. Togashi, A. Kawata, Y. Mochizuki, T. Mizutani, H. Maruyama, A. Hirano, R. Takahashi, H. Kawakami, and H. Kusaka. 2011. Optineurin is co-localized with FUS in basophilic inclusions of ALS with FUS mutation and in basophilic inclusion body disease. *Acta Neuropathol* 121 (4):555-7.

Johnston, J. A., M. J. Dalton, M. E. Gurney, and R. R. Kopito. 2000. Formation of high molecular weight complexes of mutant Cu, Zn-superoxide dismutase in a mouse model for familial amyotrophic lateral sclerosis. *Proc Natl Acad Sci U S A* 97 (23):12571-6.

Kalmar, B., S. Novoselov, A. Gray, M. E. Cheetham, B. Margulis, and L. Greensmith. 2008. Late stage treatment with arimoclomol delays disease progression and prevents protein aggregation in the SOD1 mouse model of ALS. *J Neurochem* 107 (2):339-50.

Kamel, F., D. M. Umbach, T. L. Munsat, J. M. Shefner, and D. P. Sandler. 1999. Association of cigarette smoking with amyotrophic lateral sclerosis. *Neuroepidemiology* 18 (4):194-202.

Kashiwagi, S., I. Kuraoka, Y. Fujiwara, K. Hitomi, Q. J. Cheng, J. O. Fuss, D. S. Shin, C. Masutani, J. A. Tainer, F. Hanaoka, and S. Iwai. 2010. Characterization of a Y-Family DNA Polymerase eta from the Eukaryotic Thermophile Alvinella pompejana. *J Nucleic Acids* 2010.

Kato, S., H. Sumi-Akamaru, H. Fujimura, S. Sakoda, M. Kato, A. Hirano, M. Takikawa, and E. Ohama. 2001. Copper chaperone for superoxide dismutase co-aggregates with superoxide dismutase 1 (SOD1) in neuronal Lewy body-like hyaline inclusions: an immunohistochemical study on familial amyotrophic lateral sclerosis with SOD1 gene mutation. *Acta Neuropathol* 102 (3):233-8.

Kieran, D., M. Hafezparast, S. Bohnert, J. R. Dick, J. Martin, G. Schiavo, E. M. Fisher, and L. Greensmith. 2005. A mutation in dynein rescues axonal transport defects and extends the life span of ALS mice. *J Cell Biol* 169 (4):561-7.

Kiernan, M. C., S. Vucic, B. C. Cheah, M. R. Turner, A. Eisen, O. Hardiman, J. R. Burrell, and M. C. Zoing. 2011. Amyotrophic lateral sclerosis. *Lancet* 377 (9769):942-55.

Kim, S. H., N. P. Shanware, M. J. Bowler, and R. S. Tibbetts. 2010. Amyotrophic lateral sclerosis-associated proteins TDP-43 and FUS/TLS function in a common biochemical complex to co-regulate HDAC6 mRNA. *J Biol Chem* 285 (44):34097-105.

Kuhnlein, P., H. J. Gdynia, A. D. Sperfeld, B. Lindner-Pfleghar, A. C. Ludolph, M. Prosiegel, and A. Riecker. 2008. Diagnosis and treatment of bulbar symptoms in amyotrophic lateral sclerosis. *Nature Clinical Practice Neurology* 4 (7):366-374.

Kwiatkowski, T. J., Jr., D. A. Bosco, A. L. Leclerc, E. Tamrazian, C. R. Vanderburg, C. Russ, A. Davis, J. Gilchrist, E. J. Kasarskis, T. Munsat, P. Valdmanis, G. A. Rouleau, B. A.

Hosler, P. Cortelli, P. J. de Jong, Y. Yoshinaga, J. L. Haines, M. A. Pericak-Vance, J. Yan, N. Ticozzi, T. Siddique, D. McKenna-Yasek, P. C. Sapp, H. R. Horvitz, J. E. Landers, and R. H. Brown, Jr. 2009. Mutations in the FUS/TLS gene on chromosome 16 cause familial amyotrophic lateral sclerosis. *Science* 323 (5918):1205-8.

Kwong, L. K., K. Uryu, J. Q. Trojanowski, and V. M. Lee. 2008. TDP-43 proteinopathies: neurodegenerative protein misfolding diseases without amyloidosis. *Neurosignals* 16 (1):41-51.

Lagier-Tourenne, C., and D. W. Cleveland. 2009. Rethinking ALS: the FUS about TDP-43. *Cell* 136 (6):1001-4.

Lagier-Tourenne, C., M. Polymenidou, and D. W. Cleveland. 2010. TDP-43 and FUS/TLS: emerging roles in RNA processing and neurodegeneration. *Hum Mol Genet* 19 (R1):R46-64.

Lai, C., C. Xie, S. G. McCormack, H. C. Chiang, M. K. Michalak, X. Lin, J. Chandran, H. Shim, M. Shimoji, M. R. Cookson, R. L. Huganir, J. D. Rothstein, D. L. Price, P. C. Wong, L. J. Martin, J. J. Zhu, and H. Cai. 2006. Amyotrophic lateral sclerosis 2-deficiency leads to neuronal degeneration in amyotrophic lateral sclerosis through altered AMPA receptor trafficking. *J Neurosci* 26 (45):11798-806.

Lange, D. 2008. Abstract C46: pyrimethamine as a therapy for SOD1 associated FALS: Early findings. *Amyotroph. Lateral Scler.* 9 ((Suppl. 1)):45-47.

Law, W. J., K. L. Cann, and G. G. Hicks. 2006. TLS, EWS and TAF15: a model for transcriptional integration of gene expression. *Brief Funct Genomic Proteomic* 5 (1):8-14.

Lee, H. P., G. Casadesus, X. Zhu, H. G. Lee, G. Perry, M. A. Smith, K. Gustaw-Rothenberg, and A. Lerner. 2009. All-trans retinoic acid as a novel therapeutic strategy for Alzheimer's disease. *Expert Rev Neurother* 9 (11):1615-21.

Leigh, P. N., H. Whitwell, O. Garofalo, J. Buller, M. Swash, J. E. Martin, J. M. Gallo, R. O. Weller, and B. H. Anderton. 1991. Ubiquitin-immunoreactive intraneuronal inclusions in amyotrophic lateral sclerosis. Morphology, distribution, and specificity. *Brain* 114 (Pt 2):775-88.

Li, T. M., E. Alberman, and M. Swash. 1988. Comparison of sporadic and familial disease amongst 580 cases of motor neuron disease. *J Neurol Neurosurg Psychiatry* 51 (6):778-84.

Ling, S. C., C. P. Albuquerque, J. S. Han, C. Lagier-Tourenne, S. Tokunaga, H. Zhou, and D. W. Cleveland. 2010. ALS-associated mutations in TDP-43 increase its stability and promote TDP-43 complexes with FUS/TLS. *Proc Natl Acad Sci U S A* 107 (30):13318-23.

Lomen-Hoerth, C. 2008. Amyotrophic lateral sclerosis from bench to bedside. *Semin Neurol* 28 (2):205-11.

Ludolph, A. C., and U. Knirsch. 1999. Problems and pitfalls in the diagnosis of ALS. *Journal of the Neurological Sciences* 165 Suppl 1:S14-20.

Mackenzie, I. R., R. Rademakers, and M. Neumann. 2010. TDP-43 and FUS in amyotrophic lateral sclerosis and frontotemporal dementia. *Lancet Neurol* 9 (10):995-1007.

Maenpaa, H., M. Mannerstrom, T. Toimela, L. Salminen, P. Saransaari, and H. Tahti. 2002. Glutamate uptake is inhibited by tamoxifen and toremifene in cultured retinal pigment epithelial cells. *Pharmacol Toxicol* 91 (3):116-22.

Malinowski, D. P., and I. Fridovich. 1979. Subunit association and side-chain reactivities of bovine erythrocyte superoxide dismutase in denaturing solvents. *Biochemistry* 18 (23):5055-60.

Mann, T., and D. Keilin. 1938. Haemocuprein and hepatocuprein, copper-protein compounds of blood and liver in mammals. *Proceedings of the Royal Society of London Series B-Biological Sciences* 126 (844):303-315.

Mantovani, V., P. Garagnani, P. Selva, C. Rossi, S. Ferrari, M. Cenci, N. Calza, V. Cerreta, D. Luiselli, and G. Romeo. 2007. Simple method for haplotyping the poly(TG) repeat in individuals carrying the IVS8 5T allele in the CFTR gene. *Clin Chem* 53 (3):531-3.

Manuel, M., and C. J. Heckman. 2011. Stronger is not always better: could a bodybuilding dietary supplement lead to ALS? *Exp Neurol* 228 (1):5-8.

McCombe, P. A., and R. D. Henderson. 2010. Effects of gender in amyotrophic lateral sclerosis. *Gend Med* 7 (6):557-70.

McCord, J. M., and I. Fridovich. 1969. Superoxide dismutase. An enzymic function for erythrocuprein (hemocuprein). *J Biol Chem* 244 (22):6049-55.

Miana-Mena, F. J., E. Piedrafita, C. Gonzalez-Mingot, P. Larrode, M. J. Munoz, E. Martinez-Ballarin, R. J. Reiter, R. Osta, and J. J. Garcia. 2011. Levels of membrane fluidity in the spinal cord and the brain in an animal model of amyotrophic lateral sclerosis. *J Bioenerg Biomembr* 43 (2):181-6.

Miller, R. G., J. D. Mitchell, M. Lyon, and D. H. Moore. 2007. Riluzole for amyotrophic lateral sclerosis (ALS)/motor neuron disease (MND). *Cochrane Database Syst Rev* (1):CD001447.

Miranda, M. L., M. Alicia Overstreet Galeano, E. Tassone, K. D. Allen, and R. D. Horner. 2008. Spatial analysis of the etiology of amyotrophic lateral sclerosis among 1991 Gulf War veterans. *Neurotoxicology* 29 (6):964-70.

Mulder, D. W., L. T. Kurland, K. P. Offord, and C. M. Beard. 1986. Familial adult motor neuron disease: amyotrophic lateral sclerosis. *Neurology* 36 (4):511-7.

Mulder, D. W., L. T. Kurland, K. P. Offord, and C. M. Beard. 1986. Familial Adult Motor-Neuron Disease - Amyotrophic-Lateral-Scelerosis. *Neurology* 36 (4):511-517.

Munch, C., A. Rosenbohm, A. D. Sperfeld, I. Uttner, S. Reske, B. J. Krause, R. Sedlmeier, T. Meyer, C. O. Hanemann, G. Stumm, and A. C. Ludolph. 2005. Heterozygous R1101K mutation of the DCTN1 gene in a family with ALS and FTD. *Ann Neurol* 58 (5):777-80.

Munch, C., R. Sedlmeier, T. Meyer, V. Homberg, A. D. Sperfeld, A. Kurt, J. Prudlo, G. Peraus, C. O. Hanemann, G. Stumm, and A. C. Ludolph. 2004. Point mutations of the p150 subunit of dynactin (DCTN1) gene in ALS. *Neurology* 63 (4):724-6.

Murphy, J., R. Henry, and C. Lomen-Hoerth. 2007. Establishing subtypes of the continuum of frontal lobe impairment in amyotrophic lateral sclerosis. *Arch Neurol* 64 (3):330-4.

Murros, K., and R. Fogelholm. 1983. Amyotrophic lateral sclerosis in Middle-Finland: an epidemiological study. *Acta Neurol Scand* 67 (1):41-7.

Neumann, M., D. M. Sampathu, L. K. Kwong, A. C. Truax, M. C. Micsenyi, T. T. Chou, J. Bruce, T. Schuck, M. Grossman, C. M. Clark, L. F. McCluskey, B. L. Miller, E. Masliah, I. R. Mackenzie, H. Feldman, W. Feiden, H. A. Kretzschmar, J. Q. Trojanowski, and V. M. Lee. 2006. Ubiquitinated TDP-43 in frontotemporal lobar degeneration and amyotrophic lateral sclerosis. *Science* 314 (5796):130-3.

Nishitoh, H., H. Kadowaki, A. Nagai, T. Maruyama, T. Yokota, H. Fukutomi, T. Noguchi, A. Matsuzawa, K. Takeda, and H. Ichijo. 2008. ALS-linked mutant SOD1 induces ER stress- and ASK1-dependent motor neuron death by targeting Derlin-1. *Genes Dev* 22 (11):1451-64.

Okamoto, K., T. Kihira, T. Kondo, G. Kobashi, M. Washio, S. Sasaki, T. Yokoyama, Y. Miyake, N. Sakamoto, Y. Inaba, and M. Nagai. 2009. Lifestyle factors and risk of amyotrophic lateral sclerosis: a case-control study in Japan. *Ann Epidemiol* 19 (6):359-64.

Olivares, L., E. S. Esteban, and M. Alter. 1972. Mexican "resistance" to amyotrophic lateral sclerosis. *Arch Neurol* 27 (5):397-402.

Olney, R. K., J. Murphy, D. Forshew, E. Garwood, B. L. Miller, S. Langmore, M. A. Kohn, and C. Lomen-Hoerth. 2005. The effects of executive and behavioral dysfunction on the course of ALS. *Neurology* 65 (11):1774-7.

Parge, H. E., R. A. Hallewell, and J. A. Tainer. 1992. Atomic structures of wild-type and thermostable mutant recombinant human Cu,Zn superoxide dismutase. *Proc Natl Acad Sci U S A* 89 (13):6109-13.

Pasinelli, P., and R. H. Brown. 2006. Molecular biology of amyotrophic lateral sclerosis: insights from genetics. *Nature Reviews Neuroscience* 7 (9):710-723.

Perry, J. J. P., D. S. Shin, and J. A. Tainer. 2010. Amyotrophic Lateral Sclerosis. *Diseases of DNA Repair* 685:9-20.

Perry, J. J., D. S. Shin, E. D. Getzoff, and J. A. Tainer. 2010. The structural biochemistry of the superoxide dismutases. *Biochim Biophys Acta* 1804 (2):245-62.

Piccino, P., F. Viard, P. M. Sarradin, N. Le Bris, D. Le Guen, and D. Jollivet. 2004. Thermal selection of PGM allozymes in newly founded populations of the thermotolerant vent polychaete Alvinella pompejana. *Proceedings of the Royal Society of London Series B-Biological Sciences* 271 (1555):2351-2359.

Porter, H., and J. Folch. 1957. Cerebrocuprein I. A copper-containing protein isolated from brain. *J Neurochem* 1 (3):260-71.

Rabbitts, T. H., A. Forster, R. Larson, and P. Nathan. 1993. Fusion of the dominant negative transcription regulator CHOP with a novel gene FUS by translocation t(12;16) in malignant liposarcoma. *Nat Genet* 4 (2):175-80.

Radunovic, A., D. Annane, K. Jewitt, and N. Mustfa. 2009. Mechanical ventilation for amyotrophic lateral sclerosis/motor neuron disease. *Cochrane Database Syst Rev* (4):CD004427.

Reaume, A. G., J. L. Elliott, E. K. Hoffman, N. W. Kowall, R. J. Ferrante, D. F. Siwek, H. M. Wilcox, D. G. Flood, M. F. Beal, R. H. Brown, Jr., R. W. Scott, and W. D. Snider. 1996. Motor neurons in Cu/Zn superoxide dismutase-deficient mice develop normally but exhibit enhanced cell death after axonal injury. *Nat Genet* 13 (1):43-7.

Renton A.E., E. Majounie, A. Waite, J. Simón-Sánchez, S. Rollinson, J.R. Gibbs, J.C. Schymick, H. Laaksovirta, J.C. van Swieten, L. Myllykangas, H. Kalimo, A. Paetau, Y. Abramzon, A.M. Remes, A. Kagnovich, S.W. Scholz, J. Duckworth, J. Ding, D.W. Harmer, D.G. Hernandez, J.O. Johnson, K. Mok, M. Ryten, D. Trabzuni, R.J. Guerreiro, R.W. Orrell, J. Neal, A. Murray, J. Pearson, I.E. Jansen, D. Sondervan, H. Seelaar, D. Blake, K. Young, N. Halliwell, J.B. Callister, G. Toulson, A. Richardson, A. Gerhard, J. Snowden, D. Mann, D. Neary, M.A. Nalls, T. Peuralinna, L. Jansson, V.M. Isoviita, A.L. Kaivorinne, M.Hölttä-Vuori, E. Ikonen, R. Sulkava, M. Benatar, J. Wuu, A. Chiò, G. Restagno, G. Borghero, M. Sabatelli; The ITALSGEN Consortium, D. Heckerman, E. Rogaeva, L. Zinman, J.D. Rothstein, M. Sendtner, C. Drepper, E.E. Eichler, C. Alkan, Z. Abdullaev, S.D. Pack, A. Dutra, E. Pak , J. Hardy, A. Singleton, N.M. Williams , P. Heutink, S. Pickering-Brown, H.R. Morris, P.J. Tienari and B.J. Traynor. 2011. A Hexanucleotide Repeat Expansion in C9ORF72 Is the Cause of Chromosome 9p21-Linked ALS-FTD. *Neuron*. Epub Sept 21.

Rosen, D. R. 1993. Mutations in Cu/Zn superoxide dismutase gene are associated with familial amyotrophic lateral sclerosis. *Nature* 364 (6435):362.

Sanz, M. A. 2006. Treatment of acute promyelocytic leukemia. *Hematology Am Soc Hematol Educ Program*:147-55.

Sathasivam, S. 2010. Motor neurone disease: clinical features, diagnosis, diagnostic pitfalls and prognostic markers. *Singapore Medical Journal* 51 (5):367-373.

Schmidt, S., L. C. Kwee, K. D. Allen, and E. Z. Oddone. 2010. Association of ALS with head injury, cigarette smoking and APOE genotypes. *Journal of the Neurological Sciences* 291 (1-2):22-9.

Schutz, B., J. Reimann, L. Dumitrescu-Ozimek, K. Kappes-Horn, G. E. Landreth, B. Schurmann, A. Zimmer, and M. T. Heneka. 2005. The oral antidiabetic pioglitazone protects from neurodegeneration and amyotrophic lateral sclerosis-like symptoms in superoxide dismutase-G93A transgenic mice. *J Neurosci* 25 (34):7805-12.

Scott, S., J. E. Kranz, J. Cole, J. M. Lincecum, K. Thompson, N. Kelly, A. Bostrom, J. Theodoss, B. M. Al-Nakhala, F. G. Vieira, J. Ramasubbu, and J. A. Heywood. 2008. Design, power, and interpretation of studies in the standard murine model of ALS. *Amyotroph Lateral Scler* 9 (1):4-15.

Sharma, R., S. Hicks, C. M. Berna, C. Kennard, K. Talbot, and M. R. Turner. 2011. Oculomotor dysfunction in amyotrophic lateral sclerosis: a comprehensive review. *Arch Neurol* 68 (7):857-61.

Shin, D. S., M. Didonato, D. P. Barondeau, G. L. Hura, C. Hitomi, J. A. Berglund, E. D. Getzoff, S. C. Cary, and J. A. Tainer. 2009. Superoxide dismutase from the eukaryotic thermophile Alvinella pompejana: structures, stability, mechanism, and insights into amyotrophic lateral sclerosis. *J Mol Biol* 385 (5):1534-55.

Siddique, T., and H. X. Deng. 1996. Genetics of amyotrophic lateral sclerosis. *Human Molecular Genetics* 5:1465-1470.

Silani, V., S. Messina, B. Poletti, C. Morelli, A. Doretti, N. Ticozzi, and L. Maderna. 2011. The diagnosis of Amyotrophic lateral sclerosis in 2010. *Arch Ital Biol* 149 (1):5-27.

Smith, R. A., T. M. Miller, K. Yamanaka, B. P. Monia, T. P. Condon, G. Hung, C. S. Lobsiger, C. M. Ward, M. McAlonis-Downes, H. Wei, E. V. Wancewicz, C. F. Bennett, and D. W. Cleveland. 2006. Antisense oligonucleotide therapy for neurodegenerative disease. *J Clin Invest* 116 (8):2290-6.

Soto, C. 2001. Protein misfolding and disease; protein refolding and therapy. *FEBS Lett* 498 (2-3):204-7.

Spuler, S., A. Stroux, F. Kuschel, A. Kuhlmey, and F. Kendel. 2011. Delay in diagnosis of muscle disorders depends on the subspecialty of the initially consulted physician. *BMC Health Serv Res* 11:91.

Steele, J. C., and P. L. McGeer. 2008. The ALS/PDC syndrome of Guam and the cycad hypothesis. *Neurology* 70 (21):1984-90.

Strong, M. J. 2010. The evidence for altered RNA metabolism in amyotrophic lateral sclerosis (ALS). *J Neurol Sci* 288 (1-2):1-12.

Strong, M. J., K. Volkening, R. Hammond, W. Yang, W. Strong, C. Leystra-Lantz, and C. Shoesmith. 2007. TDP43 is a human low molecular weight neurofilament (hNFL) mRNA-binding protein. *Mol Cell Neurosci* 35 (2):320-7.

Suzuki, H., K. Kanekura, T. P. Levine, K. Kohno, V. M. Olkkonen, S. Aiso, and M. Matsuoka. 2009. ALS-linked P56S-VAPB, an aggregated loss-of-function mutant of VAPB, predisposes motor neurons to ER stress-related death by inducing aggregation of co-expressed wild-type VAPB. *J Neurochem* 108 (4):973-985.

Swarup, V., D. Phaneuf, C. Bareil, J. Robertson, G. A. Rouleau, J. Kriz, and J. P. Julien. 2011. Pathological hallmarks of amyotrophic lateral sclerosis/frontotemporal lobar degeneration in transgenic mice produced with TDP-43 genomic fragments. *Brain.*

Swash, M. 1998. Early diagnosis of ALS/MND. *Journal of the Neurological Sciences* 160 Suppl 1:S33-6.

Tainer, J. A., E. D. Getzoff, K. M. Beem, J. S. Richardson, and D. C. Richardson. 1982. Determination and analysis of the 2 A-structure of copper, zinc superoxide dismutase. *J Mol Biol* 160 (2):181-217.

Tainer, J. A., E. D. Getzoff, J. S. Richardson, and D. C. Richardson. 1983. Structure and mechanism of copper, zinc superoxide dismutase. *Nature* 306 (5940):284-7.

Talbot, K. 2009. Motor neuron disease: the bare essentials. *Pract Neurol* 9 (5):303-9.

Talbot, K. 2010. Do twin studies still have anything to teach us about the genetics of amyotrophic lateral sclerosis? *J Neurol Neurosurg Psychiatry* 81 (12):1299-300.

Testa, D., R. Lovati, M. Ferrarini, F. Salmoiraghi, and G. Filippini. 2004. Survival of 793 patients with amyotrophic lateral sclerosis diagnosed over a 28-year period. *Amyotroph Lateral Scler Other Motor Neuron Disord* 5 (4):208-12.

Ticozzi, N., C. Tiloca, C. Morelli, C. Colombrita, B. Poletti, A. Doretti, L. Maderna, S. Messina, A. Ratti, and V. Silani. 2011. Genetics of familial Amyotrophic lateral sclerosis. *Arch Ital Biol* 149 (1):65-82.

Traynor, B. J., L. Bruijn, R. Conwit, F. Beal, G. O'Neill, S. C. Fagan, and M. E. Cudkowicz. 2006. Neuroprotective agents for clinical trials in ALS: a systematic assessment. *Neurology* 67 (1):20-7.

Traynor, B. J., M. B. Codd, B. Corr, C. Forde, E. Frost, and O. Hardiman. 2000. Amyotrophic lateral sclerosis mimic syndromes - A population-based study. *Archives of Neurology* 57 (1):109-113.

Turner, M. R., M. C. Kiernan, P. N. Leigh, and K. Talbot. 2009. Biomarkers in amyotrophic lateral sclerosis. *Lancet Neurol* 8 (1):94-109.

Udan, M., and R. H. Baloh. 2011. Implications of the prion-related Q/N domains in TDP-43 and FUS. *Prion* 5 (1):1-5.

Urushitani, M., A. Sik, T. Sakurai, N. Nukina, R. Takahashi, and J. P. Julien. 2006. Chromogranin-mediated secretion of mutant superoxide dismutase proteins linked to amyotrophic lateral sclerosis. *Nat Neurosci* 9 (1):108-18.

Vance, C., B. Rogelj, T. Hortobagyi, K. J. De Vos, A. L. Nishimura, J. Sreedharan, X. Hu, B. Smith, D. Ruddy, P. Wright, J. Ganesalingam, K. L. Williams, V. Tripathi, S. Al-Saraj, A. Al-Chalabi, P. N. Leigh, I. P. Blair, G. Nicholson, J. de Belleroche, J. M. Gallo, C. C. Miller, and C. E. Shaw. 2009. Mutations in FUS, an RNA processing protein, cause familial amyotrophic lateral sclerosis type 6. *Science* 323 (5918):1208-11.

Veltema, A. N., R. A. Roos, and G. W. Bruyn. 1990. Autosomal dominant adult amyotrophic lateral sclerosis. A six generation Dutch family. *J Neurol Sci* 97 (1):93-115.

Waibel, S., A. Reuter, S. Malessa, E. Blaugrund, and A. C. Ludolph. 2004. Rasagiline alone and in combination with riluzole prolongs survival in an ALS mouse model. *J Neurol* 251 (9):1080-4.

Wang, H., E. J. O'Reilly, M. G. Weisskopf, G. Logroscino, M. L. McCullough, M. J. Thun, A. Schatzkin, L. N. Kolonel, and A. Ascherio. 2011. Smoking and risk of amyotrophic lateral sclerosis: a pooled analysis of 5 prospective cohorts. *Arch Neurol* 68 (2):207-13.

Wang, J., G. W. Farr, C. J. Zeiss, D. J. Rodriguez-Gil, J. H. Wilson, K. Furtak, D. T. Rutkowski, R. J. Kaufman, C. I. Ruse, J. R. Yates, 3rd, S. Perrin, M. B. Feany, and A. L. Horwich. 2009. Progressive aggregation despite chaperone associations of a mutant SOD1-YFP in transgenic mice that develop ALS. *Proc Natl Acad Sci U S A* 106 (5):1392-7.

Wanker, E. E. 2000. Protein aggregation in Huntington's and Parkinson's disease: implications for therapy. *Mol Med Today* 6 (10):387-91.

Wicklund, M. P. 2005. Amyotrophic lateral sclerosis: possible role of environmental influences. *Neurol Clin* 23 (2):461-84.

Wicks, P. 2007. Excessive yawning is common in the bulbar-onset form of ALS. *Acta Psychiatr Scand* 116 (1):76; author reply 76-7.

Wiedau-Pazos, M., J. J. Goto, S. Rabizadeh, E. B. Gralla, J. A. Roe, M. K. Lee, J. S. Valentine, and D. E. Bredesen. 1996. Altered reactivity of superoxide dismutase in familial amyotrophic lateral sclerosis. *Science* 271 (5248):515-8.

Williams, D. B., D. A. Floate, and J. Leicester. 1988. Familial motor neuron disease: differing penetrance in large pedigrees. *Journal of the Neurological Sciences* 86 (2-3):215-30.

Wong, P. C., and D. R. Borchelt. 1995. Motor neuron disease caused by mutations in superoxide dismutase 1. *Curr Opin Neurol* 8 (4):294-301.

Worms, P. M. 2001. The epidemiology of motor neuron diseases: a review of recent studies. *J Neurol Sci* 191 (1-2):3-9.

Wright, P. D., M. Huang, A. Weiss, J. Matthews, N. Wightman, M. Glicksman, and R. H. Brown, Jr. 2010. Screening for inhibitors of the SOD1 gene promoter: pyrimethamine does not reduce SOD1 levels in cell and animal models. *Neurosci Lett* 482 (3):188-92.

Xu, L., J. Yan, D. Chen, A. M. Welsh, T. Hazel, K. Johe, G. Hatfield, and V. E. Koliatsos. 2006. Human neural stem cell grafts ameliorate motor neuron disease in SOD-1 transgenic rats. *Transplantation* 82 (7):865-75.

Yamanaka, K., C. Vande Velde, E. Eymard-Pierre, E. Bertini, O. Boespflug-Tanguy, and D. W. Cleveland. 2003. Unstable mutants in the peripheral endosomal membrane component ALS2 cause early-onset motor neuron disease. *Proc Natl Acad Sci U S A* 100 (26):16041-6.

Zhang, F., A. L. Strom, K. Fukada, S. Lee, L. J. Hayward, and H. Zhu. 2007. Interaction between familial amyotrophic lateral sclerosis (ALS)-linked SOD1 mutants and the dynein complex. *J Biol Chem* 282 (22):16691-9.

Zhang, H., J. Joseph, M. Gurney, D. Becker, and B. Kalyanaraman. 2002. Bicarbonate enhances peroxidase activity of Cu,Zn-superoxide dismutase. Role of carbonate anion radical and scavenging of carbonate anion radical by metalloporphyrin antioxidant enzyme mimetics. *J Biol Chem* 277 (2):1013-20.

Zoccolella, S., A. Santamato, and P. Lamberti. 2009. Current and emerging treatments for amyotrophic lateral sclerosis. *Neuropsychiatr Dis Treat* 5:577-95.